Lee's
Synopsis of Anaesthesia

D1610557

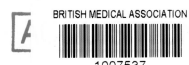

Lee's
Synopsis of Anaesthesia

FOURTEENTH EDITION

Edited by

J. N. Cashman BSc BA MD FRCA FFPMRCA
Consultant Anaesthetist
St George's Hospital, London, UK

J. E. Dinsmore MB BS FRCA
Consultant Anaesthetist
St George's Hospital, London, UK

ELSEVIER

ELSEVIER

RELX India Pvt. Ltd.
Registered Office: 818, 8th Floor, Indraprakash Building, 21, Barakhamba Road, New Delhi 110001
Corporate Office: 14th Floor, Building No. 10B, DLF Cyber City, Phase II, Gurgaon-122002, Haryana, India

Notice

Knowledge and best practice in this field are constantly changing. As new research and experience broaden our understanding, changes in research methods, professional practices, or medical treatment may become necessary.

Practitioners and researchers must always rely on their own experience and knowledge in evaluating and using any information, methods, compounds, or experiments described herein. In using such information or methods they should be mindful of their own safety and the safety of others, including parties for whom they have a professional responsibility.

With respect to any drug or pharmaceutical products identified, readers are advised to check the most current information provided (i) on procedures featured or (ii) by the manufacturer of each product to be administered, to verify the recommended dose or formula, the method and duration of administration, and contraindications. It is the responsibility of practitioners, relying on their own experience and knowledge of their patients, to make diagnoses, to determine dosages and the best treatment for each individual patient, and to take all appropriate safety precautions.

To the fullest extent of the law, neither the Publisher nor the authors, contributors, or editors, assume any liability for any injury and/or damage to persons or property as a matter of product liability, negligence or otherwise, or from any use or operation of any methods, products, instructions, or ideas contained in the material herein.

Although all advertising material is expected to conform to ethical (medical) standards, inclusion in this publication does not constitute a guarantee or endorsement of the quality or value of such product or of the claims made of it by its manufacturer.

Please consult full prescribing information before issuing prescription for any product mentioned in this publication.

Manager - Content Strategy: Renu Rawat
Content Strategist: Sheenam Aggarwal
Sr Project Manager—Education Solutions: Shabina Nasim
Content Development Specialist: Shravan Kumar
Project Manager: Nayagi Athmanathan
Cover Designer: Milind Majgaonkar

Typeset by GW Tech India
Printed in India by Rajkamal Electric Press, Kundli, Haryana.

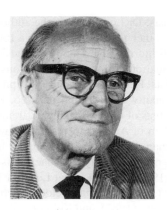

John Alfred Lee
(1906-1989)

John Alfred Lee was born in Liverpool in 1906 and qualified from the University of Durham College of Medicine in Newcastle upon Tyne in 1927 at the age of 21. He spent the next 2 years in resident appointments in Newcastle before moving to Southend-on-Sea as a general practitioner. He maintained an interest in practical anaesthesia, which he had developed in Newcastle, and in 1931 he was appointed as a general practitioner anaesthetist at the local hospital in Southend. During the second world war he became a whole-time anaesthetist in the Emergency Medical Service and served for 5 years in this capacity. In 1947 he became consultant anaesthetist to the Southend General Hospital, a post he held up until his retirement in 1971. After retirement, he continued to write, to teach and to lecture and travelled extensively, attending many regional, national and international meetings right up to the month of his death in April 1989.

His special interests included regional analgesia, and pre- and post-operative care. He rejoiced in the performance of practical skills and advocated and taught extradural block long before it became common practice. He originated one of the earliest anaesthetic outpatient clinics for the preoperative assessment of patients and organised the first Postoperative Observation (Recovery) ward adjacent to the theatres in a non-specialist hospital in the United Kingdom. This latter innovation gave him the greatest of all his satisfactions.

In 1947, following his war service, he was responsible for the first edition of *A Synopsis of Anaesthesia*, published by John Wright and Sons Ltd of Bristol. The book was soon recognised as a *vade mecum* for anaesthetists of every seniority and nationality and rapidly became a best seller. In the 70 years since the first edition the book has run to 13 editions and been translated into seven different languages. Dr Lee participated in 10 editions, being sole author of the first four editions. After his death all subsequent editions have borne the title *Lee's Synopsis of Anaesthesia* in recognition of this enormous contribution.

In addition to Synopsis, Dr Lee was also the author of many papers, wrote and edited a number of other texts and was, for a time, Assistant Editor and later Chairman of the Editorial Board of Anaesthesia. He examined for the Final Fellowship Examination, was on two occasions elected onto the Board of Faculty of Anaesthetists. He was the Faculty Joseph Clover Lecturer in 1960 and was awarded the Faculty Gold Medal in 1976. He was President of the Association of Anaesthetists of Great Britain and Ireland (1972-73). He served as President of the Section of Anaesthetics of the Royal Society of Medicine, and received its Hickman Medal in 1976. Other honours included being made Honorary Fellow of the Faculty of Anaesthetists of the Royal College of Surgeons in Ireland (1970), Gaston Labat Lecturer to the American Society of Regional Anesthesia (1985), Thomas Seldon Lecturer to the International Anesthesia Research Society (1985), and Koller Gold Medallist and Lecturer in Vienna (1984) to commemorate the centenary of local analgesia. He was also the first President of the History of Anaesthesia Society (1986–1988). He was, however, not merely active professionally but also culturally. He was a lover of opera and a life-long supporter of Newcastle United football team.

Much of the above account was written by J. Alfred Lee himself and was published after his death as part of a homage to him by the editor of Anaesthesia.

(*Source:* Lunn JN. Editorial. Anaesthesia 1989; 44: 631)

Preface to the Fourteenth Edition

In the 60 years since *A Synopsis of Anaesthesia* was first published the book had only five authors, thus ensuring a uniformity of style and approach. However, the thirteenth edition was a major break with this tradition as *Synopsis* evolved into a multi-contributor, edited book. This was a necessary response to the increasing sub-specialisation in anaesthesia. There was a complete change in layout and every chapter was substantially rewritten by a specialist in the field with the aim of providing as comprehensive an account of the topic as was possible in a 'pocket' sized book. The fourteenth edition of *Synopsis* further develops this approach with 31 new specialist contributors recruited and nearly a third of chapters written by more than one contributor. The layout remains the same but the pace of change in anaesthesia has necessitated further significant revision in almost every chapter. This is perhaps most obvious in relation to developments in perioperative medicine, airway management and within regional anaesthesia with advances in the use of ultrasound guidance. Surgical interventions have evolved with robot-assisted procedures and novel non-surgical treatments such as percutaneous heart valve insertion. In addition, the relationship between processes of care and outcome and the development of improvement science have been included with chapters on complications of anaesthesia and a new chapter on safety and standards in anaesthesia. References have been kept to a minimum whilst colour illustrations have been included wherever possible to enhance the text. All of this has been achieved without increasing the bulk of the book.

In this edition we bid farewell to Dr Nick Davies who has been associated with *Synopsis* as both author and editor since the eleventh edition, which appeared in 1993. We wish him a long, healthy and happy retirement. In association with the aforementioned changes we welcome Dr Judith Dinsmore, who brings a wealth of literary and teaching experience, as co-editor for the fourteenth edition.

The preface to the first edition stressed that *Synopsis* was not designed to take the place of larger textbooks of anaesthesia. This remains true but we hope that with the changes to the fourteenth edition *Synopsis* will continue in its appeal as a concise, general resource for anyone in the specialty of anaesthesia.

June 2017
JNC
JED

From the Preface to the First Edition

This book is not designed to take the place of larger textbooks of anaesthesia and analgesia. It is a summary of current teaching and practice, and it is hoped that it will serve the student, the resident anaesthetist, the practitioner and the candidate studying for the Diploma in Anaesthetics as a ready source of reference and a quick means of revision.

January 1947
JAL

Acknowledgements

"If I have seen further it is by standing on the shoulders of giants"
Sir Isaac Newton, 1676

We would like to pay homage to our predecessors as authors and editors of *Synopsis*; J. Alfred Lee, Dick Atkinson, Geoff Rushman and Nick Davies. In addition, we are indebted to the many distinguished colleagues from Australia, India, Saudi Arabia, Singapore and the UK who have contributed to this latest edition of *Synopsis*. We would also like to thank the publishers Elsevier for their continuing support for *Synopsis* and in particular Renu Rawat, Shravan Kumar and Nabajyoti Kar for their help with the practical aspects of publishing.

Finally, we would like to dedicate this book to our dear friend and colleague Dr Jean-Pierre van Besouw who as a clinical anaesthetist and as President of the Royal College of Anaesthetists recognised the importance of both education and clinical standards in anaesthesia.

Contributors

Adel Badr MSc FRCA
Consultant Cardiothoracic
Anaesthesia
King Faisal Specialist Hospital
Riyadh, KSA
2.8

Ravi Bhagrath BSc MB BS FRCA
Consultant Anaesthetist
St Bartholomews Hospital
London, UK
5.12

Sophie Bishop MB ChB FRCA
Consultant Anaesthetist
Wythenshawe Hospital
Manchester, UK
5.13

Peter Brooks MB ChB FRCA
Consultant in Paediatric Anaesthesia
Chelsea & Westminster Hospital
London, UK
5.6

Anna Butcher MB BS PhD
Clinical Fellow
University College Hospital
London, UK
2.7

Jeremy Cashman BSc BA MD
FRCA FFPMRCA
Consultant Anaesthetist
St George's Hospital
London, UK
2.3, 3.2

Miriam V. Chapman MB ChB
MRCP FRCA
Consultant Anaesthetist
University College Hospital
London, UK
5.10

Timothy Cook MB BS FRCA
FFICM
Consultant in Anaesthesia &
Intensive Care Medicine
Honorary Professor of Anaesthesia
(University of Bristol)
Royal United Hospital
Bath, UK
3.3

Charles Deakin MA MD FRCA
FRCP FFICM FERC
Consultant in Cardiac Anaesthesia &
Critical Care
Honorary Professor of Resuscitation
& Pre Hospital Emergency Medicine
University Hospital Southampton
Southampton, UK
2.10

Judith Dinsmore MB BS FRCA
Consultant Anaesthetist
St George's Hospital
London, UK
1.2

Simon Dolin PhD FRCA
Consultant in Pain Relief
Bignor, West Sussex, UK
6.1

Fiona Faulds BSc MB BS FRCA
Specialist Registrar
Peterborough City Hospital
Peterborough, UK
5.11

Roshan Fernando MB ChB FRCA
Consultant Anaesthetist
University College Hospital
London, UK
5.8

Richard Griffiths MD FRCA
Consultant Anaesthetist
Peterborough City Hospital
Peterborough, UK
5.11

Shubhranshu Gupta MB BS FRCA
Consultant Anaesthetist
Queen Elizabeth University Hospital
Glasgow, UK
5.4

Tim G. Hales BSc PhD FRCA
Professor of Anaesthesia
Division of Neuroscience, School of
Medicine, University of Dundee
Dundee, UK
4.1

W. Graeme Hilditch MB ChB
FRCA
Consultant Anaesthetist
Queen Elizabeth University Hospital
Glasgow, UK
5.16

Susan Hill MA PhD FRCA
Consultant Anaesthetist
University Hospital Southampton
Southampton, UK
2.4

Matthew Jackson MB ChB FRCA
FFICM
Consultant in Anaesthesia & Critical
Care
Stepping Hill Hospital
Stockport, UK
2.9

Suyogi V. Jigajinni BSc MB ChB
FRCA
Specialist Registrar, Anaesthesia &
Perioperative Medicine
University College Hospital
London, UK
5.10

Carolyn Johnston MB BCh FRCA
Consultant Anaesthetist
St George's Hospital
London, UK
7.1

Mubeen Khan MB BS FCPS FRCA
DNB
Consultant Anaesthetist
Kings College Hospital
London, UK
5.5

Andrew A. Klein MB BS FRCA
FFICM
Consultant Anaesthetist
Papworth Hospital
Cambridge, UK
2.7

Sock Koh MB ChB FRCA
Consultant Anaesthetist
Gloucestershire Royal Hospital
Gloucester, UK
3.1

Patrick Magee PhD FRCA
Consultant Anaesthetist
Royal United Hospital
Bath, UK
2.1, 2.2

Simon Maguire MB ChB, FRCA.
Consultant Anaesthetist,
Wythenshawe Hospital
Manchester, UK
5.13

Daniel Martin OBE PhD FRCA
FICM
Senior Lecturer and Honorary
Consultant
University College Hospital
London, UK
5.15

Gregory McAnulty MB BS FRCA
FFICM
Consultant in Anaesthesia & Critical
Care
Alice Spring Hospital
Alice Springs, Australia
5.14

Graeme McLeod MD FRCA
FFPMRCA
Consultant Anaesthetist and
Honorary Clinical Professor
Ninewells Hospital and Medical
School
Dundee, UK
4.1, 4.2, 4.3

James Montague MA FRCA
Consultant Anaesthetist
University Hospital Southampton
Southampton, UK
2.5

David Murray MB BS FRCA
Consultant Anaesthetist
The James Hope University Hospital
Middlesborough, UK
5.1

Ayman Mustafa MUDr FRCA
EDRA
Consultant Anaesthetist
Ninewells Hospital
Dundee, UK
4.3

Lenny Ng MB ChB FRCA
FFPMRCA
Consultant Anaesthetist
St George's Hospital
London, UK
3.2

Peter Nightingale MB BS FRCA
FRCP FFICM FRCP (Edin)
Consultant in Anaesthesia &
Intensive Care Medicine
Wythenshawe Hospital
Manchester, UK
2.8

Nicholas Pace PhD MRCP FRCA
Consultant Anaesthetist and Clinical
Director
Queen Elizabeth University Hospital
Glasgow, UK
5.4

Hemanshu Prabhakar MD PhD
Additional Professor
All India Institute of Medical
Sciences
New Delhi, India
5.7

Andrew Presland MB BS FRCA
Consultant Anaesthetist
Moorfields Hospital
London, UK
5.9

Pavan Kumar BC Raju MD FRCA
EDRA
Consultant Anaesthetist
Ninewells Hospital
Dundee, UK
4.2

Vivek Sharma MB BS FRCA
Consultant Anaesthetist
St George's Hospital
London, UK
5.2

Ian Smith BSc MD FRCA
Senior Lecturer in Anaesthesia
Royal Stoke University Hospital
Stoke-on-Trent, UK
5.3

Adrienne Stewart MB BS FRCA
Consultant Anaesthetist
University College Hospital
London, UK
5.8

Michael Swart MB BS FRCA EDIC
FFICM
Consultant Anaesthetist
Torbay Hospital
Torquay, Devon, UK
1.1

Richard J. Telford BSc MB BS
FRCA
Consultant Anaesthetist
Royal Devon and Exeter Hospital
Exeter, UK
5.17

Patrick Wong MB BS FRCA
Senior Consultant Anaesthesiologist
Singapore General Hospital
Singapore
2.6

Contents

Section 1

Preparation of the Patient for Surgery

Chapters

Chapter 1.1

Assessment and Preparation

Michael Swart

Preoperative anaesthetic assessment – all patients should have an assessment by the anaesthetist before anaesthesia to ensure the anaesthetic techniques used are both safe and acceptable to the patient. This should take place in all health care systems and involves taking a history, examining the patient and reviewing any investigations that are available.

Preoperative preparation for anaesthesia and surgery – ideally all patients should be optimally prepared for anaesthesia and surgery. This may involve nurses, physiotherapists, occupational therapists, dieticians, pharmacists and doctors. The process can take place in a pre-assessment clinic for planned surgery or in the hospital for unplanned surgery. For planned or elective surgery in developed countries, nurse-run pre-assessment clinics supported by anaesthetists usually provide this process.

Perioperative medicine clinic consultation – there are new developments in preparing patients for surgery. They involve anaesthetists providing perioperative medicine to high-risk surgery patients or elderly patients with multiple comorbidities. This may take place in an outpatient clinic or on a hospital ward.

The above three processes are described separately, but in real life they overlap.

PREOPERATIVE ANAESTHETIC ASSESSMENT

The essential first step in the assessment and preparation of a patient for anaesthesia and surgery is a preoperative visit. The reasons for this visit are to:

- Establish rapport, allay fears or anxieties that the patient might have and if necessary, prescribe premedication.
- Identify and assess existing medical conditions, note the patients physical condition and establish that the appropriate preoperative tests have been carried out and reviewed.
- Assess the risks and benefits of the various options for anaesthesia and formulate a plan for the patient.
- Provide the patient with appropriate information and obtain consent for the anaesthetic procedures.

Preoperative assessment usually begins with a careful reading of the case notes or electronic patient record detailing key aspects of the patient's medical and surgical history, treatment and current medication. Previous anaesthetic charts may record important difficulties and complications. Patient records should also contain the results of current biochemical and haematological tests and other relevant investigations, such as electrocardiography (ECG), echocardiography, pulmonary function tests (PFTs) and chest radiography (CXR).

The anaesthetist should be aware of the planned surgical procedure. Depending on the nature of surgery, blood transfusion may be required during or after the operation. Blood must be ordered and its availability checked. In some cases it will be necessary to contact the patient's general practitioner for additional information. The anaesthetist should introduce themselves to the patient and any relatives in a friendly and courteous manner, explaining the purpose of the visit and establishing whether the patient would like the interview to be conducted alone or in the presence of friends or relatives. It is best to have a systematic approach so that nothing is overlooked. Sometimes the patient has failed to fully understand the nature of the planned surgery, usually as a result of anxiety, and a brief description will usually allay fears. The surgeon should be informed if more detailed information is required.

The history taken is dictated by the complexity of any problems encountered – for a fit patient undergoing routine elective surgery, the discussion may be brief and a detailed examination unnecessary. However, in patients with complex major comorbidity, considerable time may be required assimilating copious, potentially relevant information before deciding which options are available and what further tests are necessary. The risks of proceeding with surgery should be balanced against those of postponement. In general, surgery should only be postponed if there is an opportunity to improve the patient's clinical status and thereby reduce overall chance of harm or increase the chance of a good outcome.

Template for Preoperative Assessment

There may be a local paper or electronic anaesthetic assessment record in use in your hospital that has a template for preoperative assessment. In the absence of this, Box 1.1.1 highlights what should be reviewed and documented in the patient's notes.

Systematic Assessment

Cardiovascular System

Examination and Investigations

Physical examination is extremely important and should include pulse (rate, rhythm and character), blood pressure, examination for engorgement of neck

---

BOX 1.1.1   Template for Preoperative Assessment

Anaesthetic and surgical details
Name of anaesthetist doing preoperative assessment, assessment date and time
Name of the anaesthetist providing the anaesthetic, date and time of the anaesthetic
Proposed surgery and name of the surgeon

Patient demographics
Patient's name, date of birth and hospital number

Patient's observations
Blood pressure, heart rate and oxygen saturations
Patient's height and weight

Blood results
Biochemistry results: Na, K, Urea, Creatinine, eGFR, blood glucose, HbA$_{1c}$
Haematology results: haemoglobin, platelets, INR
Blood group or cross match status

Additional investigations – ECG result, PFTs

Summary of medical history and examination
Medical conditions
Medications, adverse drug reactions, allergies, alcohol, smoking, recreational drug history

Previous anaesthetic history, adverse effects from previous anaesthetic or family history

Airway assessment
Loose teeth or dental work to teeth, upper teeth over bite, mouth opening, neck movements (extension and flexion), jaw movement (ability to protrude lower jaw), scars or previous radiotherapy, difficult airway alert cards

ASA status and urgency of surgery (Table 1.1.1)

Anaesthetic plan
Including possible complications, discussion with the patient about the anaesthetic plan, patient's response, questions or comments on this discussion, discussion with other clinicians about the anaesthetic plan

Postoperative plan for analgesia, intravenous or oral fluids, oxygen, antibiotics, venous thrombus embolism prophylaxis and restarting of regular medication

---

Notes: eGFR, estimated glomerular filtration rate; HbA$_{1c}$, glycated haemoglobin; INR, international normalized ratio; PFT, pulmonary function tests.

veins, hepatomegaly, ascites, ankle or sacral pitting oedema, basal crepitations in the lungs, cardiac murmurs and added heart sounds. An ECG should be obtained and CXR considered, together with routine haematology and biochemistry. Further tests are determined by the patient's general condition and whether the symptoms are stable. Echocardiography should be considered if

TABLE 1.1.1 ASA Classification

ASA Classification	Definition	Examples (Including, but Not Limited to)
ASA I	A normal healthy patient	Healthy, nonsmoking, no or minimal alcohol use
ASA II	A patient with mild systemic disease	Mild diseases only without substantive functional limitations, e.g. current smoker, pregnancy, obesity (30 < BMI < 40), well-controlled DM/HTN, mild lung disease
ASA III	A patient with severe systemic disease	Substantive functional limitations; one or more moderate – severe diseases, e.g. poorly controlled DM or HTN, COPD, morbid obesity (BMI ≥ 40), active hepatitis, alcohol dependence, implanted pacemaker, moderate reduction of ejection fraction, ESRD undergoing regularly scheduled dialysis, premature infant (post-conceptual age < 60 weeks), history (>3 months) of MI, CVA, TIA, CAD/stents
ASA IV	A patient with severe systemic disease that is a constant threat to life	For example, recent (<3 months) MI, CVA, TIA or CAD/stents, ongoing cardiac ischemia or severe valve dysfunction, severe reduction of ejection fraction, sepsis, DIC or ESRD not undergoing regularly scheduled dialysis
ASA V	A moribund patient who is not expected to survive without the operation	For example, ruptured abdominal/thoracic aneurysm, massive trauma, intracranial bleed with mass effect, ischemic bowel in the face of significant cardiac pathology or multiple organ/system dysfunction
ASA VI	A declared brain-dead patient whose organs are being removed for donor purposes	

Notes: If the operation is an emergency, the letter E is placed after the numerical classification. DM, diabetes mellitus; HTN, hypertension; ESRD, end stage renal disease; BMI, body mass index; MI, myocardial infarction; TIA, transient ischaemic attack; CAD, coronary artery disease; DIC, disseminated intravascular coagulation.

abnormal heart sounds are heard or for symptoms and signs of heart failure. If a new cardiac disease is suggested by history or investigations this may trigger a discussion with or referral to a cardiologist. Discussion with a cardiologist may lead to additional cardiac investigations such ambulatory or continuous ECG monitoring, cardiac MRI or cardiac CT and coronary angiography.

Heart Failure

Look for a history of heart failure, left ventricular failure or congestive cardiac failure in the medical records. Symptoms include shortness of breath, orthopnea (how many pillows they sleep with?) and paroxysmal nocturnal dyspnoea. Signs include oedema (swollen ankles or sacrum), raised jugular venous pressure and third heart sound. Abnormal investigations may include left ventricular hypertrophy on ECG, an enlarged heart on CXR, echocardiography may reveal ventricular hypertrophy, reduced ejection fraction, reduced diastolic relaxation, a dilated atrium or a dilated ventricle. Serum brain natriuretic peptide (BNP) is raised in both acute and chronic heart failure.

Myocardial Infarction (MI)

Check the medical records for a history of non-ST elevated MI or ST elevated MI. Symptoms of an MI include sudden onset central chest pain radiating to the left arm or neck, feeling clammy and sick. Investigations to review are ECGs, serum cardiac enzymes, echocardiography and coronary artery angiography. The date of the infarct in relation to the time of the proposed surgery is important. Treatment received for the infarction: no treatment, thrombolysis, coronary artery angioplasty or coronary artery stenting may be important in terms of extent of myocardial muscle damage. Check the time from MI to treatment; the quicker the treatment, the better the outcome. Check if coronary artery stents have been used and if they are bare metal or drug eluting. This will influence the choice of antiplatelet treatment and the duration of the antiplatelet treatment. There may need to be a joint discussion between the anaesthetist, cardiologist and surgeon on the timing of the surgery and the management of the antiplatelet treatment.

Angina

Symptoms of angina should be reviewed with specific questioning to detect unstable or suboptimal treatment. An increase in frequency and duration of the angina or angina occurring at a lower level of exercise or stress may indicate unstable angina. There may be potential to improve the medical management of the angina. Check if coronary artery stents have been used and, if so, whether bare metal or drug eluting. This will influence the choice of antiplatelet treatment and the duration of the antiplatelet treatment (as above).

Hypertension

High blood pressure is associated with a reduced long-term survival and an increased chance of developing illnesses such as ischaemic heart disease, heart failure, renal failure and cerebral vascular accidents (CVA or stroke). For planned surgery, a blood pressure below 180/110 mm Hg is usually considered acceptable. The time and place of the blood pressure measurement needs to be taken into account. Normal values measured at the patient's home or by their general practitioner (GP) should be used over higher measurements taken in the hospital setting when the patient may be more anxious. Severe or poorly controlled hypertension is associated with perioperative ischaemia and CVA. However, for urgent surgery the risks of not treating the surgical pathology should be balanced against the risks from the hypertension. The chance of harm from delaying urgent surgery may be greater than the chance of harm from proceeding with hypertension. Treatment for hypertension should be continued before surgery and restarted when there is cardiovascular stability after surgery.

Peripheral Arterial Disease

Symptoms are claudication on exercise and signs are weak or absent pulses, cool peripheries and skin tissue damage. Peripheral arterial disease is associated with other cardiovascular disease and a reduced postoperative survival.

Adult Congenital Cardiac Disease

Successful treatment of childhood congenital cardiac disease has brought about improved long-term survival and lead to the development of the new cardiology subspecialty of Adult Congenital Cardiac Disease. Each patient is different – contacting the cardiologist involved in the patients care is advised. There may be a correlation between the size of the cardiology medical records and the complexity of the cardiac condition.

Atrial Fibrillation (AF), Pacemakers and Implantable Defibrillators

AF may be a new diagnosis from an ECG performed as part of the preoperative assessment. This should be communicated to the patient's GP for long-term AF management. If the heart rate is fast, rate control before surgery should be considered. DC cardioversion should be considered if the patient is symptomatic or has a reduced cardiac output. Anticoagulation solely for AF can usually be discontinued before surgery and restarted postoperatively.

The reason for the pacemaker and its type should be reviewed. The last date for checking the pacemaker function should be noted. Plans should be made to disable implantable defibrillators during surgery to prevent them discharging inappropriately from sensing the diathermy. Alternative methods of defibrillation must be available if you disable the implantable defibrillator in the operating theatre.

Respiratory System

History

Ask about previous breathing problems, lung disease, current or previous cigarette smoking (amount and duration) and work-based exposure that might cause lung disease (coal dust, asbestos). Severity of lung disease is reflected by exercise capacity, frequency of admission to hospital with breathing problems, home oxygen therapy and previous need for noninvasive or invasive ventilation. Cough, fever and sputum production both amount and type should be noted.

Examination

- Initial assessment of cyanosis and finger clubbing
- Respiratory rate and pulse oximetry
- Observation of the pattern of breathing and degree of chest expansion
- Auscultation of both lung fields for added sounds, mediastinal shift and localizing signs
- Kyphosis and scoliosis
- Surgical scars

Investigations

Peak expiratory flow rate (PEFR) is a simple, low cost, portable test that can measure expiratory flow restriction in patients with asthma or COPD. Spirometry can be used to measure forced vital capacity (FVC) and forced expiratory volume over one second (FEV_1). If PEFR or FEV_1 is reduced, the response to bronchodilator therapy should be recorded. In restrictive lung disease both FEV_1 and FVC are reduced resulting in a normal or raised FEV_1/FVC ratio with a reduced FVC. In obstructive lung disease, FEV_1 is reduced while FVC remains stable causing a reduced FEV_1/FVC ratio with a reduced FVC.

These PFTs can be compared to predicted values based on age, sex, height and weight. They can give useful information to diagnose respiratory disease, assess response to treatment and determine disease progression (Table 1.1.2). Although useful to ensure that respiratory disease is optimally treated before surgery, they do not reflect functional capacity. They are also of limited value in predicting the outcome after surgery until they become extremely abnormal – an $FEV_1 < 0.8$ L is a bad prognostic measurement for lung resection surgery. Other tests used include:

- Diffusion capacity – measures limitation in gas transfer across a thickened alveolar membrane using a gas such as carbon monoxide.
- Spiral CT – to diagnose pulmonary fibrosis.
- Arterial blood gases – may be advisable in patients with severe respiratory disease who retain carbon dioxide. This can quantify the severity of lung disease and may help in guiding postoperative ventilatory support, if required.

Upper Airway Examination

An examination of the upper airway should always be carried out to identify potential difficulties with tracheal intubation. Mouth opening, neck mobility, upper teeth overbite and radiotherapy or surgical scars should be assessed. Dentition should be examined for the presence of prominent or loose teeth, caps, crowns, veneers and bridgework, especially at the front of the mouth. Their presence should be recorded and the patient warned of possible damage.

A number of scoring systems have been developed in recent years to help predict difficult intubation. The most widely used is the Mallampati score,

TABLE 1.1.2 Pulmonary Function Tests

Test	Normal Value	Use
Total lung capacity (TLC) – maximum lung volume	5–6 L	Distinguishes between restrictive (decreased TLC) and obstructive (increased TLC) disease age, sex, height and weight dependant
Forced vital capacity (FVC)	4–5 L	Measure of ventilatory reserve Reduced in both obstructive and restrictive lung disease and in neuromuscular impairment age, sex height and weight dependant
Residual volume (RV) – minimum lung volume	33% of TLC	Increased in emphysema
Forced expiratory volume in 1 second (FEV$_1$)	75% of FVC	Effort dependent. Reduced in both obstructive and restrictive lung disease
FEV$_1$/FVC ratio	>75%	Reduced in obstructive lung disease
Peak expiratory flow rate (PEFR)	450–650 L/min	Good measure of respiratory obstruction. Severe obstruction if <120 L/min
Maximal voluntary ventilation (MVV)	70–100 L/min	Index of total cardiorespiratory function
Diffusion capacity for carbon monoxide (D$_L$CO)	>80%	Decreased in emphysema and in lung fibrosis. Represents the functional alveolar area

which assesses the extent to which intraoral structures can be visualized on maximal mouth opening:

● Grade 0 – tip of the epiglottis visible
● Grade 1 – soft palate, faucial pillars and uvula visible
● Grade 2 – soft palate and faucial pillars visible, but uvula obscured by base of tongue
● Grade 3 – only soft palate visible
● Grade 4 – only hard palate visible

Other indicators of difficult intubation include a thyromental distance less than 6.5 cm and a sternomental distance less than 12.5 cm (see Chapter 2.6).

Asthma

Patients who have asthma should be assessed using PEFR or spirometry to establish a baseline, assess airway reversibility and optimize this, where possible, using bronchodilator therapy. Patients with asthma may have specific triggers that should be avoided, e.g. nonsteroidal anti-inflammatory drugs (NSAIDs). Patients have an increased risk of bronchospasm during intubation and extubation.

Chest Infection

Acute infections should be treated and elective surgery postponed until the patient recovers. The diagnosis is made from a history of pyrexia and productive sputum. Auscultation and a CXR may be abnormal. Blood cultures and sputum cultures should be obtained to try and identify any bacterial cause and guide treatment.

Chronic bronchitis is usually defined as a recurrent productive cough for 3 months of the year, over 2 consecutive years. Patients usually have seasonal fluctuations in symptoms with characteristic winter exacerbations. This may influence the timing of surgery. The presence of a productive cough is important, as is the colour and consistency of the expectorate. If active infection is suspected, antibiotic therapy should be commenced after sampling of sputum.

Chronic Obstructive Pulmonary Disease (COPD)

COPD or emphysema is dilatation of the air spaces distal to the terminal bronchioles with destruction of their walls. If active infection is suspected, antibiotic therapy should be commenced after sampling of sputum. Patients who have COPD should be assessed using spirometry to establish a baseline, to monitor the degree of airway reversibility and if possible optimize this using bronchodilator therapy.

Cigarette Smoking

Cigarette smoking is important in the aetiology of chronic lung disease and lung cancer. Current consumption along with previous smoking habits should be recorded. Even without chronic bronchitis, many smokers have increased sputum production and airway sensitivity that can cause difficulties in the perioperative period. In addition, they are at higher risk of postoperative pneumonia and poor wound healing. Smokers should be advised to avoid smoking for as long as possible preoperatively. The proposed surgery can be used as an opportunity to make an impact on long-term health and survival by referring them to any available smoking cessation service.

Renal System

Chronic renal failure is treated with dialysis and renal transplantation; most patients presenting for elective surgery are well controlled. Renal transplant patients will be on anti-rejection agents and these should be continued peri-operatively. Contacting the renal transplant team to discuss perioperative care should be considered. It is important to note the presence of any fistulae used for dialysis access, which must be carefully protected during surgery.

Plasma creatinine and urea levels remain within normal limits even if the glomerular filtration rate (GFR) is reduced to about 40 mL/min (one-third of normal). Thus, a modest increase in creatinine may indicate a significant reduction in GFR, and a high value demonstrates a serious reduction in renal reserve. Creatinine can be reduced by peripheral artery disease, malnourish-ment, reduced muscle mass and liver failure. This can lead to an under estimate of renal impairment.

Electrolytes (especially potassium), acid–base and fluid status must be care-fully checked. Hyperkalaemia may cause serious cardiac arrhythmias, especially if suxamethonium is used. A patient with established renal failure should also be assessed for anaemia, evidence of weight loss and malnourishment, neuropathy and hypo or hypercalcaemia. Uraemic pericarditis is a rare complication.

Renal impairment can deteriorate postoperatively if nephrotoxic drugs such as NSAIDs are used or if there is hypotension in the perioperative period.

Gastrointestinal System

Liver Disease

A history of liver disease or jaundice should be noted. The underlying cause may be clear (cholecystitis, gallstones or alcohol). In the case of hepatitis, a more detailed history may be required. Hepatitis serology can clarify the cause of the liver disease. Liver function tests, bilirubin, albumin and a clotting screen should be obtained. A patient with hepatitis from intravenous drug abuse may also be HIV-positive. Other causes of jaundice include adverse drug reactions. If this has occurred after anaesthesia, it may be related to the volatile agent, particularly halothane. Steps should be taken to determine the nature of the anaesthetic, the clinical course and whether a definitive diagnosis was made at the time. Volatile agents other than halothane may cause jaundice, and crossover reactions have been documented.

Risk assessment of patients with hepatic disease can be undertaken using the Child–Pugh Risk Index (Table 1.1.3). This is a useful guide to operative risk in a cirrhotic patient. The assessment is based on the sum of a number of key clinical features. Grade A corresponds to low risk (0–10%). Grade B patients should be optimized preoperatively. Grade C patients should only undergo elective sur-gery after careful consideration of the chance of benefit or harm.

Where necessary the jaundiced patient should be commenced on vitamin K. Ascites may impair respiration. The development of renal failure (hepatorenal syndrome) and decompensated liver failure can occur postoperatively in patients with severe liver disease. They may experience an exaggerated and prolonged effect of sedative drugs and some are resistant to the effects of muscle relaxants due to an increased volume of distribution.

TABLE 1.1.3 Child–Pugh Scoring System for Liver Disease

	Child Grade		
	A	B	C
Bilirubin (μmol/L)	<35	35–60	>60
Albumin (g/L)	>35	28–35	<28
Prothrombin time (seconds prolonged)	1–4	4–6	>6
Encephalopathy grade	none	1–2	3–4
Ascites	None	Mild	Moderate–Severe
Nutritional status	Excellent	Good	Poor
Operative mortality (approximate %)	0–10	4–31	19–76

Gastro Oesophageal Reflux

Patients should be asked whether they have a hiatus hernia or symptoms of heartburn or acid reflux. Severity, current treatment and precipitating factors should be assessed, in particular: obesity, inability to lie flat or use of several pillows while sleeping will help determine the need for antacid prophylaxis and rapid sequence intubation (RSI). Where symptoms are mild and especially if the anatomy suggests a possible difficult intubation, the inherent risks of an RSI should be carefully considered.

Postoperative Nausea and Vomiting

Postoperative nausea and vomiting (PONV) is one of the most feared complications of anaesthesia. For some patients PONV is more distressing than postoperative pain. Precipitating factors can be divided into:

- Operative factors – ear, eye, gynaecological surgery
- Patient factors – women, children, history of travel sickness
- Anaesthetic factors – excess gas in the stomach, nitrous oxide, volatile agents and opioids

Independent predictors of PONV include:

- Female gender
- Nonsmoker
- History of PONV or motion sickness
- Predicted opioid use

If more than one factor is present prophylactic anti-emetics should be considered.

Neurological System

Dementia is common among the elderly and is normally apparent. However, the early stages may be subtle with short-term memory loss as the only manifestation. Patients with more severe dementia cannot give a history or consent for operation; this should be sought from a responsible relative or carer. A potential deterioration in cognitive function after anaesthesia and surgery should be discussed with the patient and their carers. The cause of this is unclear but there is an association. Postoperative delirium is more common in patients with dementia or who have had a previous episode of postoperative delirium.

Patients with psychosis may be treated with lithium or monoamine oxidase inhibitors and these drugs may interact with anaesthetic drugs.

In a wide variety of neurological disorders, such as multiple sclerosis, myasthenia gravis and poliomyelitis, there may be concerns about ventilatory function. This may be checked preoperatively by spirometry and used as a baseline for the postoperative period. Special attention should be paid to neuromuscular monitoring if relaxants are to be used.

Epilepsy

Patients with epilepsy should continue anticonvulsant medication perioperatively. Enzyme induction and resistance to competitive neuromuscular blocking agents should be anticipated. Patients with a history of seizures should not be given epileptogenic agents such as enflurane, methohexitone or ketamine where alternatives are available.

Parkinson Disease

Patients with Parkinson disease must continue their medication, as normal, perioperatively – even short delays in restarting drugs can lead to a deterioration in symptoms, resulting in rigidity and reduced mobility. Specialist advice should be sought if the patient is unable to take oral drugs.

Haematological System

Anaemia

Anaemia may be suspected from the history or clinical examination. This can be confirmed by a full blood count. Unexpected anaemia is a common finding at pre-assessment and should be communicated to the patient's general practitioner for further investigation. Iron deficiency (low haemoglobin, MCV and serum ferritin) is usually related to poor diet, blood loss (menorrhagia or occult faecal loss) or chronic disease. This can be treated with oral iron. If there is limited time before surgery, intravenous iron can be used – new preparations have a much lower incidence of anaphylaxis than the older products. Oral or intravenous iron can reduce the need for intra and postoperative blood transfusion. Other causes of anaemia can be diagnosed by measuring serum folate and vitamin B_{12} levels.

Clotting Disorders

Abnormal or inappropriate bleeding or bruising should be asked about. Routine screening for clotting abnormalities is not recommended. The clotting status of patients on long-term warfarin for whatever cause should be assessed with an INR (international normalized ratio). For major surgery, warfarin is normally stopped five days preoperatively and, where necessary, covered with perioperative low molecular weight heparin (LMWH). The newer oral anticoagulants have a shorter half-life and a shorter stopping time.

Thromboembolism

Risk factors for thromboembolic disease include:

- Previous thromboembolism
- Obesity
- Major orthopaedic, abdominal or gynaecological surgery
- Prolonged immobilization
- Old age
- Malignancy
- Pregnancy
- Dehydration
- Polycythaemia
- Combined oral contraceptives
- Malignancy
- Factor V Leiden or other causes of protein C deficiency

Morbidity and mortality can occur after any surgery. All patients should be kept well hydrated and mobilized as soon as possible. An approach to thromboembolism prophylaxis is shown in Box 1.1.2.

LMWH should not be given less than 12 h before the performance of neuraxial block to minimize the risk of epidural haematoma formation.

Sickle Cell Disease

Sickle cell disease is a congenital haemoglobinopathy where sickle cell haemoglobin (HbS) leads to sickling of red cells under hypoxic, hypothermic or acidotic conditions. It is thought to confer a biological advantage against malaria

---

BOX 1.1.2 Thromboembolism Prophylaxis According to Risk

Low risk – compressive stockings unless contraindicated

Medium risk – compressive stockings or an intermittent compressive device and LMWH

High risk – compressive stockings or an intermittent compressive device and LMWH; maintain anticoagulation with an oral anticoagulant for up to 6 weeks

and is prevalent among black Africans and their descendants. Individuals may be homozygous (sickle cell disease) or more commonly, heterozygous (sickle cell trait). Patients of African or Afro-Caribbean descent should be considered for screening before surgery with a Sickledex test. If this is positive haemoglobin electrophoresis is indicated to distinguish between the homozygous and the heterozygous state and to exclude other haemoglobinopathies such as HbSC or HbS thalassaemia.

Diabetes Mellitus

Overall control and stability of blood sugar should be assessed at the preoperative visit, together with current treatment, including amount and type of insulin and the presence and severity of complications. An HbA1c level may give information on long-term glucose control. Particular areas of concern are the cardiovascular, renal and nervous systems. Autonomic dysfunction should be excluded, particularly if the patient has peripheral neuropathy. This may be manifest by impotence, lack of sweating, postural hypotension, drop attacks, painless myocardial ischaemia and gastroparesis. A simple screening test is lack of R–R variability on an ECG strip and a lack of pulse rate change with deep inspiration. If autonomic dysfunction is suspected, it may be confirmed by observing an abnormal response to a Valsalva manoeuver, particularly a lack of the characteristic bradycardia following release of the manoeuvre.

Inherited Risk Factors

Genetically determined risk factors for disease are increasingly being recognized. Some of these are single gene abnormalities, usually disclosed by a careful family history. Many have implications for the anaesthetist including:

- Malignant hyperthermia
- Suxamethonium sensitivity
- Factor V Leiden
- Sickle cell disease
- Thalassaemia
- Haemophilia
- Duchene muscular dystrophy
- Dystrophia myotonica

Malignant Hyperthermia

Malignant hyperthermia, resulting from an abnormality of the ryanodine gene, is a preventable cause of anaesthetic related death. There is usually a family history and siblings should undergo screening before anaesthesia. Screening previously required a muscle biopsy with in-vitro assessment of striated muscle sensitivity to caffeine and halothane. Genotyping is now available for many, avoiding the need for a muscle biopsy.

Rheumatoid Arthritis

Rheumatoid arthritis is a multisystem disorder with a number of anaesthetic implications. Many patients are on immunosuppressive agents. Immunosuppression may increase the risk of postoperative infection but stopping treatment may result in deterioration in the arthritis. The evidence on stopping or continuing the drugs is limited. The time to stop a drug before surgery is usually based on 3–5 times the half-life of the drug (see Box 1.1.3).

Special attention should be paid to:

- Skin – which is delicate and easily traumatized
- Anaemia – which does not always respond to iron
- Lungs – for nodules and fibrosis
- Musculoskeletal system – for osteoporosis and painful joints
- Airway – poor mouth opening, an immobile neck and atlanto-occipital instability
- Drugs – corticosteroids and immunosuppressive agents

Obesity and Malnutrition

The body mass index (BMI) (weight in kg/height in m^2) should be recorded. A BMI $>$ 35 represents morbid obesity. Obesity may cause difficulties with lifting

---

BOX 1.1.3 Stop Time for Immunosuppressive Drugs

Drug	Trade Name	Mechanism	Half-Life	Stop Time before Surgery
Adalimumab	Humira	Anti TNF	14 days	6 weeks
Certolizumab	Cimzia	Anti TNF	14 days	6 weeks
Etanercept	Enbrel	Anti TNF	3–5 days	2 weeks
Golimumab	Simponi	Anti TNF	10–15 days	6 weeks
Infliximab	Remicade	Anti TNF	9–10 days	4 weeks
Anakinra	Kineret	IL-1	4–6 h	7 days
Tocilizumab	Ro-Actemra	IL-6	13 days	4–6 weeks
Secukinumab	Cosentyx	IL-17	27 days	12 weeks
Ustekinumab	Stelara	IL-12/23	21 days	9 weeks
Rituximab	Mabthera	B cell	19 days	3 months
Abatacept	Orencia	T cell	14 days	6 weeks
Apremilast	Otezla	PDEA4 inhibitor	9 h	3 days (limited evidence)

and positioning in theatre. The morbidly obese may require special lifting equipment and an extra wide operating table. The venous system should be examined for ease of cannulation. Obese patients have an increased risk of death from stroke, cardiovascular disease and thromboembolic disease. They are at risk of perioperative hypoxia because of hypoventilation and decreased Functional Residual Capacity (FRC) due to a position-dependent restriction of diaphragmatic excursion. Chest compliance is greatly reduced. Obese patients may also have a history of hypertension, sleep apnoea, gout, diabetes mellitus, hiatus hernia and gastric reflux. Obstructive sleep apnoea can progress to Pickwickian syndrome, daytime sleepiness and chronic right heart failure. Tracheal intubation may be difficult, and provision should be made for this. Arterial cannulation may be needed to measure blood pressure accurately. Limb cuffs can be difficult to apply; a large arm and small cuff can lead to an overestimation of the true pressure.

If a neuraxial block is planned, check for a history of osteoarthritis, backache, disc prolapse or sciatica and a history of surgery on the spine. Long spinal needles should be available. The volume of the epidural space is decreased, reducing the requirement for local anaesthetics.

Premedication

Traditionally, premedication consisted of opioid analgesia with an antisialogogue such as atropine or hyoscine. Modern anaesthetic agents have reduced the need for antisialogogues. Oral benzodiazepine sedatives such as temazepam have replaced the subcutaneous injection of opiates. Increased day case or ambulatory surgery, the introduction of enhanced recovery – enabling early mobilization, eating, drinking and hospital discharge have all greatly reduced the use of sedative premedication. Most patients now walk to the anaesthetic room or operating theatre.

There is still a role for premedication in specific situations:

- To reduce regurgitation risk– antacid and H_2 antagonists
- To reduce anxiety – benzodiazepines
- To reduce sympathetic tone – benzodiazepines
- To reduce vagal tone – atropine or glycopyrronium bromide
- To reduce secretions – antisialogogue
- To reduce pain from cannulation – topical local anaesthetic cream (EMLA®, amethocaine)
- To reduce bronchospasm – inhaled bronchodilators
- To reduce postoperative pain – opiates, NSAIDs, paracetamol, gabapentin

Perioperative Drug Management

With an aging surgical population, the number of comorbidities increases, as does the number of drugs taken to treat these conditions. There is wide variation in the practice of stopping and restarting drugs perioperatively – due to a lack of clear evidence, contradictory evidence or different interpretations of the evidence available. The chances of benefit or harm from stopping or continuing a drug change with different surgical procedures, degrees of organ dysfunction, severity and combinations of comorbidities that a patient may have. The same drug can be used to treat different conditions, e.g. aspirin can be used as primary prevention for ischaemic heart disease or as part of the secondary prevention for ischaemic heart disease after inserting drug eluting coronary stents.

A full medical and drug history should be taken, including the reason for starting a drug, when it was started and by whom. Local or national guidelines may be useful – if in doubt seek advice. In complex cases there may need to be discussion between the anaesthetist, surgeon and another medical specialty. The patient's perspective on chance of benefit or harm in stopping or restarting a drug should always be considered.

Restarting or continuing drugs after surgery may need a re-evaluation, e.g. deterioration in renal function or low blood pressure may influence decision-making. Table 1.1.4 illustrates some of the issues in preoperative decision-making.

TABLE 1.1.4 Issues in Preoperative Decision-Making and Medications

Type of Drug (Example)	Preoperative Plan	Reason	Comment
Alpha adrenergic agonist (clonidine)	Continue	Rebound hypertension on stopping	May cause sedation
Alpha adrenergic blockers (doxazosin)	Continue		
Angiotensin II receptor blockers (losartan)	Continue (some clinicians stop)	Continuing may cause hypotension, stopping may cause hypertension	Variation in practice
ACE inhibitors (lisinopril)	Continue (some clinicians stop)	Continue may cause hypotension, stopping may cause hypertension	Variation in practice Stopping may impact on heart failure, continuing may impact renal function
Anxiolytics (benzodiazepines, antidepressants)	Continue	Abrupt withdrawal may precipitate anxiety	

TABLE 1.1.4 Issues in Preoperative Decision-Making and Medications—cont'd

Type of Drug (Example)	Preoperative Plan	Reason	Comment
Antiarrhythmics (digoxin, amiodarone)	Continue	Withdrawal may precipitate or worsen arrhythmia	Check serum K^+ TFT if on amiodarone for >6 months
Anticoagulants	Stop	Increased surgical bleeding	May need alternative treatment, timing of stopping depends on the drug used
Antidepressants	Continue		MAOI
Anti-epileptics	Continue	Prevent seizures	
Anti-mania (lithium)	Continue	Prevent mania	
Anti-Parkinson (levodopa, benzatropine, orphenadrine)	Continue	Prevent deterioration in Parkinson	Consider NG tube to give drugs if prolonged surgery or no oral drugs postoperative
Antiplatelets (aspirin, dipyridamole, clopidogrel)	Continue or stop	Increased surgical bleeding or increased medical complications	Follow local protocols, if complex discuss
Antipsychotic	Continue	Prevent psychosis	
Beta adrenergic blockers (atenolol, bisoprolol)	Continue	Stopping may result in tachycardia, hypertension, angina	
Bronchodilators	Continue	Prevent bronchospasm	
Calcium channel blockers (nicardipine, amlodipine)	Continue (some clinicians stop)	Continue may cause hypotension, stopping may cause hypertension	Variation in practice
Contraceptive pills containing oestrogen	Major surgery stop	Increased chance thromboembolism If continued review thromboembolism prevention	Less major surgery balance chance of pregnancy with chance of thromboembolism

Continued

TABLE 1.1.4 Issues in Preoperative Decision-Making and Medications—cont'd

Type of Drug (Example)	Preoperative Plan	Reason	Comment
Corticosteroids (oral predniso-lone, inhaled beclomethasone)	Continue	Adrenal insuf-ficiency	Corticosteroids see text below
Diuretics (furosemide, bumetanide)	Continue (some clinicians stop)	Increased hypotension if taken, increased hypertension and heart failure if not taken	Check serum electrolytes
Hormone replace-ment treatment	Continue	Increased risk of thromboembo-lism low	Review throm-boembolism prophylaxis
Oral hypoglyce-mics (gliclazide, metformin)	Stop	Increased risk hypoglycaemia	Restart when eating
Insulins	Stop long acting, review short acting	Increased risk hypoglycaemia	Restart or modi-fied dose once eating
Nitrates (GTN, ISMN)	Continue	Prevent ischaemia	
Opiates	Continue	Prevent pain or withdrawal	Refer to acute pain team
Anti-thyroid	Continue		

Notes: TFT, thyroid function test; MAOIs, monoamine oxidase inhibitors; NG, nasogastric tube; ISMN, isosorbide mononitrate.

Antihypertensive drugs are normally continued up to the time of surgery. Some prefer to omit angiotensin-converting enzyme (ACE) inhibitors or angiotensin-II receptor blockers because of intra and postoperative hypotension. If on multiple drugs, consider restarting one at a time postoperatively observing effect on blood pressure. Anti-angina drugs should be continued perioperatively; transdermal glyceryl trinitrate patches can be used if the oral route is not possible. Sublingual glyceryl trinitrate spray may be used for a fast onset of action.

Monoamine Oxidase Inhibitors

Monoamine oxidase (MAO) type A occurs mainly in the brain, and type B mainly in the lungs and liver. Older, nonselective drugs MAO inhibitors such as phenelzine, isocarboxazid and tranylcypromine irreversibly inhibit both MAO-A and B and should be discontinued 2 weeks before elective surgery. These also have anticholinergic properties. Adverse reactions to pethidine (and to a much lesser extent to fentanyl and morphine) have been reported with seizures, coma, muscle twitching, hypertension, ataxia and ocular palsies; deaths have occurred. Relief has been obtained following administration of 25 mg chlorpromazine. Not all patients have adverse reactions – small test doses of pethidine have been given while monitoring pulse and blood pressure. A combination of chlorpromazine and codeine has been successfully used for postoperative analgesia, as have regional blocks and NSAIDs. Severe hypertension and even death may occur when pressor drugs (e.g. epinephrine in local analgesic solutions) are given to patients on MAO inhibitors. This can be treated with phentolamine. The same reaction occurs when cheese containing tyramine is ingested.

The reversible specific MAO-A inhibitors (moclobemide) and MAO-B inhibitors (selegiline) are less of a risk during anaesthesia and may be continued up to the day before surgery. Caution is still needed. Pethidine and sympathomimetic drugs should be avoided. Selegiline is used in the treatment of Parkinson disease.

Corticosteroid Therapy

Normal secretion of cortisol (hydrocortisone) from the adrenal cortex is about 25 mg per day but can rise as high as 300–500 mg a day in response to the stress of trauma or surgery. Corticosteroid therapy suppresses adrenocorticotrophic hormone (ACTH) production by the anterior pituitary. In time, the adrenal cortex atrophies and is therefore unable to increase its secretion in response to the stress of surgery. This can result in perioperative hypotension and a reduced response to treatment with catecholamines. It is normally assumed that low-dose corticosteroid therapy (<10 mg prednisone per day) has little effect. For higher-dose corticosteroid therapy consider increasing the dose of oral prednisolone or giving additional intravenous hydrocortisone.

Over-the-Counter Remedies

Many herbal treatments are available, which may not be recorded in the patient's medical records and may interact with other drugs (Table 1.1.5). The drug history should include asking about herbal or alternative treatments and there may be benefit in stopping these up to two weeks before surgery to avoid adverse drug interactions. Adverse effects will depend on the dose of the herbal remedy and the amount of active ingredient may not be quantifiable. There is uncertainty on some of the evidence of harm on postoperative outcome and this should be acknowledged when advising patients on their treatment options.

PREOPERATIVE PREPARATION FOR ANAESTHESIA AND SURGERY

Until the 1980s, most surgical patients were admitted a day or more before surgery. A doctor in their first year of professional practice took a history, examined

TABLE 1.1.5 Herbal Remedies and Possible Interactions

Herbal Remedy	Potential Perioperative Concern
Echinacea	Reduced effectiveness of immunosuppressants
Ephedra	Increased risk of myocardial ischaemia and stroke Life-threatening interaction with older MAOI (see above)
Garlic	Possible increased risk of bleeding with antiplatelet drugs
Gingko	Possible increased risk of bleeding with antiplatelet drugs
Ginseng	Possible increased risk of bleeding, reduced anticoagulant effect of warfarin and hypoglycaemia
Kava	Possible increased sedative effects of anaesthesia
St John's wort	Interacts with many drugs: warfarin, steroids, cyclosporine, protease inhibitors
Valerian	Possible increased sedative effects of anaesthetics, withdrawal syndrome

the patient, took blood samples and organized and collated what were thought to be the appropriate preoperative investigations. The preoperative preparation process reflected the individual preference of the consultant surgeon in charge of the firm and that surgeon's regular consultant anaesthetist. The patient was then seen and assessed by an anaesthetist the night before surgery; this was usually a trainee anaesthetist.

In the 1980s, stand-alone day units were set up where much of the preoperative work was undertaken by appropriately trained nurses rather than doctors. The number of patients presenting for surgery is increasing; between 1980 and 2012 the number of surgical procedures performed in the English NHS in a year increased from 12 million to 18 million. At the same time, the proportion of elective procedures performed as a day-case also increased from 12% to 78%. Similar changes are reflected worldwide.

Nurse-based preoperative assessment continued to increase with the development of enhanced recovery for surgery. Enhanced recovery is a set of pre, intra and postoperative pathways designed to help patients to recover faster and go home sooner. To enable both this and admission on the day of surgery, patients must be better prepared for both anaesthesia and surgery. Nurse-based clinics target both patient preparation and the anaesthetic assessment using a multi-disciplinary team in the pre-assessment clinic. This preparation could involve provision of information to the patient and their family, identification of conditions that could be optimized or factors that might increase the chance of perioperative complications and information to help the hospital ward staff care of the patient.

Examples of Preoperative Preparation

Information from Primary Care

A referral matrix can be mandated as part of the documentation required from primary care before a referral for possible surgery is accepted by secondary care:

- Height and weight
- Pulse rate and regular or irregular
- Blood pressure
- Hb
- HbA_{1c} if a diabetic
- Drug history
- Copy of GP electronic patient record

Lifestyle

Lifestyle factors can be assessed and interventions begun using any existing resources:

- Smoking – refer to smoking cessation clinic, provide advice and information
- Alcohol – refer to alcohol and addiction services, provide advice and information, prescribe vitamin B and plan alcohol withdrawal treatment on admission
- Exercise – signpost to available community exercise resources, provide exercise training

Opportunity for Interventions in 'Difficult to Manage' Postoperative Pain

A postoperative pain risk assessment can be made to identify patients at a higher risk of postoperative pain problems. This can be used to alert the anaesthetist who will be providing the anaesthetic. It can also trigger a referral to the acute pain team for them to review the patient after surgery too. An example of a simple postoperative pain risk assessment and how it may be used is shown in Box 1.1.4.

BOX 1.1.4 Postoperative Pain Risk Assessment

- No risk factors: 19 points
- Anxiety over postoperative pain: 20 points
- Previous experience of difficult postoperative pain management: 20 points
- Established chronic pain syndrome: 20 points
- On medication for neuropathic pain: 20 points
- On long-term opioid treatment: 40 points
- Total score and treatment plan: <20 no action, 20–40 advice and patient information, >60 pain team referral

> **BOX 1.1.5 Malnutrition Universal Screening Tool (MUST) Score**
> - MUST 1   low risk, continue
> - MUST 2   medium risk, give dietary advice
> - MUST 3   refer to dietician

Malnourishment

Nutritional assessment can be done by recording the patient's height, weight and BMI. Malnutrition scores are available, e.g. Malnutrition Universal Screening Tool (MUST) developed by the British Association of Parenteral and Enteral Nutrition (BAPEN) and available at http://www.bapen.org.uk/screening-and-must/must-calculator on the BAPEN website (Box 1.1.5). In addition, special dietary needs and food intolerances should be recorded.

Additional Information

Patients may have special needs or there may be important additional information that should be identified in the preoperative assessment clinic and documented to help ward staff manage the patient when they are admitted on the day of surgery. These include:

- Skin condition (leg ulcers, pressure sores)
- Sleep needs
- Elimination (colostomy, ileostomy, incontinence)
- Mobility (stick, crutches, frame, wheel chair, hoist)
- Appendages (false teeth, false eyes, contact lenses, glasses, hearing aids, piercings, wigs, joint replacements and prosthetic limbs)
- Impaired sight, hearing or speech
- Language or communication difficulties
- Learning difficulties
- Risk of falls (delirium, dementia, unsteady on their feet, history of falls in the last year)
- Possibility of being pregnant
- Infection risk – previous methicillin-resistant *Staphylococcus aureus* (MRSA) or vancomycin-resistant *Enterococcus* (VRE)

Obstructive Sleep Apnoea (OSA)

OSA increases the risk of postoperative hypoxia, aggravated by the use of opiates to treat postoperative pain. Severe OSA can lead to heart failure and pulmonary hypertension and this may reduce survival after surgery. An assessment tool for OSA, the STOP BANG score, can be used to assess the severity of the OSA and is available on the internet (http://www.stopbang.ca). A score of five points or more indicates significant sleep apnoea (see Box 1.1.6). OSA can be treated with mask or nasal continuous airway pressure (CPAP). Those patients on CPAP at home should be asked to bring their CPAP machine with them to

---

BOX 1.1.6 STOP BANG Score

Score 1 for each positive answer, high risk variously reported as ≥3 or ≥5
Snoring: Heavy, audible in next room
Tired: Daytime somnolence
Observed: Apnoea during sleep
Blood Pressure: Hypertension
BMI: >35 kg/m^2
Age: >50 years
Neck collar: >40 cm/16 inch
Gender: Male

Source: Adapted from Chung F, Yegneswaran B, Liao P, et al. STOP questionnaire: A tool to screen patients for obstructive sleep apnea. Anesthesiology 2008;108:812–21.

hospital. The diagnosis is confirmed by sleep studies using nocturnal continuous oximetry to measure dips in oxygen saturation and their duration.

The main symptom used to identify benefit from CPAP is daytime somnolence. Patients who have STOP BANG score ≥ 5 should be assessed using the Epworth Sleepiness Scale (ESS).

Epworth Sleepiness Score

How likely are you to doze off or fall asleep in the following situations? Use the following scale to choose the most appropriate number for each situation (situations mentioned in Box 1.1.7): 0 = would never doze, 1 = slight chance of dozing, 2 = moderate change of dozing, 3 = high chance of dozing.

Delayed Hospital Discharge

One of the challenges to admitting patients to hospital for surgery is getting them safely back home. Inability to discharge a patient from hospital prevents the admission of new surgical patients into the hospital. The discharge process

---

BOX 1.1.7 Epworth Sleepiness Score

- Sitting and reading   0, 1, 2 or 3 points
- Watching TV   0, 1, 2 or 3 points
- Sitting, inactive in a public place (e.g. a theatre or a   0, 1, 2 or 3 points
  meeting)
- As a passenger in a car for an hour without a break   0, 1, 2 or 3 points
- Lying down to rest in the afternoon when circum-   0, 1, 2 or 3 points
  stances permit
- Sitting and talking to someone   0, 1, 2 or 3 points
- Sitting quietly after a lunch without alcohol   0, 1, 2 or 3 points
- In a car, while stopped for a few minutes in the traffic   0, 1, 2 or 3 points

---

Note: An ESS of 12 or more may indicate the need for sleep studies.

should begin in the pre-assessment clinic. Many factors can prevent a patient's safe discharge including housing, social support, mobility, age, frailty, activities of daily living and comorbidities. These can be identified and used to inform the hospital discharge team and social services.

Factors that might predict an increased chance of delayed hospital discharge after recovery from anaesthesia and surgery are shown in Table 1.1.6.

Patients with scores < 6 are expected to leave the hospital without needing additional support, scores of 7–10 should be considered for referral to the

TABLE 1.1.6 Discharge Risk Assessment Tool

Age		Lives with		Housing		Mobility		Needs Help with	
0–55	0	Spouse	0	No stairs	1	Independent	0	Independent	0
56–64	1	Elderly spouse	1	Stairs	2	Slow on stairs	1	Prompt supervision	1
65–79	2	Family or friend as carer	2	Warden	1	Walking aids	2	Continent	0
80–90	3	Alone with social services support	3	Nursing home	3	Unsteady standing	3	Incontinent	2
91+	4	Alone no support	4	Homeless	4	One to transfer	4	Double incontinent	3
				Poor heating	1	Two to transfer	5	Meal preparation	1
								Medication	1

Mental State		Sensory Defects		Hospital Admissions	Number of Diagnosis		Number of Drugs	
Orientated	0	None	1	0 in 3 months	0–2	0	0–2	0
Confused	3	Hearing	1	1 in 3 months	3–5	2	3–5	2
Wandering	2	Sight	1	2 in 3 months	6 or more	3	6 or more	3
Agitated	3	Speech	1	3 or more				
Psychiatric history	1							

hospital discharge team and a referral to both the hospital discharge team and social services should be made for scores > 11.

Fasting Guidelines

Fasting guidelines vary widely. The most commonly used guidance is to allow clear fluids until 2 h before anaesthesia and to stop solid food 6 h before anaesthesia. There should be local guidelines to use and patient information leaflets on fasting. There is a trend to being more liberal with some now allowing small amounts of milk in coffee or tea and allowing patients to still drink water up to 20–30 min before anaesthesia. The European Society of Anaesthesiology guidelines and the evidence on which they are based is available on the Internet (http://www.aagbi. org/sites/default/files/Perioperative_fasting_in_adults_and_children__.4.pdf)

Routine Preoperative Tests

The nursing staff should be given guidelines on what tests or investigations to perform on patients in the preoperative assessment and preparation clinic. Many hospitals have their own guidelines. The UK National Institute for Health and Care Excellence (NICE) has published guidance on this topic (Routine preoperative tests for elective surgery NICE guideline [NG45], https://www.nice.org. uk/guidance/ng45).

PERIOPERATIVE MEDICINE CLINIC CONSULTATION

Anaesthetic involvement in perioperative medicine and specialist preoperative assessment clinics is not new. J. Alfred Lee, the original author of this book, described his anaesthetic outpatient clinic in 1949.[1] While some aspects of patient care have changed over the years, much of what he described 75 years ago remains the same today.

Patients undergoing surgery today are older and many have multiple medical conditions; 65% of patients aged 65–84 years and 85% of patients more than 85 years old will have more than one comorbidity.[2] The standard surgical or nurse-based preoperative assessment is often inadequate for these patients. In addition some patients with previous anaesthetic complications or anticipated anaesthetic complications will need to be seen before the day of surgery. Patients attending the clinic fall into two broad groups. The first is a patient with an anaesthetic or medical problem, the second is the high-risk surgical patient attending for an assessment of risk and a shared decision-making consultation. In a general hospital with about 10,000 elective surgical patients per year, attending a nurseled generic multidisciplinary preoperative clinic, approximately 300 patients will subsequently have an additional medical consultation with an anaesthetist, primarily to assess medical and anaesthetic issues. In addition, a further 900 higher risk surgical patients attend a high risk assessment and shared decision-making clinic. Table 1.1.7 indicates which patients who are considering a hip or knee replacement should be referred to the perioperative medicine clinic.

TABLE 1.1.7 Perioperative Medicine Clinic Assessment for Hip and Knee Replacement Surgery

Risk	1	2		3
	Nurse Consultation	Refer for Notes Review	Anaesthetic Clinic	Shared Decision-Making ± CPET
	Age < 75	Age 75–84		Age > 85
Investigations		Abnormal investigations (ECG, bloods)		
CVS		CABG or coronary stents		MI/NSTEMI Angina Frequent angina Heart failure Peripheral arterial disease
Respiratory		Problems with SOB		
Renal		Abnormal creatinine (Cr)		Cr > 130
Neurological		TIA Dementia History of POD Recurrent falls Frailty		CVA 2X TIA Dementia POD
Haematological		PE		
Oncology		Malignancy		
Surgical factors				Revision surgery Bilateral surgery
Anaesthetic factors		Recent ICU admission (within 6–12 months)	Airway issues Intraoperative complications	
Patient factors		Previous perioperative issues Patient concerns	Patient worried Patient request	Previous postoperative metaraminol

TABLE 1.1.7 Perioperative Medicine Clinic Assessment for Hip and Knee Replacement Surgery—cont'd

Risk	1	2	3	
	Nurse Consultation	*Refer for Notes Review*	*Anaesthetic Clinic*	*Shared Decision-Making ± CPET*
Concerns from notes review		E.g. OSA, BMI >45, malnourished		Concerns around 'frailty'
		If 2 ambers, consider red referral		

Notes: NSTEMI, non-ST elevation myocardial infarction; SOB, shortness of breath; TIA, transient ischaemic attack; CABG, coronary artery bypass grafts; POD, postoperative delirium.

Assessment of Perioperative Risk

Postoperative mortality is usually reported in the medical literature as 30-day mortality. For this reason, the epidemiology data used to generate mortality prediction models predict 30-day mortality. There are a number of validated risk stratification tools, e.g. the Physiological and Operational Severity Score for the enumeration of Mortality and morbidity (POSSUM) or the Surgical Outcome Risk Tool (SORT) (http://www.riskprediction.org.uk; http://www.sortsurgery.com). The main components used in prediction models include age, comorbidities, biological markers, type of surgery and aerobic fitness. Factors associated with an increased 30-day mortality are shown in Table 1.1.8.

In general these over predict high mortality and under predict low mortality. In addition, they need updating or recalibrating over time as the patient population changes and population survival changes with time. A long-term prediction model is validated for survival after abdominal aortic aneurysms.[3] Long-term survival, disability-free survival and postoperative morbidity are probably of more valuable outcome measures from the patient's perspective. We also need to use patient reported or patient derived outcome measures to help patients in their decision-making for anaesthesia and surgery.

The chance of postoperative morbidity is greater than postoperative mortality. Life-changing complications such as an anastomotic leak, MI or stroke that results in patients never returning to their preoperative levels of fitness is double the predicted 30-day mortality. If all possible postoperative morbidity is included, it is around ten times the predicted 30-day mortality. Fitness can be estimated by taking a history from the patient. Aerobic capacity can also be estimated by using timed exercise tests such as a 6-min walk test or a shuttle

TABLE 1.1.8 Factors Associated with an Increased 30-Day Mortality

Type of Risk Factor	Risk Factor	Relative Risk	Comment
Age			Predicted 30-day mortality for an 88-year-old male in the UK is 1 in 92 without surgery in 2016. Mortality goes up with age in adults
Comorbidity	MI	1.5	Risk diminishes over time
	Angina	1.25	
	CVA	1.5	Risk diminishes over time
	TIA	1.25	
	Heart failure	1.5	
	Renal failure	1.5	Risk increases as serum creatinine increases, a low creatinine also increases risk
	Peripheral arterial disease		
	Delirium or dementia		
Biological marker	Haemoglobin		Low increases risk
	Albumin		Low increases risk
	Weight		Low and high increases risk
Type of surgery	Emergency laparotomy	12	
	Hip fracture	10	
	Open AAA	8	
	Anterior resection	6	
	Right hemicolectomy	4	
Fitness	Aerobic capacity		Increased aerobic capacity reduces risk

exercise test. Aerobic capacity can be directly measured with a cardiopulmonary exercise test (CPET).

Cardiopulmonary Exercise Testing

CPET involves measuring oxygen consumption, carbon dioxide production and power or work using a static exercise bicycle. Simultaneously, respiratory rate and tidal volume are measured and a 12-lead exercise ECG records heart rate and analyses the ECG. The power needed to continue pedalling increases during the test. The rate of increase in work or power is set depending on the patient's fitness aiming to obtain 10 min of exercise before they have to stop. The following measurements are made or derived:

- Peak oxygen consumption ($\dot{V}O_2$ peak) – highest oxygen consumption during the test; high values indicate good aerobic fitness
- Anaerobic threshold (AT) – oxygen consumption measured in mL/kg/min at which aerobic metabolism is supplemented by anaerobic metabolism; high values indicate good aerobic fitness
- Ventilatory equivalents for carbon dioxide ($\dot{V}_E/\dot{V}CO_2$) and oxygen ($\dot{V}_E/\dot{V}O_2$) – how hard you have to breath to get CO_2 out and O_2 in (minute ventilation divided by CO_2 production and O_2 consumption, respectively); high values are caused by heart failure, pulmonary hypertension or lung disease
- Oxygen pulse (mL/beat) – reflects stroke volume and oxygen extraction; high values indicate ability to increase stroke volume

Additional measurements can be derived from the test, and graphs can be produced from the numbers, to diagnose or quantify ischaemic heart disease, heart failure and lung disease.

Normal values depend on age, sex, height and weight. Values in Box 1.1.8 are intended as a rough guide, or to indicate when to seek advice on patients having major surgery. They do not take into account age, type of surgery, emergency surgery and comorbidities.

There is a UK Perioperative Exercise Testing and Training Society website that has information on CPET and standards for performing a test (http://www.poetts.co.uk).

BOX 1.1.8 A Guide to Normal Values for CPET Testing and Implications for Patients Undergoing Major Surgery			
• Peak work W	<50 bad	120 probably OK	>150 good
• Peak O_2 mL/Kg/min	<10 bad	15 probably OK	>20 good
• AT mL/Kg/min	<8 bad	10 probably OK	>15 good
• $\dot{V}_E/\dot{V}CO_2$ ratio	>42 bad	35 probably OK	<30 good

Consent

Consent involves giving permission for something to happen. Consent must be obtained before carrying out any examination or investigation, providing treatment or involving patients in teaching or research. Patients must have capacity to give consent. There are four questions to consider when assessing capacity; can the patient:

- Understand the information
- Retain the information
- Weigh up the information
- Communicate their wishes

If you are uncertain seek advice from an experienced colleague. There will be a policy and procedures to follow if a patient is unable to give consent. In exceptional circumstances, where delay may be life-threatening, one can proceed if there is consensus that this is in the patient's best interest.

Consenting a patient involves communicating information, checking understanding of the information and responding to requests for further information and documentation of the process. It is something that is taking place continuously. Some consent is obtained during social interaction and presumed by patient compliance – an anaesthetist visits a patient on the day of surgery, introduces themselves and explains they have some questions regarding the patients' anaesthetic. If the patient complies this is consent. Similarly after explaining the reasons for a blood test to a patient if they extend their arm to assist you taking a blood sample, this is consent. If they change their mind and decline to extend their arm, that is a removal of consent to the blood test. If an investigation or procedure has a chance of harm as well as benefit, this should be communicated to the patient. Determining what harm should be communicated is influenced by the frequency of the harmful event and the severity of the harm. A general principle is that frequent but minor harm and rare but catastrophic harm should be communicated. Any additional information provided should be determined by the patient's personal choice based on what matters to them.

The signature on a surgical consent form represents a completion of the consent process for both surgery and anaesthesia. Different countries have different legal requirements. Current UK practice does not need a separate signature for anaesthetic consent. This may or may not change but the key issues are the communication of all anaesthetic options to the patient including the chances of benefit or harm from these options. There must also be the opportunity for the patient to have enough time to weigh up this information and to either ask for clarification or to obtain more information. The patient's personal preference should be identified and the whole consent process must be documented.

There has been a change in society's view on the medical profession determining what information should be provided to patients. It had been considered that if 50% of a 'reasonable body of doctors' agreed on how to treat a patient, or a patient was provided with information, that the procedure was adequate and should provide protection against litigation. This no longer applies as the judiciary values the autonomy of an individual above that of a professional body such as a medical specialty. This concept has been strengthened by the Montgomery judgement from the UK Supreme Court.[4] The information given to a patient should be determined by what 'a reasonable patient' would want to know, rather than the information that a 'reasonable doctor' would want to give. Doctors may find this uncomfortable and feel threatened by litigation over consent.

The preoperative assessment process can respond to this. Patients should be given verbal and written information and directed to internet-based information on their anaesthetic options, chance of benefits and harm. They should also be offered the opportunity to obtain additional information including a consultation with an anaesthetist before their surgery. The offer and receipt, or the decision to decline information should be documented. This can take place in the nurse-based pre-assessment clinic, the perioperative medicine clinic and in the final assessment by the anaesthetist on the day of surgery. Shared decision-making is about identifying the patient's personal preference on information and treatment and is now an essential component of consent.

Information on current UK consent practice can be found on the General Medical Council website (http://www.gmc-uk.org).

High Risk Surgery Clinic: An Example of Shared Decision-Making

A standard medical consultation is structured around history, examination and interpretation of investigations to make a diagnosis and not designed for finding out what patients want. The doctor uses 'closed questioning' to obtain information and follows a medically determined diagnostic pathway. After making a diagnosis, treatment options are discussed, based on published medical evidence. The surgical literature is incompletely suited to informing patients who are considering whether or not to have an operation – most studies omit patients who decline surgical treatment and older patients with medical comorbidity. An integral part of informed consent is the provision of understandable information about the benefits and harms of surgery and other treatments. This may encompass discussion on the probabilities of death, postoperative morbidities, functional impairment and quality of life. Discussion can be aided by data from population-based studies. Patients often want to know how this translates for them, as individuals and death, at 30 days or in the long term, may not be the primary outcome for most patients making decisions about surgery. Information on postoperative function and quality of life may be more important. Unfortunately, there is limited data on such outcomes. Similarly, there are limited data on outcomes for patients who do not have surgery. In traditional medical consultations, the doctor controls the process and the patient plays a passive role. This may be all that is needed in some cases, e.g. removing a colorectal adenocarcinoma in a fit patient. For other patients a shared decision-making consultation may be more appropriate, combining the expertise of both the doctor, in terms of the effectiveness, probable benefits and potential harms of the treatment, and the patient, in terms of their perceived health, their social circumstances, attitudes to illness, risks, values and personal preferences. Shared decision-making uses open questions to identify the patient's values and preferences and the doctor takes on the role of a coach to help the patient with their decision. The Kings Fund has published a review on shared decision-making (http://www.kingsfund.org.uk/publications/nhs_decisionmaking.html).

The consultation can be divided into four stages, which rarely progresses in a linear manner, but moves back and forth depending on the needs of the patient. The consultation stages are broken down in order to communicate the process in words. Shared decision-making is best learnt by observation of a consultation.

Stage 1. Set the Agenda or Plan the Consultation

This starts before the clinic; shared decision-making should begin in primary care and follow through every point of the patient's journey through a surgical pathway. Telephone calls, letters or websites can be used to provide information. Local or nationally prepared decision aids can be used. Start your clinic on time, allow for longer than expected consultations. If running late, apologize, give an estimate of the delay and an explanation. Introduce yourself and, with the patient's permission, invite friends or relatives into the consulting room. Introduce anyone else present. Clarify with the patient why they think they are attending the clinic. Ask about their expectations and identify their agenda. Share your agenda with them, if these differ, this needs exploration and discussion. Always address the patient's agenda before your own. Introduce the concept of choice, emphasizing individual preference. Be open about the uncertainty of information, outcomes and variations in medical opinion. Use the friends or relatives in the room to help both you and the patient. If the patient does not want to discuss decision-making, or says they have reached a decision already, explore this decision. Dealing with difficult decisions is not made easier by ignoring the difficulty.

Stage 2. Clarifying the Patient's Options and the Harms and Benefits of These Options

Ask what they understand about their options. Confirm or build on this with a list of choices. Describe the possible outcome of these choices, addressing certainty and uncertainty. As you give information check they understand. Harm and benefit are best communicated as natural frequencies, as 1 in 100 rather than 1%. Balance positive and negative outcomes: a 1 in 100 risk of harm is a 99 in 100 risk of no harm. Communicating risk is difficult – you must be careful to think about what you say, whether you are understood and how the patient has interpreted it. It may be that more time is needed to consider the information, or that input from others is needed before decisions are made. Decision tools such as patient stories, decision boards or option grids may help.

Stage 3. Clarifying the Decision or Plan

Summarize the patient's decision and allow them to confirm their choice, explaining how they have reached this choice. Keep their options open and explicitly inform them that they are allowed to change their mind if they wish. Review postoperative care plans such as critical care unit admission and end-of-life issues. Document this in the patient's medical records. Agree with the patient what you are going to do next, in terms of communication with the anaesthetist, surgeon and primary care physician usually by letter. Ask if they want a copy of the same letter, summarizing the consultation. Agree with the patient and their family what they are going to do next. If a conclusion is not reached, plan further consultations or a referral to someone else, as appropriate.

Stage 4. Finding the Patient's Perspective and Handling Difficult Consultations

One of the most common difficulties in shared decision-making is getting the patient to 'open up' and share their perspective with you; it requires open rather than closed questioning. A relationship of trust and respect is needed for someone to share personal information with you. One way to develop this is to steer the discussion towards something personal and separate from the patient's decision about treatment, e.g. when inputting a patient's date of birth into a computer you can work out the day of the week a patient was born on; giving this information usually leads on to discussions about where they were born and further information about their life. Another approach is to ask about the derivation of their surname or the origin of their accent. These consultations take time and cannot be rushed. For some high-risk surgical patients, all options may lead to a bad outcome and patients may become upset or angry. Sometimes this results in terminating and rescheduling the consultations. Usually apologizing and asking permission from the patient to explore their anger resolves these issues.

Optimization

The estimated need for surgical procedures worldwide is 321.5 million.[5] Patients are living longer and with more comorbidity. There is an association with postoperative complications and a reduction in long-term survival.[6] This is an important public health issue that preoperative assessment clinics can possibly influence through identifying high-risk surgical patients and using shared decision-making to reduce wrong patient surgery, in addition to optimizing care before surgery by assessing comorbidities and ensuring optimal treatment, e.g. cardiovascular disease, diabetes, anaemia. Smoking cessation and exercise regimes may reduce postoperative complications and may convey a long-term benefit in their own right. The estimation of postoperative 30-day mortality can be used to plan postoperative high dependency or intensive care. It can also be used to initiate discussion on end-of-life care and find out what a patient wants should they suffer postoperative complications. All of this has a potential economic and social benefit. Health care resources are limited. Postoperative complications are expensive events that patients do not want to have.

There is evidence that optimization of independent risk factors for survival after surgery such as anaemia and aerobic fitness can be improved before surgery. There is ongoing research to assess if this will then result in improving long-term survival.

REFERENCES

1. Lee JA. The anaesthetic out-patient clinic. Anaesthesia 1949;4:169–74.
2. Barnett K, Mercer SW, Norbury M, Watt G, Wykes S, Guthrie B. Epidemiology of multimorbidity and implications for health care, research, and medical education: a cross-sectional study. Lancet 2012;380:37–43.
3. Carlisle JB, Danjoux G, Kerr K, Snowden C, Swart M. Validation of long-term survival prediction for scheduled abdominal aortic aneurysm repair with an independent calculator using only pre-operative variables. Anaesthesia 2015;70:654–65.
4. UK Supreme Court. Montgomery v Lanarkshire Health Board. 11 Mar 2015. https://www.supremecourt.uk/decided-cases/docs/UKSC_2013_0136_Judgment.pdf. [accessed 11.09.2015].
5. Rose J, Weiser TG, Hider P, Wilson L, Gruen RL, Bickler SW. Estimated need for surgery worldwide based on prevalence of diseases: a modeling strategy for the WHO Global Health Estimate. Lancet Glob Health 2015;Suppl 2:S13–20.
6. Khuri SF, Henderson WG, De Palma RG, Mosca C, Healey NA, Kumbhani DJ. Determinants of Long-Term Survival After Major Surgery and the Adverse Effect of Postoperative Complications. Ann Surg 2005;242:326–43.

Additional sources of information from colleges and specialist societies

American Society of Anesthesiologists perioperative surgical home www.asahq.org/psh
Anaesthesia special issue on perioperative medicine www.onlinelibrary.wiley.com/doi/10.1111/anae.2016.71.issue-S1/issuetoc
Association of Anaesthetists of Great Britain and Ireland has guidelines on its website on preoperative assessment. They include topics such as diabetes and hypertension.
    www.aagbi.org
British Geriatric Society preoperative care for older patients undergoing surgery www.bgs.org.uk/index.php/topresources/publicationfind/goodpractice/2402-bpg-pops
British Snoring and Sleep Apnoea Association www.britishsnoring.co.uk/sleep_apnoea/epworth_sleepiness_scale.php
Joint Guidelines from the Association of Anaesthetists of Great Britain and Ireland and the British Hypertension Society www.onlinelibrary.wiley.com/doi/10.1111/anae.13348/full
Kings Fund publication on shared decision-making www.kingsfund.org.uk/publications/nhs_decisionmaking.html www.kingsfund.org.uk/publications/people-control-their-own-health-and-care
NHS Right Care an NHS website on shared decision-making www.sdm.rightcare.nhs.uk
Perioperative Exercise Testing and Training Society www.poetts.co.uk

Royal College of Anaesthetists has preoperative assessment information on its website.

www.rcoa.ac.uk

www.rcoa.ac.uk/gpas2016

www.rcoa.ac.uk/perioperativemedicine

Royal College of Physicians London information on shared decision-making www.rcplondon.ac.uk/projects/future-hospital-programme

STOPBANG www.stopbang.ca

The Health Foundation has a resource for shared decision-making www.personcentredcare.health.org.uk/person-centred-care/shared-decision-making

The UK National Institute for Health and Care Excellence (NICE) Routine preoperative tests for elective surgery NICE guideline [NG45] www.nice.org.uk/guidance/ng45

www.aagbi.org

Chapter 1.2

Medical Conditions Influencing Anaesthesia

Judith Dinsmore

CARDIOVASCULAR DISEASE

The incidence of major adverse cardiac events such as myocardial infarction (MI) after major noncardiac surgery is 2%–3.5%. Key to reducing complications is the identification of high-risk patients in advance. Cardiovascular risk is influenced by:

● Surgical factors – the type of surgery (Box 1.2.1) and relative urgency, affecting time available for assessment and optimization.
● Functional capacity – determined by reported ability to exercise, e.g. Duke Activity Status Index expressed as metabolic equivalents (METs) or clinical exercise testing. Poor functional capacity (<4 METs) is associated with worse outcome after major surgery.
● Clinical risk indices – patients are assigned to categories based on comorbidities (Box 1.2.2).

Ischaemic Heart Disease

The severity, stability and the efficacy of current treatment must be determined preoperatively. Comprehensive practice guidelines exist for both the cardiovascular assessment and investigation of adults undergoing noncardiac surgery and their perioperative management.[1,2]

Investigations

Recommended investigations include:

● 12 lead ECG – all patients with risk factors for ischaemic heart disease (IHD), asymptomatic patients undergoing major surgery.
● Echocardiography – not routinely recommended but useful to assess left ventricular function in patients with dyspnoea of unknown origin or those with known heart failure but a change in symptoms.

BOX 1.2.1 Surgical Factors and Cardiovascular Risk

High risk (cardiovascular complication rate > 5%)
Emergency major surgery (particularly the elderly)
Aortic/major vascular surgery
Prolonged surgery with large fluid shifts

Intermediate risk (cardiovascular complication rate 1%–5%)
Carotid endarterectomy
Head and neck surgery
Abdominal/thoracic surgery
Orthopaedic surgery
Prostatectomy

Low risk (cardiovascular complication rate < 1%)
Endoscopic procedures
Breast or superficial surgery
Cataract surgery

BOX 1.2.2 Risk Stratification Using Clinical Predictors (Adapted from ACC/ACH Cardiac Risk Classification[1])

Active cardiac conditions
Acute (<7 days) or recent myocardial infarction (<30 days)
Unstable or severe angina (class III–IV)
Decompensated heart failure
Significant arrhythmias
   High-grade AV block
   Symptomatic ventricular arrhythmias with underlying heart disease
   Supraventricular arrhythmias with uncontrolled rate
Severe valvular heart disease

Clinical risk factors
Diabetes mellitus
Renal dysfunction
History of ischaemic heart disease
History of cerebrovascular disease
Previous or compensated heart failure

Notes: ≥1 active cardiac condition is considered high risk — surgery may need to be delayed or cancelled unless urgent; if there are no active cardiac conditions but; ≥1 clinical risk factor patients are considered intermediate risk.

- Dynamic cardiac function – exercise or pharmacological stress testing (dipyridamole thallium scanning or dobutamine stress echocardiography) are useful in patients with elevated risk but unknown or reduced functional (<4 METs) capacity. Patients with good functional capacity (>10 METs) do not need testing.

- Coronary angiography – indicated for poorly controlled angina despite medical therapy, inducible ischaemia or extensive defects on myocardial perfusion scan. Routine referral to reduce cardiac risk is unnecessary.
- Coronary revascularization – indications prior to noncardiac surgery are identical to those in a nonsurgical setting (severe left main stem stenosis, severe triple vessel disease, proximal left anterior descending disease and impaired left ventricular function).

Implications for Anaesthesia

- Only life-saving surgery should be performed within 30 days of percutaneous coronary intervention (PCI). Nonurgent surgery within 1 year of acute coronary syndrome or stenting with drug-eluting stents should be deferred. If risks of delay outweigh those of stent thrombosis and ischaemia, it could be considered after 180 days.
- Only life-saving surgery should be performed in the first 6 weeks after MI and those who have undergone revascularization by Coronary Artery Bypass Grafting (CABG). Risks remain elevated for up to 3 months. Benefits of surgery must be weighed against the consequences of delaying surgery.
- Perioperative goals are the preservation of myocardial oxygen supply (adequate haemoglobin level, oxygen saturation and blood pressure) and reduction of demand (avoidance of hypertension and tachycardia).

Anaesthesia

Perioperative medical therapy should be optimized and cardiac medications continued. Angiotensin-converting enzyme (ACE) inhibitors have been linked to severe intraoperative hypotension but also improved survival in patients with left ventricular dysfunction, diabetes and having vascular surgery. If stopped preoperatively they should be restarted as soon as feasible. Preoperative β-blockers are associated with a reduction in cardiac events but there is little evidence that the preoperative administration reduces the risk of surgical death. There is also an association between β-blocker, bradycardia and stroke. Patients established on β-blockers should continue but the benefit of starting treatment in other high-risk patients is unclear. Evidence suggests a possible benefit of statins for high-risk patients, especially for vascular surgery. Decisions to stop dual anti-platelet therapy require discussion between the cardiologist, surgeon and anaesthetist. Management will depend upon the individual patient and type of surgery.[1]

Anxiolytic premedication may be helpful. The haemodynamic responses to laryngoscopy, intubation, emergence and extubation can be reduced by opioids or a short acting β-blocker.

No single anaesthetic technique has been shown to be superior although regional techniques may attenuate the stress response to surgery. Myocardial ischaemia is best detected with a five-lead ECG, and invasive monitoring should be considered in high-risk patients. Prevention of hypothermia and good glycaemic control may also reduce complications. Most perioperative MIs occur in the first 3 days postoperatively. High-risk patients are best managed in a high-dependency care unit.

Hypertension

Hypertension is a major risk factor for cardiovascular events, renal failure and premature death. It is common, its prevalence increasing with age (73% of those over 75 years are considered hypertensive). Hypertension may be classified according to severity (Box 1.2.3).

Implications for Anaesthesia

There is little evidence that hypertension affects postoperative outcome. However, it is a common reason to cancel or delay surgery. A recent review recommends[3]:

- Severe hypertension – increases risk of perioperative complications
- Target organ damage, such as IHD, renal dysfunction and cerebrovascular disease, is of greater importance than the blood pressure (BP) itself
- A single BP reading on admission may be artificially elevated – repeat measurements should be obtained after admission
- If BP is elevated at pre-assessment, but usually well controlled – there may be no benefit in delaying surgery to optimize control
- Elective surgery should not be postponed in patients with BP < 180/110 mm Hg
- All decisions should be made on an individual basis in consultation with GP, cardiology and surgeons; the cardiovascular risk profile, the type and urgency of surgery will all help to inform the decision

Anaesthesia

Antihypertensive medication should be given preoperatively. ACE inhibitors and angiotensin II antagonists are associated with intraoperative hypotension. If stopped preoperatively they should be restarted as soon as possible after surgery. Patients with hypertension often have a more labile haemodynamic profile during anaesthesia. Hypotension on induction may be managed with i.v. fluids

BOX 1.2.3 Classification of Hypertension		
Category	Systolic Blood Pressure	Diastolic Blood Pressure
Stage 1	140–159 mmHg	90–99 mmHg
Stage 2	160–179 mmHg	100–109 mmHg
Stage 3	180–209 mmHg	110–119 mmHg
Stage 4	≥210 mmHg	≥120 mmHg

and vasoconstrictors. The cardiovascular responses to laryngoscopy and intubation may be attenuated by short-acting opioids or β-blockers. Blood pressure should be maintained within 20% of the best estimate of preoperative pressure.

Heart Failure

Heart failure is the final common pathway for many cardiovascular disease processes. Its incidence increases steeply with age and it is a major predictor of perioperative risk – patients with heart failure undergoing vascular surgery have 12 times greater risk of cardiac death than those without. The 4-year mortality is about 50%. Features include fatigue, reduced exercise tolerance, orthopnoea and arrhythmias. It is graded using the New York Heart Association (NYHA) classification. Diagnosis requires clinical signs and objective evidence of ventricular dysfunction.

Investigations

- ECG – rarely normal, arrhythmias, especially atrial fibrillation are common.
- Echocardiography – allows quantitative assessment of cardiac structures, ejection fraction and fractional shortening to assess degree of ventricular impairment.
- Radionucleotide or cardiac magnetic resonance imaging.
- Atrial natriuretic peptide may be elevated.

Implications for Anaesthesia

- Decompensated heart failure within 6 months greatly increases risk – patients may be considered too high a risk for planned surgery.
- Cardiac resynchronization therapy with biventricular pacing can improve cardiac function.
- Automatic implantable cardioverter defibrillators (AICDs) – useful in patients with history of ventricular arrhythmias.
- Perioperative goals are to minimize tachycardia, negative inotropy and ensure careful fluid balance.

Anaesthesia

Medical therapy should be optimized to minimize symptoms and maximize functional capacity before elective surgery. Cardiac medications should be continued perioperatively, including morning of surgery. If ACE inhibitors are stopped, they should be restarted promptly. Symptomatic arrhythmias should be treated with optimization of rate control. There is little evidence for the superiority of any particular anaesthetic technique. Invasive cardiovascular monitoring and assessment of cardiac output are necessary for all major surgery. Good postoperative analgesia, supplemental oxygen and monitoring in a high-dependency environment are indicated.

Cardiomyopathy

Optimal management of patients with cardiomyopathy requires an understanding of the underlying pathophysiology, a thorough assessment and management of heart failure.

Dilated Cardiomyopathy

The most common cardiomyopathy. The condition is inherited in about one-third of patients but the cause is often unknown. It can be associated with viral infections, excess alcohol and pregnancy. It results in an enlarged, poorly contractile heart with functional mitral and tricuspid incompetence.

Implications for Anaesthesia

- Cardiac failure and arrhythmias are common.
- Embolic phenomena are common – patients are often on anticoagulants.
- Cardiac resynchronization therapy may be used.
- AICDs may be in place.
- Perioperative goals include – maintenance of sinus rhythm, preload and systemic vascular resistance.

Anaesthesia is associated with significant risk. Myocardial depression should be avoided and inotropic support may be necessary. Invasive cardiovascular monitoring is required.

Hypertrophic Obstructive Cardiomyopathy

This is inherited as an autosomal dominant condition. There is myocardial hypertrophy, particularly the ventricular septum, resulting in dynamic left ventricular outflow tract (LVOT) obstruction, often with secondary mitral regurgitation. Many patients are asymptomatic, but others are prone to arrhythmias and sudden cardiac death. An ejection systolic murmur is usually present and evidence of left ventricular hypertrophy on the ECG. Echocardiography is essential to evaluate the degree of functional obstruction, ventricular hypertrophy and valvular structure.

Implications for Anaesthesia

- Cardiac failure is treated with β-blockers, verapamil, biventricular pacing.
- Arrhythmias are common and poorly tolerated.
- AICDs may be in place.
- Perioperative goals include prevention and treatment of LVOT obstruction, arrhythmias or ischaemia by maintenance of sinus rhythm, reduction in sympathetic activity, maintenance of left ventricular filling and systemic vascular resistance.

Anaesthesia

Premedication may reduce sympathetic activity and cardiac workload. Adequate hydration will help to maintain ventricular preload. Invasive arterial monitoring prior to induction allows rapid response to haemodynamic changes. Transoesophageal echocardiography (TOE) can be helpful. Volume replacement and direct acting α-agonists such as metaraminol can be used for hypotension. Inotropic agents can worsen LVOT obstruction. Regional anaesthesia is relatively contraindicated.

Restrictive Cardiomyopathy

This is rare and associated with conditions such as cardiac amyloid, haemochromatosis or sarcoidosis. It is characterized by stiff ventricles with impaired filling; cardiac output is both preload and afterload dependent. Sudden changes can result in decompensation and cardiac arrest. A multidisciplinary approach is required with optimization of volume status and heart failure. Haemodynamic management during anaesthesia and surgery presents significant challenges. Management goals include maintenance of sinus rhythm, avoidance of bradycardia and tachycardia.

Valvular Heart Disease

Valvular disease is more common in an aging population; moderate to severe disease occurs in 13% of patients over 75 years. Severe disease is a major risk factor for anaesthesia and disease significance should be assessed in view of the proposed surgery.

The following should be considered:

● Echocardiography – recommended for moderate and severe disease if no previous echocardiography within the year, or for significant changes in clinical status.
● Patients meeting indications for valve replacement or repair on the basis of symptoms and disease severity should be referred for evaluation/intervention before elective surgery.
● Asymptomatic patients, even with severe disease, can proceed with surgery.
● For mixed valvular disease the dominant lesion should be managed.
● Patients with prosthetic heart valves or congenital lesions are predisposed to bacterial endocarditis (see Table 1.2.1) – antibiotic prophylaxis (using local guidance) should be considered before dental surgery or surgical procedures.
● Mechanical valves require lifelong anticoagulation (unlike tissue valves) – anticoagulation in the perioperative period should be planned with bridging therapy instituted where necessary.

Antibiotic prophylaxis is not recommended routinely by NICE for people undergoing dental procedures or for procedures in the upper and lower

TABLE 1.2.1 Endocarditis Risk
Endocarditis Risk and Antibiotic Prophylaxis
Patients considered high risk: • Acquired valvular heart disease with stenosis or regurgitation • Hypertrophic cardiomyopathy • Previous infective endocarditis • Structural congenital heart disease, including surgically corrected or palliated conditions but not isolated atrial septal defect, fully repaired ventricular septal defect or fully repaired patent ductus arteriosus, and closure devices judged to be endothelialized • Valve replacement

gastrointestinal tract, genitourinary tract, including urological, gynaecological and obstetric procedures, and childbirth and upper and lower respiratory tract, including ear, nose and throat procedures and bronchoscopy.[4] This differs from guidance in the rest of Europe and North America where prophylaxis against infective endocarditis is recommended in high-risk groups for dental procedures requiring manipulation of the gingival or periapical region or perforation of the oral mucosa.[5]

Aortic Stenosis

Aortic stenosis (AS) usually results from calcification, rheumatic fever or a congenital lesion, e.g. bicuspid valve. Left ventricular outflow obstruction leads to concentric left ventricular hypertrophy (LVH), decreased diastolic compliance and elevated left ventricular end diastolic pressure. Greater filling pressures and sinus rhythm are necessary with a noncompliant ventricle. Symptoms include dyspnoea, angina and syncope but may appear late. A slow rising pulse, narrow pulse pressure and systolic ejection murmur radiating to the carotids are strongly suggestive of AS. The ECG may show LVH with strain. Echocardiography determines disease severity, other structural abnormalities and LV function. Disease severity is assessed by the valve area and gradient across it (see Table 1.2.2). Significant AS is a major risk factor for perioperative complications.

Implications for Anaesthesia

- All ejection systolic murmurs warrant careful preoperative evaluation.
- Patients have a fixed cardiac output – vasodilatation may result in profound hypotension, subendocardial ischaemia or even sudden death.
- Haemodynamic goals include a low, normal heart rate, maintenance of sinus rhythm and adequate volume loading.

Anaesthesia

Premedication can attenuate catecholamine-induced tachycardia. Invasive monitoring before induction allows prompt intervention using fluids and α-agonists

TABLE 1.2.2 Disease Severity in Aortic Stenosis by Valve Area and Gradient

Disease Severity	Valve Area Reduction	LV – Aortic Gradient
Normal	2.6–3.5 cm^2	
Mild	1.2–1.8 cm^2	12–25 mm Hg
Moderate	0.8–1.2 cm^2	25–40 mm Hg
Significant	0.6–0.8 cm^2	40–50 mm Hg
Critical	<0.6 cm^2	>50 mm Hg

Note: LV, left ventricle.

such as phenylephrine or metaraminol for hypotension. Fluid balance is aided by cardiac output monitoring, central venous pressure (CVP) or TOE. Arrhythmias should be treated before decompensation. Regional blocks should be used with caution due to the risk of afterload reduction. High-dependency care is recommended for all but the most minor procedures.

Aortic Regurgitation

Aortic regurgitation (AR) may occur secondary to congenital lesions, rheumatic fever, endocarditis or connective tissue disorders such as Marfan syndrome. Abnormalities of the AV leaflets, dilation of the AV annulus or aortic root can occur. Acute regurgitation secondary to aortic dissection or endocarditis presents as an emergency with acute heart failure. However, it usually develops slowly allowing the heart to adapt to increasing volumes. Patients may be asymptomatic for years but as ventricular dilation and hypertrophy progress, irreversible LV dysfunction develops. Symptoms include pulmonary congestion, dyspnoea and palpitations. Angina can occur from poor coronary perfusion secondary to low diastolic aortic pressure. A collapsing pulse with a wide pulse pressure, Corrigan's sign (visible neck pulsation), a diastolic murmur over the right sternal edge are typical signs.

Implications for Anaesthesia

- Heart rate and afterload influence the degree of regurgitation – bradycardia and vasoconstriction should be avoided.
- Haemodynamic goals include a high, normal heart rate, adequate volume loading, a degree of vasodilatation and maintenance of contractility.

Anaesthesia

Asymptomatic patients usually tolerate surgery well unlike those with poor functional capacity. Invasive monitoring is recommended for those with severe disease. Central neuraxial blocks are well tolerated.

Mitral Stenosis

The most common cause of mitral stenosis (MS) is rheumatic fever, often result-ing in mixed mitral valve disease. The pressure and volume upstream of the ste-notic valve increase producing left atrial dilation, increased pulmonary artery pressure and pulmonary hypertension. Atrial enlargement predisposes to atrial fibrillation and thromboemboli. Pulmonary hypertension results in right-sided dilation and failure. Symptoms include fatigue, breathless and palpitations. Signs include a malar flush, peripheral cyanosis and those of right heart failure. There is a loud first heart sound, opening snap and a low-pitched diastolic mur-mur loudest at the apex. ECG classically shows P mitrale and atrial fibrillation.

Implications for Anaesthesia

- Patients may be anticoagulated.
- Left ventricular filling is best with slower heart rates; tachycardia and atrial fibrillation decrease filling time and cardiac output.
- Haemodynamic goals include a low, normal heart rate, maintenance of sinus rhythm, adequate preload, vasodilatation should be avoided.

Anaesthesia

Asymptomatic patients usually tolerate surgery well. Atrial fibrillation should be treated preoperatively. Hypercarbia, acidosis and hypoxia may exacer-bate pulmonary hypertension. The use of invasive monitoring is advisable for patients with severe disease.

Mitral Regurgitation

Mitral regurgitation (MR) usually occurs secondary to LV dysfunction. There is retrograde flow into the left atrium during systole, which will depend upon the valve size, pressure difference and heart rate. Eventually, pulmonary vas-cular congestion and pulmonary hypertension develop. Symptoms range from fatigue, dyspnoea and palpitations to severe cardiac failure. Signs include a dis-placed, forceful apex and apical pansystolic murmur radiating to the axilla. The ECG may show left atrial enlargement and atrial fibrillation.

Implications for Anaesthesia

Haemodynamic goals include a high, normal heart rate, low systemic vascular resistance and adequate preload.

Anaesthesia

Asymptomatic patients usually tolerate surgery well. Hypovolaemia should be avoided, but a careful fluid balance is recommended.

Mitral Valve Prolapse

This may present with atypical chest pain and palpitations but is usually an asymptomatic finding. The aetiology is unclear but it appears to be more common in females. Echocardiography demonstrates redundant leaflets which prolapse into the left atrium during systole. Preoperative anti-arrhythmics should be continued and antibiotic prophylaxis against endocarditis is recommended.

Congenital Heart Disease

Congenital heart disease is common and 85% of children now reach adult life, many having undergone corrective surgery. Surgical procedures in these patients carry an increased risk of perioperative complications, depending on the underlying condition, surgical procedure and urgency. Ideally, these should be performed in a regional specialist centre, especially for those at particularly high risk (e.g. a prior Fontan procedure, cyanotic disease, pulmonary hypertension, heart failure or significant dysrhythmia).

Transplanted Hearts

Increasing numbers of patients survive heart transplantation and may present to nonspecialist centres for surgery. The transplanted heart is denervated with a resting heart rate of 85–95 bpm but contractility should be normal. Long-term immunosuppressants are used, haematological abnormalities or renal dysfunction can occur. Vascular access may be difficult and strict asepsis must be observed. The transplanted heart is poorly tolerant of hypovolaemia and acidosis. If pharmacological agents are needed, direct acting agents should be used. Atropine has no effect on a denervated heart; adrenaline, noradrenaline, isoprenaline and β-blockers will work as expected. There is no evidence to support any one anaesthetic technique. Neuraxial blocks may result in marked hypotension.

Arrhythmias and Conduction Disorders

Perioperative arrhythmias are common and represent a major cause of morbidity. They may be associated with underlying cardiopulmonary disease, drug toxicity, critical illness or metabolic abnormalities. Arrhythmias should be treated preoperatively to reduce the risk of decompensation during surgery. Intraoperative treatment is indicated in the event of haemodynamic disturbance – directed initially at any underlying cause followed by specific therapies as necessary.

Supraventricular Arrhythmias

Atrial Fibrillation

Atrial fibrillation (AF) may be idiopathic, due to IHD, mitral valve disease, thyrotoxicosis or cardiothoracic surgery. Uncoordinated atrial activity occurs with the ventricular response dependent upon AV node transmission (typically

160–180 bpm). The ECG will show no P waves, chaotic baseline and an irregular ventricular rate. Atrial contraction contributes up to 30% of ventricular filling and so both stroke volume and cardiac output are reduced. Hypotension, myocardial ischaemia, cardiac failure and systemic emboli from intra-atrial thrombus may all occur.

Treatment

- Aimed at rate control – with β-blockers, e.g. bisoprolol, or calcium channel antagonists, e.g. diltiazem, verapamil
- Digoxin used infrequently now in the absence of heart failure
- Embolic complications must be prevented – the stroke risk assessed (e.g. CHA_2DS_2VASc; see www.chadsvasc.org) and anticoagulation commenced as appropriate
- Cardioversion – to restore sinus rhythm if recent onset (<48 h) or for haemodynamic compromise

Atrial Flutter

There is rapid atrial discharge (typically 300 bpm) associated with a re-entrant circuit. It often occurs with 4:1 or 2:1 block. ECG shows saw-tooth flutter waves. Treatment is aimed at restoring sinus rhythm with cardioversion or drugs as for AF.

Supraventricular Tachycardia (SVT)

This usually presents as a narrow complex tachycardia (typically 150–200 bpm). It may respond to vagal manoeuvres, adenosine (0.2 mg/kg rapidly is useful for terminating re-entry SVT), β-blockers, verapamil or amiodarone. For haemodynamic compromise the treatment is synchronized DC cardioversion.

Wolff–Parkinson–White Syndrome

A congenital accessory pathway between the atria and ventricles (bundle of Kent) permits the development of re-entry tachycardias and atrial fibrillation. ECG shows a short PR interval, wide QRS complexes with δ waves. Adenosine is a first line treatment for emergency treatment of SVT or cardioversion where there is haemodynamic compromise. Longer term management involves catheter ablation of the abnormal pathway or medical treatment, e.g. with procainamide. Digoxin and verapamil may exacerbate Wolff–Parkinson–White syndrome and are contraindicated.

Ventricular Arrhythmias

Ventricular arrhythmias carry the greatest risk of sudden death. They are more common and carry greater risk in patients with structural heart disease.

- Ventricular ectopic beats – common and rarely require treatment.
- Ventricular tachycardia (VT) – defined as a rate of >100 bpm, with three or more consecutive beats originating from the ventricles, independent of atrial

or AV conduction. It may be sustained (>30 s) or nonsustained (<30 s). There is no evidence that asymptomatic, nonsustained VT is associated with an increased incidence of perioperative MI or death.
- Symptomatic ventricular arrhythmias – these are potentially life-threatening. They may be triggered intraoperatively by hypoxia, hypotension or severe electrolyte abnormalities. Management ranges from CPR and cardioversion (ventricular fibrillation) to pharmacological treatment with antiarrhythmics such as lidocaine or amiodarone (see Chapter 2.9).

Sick Sinus Syndrome

A name used for disorders of sinoatrial node function resulting in sinus brady-cardia with episodes of sinus arrest or escape rhythms. There may be episodes of tachyarrhythmias. Symptoms such as syncope, dizziness and palpitations are treated with a permanent pacing.

Heart Blocks

- First-degree block – a delay in conduction through the AV node. The PR interval is prolonged (>0.2 s). It is asymptomatic and usually benign.
- Second-degree block
  - Mobitz type I (Wenckebach) – characterized by progressive lengthening of the PR interval followed by a dropped beat and repeat of the cycle. No treatment is needed if asymptomatic.
  - Mobitz type II – most beats are conducted normally but there is intermit-tent failure of transmission, usually through the bundle of His. This can progress to complete heart block.
- Complete heart block – there is no conduction between the atria and ven-tricles. Pacing is usually indicated.
- Bundle branch blocks – caused by a delay in depolarization of the right or left bundle branches with conduction delay and QRS widening.
  - Right bundle branch block (RBBB) – characterized by wide QRS com-plexes and RSR pattern in lead V1; often benign.
  - Left bundle branch block (LBBB) – often an indicator of heart dis-ease; further interpretation of the ECG is difficult. Hemiblock involves individual fascicles of the left bundle, e.g. left anterior and posterior hemiblock.
  - Bifascicular block – a combination of RBBB and block of the left anterior or posterior fascicle. RBBB with left posterior hemiblock is most common and is demonstrated by the 'RSR' in V1 with left axis deviation.
  - Trifascicular block is used to indicate first-degree block together with bifascicular block.

General anaesthesia may result in deterioration of heart block as most volatile agents prolong cardiac conduction. Preoperative insertion of a permanent or temporary pacemaker is indicated for complete heart block, second-degree block (Mobitz type 11) and lesser degrees of heart block if symptomatic. Chronotropic drugs such as atropine, isoprenaline or adrenaline and facilities for external pacing should be readily available.

Pacemakers

Pacemakers are indicated to both treat bradyarrhythmias and improve functional capacity in patients with severe heart failure. They are classified according to a five letter/position code (see Table 1.2.3). The first three letters/positions are used to denote the antibradycardia functions. The fourth and fifth denote additional functions and may be omitted.[6]

Implications for Anaesthesia

● Electromagnetic interference (EMI) can occur with diathermy.
● If the patient is pacemaker dependent, it may be best reprogrammed preoperatively – discuss with cardiac physiologists.
● Bipolar diathermy is safe.
● Unipolar is not recommended – if needed the ground plate should be on the side of the operating site, as far away from the pacemaker as possible, the frequency and duration of use limited and the lowest possible current used.
● Magnetic resonance imaging may cause pacemaker malfunction and permanent damage.
● Magnets have an unpredictable effect on pacemaker programming and should not be placed over pacemakers without discussion.

Anaesthesia

Indications for insertion, mode of action and the pacemaker function should be checked. A backup pacing system and chronotropic drugs such as atropine, epinephrine (adrenaline) and isoprenaline should be available in case of failure.

TABLE 1.2.3 Classification of Pacemaker Functions

Code for the Classification of Pacemaker Functions	
1 – Chamber-paced – O/V/A/D	None/ventricle/atrium/dual
2 – Chamber sensed – O/V/A/D	None/ventricle/atrium/dual
3 – Response to sensing – O/T/I/D	None/triggered/inhibited/dual
4 – Programmability, mode regulation – O/P/M/R	None/simple programmable/multi-programmable/rate modulation
5 – Anti-tachycardia functions – O/P/S/D	None/pacing/shock/dual

Automatic Implantable Cardioverter Defibrillator (AICD)

AICDs are used for recurrent tachyarrhythmias unresponsive to medical treatment. They sense ventricular tachycardia or fibrillation and defibrillate the heart. However, the device may be triggered by any EMI, including diathermy. Anti-tachycardia and defibrillation functions should be inactivated if diathermy is to be used, before lithotripsy and electroconvulsive therapy. The use of transcutaneous electrical nerve stimulation (TENS) for pain management is contraindicated. Cardiac monitoring should be used continuously during the entire period of inactivation, and external defibrillation equipment readily available.

PULMONARY DISEASE

Postoperative pulmonary complications are a major cause of morbidity and mortality; they are related to both the underlying clinical condition and the surgical procedure. Some of the factors shown to predict complications are shown in Box 1.2.4.[7]

Smoking

Along with the associated long-term comorbidities, smoking produces additional adverse effects in the perioperative period. Increased carboxyhaemoglobin levels impair oxygen carriage and delivery, which may persist for over 12 h. There are more adverse respiratory events resulting from airway hyperreactivity, mucus hypersecretion and impaired ciliary function. Patients should be advised to stop smoking preoperatively. Abstinence for 8 weeks is required to significantly improve respiratory function, but oxygen carriage will be improved after 24 h.

Acute Upper Respiratory Tract Infection (URTI)

Patients frequently present for elective surgery with, or recovering from, an URTI. For those with fever and cough, underlying pulmonary disease or having major abdominal or thoracic surgery it is advisable to delay surgery. There is

---

BOX 1.2.4 Factors Shown to Predict Pulmonary Complications

- Pre-existing lung disease
- Age > 60 years
- Smoking within 8 weeks
- BMI > 40 kg/m^2
- FEV_1 < 50% predicted
- Duration of anaesthesia (>3 h)
- Head and neck surgery
- Thoracic and upper abdominal surgery
- Use of nasogastric tube

little evidence that adults with simple URTI are at increased risk of complications. Children are more likely to develop laryngospasm or transient postoperative hypoxaemia, especially with airway instrumentation. However, postoperative sequelae are rare – an individualized approach incorporating previous history, nature and urgency of surgery is preferable. Increased airway reactivity may persist for up to 6 weeks.

Chronic Obstructive Pulmonary Disease (COPD)

COPD increases the risk of perioperative complications, with longer hospital stay and higher mortality. It is characterized by small airway inflammation (obstructive bronchiolitis) and parenchymal destruction (emphysema). The former results in obstruction, air trapping, mucus hypersecretion and productive cough. Emphysema results in dilatation of airways distal to the terminal bronchioles and over-inflation of the lungs. Smoking is the most important aetiological factor, followed by occupational exposure to dusts and atmospheric pollution. Genetic factors have been implicated. Advanced COPD ultimately leads to respiratory failure.

Implications for Anaesthesia

- Clinical assessment – exercise tolerance, specifically maximal level of exertion attainable, frequency of exacerbations, timing of recent antibiotics or steroids, hospital admissions.
- Previous requirements for ventilation/noninvasive ventilation (NIV) should be identified.
- Investigations:
  - ECG – may reveal right-sided heart disease (echocardiography can be considered), coexisting IHD.
  - CXR – if recent infection or deterioration in symptoms; may reveal malignancy or bullous disease, which increases the risk of pneumothorax.
  - Spirometry – to confirm diagnosis ($FEV_1/FVC < 0.7$, post bronchodilator) and assess disease severity.
  - Functional status – stair climbing, 6-min walk test correlate well with more formal exercise testing.
  - Baseline arterial blood gas (ABG) – $PCO_2 > 5.9$ kPa, $PO_2 < 7.9$ kPa predict worse outcome.
- Review/optimization by respiratory team – oral steroids, nebulized bronchodilators and antibiotics for infection.
- Preoperative physiotherapy – especially for patients with large volumes of sputum.
- Pulmonary hypertension – specialist review is recommended, unless the risks of delay outweigh potential benefits.
- Smoking, poor nutritional status and obesity increase perioperative risk; smoking cessation advice is mandatory before contemplating elective surgery.

Anaesthesia

Regional/local anaesthesia avoids the respiratory complications of general anaesthesia, but is not always suitable. For patients unable to lie supine – reassurance, sedation, flexibility regarding positioning or the use of NIV may help. However, most patients can be managed safely with careful general anaesthesia. For brief, minor procedures intubation can be avoided; controlled ventilation will be needed for major surgery. Pressure-controlled/limited ventilation, with a low ventilation rate and prolonged expiratory phase minimizes air trapping and barotrauma. Nitrous oxide (N_2O) is best avoided in patients with emphysema, particularly in the presence of bullae.

Patients with severe COPD, particularly undergoing major surgery, should be managed in high dependency (HDU) to allow for regular ABGs and NIV if required. Effective analgesia is essential; pain leads to hypoventilation, retained secretions, atelectasis and pneumonia. Epidural analgesia improves postoperative pulmonary function and reduces pulmonary complications after thoracic and upper abdominal surgery.[8]

Asthma

Asthma is characterized by reversible airflow obstruction with inflammation, mucosal oedema and mucus plugging, airway narrowing and hyper-reactivity. The immunologic-inflammatory pathways are complex, both triggered and modified by extrinsic and environmental factors such as allergens, respiratory infections, smoke and occupation-related exposure. Symptoms include wheeze, cough and sputum production. Treatment is with bronchodilators, usually β2-agonists and anti-inflammatory agents such as inhaled corticosteroids. Leukotriene antagonists have both anti-inflammatory and bronchodilator properties.

Implications for Anaesthesia

- Patients frequently underestimate their disease severity.
- Establish – frequency of exacerbations, triggering agents, previous perioperative exacerbations, hospital visits, need for critical care/ventilation.
- Medications – dosage and degree of benefit provide clues to the severity and control.
- Steroid therapy – inhaled versus systemic use, duration of use and side effects.
- URTIs can trigger exacerbations – recent changes in cough or sputum should raise concern.
- Serial measurements of peak flow are more useful than a single reading.
- Spirometry gives a more accurate assessment of lung function.
- Lung function should be as near to baseline as possible by optimizing medications/compliance or oral corticosteroids.

Anaesthesia

Anaesthesia should be tailored to the individual patient and procedure; regional techniques considered where appropriate. As intubation may trigger bronchospasm, it seems sensible to avoid airway instrumentation where possible. Anxiolytic premedication, adequate depth of anaesthesia, opioid cover and muscle relaxation may help. Topical lidocaine spray is not effective and may even induce bronchoconstriction. There is a lower incidence of bronchospasm with supraglottic airways (SAD) than with intubation. Volatile anaesthetics are bronchodilators and are generally well tolerated. Ketamine also has bronchodilator properties and may be useful in emergency circumstances. Histamine-releasing drugs should be avoided where possible.

Acute bronchospasm may be managed by deepening anaesthesia using a volatile agent and the administration of a bronchodilator, e.g. salbutamol 250 μg, by slow i.v. injection. Aminophylline 250 mg i.v. over 20 min may also be used. High-dose steroids and magnesium sulphate (1.2–2 g i.v.) can be helpful in difficult cases. For bronchospasm unresponsive to the above, epinephrine 1 in 10,000 may be given in 1 mL increments.

Good postoperative analgesia is essential. Nonsteroidal anti-inflammatory drugs (NSAIDs) can be used if previously tolerated but best avoided in poorly controlled asthmatics. Regular nebulized bronchodilators should be continued postoperatively. Patients with severe asthma undergoing major surgery should go to HDU.

Bronchiectasis

Bronchiectasis is the permanent dilatation and thickening of the airways associated with chronic cough, sputum production, bacterial colonization and recurrent infection. It may be idiopathic or result from severe childhood infections or genetic disorders such as cystic fibrosis. Most have few symptoms. Extensive disease is associated with frequent exacerbations, colonization by *Pseudomonas aeruginosa* and smoking. There is progressive loss of lung function, right-sided heart failure and a reduced life expectancy. Cystic fibrosis is also associated with malabsorption; patients may be malnourished. Treatment is with physiotherapy and antibiotics but bronchodilators are also useful.

Implications for Anaesthesia

- Liaison with respiratory physicians is essential.
- A preoperative sputum sample for culture and antibiotics may be needed before admission.
- Intensive physiotherapy should start preoperatively.
- Bronchodilator treatment should be maximized.
- ABGs should be checked for severe disease.

Anaesthesia

Regional/local anaesthesia should be chosen where possible. If general anaesthesia is used tracheal intubation will allow bronchial toilet. Short-acting anaesthetic agents should be used to allow prompt awakening and early extubation. Effective analgesia, regular postoperative physiotherapy and HDU are recommended for those with severe disease or having major surgery.

Obstructive Sleep Apnoea (OSA)

OSA affects 5%–10% of the adult population and is associated with obesity, smoking, diabetes and alcohol. It is more common in middle-aged males. Children can develop OSA usually secondary to adeno-tonsillary hypertrophy. Intermittent airway collapse results in airflow obstruction and periods of apnoea. Partial airway collapse results in snoring and hypopnoea. Breathing resumes due to increased O_2 and CO_2 chemo-receptor activity and increased oropharyngeal tone with greater inspiratory effort. The diagnosis can often be made from history and examination. Symptoms include snoring, disturbed sleep, headaches and daytime sleepiness. Additional diagnostic tools include questionnaires such as STOP-BANG (Box 1.2.5) and formal sleep studies.[9] Treatment is with nocturnal CPAP.

Implications for Anaesthesia

● Systemic and pulmonary hypertension may be present.
● Right-sided heart failure and respiratory failure – ECG for signs of right heart strain, echocardiography if indicated.
● Polycythaemia – secondary to chronic hypoxia, check full blood count (FBC), SaO_2.

Anaesthesia

Coexisting medical conditions should be optimized. Patients should bring their own CPAP machine for perioperative use. Sedative premedication is best

---

BOX 1.2.5 STOP BANG Questionnaire for Sleep Apnoea

STOP

Do you **S**nore loudly?
Do you often feel **T**ired, fatigued or sleepy during daytime?
Has anyone **O**bserved you stop breathing during your sleep?
Do you have or are you being treated for high blood **P**ressure?

BANG

BMI > 35 kg/m^2?
Age > 50 years?
Neck circumference > 16 inches (40 cm)?
Gender – Male?

Notes: Score 1 for every yes response. If total score 0–2 low risk, 3–4 intermediate risk, 5–8 high risk of sleep apnoea

avoided. Regional anaesthesia should be considered where possible. Short acting anaesthetic and analgesic agents will enable a prompt wake up and early extubation. HDU care is recommended postoperatively or continuous oximetry on the ward with oxygen titrated to maintain preoperative saturations.

ENDOCRINE DISEASE

See also Chapter 5.4, Endocrine Surgery.

Diabetes Mellitus

Diabetes is increasing and it now affects 10%–15% of the surgical population. Diabetics are more likely to need surgery and have more complications and greater mortality. Diagnosis is based on fasting plasma glucose >7.0 mmol/L or random plasma glucose > 11.1 mmol/L. Type-1 diabetes results from an absolute insulin deficiency. Type-2 diabetes is associated with some endogenous insulin production and insulin resistance. Perioperative management aims for optimization of perioperative glycaemic control with minimal disruption to the normal regime. Patients should be involved with their individual management plan.

Diabetes is a multisystem disorder with complications arising secondary to microvascular and macrovascular disease.

Implications for Anaesthesia

- Hyperglycaemia leads to dehydration, acidosis, delayed wound healing and increased susceptibility to infection.
- Cardiovascular – accelerated atherosclerosis and generalized microvascular disease leading to IHD (often silent), hypertension and peripheral vascular disease.
- Neurological – autonomic neuropathy (postural hypotension, gastroparesis, bladder dysfunction), peripheral neuropathy (typically glove and stocking distribution).
- Renal – 40% develop microalbuminuria, diabetic nephropathy is the commonest cause of end-stage renal failure.
- Ophthalmic – cataracts, exudative and proliferative retinopathy.
- Respiratory – increased incidence of infections, including tuberculosis.
- Stiff joint syndrome – glycosylation of soft tissue occurs; intubation may be difficult.
- Increased incidence of infections, including tuberculosis.
- Gastric stasis with reflux.

Preoperative Preparation

This should begin before referral with improved glycaemic control, recognition and optimization of comorbidities. Guidance suggests delaying elective surgery if HbA1c ≥ 69 mmol/mol to improve glycaemic control. Optimal control minimizes metabolic disturbances, end-organ damage and may result in better wound healing, lower morbidity and shorter hospital stay.

During admission, both hypo- and hyperglycaemia should be avoided. Blood glucose levels should be measured at least 2 hourly and be maintained between 6 and 10 mmol/L. The regimen used for control depends on the type of diabetes, preoperative control and the nature of proposed surgery.[10,11]

- Patients should be placed first on operating list.
- For patients with short starvation times, and likely to miss only one meal, this can be achieved by manipulating the patient's own insulin regime using guidance in Tables 1.2.4 and 1.2.5.
- Variable-rate intravenous insulin infusion (VRIII) is ideal for (i) patients who are expected to miss two or more meals; (ii) patients with type-1 diabetes undergoing surgery who have not received background insulin; (iii) patients with poorly controlled diabetes (HbA1c > 69 mmol/mol); and (iv) most diabetes patients requiring emergency surgery.
- Individual regimes are available in hospitals; careful glucose monitoring is essential.

Anaesthesia

Regional anaesthesia has obvious advantages. Preservation of consciousness allows detection of hypoglycaemic symptoms and earlier oral intake, minimizing metabolic disturbance. Regional anaesthesia also reduces the stress response to surgery. However, profound hypotension may occur in patients with autonomic neuropathy. In patients with diabetic neuropathy a detailed discussion and accurate documentation of any existing neurological deficit is essential. Blood glucose should be monitored on induction and at least hourly during general anaesthesia. Rapid sequence induction may be indicated in the presence of autonomic neuropathy, but the potential for difficult intubation should be considered. Blood pressure should be maintained to reduce the risk of further end-organ damage. Care should be taken to protect pressure areas as diabetics are at risk of skin trauma, ulceration and nerve injury.

Thyroid Disease

Hypothyroidism

Most commonly caused by autoimmune thyroiditis causing a reduction in the metabolic rate. Clinical features include fatigue, cold intolerance, weight gain, mental slowing and dry skin. Undiagnosed mild hypothyroidism is common, particularly in the elderly. Treatment is with oral L-thyroxine, which may take 7–10 days to produce a clinical effect. Tri-iodothyronine may also be used; it has a shorter half-life and may be given intravenously for emergency treatment. Careful administration of replacement thyroxine is needed especially in the elderly who are susceptible to angina and heart failure.

TABLE 1.2.4 Guideline for Perioperative Adjustment of Insulin (Short Starvation Period – No More than One Missed Meal)

Insulin	Surgery in Morning	Surgery in Afternoon	While using VRIII
Once daily			
Single morning dose	Reduce dose by 20%	Reduce dose by 20%	80% of usual dose
Single evening dose	No change	No change	80% of usual dose
Twice daily			
Single injection e.g. biphasic or ultra-long-acting	Halve usual morning dose; evening meal dose unchanged	Halve usual morning dose; evening meal dose unchanged	Stop until eating and drinking
Two injections e.g. short-acting and intermediate acting	Calculate total dose of morning insulin(s); give half as intermediate-acting only in morning; evening dose unchanged	Calculate total dose of morning insulin(s); give and drinking half as intermediate acting only in morning; evening dose unchanged	Stop until eating
Three to Five Injections	Basal bolus regimes: Omit morning and lunchtime short-acting insulin(s); keep basal unchanged[a] Pre-mixed morning insulin: Halve morning dose, omit lunch-time dose	Give usual morning insulin; omit lunch dose and drinking	Stop until eating

Source: Modified from Barker et al.[11]

[a]If a patient requires a VRIII then long-acting background insulin should be continued at 80% usual dose.

TABLE 1.2.5 Guidance for Perioperative Adjustment of Noninsulin Medication (No More than One Missed Meal)

Agent	Day of Surgery	
	Morning Surgery	*Afternoon Surgery*
Acarbose	Omit morning dose if 'nil by mouth'	Give morning dose if eating
Meglitinides (e.g. repaglinide)	Omit morning dose if 'nil by mouth'	Give morning dose if eating
Metformin (no contrast media)[a]	Omit morning dose	Omit morning dose, restart with meals
Sulphonylureas (e.g. glibenclamide, gliclazide)	Omit morning dose	Omit morning dose, restart with meals
Pioglitazone	Take as normal	Take as normal
DPP-IV inhibitors (e.g. vildagliptin, sitagliptin)	Take as normal	Take as normal
GLP-1 analogues (e.g. exenatide, liraglutide)	Omit day of surgery	Omit day of surgery

Notes: All medication can be taken as usual the day before surgery.
DPP-IV, dipeptidyl peptidase-IV; GLP-1, glucagon-like peptide-1.
Source: Modified from Barker et al.[11]
[a]If contrast media is to be used or the eGFR < 50 mL/min/1.73 m^2, metformin should be omitted on the day of surgery and for the following 48 h.

Implications for Anaesthesia

- Cardiovascular – depression of myocardial function, abnormal baroreceptor function, reduced plasma volume
- Respiratory – decreased spontaneous ventilation
- Metabolic – anaemia, hypoglycaemia, hyponatraemia
- Liver – impaired hepatic drug metabolism

Anaesthesia

Patients should be euthyroid before elective surgery. A hypometabolic state renders patients susceptible to profound hypotension. Anaesthetic agents should be chosen carefully and titrated to effect – there may be increased sensitivity to respiratory depressants; controlled ventilation may be preferred. Temperature monitoring and active warming are recommended.

Hyperthyroidism

The commonest cause is the autoimmune disorder Graves disease. Features include weight loss, heat intolerance and tremor. Treatment is with drugs that block thyroxine synthesis, such as carbimazole and propylthiouracil, or with radioactive iodine. β-Blockers such as propranolol may be used for tremor or palpitations.

Implications for Anaesthesia

- Cardiovascular effects – AF, congestive cardiac failure
- Exophthalmos – in Graves disease
- Goitre – potential airway difficulties. Chest X-ray, thoracic inlet views to assess tracheal compression; CT or MRI scan if necessary; Indirect laryngoscopy may be helpful
- Superior vena cava obstruction can occur

Anaesthesia

Patients should be euthyroid before surgery to prevent a thyroid crisis. β-blockers should be continued perioperatively. A thyroid crisis can be precipitated by any major physical stress and has a mortality of 20%–30% untreated. It is characterized by tachycardia, arrhythmias, hyperpyrexia and heart failure. Supportive treatment includes hydration, cooling, β-blockade and inotropes.

Adrenal Disorders

Primary Adrenocortical Insufficiency (Addison's Disease)

Addison's disease is caused by autoimmune disease, infection, sepsis, metastatic tumour or amyloid. Clinical features result from glucocorticoid and mineralocorticoid deficiency, including fatigue, weight loss, postural hypotension, increased skin pigmentation, hyponatraemia, hyperkalaemia and hypoglycaemia. Treatment is with oral hydrocortisone (20 mg morning, 10 mg night) and fludrocortisone 0.1 mg.

Secondary Adrenocortical Insufficiency

Insufficient adrenocorticotrophic hormone (ACTH) occurs secondary to suppression of the hypothalamo-pituitary axis from long-term exogenous corticosteroids or secondary to pituitary or hypothalamic lesions. There is glucocorticoid deficiency only.

Addisonian Crisis

Acute Addisonian crises are characterized by abdominal pain, vomiting, hypotension, hyponatraemia, hyperkalaemia and hypoglycaemia. Crises are precipitated by physiological stress in patients with chronic adrenal insufficiency and inadequate steroid replacement, pituitary apoplexy or adrenal failure (adrenal haemorrhage or infarction, e.g. Waterhouse–Friedrichsen syndrome).

Anaesthesia

Liaison with an endocrinologist is advisable. All medications should be given on the morning of surgery. Patients with adrenocortical insufficiency or taking long-term corticosteroids need perioperative corticosteroid supplementation. Surgery in undiagnosed or inadequately treated patients may precipitate an Addisonian crisis, presenting as perioperative cardiovascular collapse. Treatment is with hydrocortisone 200 mg stat followed by 100 mg, 6 hourly and intravenous saline. Vasopressors may be required.

Cushing's Syndrome

Cushing's syndrome results from excess circulating glucocorticoid usually secondary to administration of synthetic corticosteroids. Other causes include pituitary adenoma (Cushing's disease), ectopic ACTH secretion, adrenal adenoma or carcinoma. Classical features include truncal obesity, moon face and thin extremities. Diagnosis is confirmed by a high plasma cortisol, loss of diurnal variation and failure of suppression with dexamethasone 2 mg. ACTH is low with adrenal or exogenous cortisol administration and very high with ectopic ACTH secretion.

Implications for Anaesthesia

- Impaired glucose tolerance, diabetes
- Refractory hypertension, left ventricular failure (LVF), ventricular dysfunction
- OSA
- Osteoporosis, proximal myopathy, thin friable skin, striae
- Exophthalmos

Anaesthesia

Hypertension and diabetes should be optimized and metabolic abnormalities corrected. Both positioning and venous access can be difficult. Patients, especially with OSA, should be managed in HDU postoperatively.

Primary Hyperaldosteronism (Conn's syndrome)

This results from excess aldosterone production, usually from an adrenal adenoma, but also bilateral adrenal hyperplasia or carcinoma. Clinical features include severe hypertension, hypervolaemia, metabolic acidosis and hypokalaemia. Muscle weakness occurs secondary to hypokalaemia and impaired glucose tolerance is common. Secondary hyperaldosteronism may result from excessive renin secretion by a tumour or renal artery stenosis. Diagnosis is confirmed by an aldosterone to renin ratio > 400. Adrenal vein sampling, CT and MRI are used to distinguish between adrenal adenoma and hyperplasia. An adenoma is treated surgically. Otherwise, treatment is with the aldosterone receptor antagonist spironolactone.

Phaeochromocytoma

See Chapter 5.4, Endocrine Surgery.

Pituitary Disease

Pituitary disease presents with the direct effects of hormone hyper- or hypo-secretion or the mass effect of the enlarging gland. Pituitary adenomas may secrete prolactin, growth hormone (GH) or ACTH.

Acromegaly

Hypersecretion of GH after puberty causes acromegaly. Presentation is insidious, often in middle age, with local mass effect (headache and visual field defects) and an excess of GH. Diagnosis is confirmed by raised serum IGF-1 and GH value after oral glucose tolerance test. Medical treatment is with bromocriptine, a dopamine receptor agonist and/or octreotide, a somatostatin analogue. Many patients require surgery, usually trans-sphenoidal hypophysectomy. Surgery may also be required for unrelated pathology.

Implications for Anaesthesia

- Difficult airway – prognathism, macrognathia, macroglossia, thickening of oropharyngeal tissues
- Refractory hypertension, IHD, cardiomyopathy and biventricular dysfunction
- Diabetes mellitus
- OSA – 70% of patients
- Kyphoscoliosis and proximal myopathy
- Thickened skin – difficult cannulation and nerve entrapment

Anaesthesia

Comorbidities should be optimized. Anaesthetic challenges include airway management, possible difficult intubation, difficult patient positioning and vascular access. Anaesthesia should be planned accordingly. HDU care is recommended especially for those with OSA.

Carcinoid Disease

Carcinoid tumours arise from enterochromaffin cells and are most common in the gastrointestinal tract, bronchus and pancreas. Most are slow growing, although some may be aggressive with widespread metastases. About 25% of malignant lesions secrete vasoactive substances such as serotonin, bradykinin, histamine and vasoactive peptide, resulting in carcinoid syndrome. These substances are normally metabolized in the liver before reaching the systemic circulation – clinical effects only occur with liver metastases or those tumours with venous drainage directly into the systemic circulation.

Carcinoid Syndrome

Clinical manifestations include flushing, tachycardia, hypotension or hypertension, bronchospasm and diarrhoea. Medical treatment may include antihistamines, 5HT antagonists and the somatostatin analogue octreotide.

Implications for Anaesthesia

- Carcinoid heart disease – restrictive cardiomyopathy, plaque formation and fibrosis, particularly right-sided heart valves
- Electrolyte abnormalities from diarrhoea
- Bronchoconstriction

Anaesthesia

Electrolyte abnormalities should be corrected and volume deficits replaced. Cardiac failure should be optimized if present. Octreotide is given for 2 weeks prior to surgery; perioperative infusion helps prevent mediator release. Premedication with an anxiolytic is useful. All histamine releasing drugs and catecholamines should be avoided. Marked cardiovascular instability can occur intraoperatively following mechanical and/or pharmacological manipulation and release of vasoactive substances. Invasive monitoring is essential. Severe bronchoconstriction and hypotension, resistant to conventional therapy, may also occur. Intravenous octreotide has been used successfully, as has aprotinin. Delayed emergence from anaesthesia has been reported possibly related to high serotonin levels. The use of regional techniques is controversial because they may exacerbate any hypotension.

METABOLIC AND BIOCHEMICAL DISORDERS

Porphyria

The porphyrias are a heterogeneous group of disorders resulting from inherited deficiencies of the intermediary enzymes of haem synthesis. The haem biosynthetic pathway is most active in the liver and bone marrow. Any factors that increase pathway activity will lead to accumulation of substrate before the enzyme defect. Those most relevant to anaesthetists are the three acute hepatic forms which are all inherited in an autosomal manner:

- Acute intermittent porphyria (AIP) – common in Sweden
- Variegate porphyria (VP) – common in South Africa's Afrikaner community
- Hereditary coproporphyria (HCP) – rare

All defects in the acute porphyrias result in accumulation of δ-aminolaevulinic acid (ALA). In the forms above, porphobilinogen (PBG) is also elevated and can be used to diagnose acute crises. Attacks are most common in women in their 30s. They may be provoked by hormonal fluctuations, stress, dehydration, fasting and infection. Almost all have severe abdominal pain, associated with a tachycardia. Neurological symptoms including peripheral neuropathy, cranial nerve palsies, autonomic disturbance, epilepsy and neuropsychiatric symptoms may also occur. Patients with VP and HCP may present with skin lesions, e.g. blistering and photosensitivity during acute crises. The excretion of porphyrins turns urine red or dark brown on standing. Precipitating factors are commonly encountered in the perioperative period.[12]

Implications for Anaesthesia

- Most patients will never have had symptoms; all patients with a strong family history should be considered at risk.
- Biochemical tests are often normal between attacks.
- Hepatic porphyrias affect synthesis of the cytochrome P450 enzyme system – drugs causing enzyme induction may trigger a crisis.
- Many common anaesthetic drugs have the potential to trigger a crisis – expert guidance should be sought before anaesthesia; databases are available based on international experience.
- Crises can be triggered by illness or stress.

Anaesthesia

Preoperative fasting should be minimized and i.v. fluids started preoperatively. An anxiolytic premedication is useful, midazolam or temazepam are safe. Propofol is safe and can be used for induction and maintenance. Isoflurane, halothane and desflurane have been used safely. Barbiturates are contraindicated. Neuromuscular blocking drugs (NMBs) are considered safe as is neostigmine. Pentazocine is considered unsafe, but other opioids, including morphine, codeine, pethidine, fentanyl, remifentanil, alfentanil and naloxone, have been used safely. Oxycodone and diclofenac are considered unsafe. There are reports of the safe use of regional anaesthesia in patients with porphyria. Patients should be monitored after operation for symptoms and signs of a crisis.

Management of an acute crisis should be in ICU and includes withdrawal of precipitating agents, symptomatic treatment with 'safe' drugs and supportive therapy. Intravenous haem arginate therapy should be started as soon as possible, 3 mg/kg i.v. daily for 4 days.

Electrolyte Disturbance

Hyponatraemia

Hyponatraemia is defined as a serum sodium <135 mmol/L and classified according to severity:

- Mild   130–135 mmol/L
- Moderate   125–129 mmol/L
- Severe   <125 mmol/L

It is considered acute if the rate of onset <48 h and chronic if greater. The duration is often unknown and should be considered chronic, unless there is evidence otherwise (e.g. new medications or recent surgery). Hyponatraemia occurs via three basic mechanisms in relation to extracellular fluid volume:

● Reduced – gastrointestinal losses, diuretics, Addison disease
● Normal – inappropriate antidiuretic hormone (ADH) secretion
● Increased – cardiac failure, cirrhosis, nephrotic syndrome

Hyponatraemia can also be artefactual (pseudo-hyponatraemia) as a result of high serum protein, lipid levels or hyperosmolarity from severe hyperglycaemia. Severe hyponatraemia is associated with neurological symptoms and cerebral oedema, convulsions and coma can occur. Asymptomatic hyponatraemia is treated by correction of the underlying cause and fluid restriction. Symptomatic chronic hyponatraemia with hypervolaemia is treated with loop diuretics and, in the presence of low or normal volume status, i.v. normal or hypertonic saline. Correction should be no greater than 1–2 mmol/L per hour to minimize the risk of central pontine myelinolysis.

Hypernatraemia

Hypernatraemia is defined as a serum sodium >145 mmol/L and is caused by excessive salt intake, or more commonly inadequate water intake. Consideration of the patient's volume status is essential. In hospital, it is often iatrogenic from insufficient water intake or excessive sodium administration. Clinical features usually include neurological signs, e.g. irritability, lethargy, muscle twitching, spasticity and hyperreflexia. Severe hypernatraemia (>158 mmol/L) may present with hyperthermia, delirium, seizures and coma. Treatment depends on the underlying aetiology; i.v. fluids should replace any volume deficit. Correction should be undertaken slowly (>24 h) to avoid precipitating cerebral oedema and convulsions. Diabetes insipidus (DI) results in inappropriately dilute urine, raised serum osmolality and hypernatraemia due to reduced ADH secretion (central DI) or reduced responsiveness of the kidney to ADH (nephrogenic DI). Treatment is with desmopressin and fluid replacement.

Hypokalaemia

Hypokalaemia is defined as a serum potassium <3.5 mmol/L and results from:

● Depletion of intracellular potassium – inadequate intake (e.g. gastrointestinal losses) or increased loss (e.g. increased renal excretion)
● Intracellular potassium shifts – insulin, alkalosis, β-agonists

Clinical features include muscle weakness, tetany, ileus and polyuria. Characteristic ECG changes include flattened T waves, ST segment depression and U waves. Digitalis toxicity is enhanced and can induce life-threatening ventricular arrhythmias. Hypokalaemia should be corrected using oral supplements, or potassium-containing intravenous fluids. If urgent correction is required potassium may be given intravenously with continuous ECG monitoring.

Hyperkalaemia

Hyperkalaemia is defined as a serum potassium >5.5 mmol/L and results from:

- Potassium redistribution from cells into the extracellular compartment – acidosis, insulin deficiency, suxamethonium, muscle damage
- Increased intake – i.v. supplementation or blood transfusion
- Decreased renal excretion – renal failure, adrenocortical insufficiency, drugs, e.g. NSAIDs, ACE inhibitors and potassium-sparing diuretics

Clinical features include nausea, vomiting and diarrhoea, muscle weakness and acidosis. Cardiac arrhythmias such as VF and asystole can occur. Characteristic ECG changes include flattened P waves, widened QRS complexes and tented T waves. In the presence of $K^+ > 6.5$ mmol/L or ECG changes, urgent correction is necessary. Calcium stabilizes the myocardium either as calcium gluconate (5–10 mL of 10%) or chloride (3–5 mL 10%) preparations. Other treatments include insulin (10u in 50 mL 50% dextrose over 30–60 min) or sodium bicarbonate, if acidotic. β_2-agonists act by shifting potassium back into the cells. Subsequent treatment is aimed at removing the cause and eliminating excess potassium from the body with a cation exchange resin.

Hypocalcaemia

Hypocalcaemia occurs when calcium is lost from the extracellular fluid in greater quantities than can be replaced by intestine or bone. Causes include renal failure, vitamin D or magnesium deficiency, acute pancreatitis, hypoparathyroidism and massive transfusion with citrate-anticoagulated blood. Hypocalcaemia also occurs following parathyroidectomy, thyroidectomy and cardiopulmonary bypass. Falsely low levels of calcium due to hypoalbuminaemia can be excluded by measuring ionized calcium.

Symptoms depend upon the magnitude and rate of fall in calcium. Severe hypocalcaemia (< 0.50 mmol/L) produces increased neuronal irritability but can also result in respiratory and cardiovascular disturbances. Complications include hypotension, impaired cardiac contractility, cardiac arrhythmias, tetany, muscle weakness, laryngeal spasm, bronchospasm and convulsions. Treatment is with i.v. calcium (calcium gluconate 10%, 10 mL over 10 min) and correction of any coexisting hypomagnesaemia or alkalosis.

Hypercalcaemia

The commonest causes of hypercalcaemia are primary hyperparathyroidism (usually an adenoma secreting parathyroid hormone, hypercalcaemia and hypophosphataemia) and malignancy. Severe hypercalcaemia disrupts gastrointestinal, neurological, cardiovascular and renal function. Clinical features include dehydration, muscle weakness, impaired renal function, hypertension and cardiac arrhythmias. Characteristically there is a shortened QT segment on the ECG. Initial treatment is by rehydration with intravenous saline. Pamidronate is rapidly effective as is calcitonin but its effects are temporary. If further treatment is necessary, forced saline diuresis with furosemide can be considered, but cardiovascular status and electrolyte levels must be closely monitored.

LIVER DISEASE

Acute Hepatitis

The commonest cause of acute hepatic failure worldwide is viral hepatitis. In the UK, 70% of cases are a result of acetaminophen overdose; others include alcohol and drugs or toxins. Outcome is dependent upon the degree of hepatic dysfunction. Perioperative mortality is extremely high and elective surgery should be postponed until liver function tests return to normal.

Chronic Liver Disease

The commonest causes are viral hepatitis (B, C), autoimmune and alcohol. Others include cryptogenic liver disease, cholestatic conditions, e.g. primary biliary cirrhosis and sclerosing cholangitis, venous outflow obstruction, drugs, toxins and metabolic disease, e.g. Wilson's disease, haemochromatosis and alpha$_1$-antitrypsin deficiency. Mild disease (chronic persistent hepatitis) is usually asymptomatic and anaesthesia is usually well tolerated. More severe disease (chronic active hepatitis) may progress to liver fibrosis and cirrhosis.

Alcoholic Liver Disease

This may result in steatosis (fatty liver), alcoholic hepatitis and cirrhosis. Patients with steatosis generally tolerate surgery well. However, hepatitis and cirrhosis are associated with increased perioperative morbidity and mortality.

Patients with liver disease have multisystem organ dysfunction. The Child–Turcotte–Pugh classification is a commonly used scoring system for patients with liver disease. Scores are calculated from five variables: serum albumin, serum bilirubin, ascites, prothrombin time (PT) or INR, and grade of encephalopathy to place patients into three groups (Class A = score 5–6; Class B = score 7–9; Class C = score 10–15). Mortality rates for class B and C have traditionally been very high following abdominal surgery. More recently lower rates have been reported: Class A = 2%; Class B = 12%; Class C = 12%. Overall risk can be stratified using specific scoring systems, patient risk factors and type of surgery. Factors associated with perioperative complications are shown in Box 1.2.6.

Implications for Anaesthesia
- Hepatic disease – decreased metabolic function, gluconeogenesis, hyperbilirubinemia, varices, ascites and portal hypertension

> **BOX 1.2.6 Risk factors Associated with Complications and Mortality in Liver Disease[13]**
>
> **Factors associated with perioperative complications**
> *Scoring systems:*
>   Child–Turcotte–Pugh (CTP) score
>   ASA status IV or V
>
> *Patient-specific factors:*
>   Male gender
>   Age > 70 years
>   Preoperative infection
>   Cirrhosis
>   Raised creatinine
>   COPD
>   Ascites
>   Upper GI bleeding
>   Intraoperative hypotension
>
> *High-risk surgery:*
>   Abdominal
>   Cardiothoracic
>   Emergency

- Haematological – coagulopathy and thrombosis, reduced synthesis of clotting factors, thrombocytopenia and platelet dysfunction, dysfibrinogenaemia
- Cardiovascular – vasodilation, hyperdynamic circulation, cirrhotic cardiomyopathy, porto-pulmonary hypertension
- Pulmonary – aspiration risk, hepatopulmonary syndrome, atelectasis; pleural effusions
- Electrolyte or metabolic – hypoglycaemia, hyponatraemia, malnourishment
- Renal – acute kidney injury, hepatorenal syndrome
- Neurological – encephalopathy, cerebral oedema, raised intracranial pressure
- Infection – immune function is depressed
- Drug metabolism – enhanced, prolonged unpredictable effects of drugs, including opioids, benzodiazepines, neuromuscular blocker; a reduction in plasma cholinesterase activity may lead to prolonged action of suxamethonium

Anaesthesia

Tests such as bilirubin and albumin are nonspecific, FBC will detect anaemia, thrombocytopenia or raised white cell count. PT is an indicator of hepatocellular function and prognostic indicator. Electrolyte abnormalities and coagulopathy should be corrected, using vitamin K, fresh frozen plasma and cryoprecipitate. ECG and echocardiography are indicated, if risk factors for left ventricular dysfunction, cardiomyopathy, or pulmonary hypertension. CXR or ultrasound may demonstrate pleural effusions in need of drainage. Ascites may be treated with diuretics or paracentesis. For major surgery, invasive monitoring is recommended. Oesophageal Doppler may be helpful in some patients, but is contraindicated with oesophageal varices as are nasogastric tubes and oesophageal temperature probes. Invasive arterial monitoring allows assessment of ABGs, lactate, glucose, electrolytes and coagulation. Monitoring of temperature, neuromuscular block and urine output are necessary. Haemodynamic optimization and maintenance of intravascular volume are essential to achieve an adequate urine output. Loop diuretics or mannitol are occasionally used.

Choice of anaesthetic agents for induction and maintenance are less important than the care with which they are used. Agents with minimal hepatic metabolism, such as isoflurane and sevoflurane, or total intravenous anaesthesia (TIVA) with propofol and remifentanil are preferred. Atracurium is the muscle relaxant of choice. Other opioids should be administered cautiously at a reduced dose and sedatives avoided where possible. Drugs that are potentially hepatotoxic or nephrotoxic, including NSAIDs, should be avoided. Regional anaesthetic techniques may be of benefit in the absence of coagulopathy or thrombocytopenia.

RENAL DISEASE

Chronic Kidney Disease (CKD)

CKD is common. Causes include diabetes mellitus, glomerulonephritis, polycystic kidney disease, pyelonephritis and hypertension. Glomerular filtration rate (GFR) defines and classifies renal function. Severe impairment is diagnosed when GFR < 35 mL/min and dialysis is required when <15 mL/min. Patients have complex medical histories due to co-existing disease and multisystem complications and CKD is a risk factor for serious perioperative complications, especially cardiovascular and acute renal failure. Renal function may deteriorate perioperatively secondary to reductions in renal blood flow or from drug-induced nephrotoxicity.

Implications for Anaesthesia

- Cardiovascular – hypertension, LVH, IHD (often silent), conduction abnormalities, cardiomyopathy, heart failure, pulmonary oedema, pericarditis, pericardial effusions, autonomic neuropathy
- Endocrine – diabetes mellitus, secondary and tertiary hyperparathyroidism, vitamin D deficiency
- Gastrointestinal – anorexia, vomiting, delayed gastric emptying
- Haematology and haemostasis – normochromic, normocytic anaemia, prothrombotic tendency/hypercoagulation and reduced fibrinolysis, uraemic thrombocytopathy
- Fluid, electrolyte and metabolic haemostasis – salt and water retention, hyperkalaemia, volume overload, dehydration, metabolic acidosis
- Immune system – immunosuppression due to uraemia or drugs

Anaesthesia

The aetiology, stage of CKD, previous surgery should be established; systemic complications and comorbidities optimized. Ascertain last dialysis, presence of arteriovenous fistulae or peritoneal dialysis lines, patient's weight and usual dry weight. Baseline FBC, urea and electrolytes (U&Es), especially recent K^+, are essential. Platelet dysfunction or residual effect of heparin after dialysis may result in coagulopathy. Immunosuppression (especially if previous renal transplant) is common and strict asepsis is essential. Fistulae must be protected and potential construction sites avoided when establishing venous access.

Regional or general anaesthesia may be safely used. The risk of reflux is increased. Suxamethonium should be avoided in the presence of hyperkalaemia. Drug choice is affected by altered clearance, the production and accumulation of active metabolites, and the risk of aggravating renal dysfunction (see below). All drugs should be given slowly and titrated to response. A nerve stimulator must be used with NMBs. Maintain euvolaemia, normotension and cardiac output to optimize renal perfusion.

Anaesthetic Drugs in Renal Failure

The free fraction of benzodiazepines is increased and thiopental has an increased volume of distribution and reduced plasma protein binding in renal failure. The dose of both should be reduced. Propofol is considered a more suitable induction agent. Some inhalational agents are metabolized to fluoride, which is potentially nephrotoxic. Enflurane produces the highest levels and is probably best avoided. Sevoflurane is also metabolized to fluoride and degrades in soda lime to form compound A; there is no evidence of nephrotoxicity in humans. Atracurium and cisatracurium are the muscle relaxants of choice as elimination is independent of renal function. Vecuronium and rocuronium are considered safe; pancuronium should be avoided. Suxamethonium increases serum potassium by about 0.5 mmol/L, but should be safe in the absence of hyperkalaemia. The clearance of neostigmine is reduced and half-life prolonged in CKD. Sugammadex may prove useful if patients have had rocuronium. Opioid analgesics are largely metabolized in the liver, but metabolites are often renally excreted. The action of morphine may be prolonged due to the active metabolite morphine-6-glucuronide; accumulation of norpethidine, a metabolite of pethidine, may result in CNS excitation and convulsions. Alfentanil and remifentanil may be used in normal doses. Paracetamol is safe and tramadol best avoided. NSAIDs may result in further deterioration of renal function and should be avoided.[14]

NEUROLOGICAL DISEASES

Cerebrovascular Disease

Stroke is the third commonest cause of death and the leading cause of disability in the industrialized world. Cerebrovascular disease is associated with hypertension, diabetes, obesity and smoking. Its incidence increases with age. It manifests as global cerebral dysfunction (multi-infarct dementia) or a focal neurological event such as a stroke or transient ischaemic attack (TIA). Patients at high risk of stroke should be identified in advance; risks include advanced age, renal disease and history of previous stroke or TIA. For patients with recent stroke, consider delaying elective surgery until the peak autoregulatory disturbance has passed (about 1 month).[15]

Anaesthesia

Evidence suggests that continuation of aspirin in patients at risk of stroke is not indicated and may increase the risk of bleeding. Continuation of ß-blockers and statins is important. Intraoperative hypotension should be avoided; blood pressure should be maintained as close as possible to preoperative levels.

Neurology or stroke doctors must review surgical patients manifesting symptoms or signs of stroke urgently and neuroimaging is essential. Major noncardiac, nonneurological surgery is not an absolute contraindication to intravascular thrombolysis; mechanical thrombolysis is also an option for those at high risk of surgery-related haemorrhage.

Epilepsy

A diagnosis of epilepsy is based on two unprovoked seizures, at least 24 h apart. It is not a single condition with more than 40 different types. Treatment is with anticonvulsants. The goal of perioperative care is to minimize interference with usual anticonvulsant regimes and avoid physiological or pharmacological disturbances that might lower seizure threshold. It is important to establish seizure type and frequency, current drug regime and control. Most common anticonvulsants cause enzyme induction affecting the metabolism of other drugs with the exception of levetiracetam. Sodium valproate may interfere with haemostasis. Determine comorbidities, e.g. congenital syndromes or seizures after stroke.

Anaesthesia

Most induction agents are proconvulsant at low dose but anticonvulsant at doses used for general anaesthesia. Thiopental is safe, despite excitatory phenomena occasionally seen with propofol it is also considered safe – both are established treatments for refractory status epilepticus. Benzodiazepines are all potent anticonvulsants. Agents associated with seizures such as methohexitone, etomidate and enflurane are best avoided, particularly in patients with a driving licence. Most opioid analgesics have been used safely. However, alfentanil enhances EEG activity and tramadol lowers seizure threshold.

Abnormal movements in the postoperative setting may be seizures or other conditions such as shivering, dystonic drug reaction, vaso-vagal and psychogenic nonepileptic seizure. Management is with an ABC approach, determination of cause and termination of seizure with benzodiazepine. A diagnosis of first seizure should be made with caution in the perioperative setting.

Status epilepticus is defined as seizure activity lasting over 30 min without recovery of consciousness. Rapid treatment is required to prevent neuronal damage and systemic complications with an ABC approach. Lorazepam 0.1 mg/kg i.v. is considered to be the most effective initial treatment, followed by phenytoin and/or phenobarbital according to response.

Parkinson's Disease

Although the aetiology of Parkinson's disease is unknown, 'Parkinsonism' can be precipitated by a variety of causes including arteriosclerosis, diffuse degenerative disease, repeated head trauma, metabolic defects such as Wilson disease, heavy metal or carbon monoxide poisoning. Drug induced Parkinsonism results from dopamine receptor blockade by drugs including phenothiazines, butyrophenones and metoclopramide. Age is the most consistent risk factor. A loss of dopaminergic neurons in the substantia nigra of the basal ganglia produces an imbalance between the dopaminergic and cholinergic systems. It is characterized by resting tremor, muscle rigidity and bradykinesia. Treatment is usually with levodopa in combination with a peripheral DOPA-decarboxylase inhibitor to minimize peripheral side effects. Dopamine agonists (bromocriptine) and type B monoamine oxidase inhibitors (selegiline) may also be used. Surgical treatments are increasing in popularity.

Anaesthesia

The usual drug regime must be continued. If possible, a specialist physician or Parkinson nurse should assist with perioperative care. Levodopa can only be given enterally and has a short half-life. Apomorphine can be used subcutaneously but is very emetogenic. Where possible regional anaesthesia should be used. Patients with excessive salivation and pharyngeal dysfunction are at risk of regurgitation and aspiration. Postoperative atelectasis and respiratory infection may occur owing to impaired clearance of secretions and chest wall rigidity. Advanced disease is associated with autonomic dysfunction, marked postural and drug-induced hypotension. Phenothiazines, butyrophenones and metoclopramide should be avoided because they may exacerbate extrapyramidal symptoms. An increased incidence of postoperative confusion and hallucinations has been reported.

Multiple Sclerosis

Multiple sclerosis is a demyelinating disease affecting the CNS. It is thought to be autoimmune in nature, but viral and genetic factors have also been implicated. It occurs more commonly in women and in geographical clusters, e.g., Europe, North America and New Zealand. The optic nerve, brainstem and spinal cord are most often affected and progression is marked by remissions and relapses. Permanent weakness develops in some leading to severe disability. Respiratory failure and bulbar palsy may occur in end-stage disease. Pregnancy, particularly the third trimester, is often associated with an improvement in symptoms, but an increased relapse rate has been reported in the first 3 months postpartum. Treatment is with immunomodulating drugs such as interferon to modify disease course. Relapses are treated with steroids and symptoms such as spasticity or spasm with baclofen or dantrolene.

Anaesthesia

There is no evidence that general anaesthesia affects the course of the disease. Patients with severe, advanced disease will be at greater risk of complications such as respiratory infections. Spinal anaesthesia has been linked with neurological complications but the safe use has also been reported. Epidural anaesthesia also appears safe. Existing signs and symptoms must be documented before performing a regional technique, and the patient fully involved in the decision-making process. Local anaesthetic toxicity may be more likely due to disruption of the blood–brain barrier.

Motor Neuron Disease

This is characterized by degeneration of motor neurons within the motor cortex (amyotrophic lateral sclerosis), brainstem motor nuclei of the cranial nerves and anterior horn cells of the spinal cord. The disease is progressive, presenting between 50 and 70 years. Clinical features include muscle weakness, wasting, fasciculations, spasticity and hyperreflexia. Bulbar palsies are common and may lead to impairment of speech, swallowing and laryngeal reflexes. Respiratory failure develops due to inspiratory muscle weakness and inability to clear secretions effectively.

Anaesthesia

Patients with advanced disease are at considerable risk from general anaesthesia. Suxamethonium may cause severe hyperkalaemia and there is increased sensitivity to nondepolarizing NMBs. Bulbar involvement increases the risk of regurgitation and aspiration. Patients are prone to postoperative respiratory failure due to increased sensitivity to respiratory depressants and impaired ability to clear secretions. Despite concerns that exacerbations of the disease may follow the use of regional anaesthetic techniques, epidural anaesthesia has been used successfully.

NEUROMUSCULAR DISORDERS

Myasthenia Gravis (MG)

MG is an autoimmune disorder affecting the neuromuscular junction and characterized by muscle weakness and fatiguability (weakness on exertion that improves with rest). It is more common in women and is associated with other autoimmune disorders. IgG antibodies result in destruction of postsynaptic acetylcholine receptors. About 10%–15% of patients have a thymoma. Hyperplasia of the thymus is common in younger patients. The ocular, bulbar and facial muscles are commonly involved with a spectrum of features ranging from ptosis, to dysarthria, dysphagia and respiratory failure; limb weakness is usually proximal. Symptomatic treatment is with oral anticholinesterases such as pyridostigmine. Steroids or immunosuppressives are often effective in eliminating the antibody. Thymectomy is indicated in most patients under 60 years and those with a thymoma. Plasmapheresis or immunoglobulin infusions may be useful for crises.

Implications for Anaesthesia

- Increased sensitivity to nondepolarizing NMBs
- Resistance to depolarizing NMBs
- Increased sensitivity to the neuromuscular effects of volatile agents
- Risk of aspiration with bulbar weakness, postoperative respiratory failure with respiratory muscle weakness
- Risk of cholinergic crisis with excessive doses of anticholinesterases
- Effects of immunosuppressant therapy

Anaesthesia

Management depends upon disease severity, type of surgery and the requirement for muscle relaxation. The extent of muscle weakness should be assessed and treatment optimized. A bulbar palsy is predictive of the need for airway protection and possibly a nasogastric tube. Severe respiratory dysfunction will need postoperative support. Anticholinesterase treatment should be continued perioperatively and NMBs avoided if possible. Many procedures, including thymectomy, are possible without. If required, small doses (~10% of normal) of short-acting nondepolarizing NMBs and monitoring with a nerve stimulator. Avoid neostigmine if possible. Sugammadex has been used successfully. Volatile agents potentiate the effects of nondepolarizing NMBs. Maintenance of anaesthesia with propofol and remifentanil should be considered. Sevoflurane or desflurane are the volatile agents of choice for rapid emergence. Cautious use of other opioids is recommended. Nonopioid analgesics and local/regional anaesthesia should be used where possible. Early resumption of all treatment drugs is essential. Patients should be closely monitored in a HDU postoperatively. Predictors of the need for ventilatory support include:

- Major body cavity surgery
- Disease duration (>6 years)
- Co-existent respiratory disease
- Preoperative vital capacity < 2.9 L
- Dose requirements for pyridostigmine > 750 mg/day

Myasthenic Emergencies

Respiratory failure may be caused by a myasthenic or cholinergic crisis. Myasthenic crises are life-threatening episodes of respiratory or bulbar paralysis. Cholinergic crises result from excessive anticholinesterase medication leading to a depolarizing block of neuromuscular transmission. Respiratory support is necessary and anticholinergic medication withheld until the nature of the crisis is determined.

Myasthenic Syndrome (Eaton–Lambert Syndrome)

Myasthenic syndrome is a proximal weakness associated with cancer and originally described in association with small cell carcinoma of the lung. Autoantibodies to the presynaptic calcium channels cause impaired neuromuscular transmission with little response to anticholinesterases. Clinical features include weakness of the proximal lower limbs and trunk, loss of lower limb reflexes, ptosis and autonomic dysfunction. There is marked sensitivity to both depolarizing and nondepolarizing NMBs; prolonged paralysis may occur.

Myotonia

Myotonia is defined as delayed relaxation of muscle after voluntary contraction or mechanical stimulation. Dystrophia myotonica (myotonic dystrophy) is the most common dystonia. The others are myotonia congenital and paramyotonia. All are inherited in an autosomal dominant manner. It usually presents between 20 and 40 years of age. Unlike the other dystonias, it is a multisystem disease, characterized by prefrontal balding and cataracts. Clinical features include atrophy and weakness particularly of the facial, sternomastoid and peripheral muscles. Progressive skeletal, smooth and cardiac muscle atrophy results in cardiorespiratory compromise and cardiomyopathy.

Implications for Anaesthesia

● Persistent skeletal muscular contraction after stimulation – suxamethonium may produce prolonged contraction; surgical manipulation, diathermy, hypothermia and shivering may all cause myotonia
● Respiratory muscle weakness – risk of postoperative respiratory complications
● Pharyngeal muscle weakness, obstructive sleep apnoea
● Progressive bulbar palsy and oesophageal dysfunction – risk of regurgitation and aspiration
● Cardiovascular disease – arrhythmias, conduction defects and cardiomyopathy
● Endocrine dysfunction may result in diabetes, hypothyroidism, adrenal insufficiency and gonadal atrophy
● Mental decline after the second decade

Anaesthesia

The severity of respiratory dysfunction, including bulbar palsy, must be assessed preoperatively. Arrhythmias and conduction defects may require treatment. Precautions against regurgitation and aspiration are advisable. Response to induction agents is unpredictable and cautious administration is recommended. Suxamethonium must be avoided and the response to nondepolarizing NMBs is difficult to predict. Intubation may be possible without muscle relaxants but, where necessary, incremental short-acting agents and neuromuscular monitoring is recommended. Neostigmine may provoke contraction. Invasive arterial monitoring is recommended for patients with significant cardiovascular disease. Regional techniques have been used successfully but do not necessarily abolish intraoperative myotonia. Cataract surgery is usually performed under local anaesthesia. The patient must be kept warm, and HDU is recommended postoperatively.

Muscular Dystrophy

The muscular dystrophies are a group of inherited disorders characterized by progressive muscle wasting and weakness. Classification is according to mode of inheritance:

- X linked – Duchenne, Becker
- Autosomal recessive – Limb girdle, childhood, congenital
- Autosomal dominant – Facio-humeral, oculopharyngeal

Duchenne Muscular Dystrophy

Duchenne muscular dystrophy is the commonest and most severe form. Presentation is with lower limb and pelvic muscle weakness aged 2–5 years. Death is usual by the second decade secondary to cardiorespiratory complications.

Implications for Anaesthesia

- Suxamethonium and volatile agents may result in a rhabdomyolysis and hypermetabolism resembling malignant hyperthermia
- Myocardial degeneration – hypertrophic cardiomyopathy and arrhythmias are common; right heart failure may occur
- • Progressive respiratory muscle weakness – a restrictive ventilatory pattern, diminished cough progressing to respiratory failure
- Progressive kyphoscoliosis

Anaesthesia

Optimization of respiratory status is essential. Preoperative echocardiography is recommended if patient is wheelchair bound to assess ventricular and valve function. Precautions against regurgitation and aspiration are advisable. Suxamethonium is contraindicated. Volatile anaesthetic agents are controversial – they are not always accompanied by complications. However, it may be safer to avoid them. Response to nondepolarizing NMBs is variable – incremental doses and neuromuscular monitoring is recommended. The respiratory depressant effects of opioids are enhanced and patients should be closely monitored. Respiratory support may be needed postoperatively.

MUSCULOSKELETAL AND CONNECTIVE TISSUE DISORDERS

Ankylosing Spondylitis

Ankylosing spondylitis is an inflammatory arthropathy affecting primarily the spine and sacroiliac joints. There is systemic involvement and a proportion of patients develop ophthalmic, cardiovascular, respiratory and neurological complications. It is four times more common in males and associated with HLA B27 in over 95% of patients.

Implications for Anaesthesia

- Difficult intubation – cervical immobility, limited mouth opening due to temporomandibular joint involvement
- Risk of cervical fracture with minimal trauma
- Limited chest expansion and pulmonary fibrosis – postoperative respiratory complications
- Cardiovascular – aortic regurgitation and conduction defects
- Progressive kyphosis and fixation of spine – difficulty with positioning, technical difficulties with neuraxial block
- Renal impairment – amyloidosis or IgA nephropathy

Anaesthesia

Difficult intubation should be anticipated and airway adjuncts prepared. SADs or videolaryngoscopes may be useful, and awake fibre-optic intubation (AFOI) in severe disease. Care should be taken on transfer and positioning. Postoperative respiratory support may be required.

Rheumatoid Arthritis

Rheumatoid arthritis is a relatively common, chronic inflammatory disorder. It primarily affects joints; characteristically a symmetrical peripheral polyarthritis. Systemic complications occur in more than 50% of patients.

Implications for Anaesthesia

- Cervical instability – atlantoaxial subluxation (25% of those with advanced disease), may be asymptomatic; cord damage possible with cervical manipulation, particularly flexion
- Temporomandibular joint involvement – mouth opening may be limited
- Cricoarytenoid joint involvement, laryngeal deviation

- Pulmonary fibrosis, restrictive lung defect, pleural effusions or nodules
- Myocardial disease due to fibrosis, pericarditis, pericardial effusion, aortic regurgitation, systemic vasculitis
- Autonomic and peripheral neuropathy
- Immunosuppression, anaemia – of chronic disease, gastrointestinal blood loss from NSAIDs, bone marrow suppression
- Felty syndrome – splenomegaly and neutropenia

Anaesthesia

Careful preoperative assessment to identify a potential difficult airway – AFOI may be indicated. Determine systemic involvement and optimize comorbidities. Steroid supplementation may be needed and strict asepsis maintained. Ensure careful positioning and padding of vulnerable areas. Vascular access and regional techniques may be difficult.

Systemic Lupus Erythematosus (SLE)

SLE is a chronic inflammatory disorder characterized by immune-mediated tissue damage. A variety of autoantibodies are found including antinuclear antibody. The aetiology is multifactorial. It is more common in females with onset aged 30–40 years. Arthritis, often affecting the hands, and skin lesions are the commonest presenting features, but it is a multisystem disorder.

Implications for Anaesthesia

- Cardiac complications – conduction abnormalities, noninfective endocarditis of the mitral valve, myocarditis, pericarditis, coronary artery disease
- Pulmonary emboli, pleuritis, pleural effusions, pulmonary fibrosis.
- Renal dysfunction due to glomerulonephritis
- Haematological – anaemia, leucopenia, thrombocytopenia, coagulopathy
- Neurological – cranial and peripheral nerve lesions, psychosis, seizures
- Antiphospholipid antibodies – associated with risk of thrombosis and stroke

Scleroderma

Scleroderma (systemic sclerosis) encompasses a spectrum of diseases involving abnormal collagen deposition and microvascular changes in the skin and other organs. Characteristically, the skin becomes taut and shiny with a loss of skin folds. Contractures of the joints and around the mouth may develop. Raynaud phenomenon is common, and oesophageal, pulmonary, cardiac and renal complications may also occur.

Implications for Anaesthesia

- Difficult venous access
- Limited mouth opening – potential difficult intubation

- Oesophageal motility disorders – risk of regurgitation
- Cardiovascular complications – arrhythmias, conduction defects, hypertension, cardiomyopathy, pericarditis and effusions
- Pulmonary fibrosis and pulmonary hypertension
- Renal dysfunction, progressing to renal failure

HAEMATOLOGICAL DISORDERS

Anaemia

The WHO classification of anaemia is haemoglobin (Hb) $<$ 13 g/dL in men and $<$ 12 g/dL in women. It occurs in up to a third of the surgical population and is associated with worse outcomes. Causes include:

- Dietary iron, folate or vitamin B_{12} deficiency
- Acute or chronic blood loss
- Chronic illness (renal failure, malignancy)
- Bone marrow failure
- Haemolytic anaemias – inherited (sickle cell, thalassaemia), acquired (autoimmune, drugs) or physical (mechanical heart valves, marathon running)

Anaemia reduces oxygen-carrying capacity. Adverse effects depend upon the capacity for compensation. Compensatory mechanisms include an increase and redistribution of cardiac output, increased red blood cell 2,3-diposphoglycerate (2,3-DPG), a right shift of the oxygen dissociation curve and increased oxygen extraction. Symptoms include fatigue, breathlessness, palpitations and angina.

All patients should have their haemoglobin measured before listing for major elective surgery. Anaemia should be investigated and treated appropriately. Elective treatment should be postponed. Nutritional deficiencies are treated with oral or i.v. iron, folate or vitamin B_{12} therapy. Recombinant human erythropoietin (rHuEpo) may be useful for those with anaemia of chronic disease or chronic renal failure. In view of the potential hazards of transfusion and shortage of blood products, a rational approach to the transfusion is recommended. Decisions to transfuse should take into account duration of anaemia, intravascular volume, expected intraoperative blood loss and comorbidities, such as significant cardiovascular and respiratory disease. A transfusion threshold of 7 g/dL appears to be adequate in fit patients. Uncertainty remains in patients with cardiovascular disease where higher transfusion thresholds Hb 8 g/dL may be more appropriate.[16]

Haemoglobinopathies

Sickle Cell Disease (SCD)

SCD is an autosomal recessively inherited haemoglobinopathy resulting from a mutation on chromosome 11. Valine is substituted for glutamic acid on the β-globin subunit of normal adult haemoglobin A (HbA) – resulting in the formation of haemoglobin S (HbS). It occurs mostly in those of African or Southwest Asian descent, but also in some Mediterranean races. HbS is bio-chemically unstable – desaturation results in polymerization of haemoglobin, which deforms red cells into the typical sickle cells. The consequences are two-fold: small vessel obstruction (vaso-occlusive crises) and haemolytic anae-mia. Sickling is also precipitated by hypothermia, stasis, infection and dehy-dration. The more HbS, the greater the propensity to sickle. The homozygous state SS (75%–95% HbS) results in SCD, whereas heterozygotes (20%–45% HbS) have sickle cell trait. This is usually a benign condition – sickling rarely occurs and it may provide some protection against *Plasmodium falciparum* malaria. Features of SCD are not apparent until the main switch from foetal to adult haemoglobin at 3–4 months.

Implications for Anaesthesia

- Cardiovascular – cardiomegaly secondary to anaemia or cardiac failure, pul-monary hypertension secondary to recurrent pulmonary infarction
- Respiratory – dyspnoea, haemoptysis and pleuritic chest pain occur with 'acute chest syndrome'; recurrent episodes cause respiratory dysfunction
- Splenic sequestration – massive pooling of red blood cells and platelets, occurs mostly in children but can be life–threatening; recurrent splenic infarction results in hyposplenism and immunocompromise
- Gallstones – secondary to chronic haemolysis
- OSA – from adenotonsillar hypertrophy
- Marrow hyperplasia and bone infarction – skeletal deformities, e.g. frontal bossing, aseptic necrosis and skin ulcers
- Renal dysfunction is common; painful priapism may occur
- Eye changes – microvascular retinopathy, vitreous haemorrhage
- Neurological complications – thrombotic stroke, transient ischaemic attacks and haemorrhagic events
- Haematological crises – aplastic crises with temporary bone marrow fail-ure has a high mortality, haemolytic crises often accompany vaso-occlusive crises, splenic sequestration crises

Anaesthesia

Screening should be performed in at-risk populations before surgery. A Sickledex test will detect the presence of HbS > 10%; haemoglobin electro-phoresis is required to differentiate between SCD and trait. In the absence of severe hypoxia or stasis, sickle cell trait is not associated with increased peri-operative risk. SCD increases risk as a result of anaemia, sickle-related organ damage, the potential for vaso-occlusive crises and susceptibility to infection. A careful assessment of disease severity and complications is essential. The ideal haematocrit and the role of perioperative transfusion remain controversial. A conservative transfusion regimen targets a haemoglobin of 10 g/dL regard-less of the proportion of HbS present, whereas an aggressive regimen involves exchange transfusion to reduce the proportion of HbS < 30%. Haematology should be involved before admission.[17]

Preoperative intravenous fluids are advisable to ensure optimum hydration. Prophylactic antibiotics should be considered. Careful maintenance of temperature, acid–base status and fluid balance is essential. Controlled ventilation is recommended to maintain oxygenation and normocarbia. Conditions that promote local stasis of blood, e.g. vasoconstrictors and tourniquets, should be avoided. However, tourniquets have been used without complications in the presence of normal oxygenation and acid–base status. The use of cell salvage is not recommended by manufacturers. Good analgesia is important but may be difficult due to concomitant opioid use.

Haemoglobin SC Disease

Patients have both HbS and HbC. Disease is usually of intermediate severity between SCD and sickle cell trait but with significant variability. Complications include all those seen in SCD. Management principles remain the same.

Thalassaemia

The thalassaemias are a group of inherited haemoglobinopathies caused by defective synthesis of the α chain or the β chain of haemoglobin. Severity is related to the degree of impaired synthesis. It is prevalent in peoples of Mediterranean (mainly β), African (α and β) and Asian (mainly α) origin. Diagnosis is by electrophoresis and globin chain analysis. α-thalassaemia have mild or moderate disease. β-Thalassaemia is the most common form of thalassaemia. Heterozygotes (thalassaemia minor) have a mild hypochromic, microcytic anaemia. The homozygous state (thalassaemia major) results in profound anaemia due to ineffective erythropoiesis and haemolysis.

Implications for Anaesthesia

- Bone marrow expansion and extramedullary erythropoiesis – characteristic skull and facial deformities
- Potential airway problems
- Splenomegaly – thrombocytopaenia, splenectomy may be required
- Haemosiderosis – from chronic haemolysis or repeat transfusions can lead to cardiac hypertrophy, cardiomyopathy, pulmonary hypertension, cirrhosis and endocrine dysfunction

Treatment is with regular blood transfusion and desferrioxamine to chelate iron.

Glucose 6-Phosphate Dehydrogenase Deficiency

Glucose 6-phosphate dehydrogenase (G6PD) deficiency is the commonest inherited metabolic disorder of red blood cells worldwide. It is X-linked inheritance with variable penetrance. The G6PD enzyme is responsible for the production of nicotinamide adenine dinucleotide phosphate (NAPDH), necessary for the protection of the red blood cell against oxidative stresses caused by infections or certain drugs. The patient is usually asymptomatic until a drug or infection triggers haemolysis. Typically, haemolysis occurs 2–5 days after exposure with anaemia, haemoglobinaemia, haemoglobinuria and jaundice. Classically ingestion of fava beans results in haemolysis (favism).

Polycythaemia

Polycythaemia is used to describe a haemoglobin level (Hb >17.5 g/dL in males and > 15.5 g/dL in females), red cell count (6.0 and 5.5 × 10^{12}/L) or haematocrit (55% and 47%), respectively. Apparent polycythaemia (normal red cell mass) occurs due to chronic hypoxia, smoking, obesity, fluid loss and hypertension. Absolute polycythaemia (increased red cell mass) may be primary (polycythaemia vera) or secondary due to compensatory erythropoietin increase – cardiopulmonary disease, high altitude and inappropriate production of erythropoietin – renal disease, some tumours.

Polycythaemia vera is a chronic myeloproliferative disorder – often an associated leucocytosis, thrombocythaemia and splenomegaly. Presenting features include headaches, dyspnoea, hypertension, chest pain and gout. Raised blood viscosity increases the risk of thrombotic events, but bleeding problems also occur due to impaired platelet function. Treatment is with venesection and pharmaceutical myelosuppression. Elective surgery should be postponed until the condition has been medically controlled.

Abnormalities of Haemostasis

Acquired Disorders

Any imbalance between coagulation (clot formation) and fibrinolysis (clot breakdown) can lead to coagulopathy. Acquired disorders of clotting factors include:

- Decreased synthesis – liver disease, vitamin K deficiency, anticoagulant drugs.
- Increased loss or consumption – massive bleeding, DIC.
- Substances interfering with their function – drugs.

Abnormalities associated with vitamin K deficiency, liver disease and warfarin therapy may be treated with vitamin K. Rapid reversal can be achieved with prothrombin complex concentrate (PCC). Fresh frozen plasma (FFP), which contains clotting factors V, VIII and IX can be given in the presence of bleeding. Coagulopathy following massive blood transfusion is usually a combination of deficiency of clotting factors and thrombocytopenia. Treatment may include FFP, platelets and, in the presence of low fibrinogen levels, cryoprecipitate which contains fibrinogen, factor VIII and von Willebrand factor.

Disseminated Intravascular Coagulation (DIC)

Activation of the coagulation system results in widespread deposition of fibrin and microvascular thrombus formation. Consumption of clotting factors and platelets may result in severe bleeding. DIC usually results from a systemic inflammatory response (e.g. sepsis or major trauma) or the release of pro-coagulant material into the circulation (e.g. amniotic fluid embolism or malignancy). Laboratory abnormalities are variable and a haematologist should be involved with specific management, which includes treatment of the underlying cause.

Inherited Disorders

Haemophilia

Haemophilia is classified according to the clotting factor deficiency:

- Haemophilia A (VIII) is commonest.
- Haemophilia B (IX) or Christmas disease.
- Haemophilia C (XI).

Haemophilias A and B are X-linked recessive disorders, but one-third will have no family history. Presentation is usually with bleeding into weight-bearing joints or muscles. Only essential surgery should be undertaken. Patients should be evaluated for transfusion-related infections such as viral hepatitis and HIV. Management is guided by a haematologist with factor levels measured preoperatively. Factor VIII levels need 80%–100% correction before major surgery and maintained postoperatively (for 6 weeks after orthopaedic procedures). Factor IX may be helpful in Haemophilia A. Desmopressin and tranexamic acid are also useful.

Von Willebrand Disease

This is the most common of the inherited bleeding disorders and classified into three types based on quantitative or qualitative defects of von Willebrand factor (VWF). It has an autosomal inheritance, dominant or recessive depending on the subtype. VWF is required for platelet adhesion and aggregation, resulting in a prolonged bleeding time. Desmopressin is recommended for diagnostic procedures, but factor VIII concentrate is required before surgery.

COMMON PROBLEMS

The Elderly Patient

In terms of physiological parameters, there is considerable variation between individuals > 80 years is probably now a better definition than the conventional > 65 years. Patients are more likely to require emergency surgery and tend to be sicker on presentation. Surgical intervention is associated with increased perioperative morbidity and mortality due to comorbidities but also the physiological consequences of ageing (Box 1.2.7).

BOX 1.2.7 Physiological and Anatomical Consequences of Ageing

Cardiovascular

Fibrosis in the myocardium and conducting system results in an increased incidence of arrhythmias, heart block and congestive cardiac failure with diastolic dysfunction

Calcification of the heart valves

Decreased response to catecholamines

Reduced arterial compliance – elevated systolic blood pressure, slight reduction in diastolic pressure

Respiratory

Reduction in lung and chest wall compliance

Closing volume may exceed functional residual capacity, leading to alveolar and small airway collapse

Increased physiological dead space

Increased ventilation–perfusion mismatch, resulting in lower arterial oxygen tension

Reduced laryngeal sensitivity – silent aspiration may occur

Renal

Reduced renal blood flow and glomerular filtration rate

Reduced number of functioning nephrons

Loss of renal reserve

Neurological

Progressive loss of neurones

Increased incidence of cognitive impairment

Autonomic dysfunction (postural hypotension, impaired temperature regulation, tendency to urinary retention and constipation)

Deafness

Locomotor

Osteoarthritis

Osteoporosis

Pharmacokinetics

Impaired metabolism due to a decline in renal and hepatic function

Altered volume of distribution due to decreased total body water and decreased lean muscle mass

Altered protein binding due to decreased serum albumin

Implications for Anaesthesia

- Multiple comorbidities
- Multiple medications and altered pharmacokinetics – increased risk of adverse drug reactions
- Haemodynamic instability due to loss of compensatory mechanisms
- Fluid overload may easily precipitate pulmonary oedema and cardiac failure

- Impaired thermoregulation – increasing risk of hypothermia
- Increased risk of postoperative pulmonary complications
- Postoperative cognitive dysfunction (POCD) and delirium are common – risk factors include increasing age, longer surgeries, coexisting disease, infection, pre-existing cognitive dysfunction
- Increased risk of pressure sores and thromboembolism, especially with longer procedures and immobility
- Increased risk of postoperative infection – reduced immune response and poor nutrition

Anaesthesia

Anaesthesia must allow for age-related physiological changes – loss of functional reserve and reduced ability of the cardiovascular and endocrine systems to respond to external stress. A thorough assessment is required and optimization of comorbidities. There is no conclusive evidence that any one anaesthetic technique is superior. Local anaesthesia should be used where possible. Regional techniques may reduce complications such as respiratory infection, deep venous thrombosis (DVT) and POCD but profound hypotension may occur. Drugs should be titrated slowly to response with careful monitoring. Short-acting agents may be advantageous to minimize postoperative impairment. Care of pressure areas, maintenance of body temperature and attention to fluid balance are essential. Effective analgesia, early nutrition, physiotherapy and mobilization are extremely important.

Obesity

Obesity is increasing in prevalence worldwide. It is a multisystem disorder, associated with increased perioperative morbidity. Obesity is defined as BMI > 28 kg/m^2 and morbid obesity as BMI > 35 kg/m^2, where BMI is defined as weight (kg)/height^2 (m^2).

Implications for Anaesthesia

- *Respiratory system:*
  - Oxygen consumption – increased by active adipose tissue
  - FRC is reduced – decreases further with anaesthesia, encroaching on closing capacity
  - OSA, obesity hyperventilation syndrome
  - Pulmonary hypertension
- *Cardiovascular:*
  - Increased cardiac output and stroke volume
  - Hypertension and IHD
  - Dilated cardiomyopathy
- *Gastrointestinal:*
  - Hiatus hernia with reflux
  - Fatty liver

- *Endocrine:*
  - Insulin resistance, diabetes mellitus
- *Pharmacology:*
  - Altered drug metabolism – dose calculation can be difficult, altered volume of distribution, plasma protein binding, clearance

Anaesthesia

A detailed preoperative assessment is essential with attention to comorbidities. Routine prophylaxis with ranitidine or a proton-pump inhibitor is advisable. Venous access and positioning may be difficult. A suitable operating table is required – for induction and maintenance of anaesthesia. Intubation may be necessary for all but the briefest of procedures; patients may be a potentially difficult intubation. Optimal positioning is important. Pre-oxygenation is essential and airway adjuncts should be available. Invasive arterial monitoring may be required. Postoperative HDU should be available.

Substance Use Disorder

This may be defined as the use of a drug or chemical in a way that was not intended or to excess. The range of abused substances is diverse and increasing. Chronic substance abuse may result in tolerance and addiction. Complications may arise either due to the substance itself or its route of administration. Inhalational administration is associated with the complications of smoking. The intravenous route may result in thrombophlebitis, endocarditis and viral infections, e.g. hepatitis B, C or HIV. There may be additional problems from an inadequate diet, poor hygiene and infrequent medical care.

Opioid addiction, most commonly diamorphine (heroin), is associated with the highest morbidity and mortality rates. No attempt should be made to withdraw the drug perioperatively. Patients on withdrawal programmes should receive their usual dose of methadone. Local anaesthesia and nonopioid analgesics are recommended for postoperative pain where possible, but there is no justification for withholding opioid analgesia. Increased doses may be required. Stimulants such as cocaine, amphetamines and Ecstasy cause hypertension and tachycardia, often with ventricular extrasystoles. Elective anaesthesia should be postponed if there is evidence of recent intake. Adverse reactions associated with hyperthermia may occur and the principles of management are similar to those for malignant hyperpyrexia.

HIV

An estimated 38 million people are now thought to be infected with the human immunodeficiency virus (HIV) worldwide. Transmission is via blood, blood products, sexual contact and perinatal. Impaired cell-mediated immunity increases susceptibility to infections and malignant disease. There is a broad spectrum of disease which may be associated with cardiovascular, respiratory, haematological, neurological, gastrointestinal, renal and metabolic complications. Antiretroviral drugs delay disease progression and improve survival. It is estimated that 20%–25% of patients will require surgery during the course of their illness. The status of the disease, the presence of complications and the side effects of antiretroviral therapy should be determined preoperatively. Strict aseptic technique should be observed to minimize the risk of infection to the patient and universal precautions adopted to prevent the spread of infection to healthcare staff. Regional anaesthesia has the advantages of not interfering with the immune system or interacting with antiretroviral drugs, but is contraindicated in the presence of sepsis or coagulopathy.

REFERENCES

1. ACC/AHA. Guideline on Perioperative Cardiovascular Evaluation and Management of Patients Undergoing Non-cardiac Surgery. J Am Coll Cardiol 2014;64. http://dx.doi.org/10.1016/j.jacc.2014.07.944.
2. Guidelines for pre-operative cardiac risk assessment and perioperative cardiac management in non-cardiac surgery. The Task force for Preoperative Cardiac Risk assessment and Perioperative Cardiac Management in Non-cardiac surgery of the European Society of Cardiology (ESC) and endorsed by the European Society of Anesthesiology (ESA). Eur Heart J 2009;30:2769–12.
3. Hartle A, McCormack T, Carlisle J, et al. The measurement of hypertension before elective surgery. Anaesthesia 2016;71:326–37.
4. Prophylaxis against infective endocarditis: antimicrobial prophylaxis against infective endocarditis in adults and children undergoing interventional procedures. NICE clinical guideline CG64. 2016. https://www.nice.org.uk/guidance/cg64.
5. Habib G, Lancellotti P, Antunes MJ. 2015 Guidelines for the management of infective endocarditis. Eur Heart J 2015;ehv 319. doi: 10.1093/eurheartj/ehv319.
6. Stone ME, Salter B, Fischer A. Perioperative management of patients with cardiac implantable electronic devices. Br J Anaesth 2011;107(suppl 1):i16–126.
7. Clarke T. Perioperative management of respiratory disease in Core Topics in Perioperative Medicine. In: Hudsmith J, Wheeler D, Gupta A, editors. Cambridge University Press.
8. Lumb A, Biercamp C. Chronic Obstructive pulmonary disease and anaesthesia. Continuing education in Anaesthesia. Crit Care & Pain 2014;14:1–5.
9. Wolfe RM, Pomerantz J, Miller DE, Weiss-Coleman R, Solomonides T. Obstructive sleep apnoea: Preoperative screening and postoperative care. J Am Board Fam Med 2016;29:263–75.
10. Dhatariya K, Levy N, Kilvert A, et al. Diabetes UK Position Statements and Care Recommendations. NHS Diabetes guideline for the perioperative management of the adult patient with diabetes. Diabetic Med 2012;29:420–33.
11. Barker P, Creasey PE, Dhatariya K, Levy N, Lipp A, Nathanson MH, et al. Peri-operative management of the surgical patient with diabetes 2015. Anaesthesia 2015;70:1427–40.
12. Findley H, Philips A, Cole D, Nair A. Porphyrias: implications for anaesthesia, critical care and pain medicine. Continuing education in Anaesthesia, Crit Care & Pain 2012;12:128–33.
13. Kiamanesh D, Rumley J, Moitra VK. Monitoring and managing hepatic disease in anaesthesia. Br J Anaesth 2013;111(suppl i):i50–61.
14. Craig RG, Hunter JM. Recent developments in the perioperative management of adult patients with chronic kidney disease. Br J Anaesth 2008;101:296–310.

15. Mashour GA, Moore LE, Lele AV, Robicsek SA, Gelb AW. Perioperative Care of Patients at High Risk for Stroke during or after Non-Cardiac, Non-Neurologic Surgery: Consensus Statement from the Society for Neuroscience in Anesthesiology and Critical Care. J Neurosurg Anesthesiol 2014;26:273–85.
16. Klein AA, Arnold P, Bingham RM, et al. AAGBI guidelines: the use of blood components and their alternatives 2016. Anaesthesia 2016;71:829–42.
17. Wilson M, Forsyth P, Whiteside J. Haemoglobinopathy and sickle cell disease. Continuing education in Anaesthesia. Crit Care & Pain 2010;10:24–28.

Section 2

General Anaesthesia

Chapter 2.1

Anaesthetic Equipment

Patrick Magee

THE ANAESTHETIC MACHINE

The principles of gas delivery in a modern anaesthetic machine are basically unchanged since the days of the Boyle's machine. In other aspects, however, such as in monitoring and safety devices, the modern apparatus has evolved a great deal. Gases are delivered from pipelines or cylinders via pressure-reducing valves to flowmeters, where needle valves reduce pressure further and control flow, or the fresh gas passes through a set of solenoid valves. In the backbar are one or more vaporizers. Gases then pass through the common gas outlet to a breathing system. Modern anaesthetic machines, usually with integrated monitoring, are complex items of equipment that are now often dependent on electronic hardware and software. This provides a high level of redundancy in fault detection, and the user should take care not to diminish clinical watchfulness.

THE PRE-ANAESTHETIC CHECKLIST

The 2012 edition of the Association of Anaesthetists recommendations for checking anaesthetic equipment[1] emphasizes the need to understand and check any equipment used. A self-inflating bag should always be available in case other equipment fails. The following checks should be undertaken before every anaesthetic session:

- Perform the manufacturers' automated machine check.
- Ensure power supply is plugged in and switched on, and that back-up batteries are functioning.
- Check gas and suction pipelines are working by a 'tug' test; cylinders are filled and turned off; flowmeters (if applicable); hypoxic guard and oxygen flush; suction (also before every case).
- Check breathing system for patency and freedom from leaks using 'two bag' test (also before every case); alternative system available; vaporizers correctly fitted, filled; check soda lime (colour); correct machine outlet selection.

- Check ventilator function and configuration (also before every case).
- Check scavenger function and configuration.
- Check monitors' function and configuration, including appropriate alarm limits.
- Check availability and function of full range of airway equipment, with spares (also before every case).
- Check availability and function of total intravenous anaesthesia (TIVA) equipment where appropriate.
- Check availability and function of resuscitation equipment.

SUPPLY OF ANAESTHETIC GASES

In medically advanced countries, medical gases are usually supplied in hospitals by pipeline, with cylinders available as backup.

Oxygen

Vacuum Insulated Evaporator

Oxygen is usually supplied and stored on the hospital site in liquid form in a vacuum insulated evaporator (VIE). One volume of liquid yields 840 volumes of gaseous oxygen at 15°C. The VIE consists of an insulated container in which the liquid oxygen is stored at about −160°C, at a pressure between 700 and 1200 kPa. There is a vapour withdrawal line at the top of the VIE, from which oxygen vapour is heated towards ambient temperature and delivered to the pipeline. Continual evaporation keeps the VIE cold. There is also a liquid withdrawal line from the bottom of the VIE, from which liquid oxygen can be withdrawn, superheated initially to a vapour and subsequently to a gas.

Oxygen vapour is passed through a series of pressure regulators to drop the pressure down to the distribution pipeline pressure of 410 kPa. There is a pressure relief valve on top of the VIE in case lack of demand and gradual temperature rise result in a pressure rise. There is considerable wastage during filling of the VIE. The whole device is situated outside the hospital building on a hinged weighing device, protected by a caged enclosure, which also houses two banks of reserve cylinders. These take over automatically if the VIE output falls.

Cylinder Banks

In a smaller hospital, banks of large cylinders can be used to deliver piped oxygen. Appropriate valves, monitoring and alarms need to be in place to ensure that the supply automatically switches to a full cylinder. Gas pressure in a full cylinder, including the E size on the anaesthetic machine, is around 135 atmospheres (13,700 kPa). The ISO (International Organization for Standardization) colour for oxygen cylinders, indicated on the cylinder shoulder, is white, whereas the body is black.

Oxygen Concentrator

An oxygen concentrator is used in some countries. Ambient air is compressed, then passed through zeolite, an aluminium hydroxide lattice, which adsorbs nitrogen, leaving a 95% oxygen mixture at the outlet. On depressurization the nitrogen is desorbed and released to the environment. Efficiency depends on the pressure change available and the need to adsorb water vapour from air using silica before entering the zeolite.

Oxygen Failure Alarm

The oxygen failure alarm is activated when oxygen delivery pressure falls below 200 kPa. The function of the ideal device should:

- Not depend on the pressure of any gas other than the oxygen itself.
- Have an alarm system that does not use battery or mains power, and sound an audible signal of sufficient length, volume and character.
- Warn of impending failure, and warn again that failure has occurred.
- Open the breathing system to the atmosphere to supply an adequate oxygen concentration to the patient and prevent other gases flowing, and minimize the retention of carbon dioxide. It should be impossible to resume the supply of anaesthetic gases until the oxygen supply has been restored.

Nitrous Oxide

Nitrous oxide is stored as a liquid in pressurized cylinders, either in a bank or on the anaesthetic machine. It is released as vapour. The pressure of a cylinder containing a liquid reservoir is therefore the saturated vapour pressure (SVP) at room temperature, usually between 4400 and 5400 kPa. If the vapour flowrate is high, freezing of water vapour and possible obstruction of the regulator outlet can occur, due to excessive heat of vaporization demand by the nitrous oxide liquid, unless thermostatically controlled. The ISO colour for a nitrous oxide cylinder is blue.

Entonox

Entonox is a safe and effective analgesic gas mixture of 50% each of oxygen and nitrous oxide. The mixture is stored and delivered to the patient using a two-stage pressure regulator, the second incorporating a demand valve. If the cylinder temperature falls below $-6°C$, the pseudocritical temperature, the oxygen and nitrous oxide separate into layers (a process known as lamination, or the Poynting effect). The effects of lamination may be minimized either by storing the cylinders horizontally at a temperature of $5°C$ or more for 24 h before use, or by the presence of a tube from the valve housing at the top of the cylinder to a point near the bottom, which prevents the withdrawal of pure nitrous oxide.

The pressure in an Entonox cylinder is 135 atmospheres. Its ISO colour is blue and white quarters on the cylinder shoulder and a blue body.

Medical Compressed Air

Medical compressed air requires no trace of oil to be present, because of the risk of explosion. Medical air for breathing devices is supplied from the pipeline at 410 kPa. When supplied at 700 kPa, it is used to power operating tools, when the oil lubricant should be re-added. These two sources of compressed air must not be confused. If supplied by cylinder, the pressure is 135 atmospheres, and the ISO colour is black and white quarters on the cylinder shoulder and a black body.

Gas Pipelines

The union between gas hoses and the anaesthetic machine should be permanent. The connection of hoses to the appropriate wall outlet is via a gas-specific, non-interchangeable Schräder valve, making it theoretically impossible to connect hoses incorrectly. The routine anaesthetic machine check will detect any such faults. Hoses are colour coded: white for oxygen, blue for nitrous oxide, black for air and yellow for suction vacuum. When repairs are necessary, they should only be carried out by a trained engineer, and a complete hose assembly is usually provided, rather than piecemeal repair.

Piped Medical Vacuum

A medical suction device is connected to a vacuum source by a yellow colour-coded hose. The outlet on the wall supplying a vacuum is one of many on a ring main, whence the pipe work goes via drainage, filtering and valve mechanisms towards a vacuum reservoir. Materials that have been suctioned then go through bacterial filters towards a vacuum pump. Flexible hoses are used for this transmission to reduce noise. Duty and standby pumps are in the system. The pump output is passed through a silencer.

Gas Cylinders

Gas cylinders are made from steel alloyed with molybdenum, which is resistant to corrosion. Cylinders are subject to regular testing. Oxygen, nitrogen, air and helium are stored in cylinders as gases. Nitrous oxide, carbon dioxide and cyclopropane (no longer available for anaesthesia in the UK) are stored as liquids in equilibrium with their saturated vapour.

A 'full' nitrous oxide cylinder contains liquid up to a maximum of 80% of its volume. The ratio of the weight of nitrous oxide to the weight of water that would fill the cylinder is the filling ratio, usually 0.75 in temperate climates, 0.67 in tropical climates.

Cylinder outlet valves use the pin index system (ISO 407:2004, reviewed 2013) which makes it impossible to connect cylinders to the wrong yokes. Yokes for stand-alone cylinders are connected to flowmeters via noninterchangeable screw-threaded (NIST) connectors.

Before connection to the yoke, the cylinder valve is opened briefly to flush out inflammable dust and the presence of a Bodok seal checked.

After connection, the cylinder valve is slowly opened 2.5 turns. Machine backflow check valves prevent cross-filling of cylinders, but if a cylinder yoke is empty, it must be blanked off to prevent leakage from other cylinders. Table 2.1.1 shows cylinder sizes and capacities in current use.

Pressure-Reducing Valves (Pressure Regulators) and Other Valves

Pressure-reducing valves minimize danger to patients and damage to the downstream flowmeters. Between an oxygen cylinder and the anaesthetic machine, the pressure is reduced from 13,700 to 420 kPa, or lower in some countries.

The classic reducing valve is the Adams valve, in which a toggle mechanism occludes the high-pressure outlet when the downstream pressure rises.

The pressure is further reduced at the entrance to the flowmeter by the needle valve operating the flow controller to the flowmeter, or by a set of solenoid valves controlling total flow (see "Flowmeters" below).

Distal to the flowmeters, backbar pressure ranges from 1 to 8 kPa. The backbar has a pressure-relief valve, which activates at about 40 kPa.

Automatic pressure-limiting (APL) valves and expiratory valves on breathing systems are spring-loaded valves designed to open at preset pressures.

Flowmeters

Traditionally the flowmeters on anaesthetic machines have been of the rotameter type, giving a direct visual reading. In recent years, modern anaesthetic

TABLE 2.1.1 Cylinder Sizes and Capacities

	Cylinder Size					
	C	D	E	F	G	J
Oxygen capacity (L)	170	340	680	1360	3400	6800
N_2O capacity (L)	450	900	1800	3600	9000	–
Entonox capacity (L)	–	500	–	2000	5000	–
Air capacity (L)	–	–	–	–	3200	6400
CO_2 capacity (L)	450	900	1800		–	–

Notes: CO_2, carbon dioxide; N_2O, nitrous oxide.

machines merely show an iconic representation of a rotameter on a monitoring screen.

Rotameters

A traditional rotameter is a variable-orifice, constant-pressure flowmeter. Gas is led to the base of a machined glass tube with a tapering cross-section.

A metal bobbin rides the gas jet, rotating in the flow, the gas escaping between the bobbin and the walls of the glass tube. As the bobbin rises with increased flow, the size of the annular gap between it and the glass tube increases. The height to which the bobbin rises indicates the flow rate.

Calibration accounts for both gas density and viscosity. At low flows, gas flow around the bobbin behaves like laminar flow through a tube (width of annulus less than length). At high flows, it is turbulent through an orifice (width of annulus greater than length). Hence, a rotameter calibrated for carbon dioxide will not read true in the laminar range for cyclopropane, because although their densities are similar (44:42), their viscosities are different (1:0.6).

The needle valve control knob carries the name of the gas and is colour coded. The oxygen control knob commonly protrudes further than the others, and feels different to touch, to assist recognition. The needle valve which controls flow through the rotameter may be upstream of the rotameter (UK), or downstream (USA), which maintains a more constant pressure in the glass tube and avoids error due to ventilator backpressure. The bank of rotameter tubes may have oxygen on the left (UK) or on the right (USA).

Antihypoxic Device

The antihypoxic device limits the flow of nitrous oxide if the delivery pressure or flow of oxygen falls or fails, to prevent delivery of a hypoxic mixture. Such devices include the Ohmeda chain link between the oxygen and nitrous oxide flowmeter controls, and the Dräger device, which uses a hydraulically coupled valve.

Oxygen Flush Button

A button connected directly to the high-pressure oxygen source allows delivery of oxygen (oxygen flush) at more than 35 L/min. Safety dictates that the button should not be lockable in the depressed position.

Effect of Barometric Pressure

Rotameters are calibrated for use at sea level in terms of litres the gas will occupy (per unit time) after discharge to atmospheric pressure; if used at altitudes or in hyperbaric chambers they are inaccurate. Similarly, if the outlet is restricted, or when a ventilator is used downstream and the pressure rises, the flow is greater than indicated with variable orifice rotameters. These inaccuracies can be corrected by placing the control valve at the downstream end of the rotameter, when the pressure in the flowmeter is the same as that in the supply line.

Inaccuracies and Dangers of Rotameters

The following inaccuracies and dangers are associated with rotameters:

- Static electricity and dirt can cause sticking of the bobbin, especially when low flows are used, leading to inaccuracy as high as 35%. The bobbin must rotate freely.
- A leak through a cracked glass tube may cause a hypoxic mixture. This is less likely if the oxygen enters the backbar last. An internal baffle at the top of the rotameter bank achieves this even when the oxygen rotameter is upstream on the left.
- A defect in the top sealing washer of a rotameter can cause hazardous hypoxia.
- The rotameter tube must be vertical.
- Backpressure from a ventilator can give a falsely low flow reading.
- A wire stop at the top keeps the bobbin in sight. This prevents a small bobbin jamming there with the anaesthetist unaware that gas is flowing.

Solenoid Valve Flow Controllers

Modern anaesthetic machines with integrated electronic control systems have merely a rotameter icon on a monitoring screen, the flow being controlled through a series of solenoid valves. The manually operated flow control knob appears the same, but is connected to a series of eight solenoid valves, each of which double the flow of the previous one, the opening of each valve being controlled by a digital signal.

VAPORIZERS

Plenum Vaporizers

When the carrier gas enters a vaporizer, part of it goes through the vaporization chamber, whereas the remainder bypasses it. The vaporizer control knob determines the ratio of these two flows, the splitting ratio. Thus, for an ordinary anaesthetic volatile agent with a relatively high boiling point (e.g. Isoflurane, Sevoflurane) the vapour has a partial pressure equal to its SVP at room temperature and is diluted by the carrier gas, so the emerging mixture contains an accurately dialled fractional vapour concentration. Full vaporization within the chamber may be ensured by use of a wick, a cowl, multiple baffles and a nebulizer. A keyed filling port prevents filling with the wrong agent. The vaporizer should not be overfilled. Output has been shown to vary by more than $\pm 15\%$, but the user has access to calibration curves. In anaesthetic machines incorporating integral agent monitoring, a servo-controlled closed-loop feedback mechanism changes the splitting ratio if the measured output differs from the dialled output.

Temperature Compensation

The SVP is kept constant by attaching the vaporizer to a metal jacket to minimize the temperature fall. Other methods of temperature compensation, to prevent a fall in output if temperature falls, include:

- A bimetallic strip, acting as a cap over the gas entry port to either the bypass or the vaporizing chamber
- Aneroid bellows in the vaporization chamber, which reduces the bypass flow if temperature falls

Pressure Compensation

If downstream pressure increases (e.g. owing to the presence of a ventilator), there may be retrograde movement of vapour-rich gas into the vaporizer. This pumping effect will increase the resultant vapour concentration. It may be prevented by including either a one-way valve or an additional length of tubing downstream of the vaporizer.

Altitude

At altitude the volume concentration fractional output from a vaporizer is increased because the carrier gas is less dense. The SVP is independent of ambient pressure, so its partial pressure in the vaporizing chamber is unchanged for a given position of the control knob, as long as temperature remains constant. Partial pressure, rather than volume concentration, is the important variable pharmacologically in determining its clinical effect.

Desflurane Plenum Vaporizer

A plenum vaporizer for an agent with a low boiling point close to room temperature, such as Desflurane, uses an integrated heater to ensure aliquots of agent are fully and controllably vaporized before mixing with carrier gas.

Drawover Vaporizers

Plenum vaporizers are mounted on a continuous-flow anaesthetic machine with a pressurized gas supply, and resistance to gas flow is not considered important. When the patient inhales air through a vaporizer, either spontaneously or with intermittent positive-pressure ventilation (IPPV), the resistance to gas flow must be designed to be as low as possible. This is called a drawover vaporizer.

ANAESTHETIC BREATHING SYSTEMS

A breathing system consists of a fresh gas limb, inspiratory and expiratory limbs (which may coincide), a pressure limiting valve and a reservoir bag. It may also have one or more unidirectional valves and a CO_2 absorber. The simpler systems have fewer components and usually involve some rebreathing.

The ability to minimize rebreathing at a low fresh gas flow is a measure of the breathing system's efficiency and depends on design and whether the patient is breathing spontaneously or being ventilated. More complex systems (circle systems) ensure minimum rebreathing by the use of unidirectional valves and CO_2 absorption while allowing more economical use of fresh gas and volatile agent.

Semi-Closed Rebreathing Systems

Mapleson A System

The Mapleson A system (Fig. 2.1.1) is also known as the Magill system and is economical in spontaneous breathing. The last gas inhaled on inspiration is fresh gas, which therefore resides in the patient's dead space, becomes the first gas exhaled on expiration and is stored for the next breath. As expiration proceeds, the expiratory valve opens and alveolar gas is preferentially vented. No significant rebreathing occurs when the fresh gas flow falls as low as alveolar ventilation (70 mL/kg/min or 70% of minute ventilation). This efficiency is unrelated to the respiratory pattern.

Efficiency during controlled ventilation is relatively poor. The design, which, in spontaneous breathing, preferentially vents alveolar gas and stores fresh gas, does the opposite when intermittent positive pressure ventilation (IPPV) is used. When the reservoir bag is squeezed, the partially closed expiratory valve opens and fresh gas is preferentially vented, although some will go to the patient. On expiration, the system preferentially fills with alveolar gas, ready to be rebreathed on the next inspiration. The Mapleson A system is the least appropriate for IPPV when a fresh gas flow of up to three or four times minute ventilation is required to prevent rebreathing.

The efficiency of the Mapleson A system during IPPV can be improved with the Miller modification, which prevents the

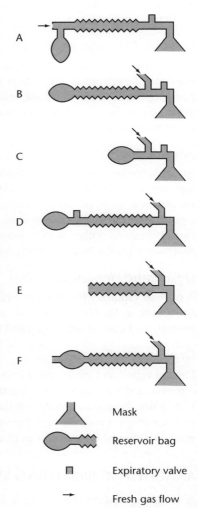

Mask

Reservoir bag

Expiratory valve

Fresh gas flow

FIGURE 2.1.1 Mapleson classification of semi-closed rebreathing systems.

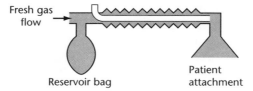

FIGURE 2.1.2   Coaxial Mapleson A system – the Lack system.

escape of fresh gas during inspiration by enclosing the expiratory valve in a shroud, pressurized by the positive pressure used to compress the reservoir bag. This is an example of an enclosed afferent rebreathing (EAR) system.

Lack System

The Lack system (Fig. 2.1.2) is a coaxial variant of the Mapleson A system. It allows inspiration to occur through the outer tube and expiration down the inner tube. Therefore, the diameter of the tubing is wider than standard 22 mm tubing. It is functionally identical to the Magill and probably as efficient. In the parallel Lack system the tubes lie side by side.

Mapleson B and C Systems

The Mapleson B and C systems are seldom used these days and form the basis of modern systems used for resuscitation purposes.

Mapleson D, E and F Systems

The Mapleson D, E and F systems are all known as T pieces because fresh gas is delivered at a T junction close to the patient. Functionally, all T pieces have common performance characteristics. In the early part of inspiration, fresh gas flow exceeds the inspiratory requirement, allowing some to be stored in the system. Their efficient performance is highly dependent on a long expiratory pause. They are much less efficient than Mapleson A systems for spontaneous breathing, and a fresh gas flow of at least twice minute ventilation is needed. For IPPV, a fresh gas flow of 70–100 mL/kg/min will give normocapnia, provided minute ventilation is sufficiently high (120–150 mL/kg/min).

Bain System

The Bain system (Fig. 2.1.3) is a coaxial variant of the Mapleson D system. Although superficially it resembles the Lack system, fresh gas is delivered down the relatively narrow-bore inner tube to a point close to the patient. Expiration occurs down the standard 22 mm diameter outer tube. Care must be taken that the inner coaxial tube does not become detached at either end or the circuit dead space becomes much larger. It may not be as efficient as the orthodox Mapleson D system, because the coaxial arrangement at the patient end may encourage gas mixing. If it is necessary to ventilate patients from a distance, as for magnetic resonance imaging, a long Bain system may be used. The additional length increases its compliance and resistance, so smaller tidal volumes and higher end-expiratory pressures result.

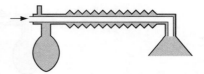

FIGURE 2.1.3 Coaxial Mapleson D system – the Bain system.

Mapleson E and F Systems

Mapleson E and F systems are otherwise known, respectively, as the Ayre's T piece and its Jackson Rees modification. A reservoir tube with a volume one-third of the patient's tidal volume is needed to prevent both rebreathing and dilution. The valveless system is simple and provides low resistance to spontaneous breathing for small children.

The Jackson Rees modification is the addition of an open-tailed reservoir bag to allow visible monitoring of breathing as well as a means of manual controlled ventilation. During spontaneous respiration, the fresh gas flow required to avoid rebreathing is twice the child's minute ventilation. During IPPV, as with the Mapleson D system, much less is needed, e.g. 1000 mL/min + 200 mL/kg/min.

Humphrey ADE System

The Humphrey ADE system was designed so that, at the turn of a lever, a system with Mapleson A characteristics could be used for spontaneous ventilation, and a system with D and E characteristics is available for controlled ventilation. It may also be used in children.

The Circle System

The circle system (Fig. 2.1.4) is a more complex system in which exhaled gas is recirculated to enhance economy and to reduce pollution. It incorporates unidirectional valves and a means of absorbing CO_2. The fresh gas flow can be as low as 500 mL/min or less of both oxygen and nitrous oxide. There are a number of components and connections. Inspired anaesthetic gas and vapour concentrations are lower than those in the fresh gas input, particularly at low fresh gas flows, because of uptake into the patient's tissues. Gas and vapour monitoring is particularly important. At higher fresh gas flows, above about 3 L/min, a circle system behaves more like a semi-closed rebreathing system and the CO_2 absorber may be unnecessary. High fresh gas flows at the beginning of an anaesthetic enhance gas uptake and denitrogenation, after which they may be reduced. The response time of a circle system is inversely proportional to gas inflow and directly proportional to system volume.

Circle systems can be used for paediatric anaesthesia, using a 1 L reservoir bag and smaller-bore tubing. The work of breathing is acceptable.

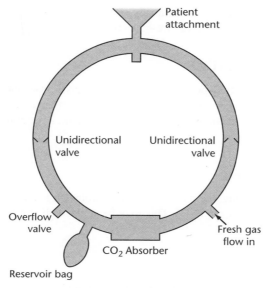

FIGURE 2.1.4   Circle system.

Carbon Dioxide Absorption

A low-resistance absorber is an important part of a circle system. Two absorbents in common use are soda lime and baralyme. Soda lime consists of 4% sodium hydroxide, 1% potassium hydroxide, 14%–19% water and the balance is calcium hydroxide. There are additional small amounts of silica for drying, kieselguhr for hardening and dye indicators to show when the crystals are spent. Ethyl violet is one such indicator, although its activity can be impaired by fluorescent lighting. The water is essential for CO_2 absorption, thus:

$$CO_2 + H_2O \rightarrow H_2CO_3$$
$$2NaOH + 2H_2CO_3 + Ca(OH)_2 \rightarrow CaCO_3 + Na_2CO_3 + 4H_2O$$

The heat and water liberated by these reactions provide useful warmth and humidity for the patient.

Baralyme is a mixture of 20% barium hydroxide, 80% calcium hydroxide and a small amount of potassium hydroxide. The water for the reaction is present as the octahydrate of barium hydroxide.

In both cases, the monovalent hydroxides are more reactive than the divalent $Ca(OH)_2$. Where the absorbent crystals have been allowed to dry out, these highly reactive monovalent hydroxides can also produce significant amounts of carbon monoxide and formaldehyde. Absorbents also tend to absorb volatile agents, which was hazardous when the (now largely obsolete) volatile agent trichloroethylene was used. This reacted with soda lime to produce dichloroacetylene gas or phosgene, a neurotoxin. Sevoflurane reacts with soda lime to produce Compound A, a renal toxin, although this is not clinically significant. Nevertheless, regulations in the USA recommend a minimum fresh gas flow of 3 L/min to minimize this.

SCAVENGING SYSTEMS

Scavenging systems transport waste anaesthetic gases from the breathing system to the atmosphere to avoid local pollution. Systems can be active or passive. They consist of a collecting system, a transfer system, a receiving system and a disposal system.

Active Scavenging

With active scavenging, the patient should be protected from negative pressures greater than 100 Pa (1 cm H_2O). This may be achieved by an open T-piece reservoir or an air break.

Passive Scavenging

With passive scavenging, total flow resistance should not exceed 50 Pa (0.5 cm H_2O) at 30 L/min. Copper pipes of 28–35 mm outer diameter are satisfactory. The discharge point should avoid wind pressures. A T termination with a downward right-angle bend at each end is preferred, placed above a flat roof.

VENTILATORS

Modern ventilators can act as constant or nonconstant generators of either pressure or flow. The ventilator has to execute an inspiratory phase, cycle from inspiration to expiration, allow expiration and an expiratory pause, and then cycle back to inspiration.

Pressure Generator

A pressure generator delivers a preset pressure to the patient. The flow (and hence the tidal volume) depends on airway resistance and lung compliance. It may be thought of as weighted bellows.

Flow Generator

A flow generator delivers a preset flow pattern, which is maintained whatever the airway resistance and lung compliance. Under adverse circumstances, airway pressure may rise high enough to cause barotrauma.

Constant flow generation may be achieved by forcing gas at high pressure through a nozzle, whereas other flow patterns may be achieved by a sinusoidal or positive displacement pump.

Power

Power is required during the inspiratory phase, typically about 20 W. Peak power production must exceed peak airway pressure times peak flow rate, plus any energy losses. A high proportion of the required power is spent overcoming the internal resistance of the ventilator. The power provided may be from the fresh gas flow itself in minute volume dividers (e.g. Manley ventilator), electrical power or compressed gas, usually oxygen.

Cycling

Cycling is initiated by time, volume, pressure, flow or patient triggering.

Expiration

Expiration is generally passive release to the atmosphere. Patients with acute lung injury often benefit from positive end-expiratory pressure (PEEP) to recruit alveoli and improve oxygenation.

Safety Features

All users of ventilators should have a low threshold of suspicion for faults. Numerous variables are monitored on a ventilator and there should be appropriate alarms on these monitors, especially to detect inadequate or excessive volume or airway pressure before the patient is harmed. The function of low-pressure (disconnection) alarms should be checked by disconnecting at the patient end of the circuit, in case the threshold pressure is set inappropriately low.

Testing

Before being put into clinical use, all ventilators are rigorously tested on a lung model. Testing to a number of ISO standards includes tests of endurance, waveform and volume performance, and internal compliance.

Paediatric Ventilators

Paediatric ventilators need to offer respiratory rates between 15 and 40 per min, and tidal volumes between 16 and 500 mL. Lung compliance and airways resistance in babies can vary tenfold. Neonates may require an inspiratory time as short as 0.5 s, inspiratory flow as low as 2 L/min and peak airway pressure limited to 6–7 cm H_2O. Appropriate alarms should be available and used to respond to the tight constraints of excessive or inadequate measured values of important variables. Adequate humidification is mandatory.

AIRWAY MANAGEMENT DEVICES

See Chapter 2.6, Airway Management.

INTRAVENOUS PUMPS AND SYRINGE DRIVERS

Programmable volumetric intravenous pumps and syringe drivers are used to deliver intravenous anaesthesia, patient-controlled anaesthesia and epidural infusions. Some pumps control the flow rate by a photoelectric drip-rate detector in conjunction with a microprocessor-controlled occlusion device.

Syringe drivers give a continuous, pulsatile flow to an accuracy of 2%–5%. Some syringe drivers are driven by clockwork motors, others by a battery-powered motor, which is intermittently on and off. The syringe driver should not be positioned above the patient to avoid siphoning. Modern syringe drivers are usually sufficiently accurate, but there may be a delay before the infusion is initiated. Where the bolus to be delivered is small, say 0.5 mL from a patient-controlled analgesia (PCA) pump, the accuracy of the delivered bolus becomes questionable.

Volumetric pumps enable constant volumetric delivery despite variation in resistance to flow and use either a peristaltic pump, a reservoir or syringe-type cassettes to drive the flow, and have an accuracy of 5%–10%. Safety problems with these devices include infusion of air, power failure, disturbance of the infusion by a secondary infusion and software corruption.

Target-controlled infusion pumps with advanced software have been developed which allow patient characteristics and desired drug plasma concentration to be entered. A multi-compartment pharmacokinetic mathematical model is used to control the pump.

STERILIZATION OF EQUIPMENT

Disinfection is the killing of nonsporing microorganisms. Sterilization is the killing of all microorganisms, including viruses, fungi and any spores. Disposable equipment meant for single use only is increasingly used in both anaesthetic and surgical practice.

Methods of Sterilization

Moist Heat

Moisture increases cellular permeability and heat coagulates protein. Boiling (100°C) for 15 min kills bacteria, but spores may escape destruction. Increased pressure makes it possible to produce higher temperature.

In the modern autoclave, air is replaced by steam at 134°C and 2 bar pressure for 3½ min. To remove moisture, the steam is evacuated and replaced by sterile air. The cycle takes about 10 min. It is useful for metal objects and fabrics.

This will kill all living organisms provided the material treated is properly wrapped to allow penetration. Deterioration of rubber and plastics is hastened by this method and exposure for 15 min to a temperature of 121°C may be substituted. Sharp instruments may become dulled.

Low-temperature (73°C) steam sterilization (290 mmHg pressure) takes just over 2 h. If formaldehyde is added spores are also killed. This may be used for materials harmed by steam at higher temperatures.

Chemical Sterilization

Chemical sterilization is useful for objects that will not withstand heat (e.g. endoscopes). Chemicals kill by coagulation or alkylation of proteins. Nonsporing bacteria, viruses, the tubercle bacillus and spores are resistant to destruction (in ascending order). Chemicals only act on exposed surfaces, some react with metals and some impregnate materials (e.g. rubber) and remain as a source of mucosal irritation.

Formaldehyde

Formaldehyde can be used for endoscopic equipment, catheters, etc. Residual formaldehyde may persist after prolonged airing and harm the skin or in favour of more urgent cases irritate the operator's eye.

Ethylene Oxide

Ethylene oxide (C_2H_4O) is a colourless gas and a good bactericidal agent, although toxic to inhale. It has good penetrability and few materials are harmed; it is effective against all organisms, but is slow (8–12 h).

Ethylene oxide is explosive at a concentration above 3% in air, and it is necessary to use 10% in CO_2 at a relative humidity of 30%–50%. This is a good method for sterilizing complicated and delicate apparatus (e.g. oxygenators, prostheses, ventilators and respiratory equipment), although expensive and time consuming. The accepted method of removing adsorbed ethylene oxide by allowing 7 days' shelf-life is inadequate, and the pulling of six post-sterilization vacuums is advised. The cylinders containing the mixture are identified by aluminium paint: the shoulder is red and below it is a circular band of yellow paint.

Liquids

Liquids used for chemical sterilization are as follows:

- Phenol (1%–5%) – used to clean surfaces of apparatus. It should not be used on equipment that comes into contact with the patient and does not kill spores.
- Iodine (0.5%–2% in alcohol) – which may irritate or burn the skin. Povidone-iodine 10% is less irritant.
- Ethyl alcohol 70%–80% is more efficient than absolute (100%) alcohol. Isopropyl alcohol 50%–70% can be used.

● Chlorhexidine 2% in 70% ethyl alcohol for skin sterilization; 0.5% should be used for skin sterilization prior to central neuraxial blockade.
● Glutaraldehyde – commonly used for endoscopes – a 2% solution made alkaline by the addition of 0.3% sodium carbonate. This will kill bacteria in 15 min and spores in 3 h.

Gamma Rays (Ionizing Radiation)

2.5 Mrad is bactericidal.

Filtration

Filters are used to prevent contamination by organisms and can remove 99.99% of particles over 0.5 μm diameter. The filters themselves can be autoclaved. Disposable filters are used for bolus injections or infusions through epidural catheters.

REFERENCES

1. Association of Anaesthetists of Great Britain and Ireland. Checking anaesthetic equipment. Anaesthesia 2012;67:660–68.

FURTHER READING

Magee P, Tooley M. The Physics, Clinical Measurement and Equipment of Anaesthetic Practice for the FRCA. 2nd edition. Oxford; Oxford University Press, 2011.

Monitoring

Patrick Magee

GENERAL PRINCIPLES

Monitoring is intended to measure and record deviations from normal values and warn of adverse events. Standards have been agreed in many countries, and those in the UK are published and updated by the Association of Anaesthetists.[1] It is necessary to monitor both the patient and the anaesthesia delivery system.

Clinical Monitoring

The most important factor for clinical monitoring is the continual presence of a trained and competent anaesthetist. This applies to general and regional anaesthesia, sedation with multiple drugs and the early phase of recovery. The experienced anaesthetist will monitor:

- The circulation – pulse rate, rhythm and quality, vein filling, skin elasticity and temperature, and urine output (if catheterized)
- Respiration – effort, pattern, tidal volume, frequency, reservoir bag movement
- Oxygenation – skin, mucous membrane and blood colour
- Depth of anaesthesia – pupillary signs (after Guedel), lacrimation, sweating, muscle movement

Instrumental Monitoring

Of the Patient

In this age of numerical recording of variables, it is important to make use of simple and well-established technology to monitor the patient's physiology, which should be applied immediately before the induction of anaesthesia and maintained until the patient has recovered, as follows:

- Circulation – noninvasive blood pressure, electrocardiogram (ECG), pulse oximetry
- Respiration – pulse oximetry, airway pressure, especially during intermittent positive-pressure ventilation (IPPV), ventilatory volume, inspired and

expired carbon dioxide and volatile agent concentrations, expired carbon dioxide waveform
- Neuromuscular transmission – nerve stimulators whenever relaxants are used
- Metabolic monitoring – sometimes indicated (e.g. temperature, blood glucose, acid–base balance)
- Increasing use being made of depth of anaesthesia monitoring

Of the Anaesthetic Machine

Instrumental monitoring of the anaesthetic machine is also necessary to ensure patient safety. Some of the monitors already listed as physiological monitors perform some of these functions, but others are also needed as follows:

- Loss or reduction of gas supply – gas pressure, gas concentration (particularly oxygen), oxygen failure warning device
- Breathing system disconnection or ventilator failure – airway pressure, inspired and expired carbon dioxide concentrations, gas volumes
- Vaporizer malfunction – inspired and expired volatile agent concentrations

Additional Monitoring

In many major surgical operations, invasive monitoring of the circulation is sometimes required, such as:

- Invasive measurement of arterial pressure, central venous pressure, pulse contour analysis (PiCCO, Pulsion Medical Systems, Munich, Germany; LiDCO, Cambridge, UK) to estimate cardiac output. Pulmonary arterial catheterization has declined in popularity due to its highly invasive nature. Noninvasive monitoring of cardiac output using transthoracic electrical bioimpedance or echocardiography is now preferred; the probe for echocardiography can be usefully incorporated in the tip of an endotracheal tube.
- Urinary catheter to measure urine output.
- Coagulation testing.
- Haemoglobin and electrolytes, which are readily obtainable with modern blood gas analysers.

All monitors have limitations. Pulse oximeter probes become detached, gas sampling lines become blocked, a gas-pressure alarm can fail to detect a disconnection if the sensor is placed inappropriately. The anaesthetist's clinical sense and experience should always be paramount.

Noninvasive and minimally invasive monitoring are preferred if they give information that is as accurate or useful as invasive monitors. It is difficult to determine with certainty the effect that additional instrumental monitoring has on patient safety. No study to do this would be ethical.

It has been shown that over 90% of critical incidents which can occur during anaesthesia are detectable when both carbon dioxide monitoring and pulse oximetry are used, strongly supporting the use of both these monitors. Nonetheless, if resources are limited a high level of safety may be achieved by a careful, conscientious anaesthetist.

The information available from clinical observation and monitors must be accurately and contemporaneously recorded. This is usually done manually, but can be now automatically downloaded to a printer.

Transfers

Critically ill or anaesthetized patients who need to be transferred within or between hospitals should be monitored to the same standards outlined above.

Alarms

Alarms should not be turned off and appropriate limits for the case set by the anaesthetist. This includes infusion pumps, if used to administer anaesthetic drugs.

Modern monitors have vastly increased the amount of information available to the anaesthetist. This can result in multiple alarm noises, making alarm systems unpopular and risking their non-use. It is important that alarm systems are designed with the intended users in mind.

CARDIOVASCULAR MONITORING

Pulse Oximetry

The human eye has difficulty in detecting cyanosis, and the pulse oximeter has undoubtedly improved the ability to monitor oxygenation. It uses both plethysmography and infrared spectroscopy.

The pulse oximeter probe consists of a light source on one side, capable of delivering both red and infrared light, and a photodetector on the other side. The probe is placed either on a digit or an earlobe. The light source emits alternating red and infrared light separated by a time gap, at a frequency of 400 Hz. The wavelengths used are 660 nm and 940 nm, these being wavelengths on the absorption spectra of reduced and oxygenated haemoglobin at which the absorptions of these two haemoglobins are, respectively, widely separated and nearly equal. This allows the device to take account of the total amount of haemoglobin present as well as the proportion of oxygenated haemoglobin present. Signals from non-pulsatile sources are electronically filtered out. The software contains a calibration curve constructed from a series of blood samples from volunteers, which calculates arterial oxygen saturation from the absorption data. The amplitude of the plethysmographic signal should not be thought of as a quantitative indicator of the pulse signal because it is variably amplified by the device.

Sources of Error in Pulse Oximetry

These include the following:

- A poorly fitting probe.
- Poor pulsatile arterial flow (e.g. vasoconstriction).
- Pulsatile venous flow (e.g. tricuspid regurgitation).
- Electrical or mechanical interference (e.g. strong ambient light, diathermy, vibration and movement).
- Presence of other haemoglobin variants. Carboxyhaemoglobin has a similar absorption spectrum to oxygenated haemoglobin in red light. Sulphaemoglobin or methaemoglobin, caused by drugs such as prilocaine, have similar absorption spectra to reduced haemoglobin causing the oximeter to read around 85%. Foetal haemoglobin does not alter the accuracy of pulse oximetry.
- Dyes, such as methylthioninium chloride (methylene blue). Bilirubin does not significantly absorb light in this bandwidth to corrupt pulse oximetry but does affect the accuracy of a co-oximeter that uses a greater range of wavelengths. Dark nail polish interferes with the probe, but skin colour does not.
- There is a delay in the response to changes in arterial saturation, which is longer for digital probes than for ear probes. There is a further delay caused by electronic averaging of several heart beats.
- Readings outside the calibrated range (usually $< 85\%$) are extrapolated and should not be relied upon.

Arterial Blood Pressure

Blood pressure was first measured invasively by arterial cannulation in an animal by Hales in 1733. Noninvasive methods were introduced into clinical practice in the late 19th century, and remain a primary means of monitoring the circulation. All monitors can measure systolic and diastolic pressures and deduce mean arterial pressure, or deduce diastolic pressure from the other two.

Noninvasive Measurement

A single compression cuff or double cuff is wrapped around a limb, usually the upper arm, and inflated above systolic pressure. The onset of pulsations is detected as the cuff is deflated. This can be a manual or an automatic process.

The dimensions of a single compression cuff are important in determining the accuracy of measurement, particularly in children or in obese patients. The American Heart Association stipulates that the width (of the inflatable bladder part) of the cuff should be 40% of the mid-circumference of the limb, and the length of the cuff should be twice this width. Recommended cuff widths are:

- Neonate 2.5 cm
- 1–4 years 6.0 cm
- 4–8 years 9.0 cm
- Adult 12–14 cm (15 cm for the adult leg)

A narrow cuff gives a falsely high reading whereas a wide cuff gives a falsely low reading. A cuff reading may not correlate with intra-arterial measurement across the whole range of pressures because there is a nonlinear relationship between the pressure in a cuff and its internal diameter around a limb.

Morbidity from cuffs includes skin and underlying tissue damage, and possible ulnar nerve damage when used on the arm too close to the elbow.

Manual Measurement

The cuff is compressed by inflating a bulb that is connected to the cuff and to either a mercury column or an aneroid barometer and a pressure gauge. As the system is decompressed, the return of pulsations in the downstream artery is detected, usually by palpation or auscultation of the Korotkoff sounds.

The Von Recklinghausen oscillotonometer has a double cuff. The upper cuff is a narrower, occluding cuff connected to the inside of a sealed box, the pressure inside which is measured by an aneroid barometer. The lower cuff is wider for sensing the return of pulsations on deflation of the occluding cuff and is connected to a more sensitive aneroid baromet er inside the sealed box. An inflation bulb and a small lever allow inflation and deflation of the cuff, and detection of the onset of systolic and diastolic pressures.

Automatic Measurement

Oscillometry uses a single cuff, which allows the process to be automated using microprocessor technology. Automated, controlled hydraulics allow the cuff to be inflated to above systolic pressure and then deflated in a stepwise fashion. On deflation of the cuff, arterial pulsations are detected by the cuff as the systolic value is reached. As mean pressure is reached, these pulsations reach maximum amplitude. At diastolic pressure the pulsations diminish and disappear. A single pressure transducer continuously detects both the cuff pressure and the arterial pulsations.

These signals are digitized, filtered and electronically processed to display systolic, mean and diastolic pressures. The electronic algorithm crosschecks the relationship between the three pressures.

Accuracy is maximized if the system volume is kept to a minimum. Extreme hypotension, excessive cuff movement, rapid changes in blood pressure, abnormal pulse rhythms and interchanging cuffs can all be causes of inaccuracy. Otherwise, these devices have been shown to be convenient and reasonably accurate.

Invasive Measurement

Direct measurement of blood pressure using an arterial cannula allows a continuous, real-time arterial waveform to be obtained. It is potentially the most accurate method and is indicated in the following circumstances:

- Critically ill patients
- Where the cardiovascular system may be compromised or unstable

- In patients who require physiological or pharmacological manipulation of blood pressure (e.g. cardiopulmonary bypass or hypotensive anaesthesia)
- As a convenient means for analysing blood gases

The radial artery is usually cannulated, using a 20 G or 22 G cannula connected to the transducer system. Although the vessel might become partially thrombosed by cannulation, the hand is protected by the arterial arcade supplied by both radial and ulnar arteries. Other arterial choices include the brachial artery and the dorsalis pedis artery.

A fluid-filled catheter connects the arterial cannula to the transducer and a means of processing and displaying the resulting electronic signal. The catheter must be reasonably stiff and straight. The fluid is assumed to be incompressible and must not contain any air bubbles. The pressure transducer consists of a diaphragm separating the catheter connecting system from the electronic measuring system. The diaphragm usually contains four strain gauges, which transduce the mechanical movement of the diaphragm into an electrical signal. These are connected to a bridge circuit to minimize errors.

The accuracy of this system depends on its natural frequency being well above those of the waveform to be measured to avoid resonance, as well as providing optimal damping to the waveform displayed. The whole system must be properly calibrated, usually at manufacture, and then levelled and zeroed at the chosen reference level (usually the heart) by the user.

Cardiac Filling Pressures

Central Venous Pressure

Normal central venous pressure (CVP) when the patient is breathing spontaneously is only a few mm Hg, and therefore accurate zeroing of the measurement system is important. A mean value is usually quoted because the pulsatile component is relatively small. A U-tube manometer may suffice or a strain gauge transducer if available. The CVP represents the filling pressure of the right side of the heart. Nevertheless, unless there is cardiorespiratory disease, a relationship is assumed to exist between right atrial pressure and left ventricular filling pressure. In general, CVP measurements are interpreted in the light of trends in values rather than the actual values themselves. Problems with CVP measurement occur when:

- The catheter is too short and therefore does not reach the thoracic cavity.
- The catheter is too long and therefore in the right ventricle, where it may also cause arrhythmias.
- The catheter is being used simultaneously to deliver fluids.
- There is compression of intrathoracic veins by IPPV, especially if positive end-expiratory pressure (PEEP) is applied, when vein compression gives falsely high readings.

Pulmonary Artery Pressure and Pulmonary Capillary Wedge Pressure

When more precise knowledge of left ventricular function is needed, a pulmonary artery (PA) catheter may be used, introduced via a central vein, usually the jugular vein. The catheter is advanced through the right ventricle and into a pulmonary artery; wedging the tip of the catheter and measuring the mean pressure can give an estimate of left atrial pressure. However, in recent years use of the PA catheter has declined due to its invasive nature, complications in its use and the availability of less invasive means of measuring cardiac output.

It is also possible to sample mixed venous blood from a PA catheter to measure the mixed venous oxygen saturation. This gives useful information about oxygen usage by cells and is characteristically low in sepsis.

Complications associated with the use of PA catheters, include:

- Arrhythmias (as with any intracardiac catheter)
- Damage to the PA, lung tissue and right ventricle
- Infection and thromboembolism
- Obstruction of venous return during cardiopulmonary bypass
- Balloon rupture, knotting or migration of the catheter

Cardiac Output Measurement

Echocardiography

Doppler ultrasound measures the mean velocity of blood through the aorta, and multiplication by the aortic cross-sectional area gives blood flow or cardiac output. The technique can also be used to measure blood flow in vessels other than the aorta.

The Doppler probe is used to measure cardiac output continuously. It can be:

- Inserted into the oesophagus
- Situated on the tip of an endotracheal tube
- Placed noninvasively on the suprasternal notch

The ultrasonic waves from the end of the probe are produced by a piezoelectric crystal in the range 2.5–5.0 MHz. The same transducer alternately transmits the wave for 1 μs and detects the reflected waves for 250 μs. Cardiac output measured by Doppler can be as accurate as thermodilution even when used intraoperatively in the presence of cardiac disease, although the user must be appropriately trained.

Echocardiography can also be used to look at cardiac structure and function (e.g. valvular area) or dysfunction: abnormal wall movement in ischaemic regions, end-diastolic and systolic volumes, ejection fraction and the detection of thrombus, air embolus and aortic dissection. Bernoulli's theorem is used to calculate any pressure gradient across the aortic valve.

Pulse Contour Analysis (PiCCO, LiDCO, FloTrac/Vigileo)

An alternative technique for measurement of cardiac output is the use of algorithms to analyse the pulse contour of the arterial pressure waveform and produce a volume waveform. Algorithms also require demographic data and can then be used to display a range of physiological variables including stroke volume, systemic vascular resistance and cardiac output. In addition, information can be obtained on stroke volume variation (SVV) with respiration as an indicator of fluid responsiveness. Algorithms require regular calibration in the clinical situation. PiCCO (Pulsion Medical Systems, Munich, Germany) uses a thermodilution technique for this (see below). It is assumed that a CVP line and a femoral arterial line is already in place; a cold bolus of fluid is injected into the CVP line and temperature change is measured at the femoral artery, and the algorithm is updated for that patient. This transpulmonary thermodilution (somewhat different from the technique used with a PA catheter) is adequate for this purpose. LiDCO (LiDCO, Cambridge, UK) uses lithium as the indicator, when a dilute concentration of lithium is injected into a central line and a blood sample is drawn from a peripheral artery where the arterial line is sited. There may be some inaccuracy in the presence of lithium therapy and the metabolites of non-depolarizing neuromuscular blockers interfere with lithium detection. The FloTrac/Vigileo system (Edwards Lifesciences, Irvine, CA, USA) does not require external calibration.

Thermodilution

Traditionally a PA catheter is introduced through a central vein (internal jugular). A bolus of cold dextrose, injected through a proximal hole of the catheter situated in the right atrium, mixes with the circulation, and the change in blood temperature is measured by a thermistor at the catheter tip. As described above, when a PA catheter is not used, it is possible to inject the bolus into a central vein and detect changes at the femoral artery. The associated microprocessor plots a curve of blood temperature with respect to time, and the cardiac output is inversely proportional to the area under this curve. Room temperature fluid can be as accurate as iced infusate. An average of three estimates is normally taken. A change of more than 15% suggests a real change of cardiac output. A variant on this technique allows continuous cardiac output measurement by using a constant infusion instead of a bolus injection.

Errors in the method include variations in temperature of the PA blood and overestimation of a low cardiac output due to the increase in cardiac preload caused by the injected bolus.

For many years, the PA catheter was the gold standard for cardiac output measurement against which all other methods were compared. More recently, factors that have contributed to its lesser use include not only those mentioned above but also:

● Difficulty demonstrating significant improvement in outcome from life-threatening conditions such as septic shock after years of use of the PA catheter

- The development of noninvasive methods of assessing cardiac output, in particular echocardiography

Nevertheless, thermodilution, lithium dilution or the use of any indicator which uses Fick's principle remain an important means of calibration of noninvasive techniques for cardiac output measurement.

Transthoracic Electrical Bioimpedance

An electrical signal of 100 kHz frequency is applied across electrodes attached round the body at the upper and lower limits of the thorax. The output signal from the thorax is amplified and processed to give electrical impedance. Some change occurs with respiration, but the majority is associated with changes in blood distribution within the thorax. The method has a variance of more than 20%. However, better accuracy with this method has been found using the phase shift in the reactance component of the impedance signal.

Electrocardiogram

The ECG is a noninvasive monitor of cardiac rate and rhythm and especially of unexpected cardiac events. It also monitors R–R interval variability, which is a useful index of autonomic activity.

The ECG is a surface reflection of the depolarizing and repolarizing electrical activity of various parts of the heart. It does not measure the heart's mechanical activity. In fact, normal electrical activity may occur when there is no cardiac output.

Excitation of the atria gives rise to the P-wave, but an atrial recovery wave is rarely seen because it is obscured by ventricular excitation, which is signalled by the QRS-wave. Recovery of the ventricles is preceded by the T-wave.

For routine operating room monitoring three electrodes are placed on the chest, as near to the heart as convenient to increase the signal-to-noise ratio. Because about 75% of ischaemic ECG patterns are best detected in the V5 lead, the positive electrode should be placed in this position (CM5) if possible.

Electrical interference from the mains can be minimized by ensuring good electrode contact, high-quality lead screening and a high common mode rejection ratio in the associated differential amplifier. Electronic filtering can give a bandwidth of 0.5–40 Hz, which removes most interference and is usually adequate for operating room use.

Measurement of Blood Loss

Gravimetric Method

The gravimetric method is the simplest and most commonly used method for measuring blood loss. Blood loss is estimated by measurement of the gain in weight of swabs, together with the measurement of the contents of suction bottles. It is assumed that 1 mL of blood weighs 1 g. The weight gain of swabs is said to underestimate blood loss by 25%. In operations involving complex exchanges of blood (e.g. extracorporeal circulation), it may be useful to weigh the whole patient before and after operation.

Colorimetric Method

In the colorimetric method, swabs and towels are mixed thoroughly with a large known volume of water, and the change in colour is estimated by infrared absorption. Errors may occur owing to incomplete extraction of blood or contamination with bile. The patient's haemoglobin must be known.

RESPIRATORY MONITORING

Respiratory Gas Analysis

Different gas analysers capitalize on different physicochemical properties of the gas or vapour.

The response time of any analyser depends on the time taken for the gas to be sampled (delay time) and the time taken for the device to measure the gas concentration (response time). The sampling flow rate is usually about 100–200 mL/min. Response time is often expressed as the time taken to produce a 90% or 95% response to a step or square wave input change. Zeroing and calibration of the analyser are important because they are all prone to drift in both zero and gain.

Breath-by-breath analysis of respiratory gases has a number of clinical uses.

Oxygen analysis at the common gas outlet of the anaesthetic machine identifies adequate oxygen delivery and oxygen supply failure. In the breathing system, it fulfils the same role, which is particularly important in low-flow anaesthesia and also gives data on oxygen consumption.

Volatile anaesthetic agent analysis confirms correct functioning of the vaporizer and is particularly useful in low-flow anaesthesia.

Carbon dioxide analysis (capnography) has particularly important applications, including clinical decision-making in:

- Confirming successful tracheal intubation and avoiding unintentional oesophageal or endobronchial intubation
- Detecting the breathing system or ventilator disconnection, or failure of other breathing system components, such as unidirectional valves or coaxial tubing
- Determining the adequacy of ventilation or the presence of rebreathing
- Detecting changes in the circulation, such as a fall in cardiac output, the presence of a pulmonary embolus, or other causes of ventilation–perfusion mismatch
- Detecting the presence of metabolic changes, such as malignant hyperthermia or the respiratory response to metabolic acidosis

- Detecting bronchospasm
- Detecting the offset of neuromuscular blockers

Oxygen

Paramagnetic Oxygen Analyser

In contrast to most other molecules, which are diamagnetic, oxygen and nitric oxide are attracted into a magnetic field and are paramagnetic. This enables oxygen concentration to be analysed breath by breath.

The original paramagnetic oxygen analyser contained a pair of glass spheres filled with nitrogen, suspended between the poles of a magnet by a thread. When a gas mixture containing oxygen is drawn through the analyser, oxygen is attracted into the magnetic field, resulting in a measurable displacement of the nitrogen-filled spheres. The detection system was either by a deflection measurement or a null deflection type. These devices are accurate to within 0.1% oxygen but are adversely affected by pressurization, vibration, water vapour and high flow rates. There is also a slow response time of up to 1 min.

A modern development of the analyser contains an electromagnet, which produces an alternating magnetic field at a frequency of 110 Hz. A bifurcated gas sample tube passes through the field. A reference gas enters one arm of the sample tube, and the gas for analysis enters the opposite arm. Vibrations in the gas molecules caused by the alternating magnetic field are detected and measured by a pressure transducer. The difference between them causes 2–5 Pa pressure oscillations, which are transduced into a sound signal, the amplitude of which is directly proportional to the oxygen concentration. Desflurane interferes with the accuracy of this type of analyser.

Polarographic Electrodes and Fuel Cells

The Clarke polarographic electrode consists of a cellophane-covered platinum cathode and Ag/AgCl anode in a phosphate and KCl electrolyte buffer, between which a potential difference of –0.6 V is applied by a battery. The gas sample is separated from the device by a membrane permeable to oxygen. At the cathode the following reaction takes place:

$$O_2 + 2H_2O + 4e^- = 4OH^-$$

At the anode the following oxidative reaction takes place:

$$4Ag^+ + 4Cl^- + 4e^- = 4AgCl$$

The current generated is proportional to the PO_2 of the gas sample.

A fuel cell consists of a gold cathode and a lead anode. The same reaction occurs at the cathode as in the polarographic electrode and no polarizing voltage is required.

For both devices the response time is comparatively slow, making them acceptable but less suitable for breath-by-breath analysis than other methods.

Carbon Dioxide and Volatile Anaesthetic Agents

Infrared Absorption Spectroscopy

The interatomic bonds between dissimilar atoms of polyatomic molecules such as nitrous oxide (N_2O), carbon dioxide (CO_2), water vapour and the volatile anaesthetic agents absorb infrared (IR) radiation, whereas oxygen, nitrogen and helium do not.

Different polyatomic species absorb maximally at characteristic wavelengths, making it possible to identify the gas molecule as well as quantify the gas concentration.

In a typical Luft analyser a source emits IR with wavelengths between 1 and 15 μm and filters allow through IR to match the wavelength of maximum absorption of the gas under study. For example, the filters transmit a wavelength of 3.3 μm for halothane, isoflurane and enflurane, 4.3 μm for CO_2 and 4.5 μm for N_2O.

The light passes through to a reference chamber and a sample chamber. Transmitted (non-absorbed) light is passed to a pair of air-filled detector chambers, separated by a diaphragm. The diaphragm oscillates and produces a signal proportional to the gas concentration.

Although CO_2, N_2O and carbon monoxide (CO) absorb IR light maximally at 4.3, 4.5 and 4.7 μm, respectively, there is considerable overlap in their absorption spectra, which can result in error. There is also the phenomenon of collision broadening, where the presence of one gas may broaden the IR absorption spectrum of another. Electronic correction factors in the analysers try to allow for this. For example, in a gas mixture containing 79% helium in oxygen, an IR analyser under-reads CO_2 values. Desflurane, cyclopropane, acetone and alcohol all produce errors in IR spectroscopy.

Water is a strong absorber of IR across the bandwidths of interest and must be eliminated in the sampling process, which produces some inaccuracy.

Some analysers use the 8–13 μm bandwidth to detect volatile agents, e.g. to detect sevoflurane and desflurane, where there is less chance for interference between absorption spectra.

Infrared spectroscopy is a means for determining partial pressure, so error can be introduced if the pressure of the gas sample changes or if ambient pressure changes. If the gas sample pressure changes, the partial pressure of the gas being analysed will change, without there being a real change in the fractional concentration. Similarly, if the device is calibrated at sea level and subsequently used at altitude, there will be an error in calculating gas concentration.

The 90%–95% response time of IR analysers to a step change is 150 ms. Most devices either have a water trap or use sample tubing, which absorbs water vapour. IR capnographs are accurate to about 0.1% in a range of CO_2 up to 10%.

A variant of the IR analyser described above uses a combination of IR and photo-acoustic spectroscopy. Oscillating pressure waves from the IR heated gas sample, separated into its components by a chopper wheel and filters, produce audible pressure waves detectable by microphone. The advantages of photo-acoustic IR spectroscopy over conventional IR spectroscopy include stability, zero drift, reduced need for calibration over prolonged periods and fast response time.

All Gases

Mass Spectrometry

Mass spectrometry identifies gas molecules by bombarding them with electrons and separating them in a magnetic field according to the ratio of mass and charge. The method can identify and quantify all molecular species. It is considered the gold standard of gas monitoring techniques.

The device consists of three stages:

- In the first, the gas sample is drawn into a very low-pressure chamber (about 1 mm Hg).
- In the second, which is the main part of the device, the sample diffuses into an ionization chamber with an even lower pressure (about 10^{-6} mm Hg), where the gas molecules are bombarded with electrons and the resulting ions are accelerated into a dispersion chamber.
- In the third stage, the ions are deflected by a magnetic field to different extents dependent on their mass, the separated beams of ions are detected and the signal is processed and displayed.

The respiratory mass spectrometer is accurate and requires only 20 mL/min gas sampling rate, with a 100 ms response time. However, if the device itself is at some distance from the sampling site, significant delay time may be added to the response time. Water condensation can be avoided by heating the sampling tube.

Some molecules lose two electrons rather than one in the ionization process and therefore become doubly charged ions. They then behave within the magnetic field like an ion with half the mass, which can make interpretation difficult. Furthermore, ionization can lead to fragmentation of a molecule, so that a mass spectrum appears at the output rather than a single peak.

This anomaly is useful to distinguish gas components with the same molecular weight, such as N_2O and CO_2 (44 Da), or N_2 and CO (28 Da). N_2O is fragmented into NO, O_2, N_2, N and O and can be detected at the subordinate peak for NO (30 Da). CO_2 is fragmented into O_2, C_2, C and O and can be detected at the peak for C (12 Da). Because the fragmentation is predictable, the amplitude of the subordinate peak can be used to measure gas concentration.

Raman Spectroscopy

A small fraction of incident light reflected from the surface of a molecule, about 10^{-6}, is scattered with a loss of energy and a change of wavelength characteristic of the molecule off which the light is being reflected. This is Raman scattering.

To be useful in a clinical setting, Raman spectroscopy requires powerful laser light sources and sensitive photocell detectors. A Raman spectroscope incorporates an argon laser source of wavelength 485 nm, high reflectance mirrors to concentrate the laser beam, a gas sampling chamber, appropriate optics, a detection system and a microprocessor and display system. If plotted graphically, the amplitudes of the frequency shifted peaks are proportional to the gas concentrations.

In Raman spectroscopy each gas is analysed independently, including CO_2, N_2O, volatile agents, O_2, N_2 and water vapour. The response time is 100 ms. The sample is not altered by the process and can therefore be returned to the breathing system, an advantage in low-flow anaesthesia, although there is some overlap between gas species. However, the devices are power consumptive and noisy.

Blood Gas Analysis

A heparinized blood sample, 100–300 μL, is passed through four electrodes simultaneously. Partial pressure of blood O_2 is measured using a Clarke electrode, CO_2 using a Severinghaus electrode and pH with a conventional glass electrode. The fourth electrode is a reference electrode.

A blood gas analyser frequently measures haemoglobin concentration and biochemical parameters, as well as deriving such values as O_2 saturation and content, bicarbonate, base excess and total CO_2. The sample is usually from an artery, but might also be capillary, or taken from a PA catheter as a mixed venous sample. Intravascular, micro-miniaturized versions of these devices are being developed.

Clarke Polarographic Electrode

The Clarke polarographic electrode for measuring PO_2 has been described earlier (see page 119). It is suitable for both gas and blood analysis. The membrane covering the electrode is designed to allow only oxygen to cross it, rather than blood.

pH Electrode

The pH electrode consists of two half electrochemical cells. One half consists of an Ag/AgCl electrode and the other of an $Hg/HgCl_2$ (calomel) electrode, each maintaining a fixed potential. The Ag/AgCl electrode is immersed in a buffer solution of known pH, surrounded by pH-sensitive glass. Outside the glass membrane is the blood sample. The potential difference across the glass, between these two solutions, is variable. The blood sample is separated from the calomel electrode by a porous plug and a potassium chloride salt bridge to minimize diffusion. The potential difference across the system is about 60 mV per unit of pH change at 37°C. The electrode is calibrated against standard buffer solutions of pH 6.841 and 7.383.

PCO_2 (Severinghaus) Electrode

The PCO_2 (Severinghaus) electrode is similar to a pH electrode. The H^+-sensitive glass membrane is itself covered with a membrane, which is selectively permeable to CO_2. There is a dynamic equilibrium between H^+ and CO_2, described by the Henderson–Hasselbalch equation:

$$pH = pK_a + \log_{10} \frac{[HCO_3^-]}{\alpha.PCO_2}$$

This electrode therefore allows a change in PCO_2 to generate a change in pH, which is measured by the electrode.

Temperature and Blood Gas Analysis

Analysers measure blood gas variables at 37°C. Hypothermia itself does not alter blood gas values at 37°C, and arterial blood taken at lower temperatures should be corrected by the analyser software to 37°C before clinical decisions are made on the results.

Transcutaneous Blood Gas Analysers

Modified electrodes can be used to measure PO_2 and PCO_2 transcutaneously. A common O_2 and CO_2 permeable membrane and electrolyte solution is used, ensuring a common pH for both measurements. Measured values are not particularly accurate, but trends are clinically useful, especially in babies.

Respiratory Gas Volumes and Flow Rates

Fleisch Pneumotachograph

The Fleisch pneumotachograph is a variable pressure drop, fixed-orifice flowmeter. It depends on a reasonably linear relationship between pressure and flow during laminar flow. Gas flow through the device is divided into a large number of parallel small-diameter tubes, thus ensuring laminar flow through each. Accuracy depends on the extent to which this has been achieved. The pressure difference between the inlet and outlet is measured and is directly related to flow. Variations use a mesh rather than tubes, which does not result in laminar flow but is adequate for clinical use. The flow signal is integrated to give volume. Further software uses airway pressure measurement and the volume calculation to draw a pressure–volume loop for each breath.

Hot Wire Anemometry

If a heated wire is placed in a gas stream, the degree of its cooling by the gas flow depends on gas temperature, specific heat and flow rate.

Ultrasonic Flow Transducer

The ultrasonic flow transducer is based on ultrasonic detection of vortex formation behind a partial obstruction to gas flow. It is not affected by temperature or gas composition, but may only detect vortices above a critical flow rate.

Respiratory Inductance Plethysmography

A pair of electrical inductance coils is wrapped around the chest and abdomen. Respiration and change in chest volume alters the inductance between them, a change which is therefore related to tidal volume.

Positive Displacement Flowmeter

The positive displacement flowmeter consists of a pair of low-friction cogwheels within the gas volume measurement tube. The gas flow rotates the cogwheels and a small metal button on one of them acts as a magnetic revolution counter.

OTHER MONITORING

Neuromuscular Junction Monitoring

A supramaximal electrical stimulus of between 10 and 50 mA is applied to an accessible peripheral motor nerve (e.g. ulnar or facial nerve) and the response of the appropriate muscle group is assessed. The stimulus may be delivered as a single stimulus, a train-of-four stimuli at 2 Hz, a tetanic stimulus at 50 Hz or a double-burst stimulation, which is two 40 ms tetanic bursts 750 ms apart. The stimulus has a square waveform of width 0.2 ms. The nerve stimulator should have a constant current output.

Assessment of the responding muscle group is usually visual (e.g. levator palpebrae superioris in the case of the facial nerve, or adductor pollicis longus with the ulnar nerve).

Electromyographic assessment is now more commonly available.

Electroencephalography and Depth of Anaesthesia Monitoring

Electroencephalography (EEG) is a surface recording of cortical neuronal activity and is made up of frequencies up to around 40 Hz, commonly divided into four frequency bands δ (<4 Hz), θ (4–7 Hz), α (8–13 Hz) and β (13–40 Hz).

α-Activity occurs during relaxation with the eyes closed. Mental activity or eye opening results in a higher frequency, lower amplitude wave form. The normal EEG amplitude is 10–50 μV, with the range 1–100 μV. Anaesthetics affect the EEG, as do other factors such as blood pressure, PO_2, PCO_2, temperature and stimulation.

The raw EEG signal can be analysed with respect to time or frequency, but this has proved challenging with such a complex set of waveforms. Frequency analysis by Fourier transform yields a frequency spectrum and the power within each frequency band. It is quantified by indices such as the median power frequency (50% power below this frequency) and spectral edge frequency (95% power below this frequency).

It has been found that there is decreasing amount of disorder in the EEG associated with anaesthesia, with coupling of electrical sources in neurons. Some devices use algorithms to analyse the decrease in extent of neuronal electrical disorder (entropy) to assess depth of anaesthesia. The bispectral index (BIS) monitor looks at a number of aspects of the power spectrum of the EEG but also examines the BIS, which includes consideration of the phase relationships of the different component waves of the EEG. The device uses frontotemporal electrodes and calculates a dimensionless number between 0 (deeply unconscious) and 100 (wide awake), which is meant to be drug independent. A value of 40–60 correlates with surgical anaesthesia, and a value of 60–85 with sedation. However, it is found not to be reliable during ketamine anaesthesia, and its accuracy is questionable in the presence of nitrous oxide anaesthesia and high dose opioids.

Instead of monitoring the spontaneous EEG, it is possible to input a sensory stimulus to the patient and monitor the evoked potential. The stimulus can be visual, auditory or somatosensory and is repeated to allow temporal summation of the evoked potentials. The auditory evoked potential is a composite waveform, which can be plotted against time. The early cortical waves, Pa and Nb, occurring 10–50 ms after an auditory stimulus, seem to be most suitable when attempting to monitor depth of anaesthesia. Increasing depth lowers their amplitude and increases their latency.

Temperature

Formerly temperature was measured using a glass thermometer containing either mercury or alcohol. A thermistor is a semiconductor device whose electrical resistance changes with temperature and is the basis of the nasopharyngeal temperature probe.

A thermocouple generates a potential difference between the two junctions formed at the connections of two dissimilar metals, proportional to the difference in temperature between them. This is the Seebeck effect.

The infrared tympanic thermometer consists of a thermopile, a series of thermocouples that detect the infrared radiation from the tympanic membrane. The thermopile generates a potential difference proportional to tympanic membrane temperature.

Liquid crystal displays may be made of materials that change colour with temperature. They exhibit hysteresis and are sensitive to draughts.

REFERENCES

1. Association of Anaesthetists of Great Britain and Ireland. Recommendations for standards of monitoring during anaesthesia and recovery. Anaesthesia 2016;71:85–93.

FURTHER READING

Magee P, Tooley M. The Physics, Clinical Measurement and Equipment of Anaesthetic Practice for the FRCA. 2nd ed. Oxford; Oxford University Press, September 2011.

Chapter 2.3

Inhalational Anaesthesia

Jeremy Cashman

In 1799, Sir Humphrey Davy inhaled nitrous oxide and noted strange effects that included euphoria mixed with uncontrollable laughter and sobbing, finally leading to loss of consciousness. He called it 'laughing gas'. This was the year in which 'anaesthesia' was born, although the term did not enter common usage until the 1840s.

In 1844, the value of 'laughing gas' in surgery was established when Horace Wells had one of his teeth extracted painlessly. Just 2 years later in 1846, William Morton demonstrated ether anaesthesia at Massachusetts General Hospital in Boston for the surgical removal of a lump from under the jaw of a patient. This was the year in which the value of 'anaesthesia' was recognized.

During the second half of the 19th century and the course of the 20th century, a succession of inhalational anaesthetic agents have been developed. Over the same period, many agents have been discarded (Table 2.3.1). At the time of writing there are no new agents planned, and although inhalational agents remain at the centre of general anaesthesia worldwide, total intravenous techniques are slowly displacing them, at least in westernized countries.

TABLE 2.3.1 Inhalational Anaesthetic Agents

Agents in Clinical Use (Year of Introduction)	Agents of Historical Interest (Year of Introduction)
Nitrous oxide (1844)	Diethyl ether (1846)
Halothane (1956)	Chloroform (1847)
Methoxyflurane (1960)[a]	Ethyl chloride (1848)
Enflurane (1973)	Amylene (1856)
Isoflurane (1980)	Ethylene (1864)
Sevoflurane (1990)	Cyclopropane (1925)
Desflurane (1994)	Trichloroethylene (1930)
Xenon (1997)	Fluoxene (1951)

[a]Reintroduced for use as an analgesic in 2015.

GENERAL PRINCIPLES OF INHALATIONAL ANAESTHESIA

Uptake of Anaesthetic Gases and Vapours

The uptake and distribution of an inhaled anaesthetic from the inspired gas through the body to a site of action is principally determined in any individual by the physicochemical properties of the agent. Ultimately, general anaesthesia is the result of a rise in the partial pressure of the agent in the central nervous system (CNS). Provided the partial pressure of the agent is higher in the alveoli than it is in the brain, the flux of the agent will be down a pressure gradient in that direction. If the partial pressure in the alveoli is reduced below that in the brain, the flux is reversed. To study this flux, three areas require consideration:

● Partial pressure of the agent in the alveoli
● Partial pressure of the agent in the circulation
● Partial pressure of the agent in the brain and other organs

Partial Pressure of Anaesthetic Agent in the Alveoli

Concentration of the Agent in the Inspired Gas

According to Dalton's law of partial pressures, the concentration by volume of the agent in inspired gas determines its partial pressure. The concentration and partial pressure of the agent in the alveoli are slightly less than in the inspired fresh gas because:

● There is dilution by carbon dioxide (CO_2) and nitrogen.
● The agent is removed into the pulmonary capillary circulation.

Increasing the inspired concentration will speed induction of anaesthesia provided that it does not cause breath-holding or laryngeal spasm.

If the inspired concentration requirement of the agent is high, such as with N_2O, rapid uptake into the blood allows more fresh gas to enter the lungs. This shortens the time of induction and is called the concentration effect. The alveolar partial pressure of any accompanying volatile agent also rises more quickly, the second gas effect, and induction with a volatile agent is therefore more rapid in the presence of N_2O.

Alveolar Ventilation

The alveolar concentration of the anaesthetic agent will rise more quickly if alveolar ventilation is increased, and more slowly if it is reduced by respiratory depression or airway obstruction.

Partial Pressure of Anaesthetic Agent in the Circulation

Blood/Gas Partition Coefficient

The blood/gas partition coefficient is the ratio of the concentration of agent in blood to that in gas at equilibrium.

A high value indicates high solubility in blood, and that the partial pressure of the agent in blood will therefore rise slowly owing to the agent being continuously dissolved. In consequence, the alveolar partial pressure will also rise slowly because the agent continues to be absorbed and dissolved.

Correspondingly, the alveolar concentration of a poorly soluble agent will rise towards the inspired value more rapidly, and also decay more rapidly when withdrawn at the end of surgery.

In summary, agents with low blood/gas partition coefficients are characterized by alveolar, arterial and hence brain partial pressures that respond rapidly to changes in the inspired vapour concentration and *vice versa*.

Cardiac Output or Pulmonary Blood Flow

An increased cardiac output removes agent from the lungs more quickly, thus reducing the alveolar partial pressure. This delays induction of anaesthesia. This effect is compounded where more soluble agents are concerned. Correspondingly, a low cardiac output will decrease induction time (within the limitations of the increased lung/brain circulation time) although this may be offset by the longer lung/brain circulation time.

Ventilation–Perfusion Relationships

Where pulmonary ventilation and perfusion are within normal limits, there is no barrier to the diffusion of anaesthetic agents from alveolar gas into pulmonary capillary blood. The agents are then distributed in the arterial circulation. Areas of ventilation–perfusion mismatch and certain lung diseases, such as pulmonary fibrosis and emphysema, delay the uptake of anaesthetic agents from the alveoli into the circulation and slow the induction of anaesthesia.

Partial Pressure of Anaesthetic Agent in the Brain and Other Tissues

Cerebral Blood Flow

Although the brain comprises only 2% of the body weight, it receives 14% of the cardiac output. Depth of anaesthesia depends on the partial pressure of agent in the brain and rises more quickly with increased cerebral blood flow (CBF). In health, the CBF is maintained until the mean blood pressure has fallen to 40–50 mm Hg. However, CBF then assumes a greater proportion of the cardiac output, and equilibration of the partial pressures of agent in the blood and brain is reached more quickly. A similar situation occurs with intravenous anaesthetics.

Oil/Gas Partition Coefficient

The oil/gas partition coefficient is the ratio of the concentration of agent in fat to that in gas and is a measurement of fat solubility, and therefore solubility in the fat-rich tissues of the CNS. This equates with the potency of individual agents. There is a direct relationship between the minimum alveolar concentration (MAC) value

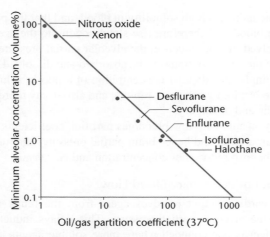

FIGURE 2.3.1   Meyer–Overton correlation between lipid solubility and anaesthetic potency, both plotted logarithmically.

of inhaled anaesthetic agents and lipid solubility in terms of the oil/gas partition coefficient according to the Meyer–Overton theory (Fig. 2.3.1).

Relative Blood Supply to Different Tissues

Under basal conditions 75% of the cardiac output goes to the brain, heart, liver, kidneys and endocrine glands – the so-called vessel-rich group of organs, although collectively these account for only 7% of the body weight.

Muscle and skin receive less than 20% of the cardiac output and constitute an intermediate group.

The vessel-poor group of tissues (fat, bone, ligament and cartilage) comprise 25% of the body weight, but receive only a small blood flow. However, fat has a great affinity for anaesthetic vapours because of their high oil/gas partition coefficients. This slows induction and recovery from anaesthesia in obese patients.

In general, the speed of equilibration of an anaesthetic agent between the alveolar concentration and any tissue of the body depends upon a rich blood supply combined with a low agent solubility in that tissue. The time constant for N_2O in brain tissue is just over 1 min but is 100 min in fat. For halothane the respective figures are 3.3 and 2720 min.

Minimum Alveolar Concentration

The potency of anaesthetic vapours may be compared by determining the MAC of an anaesthetic agent, which produces a lack of reflex movement in 50% of nonparalysed subjects when skin is incised.

Alveolar partial pressure rather than inspired concentration is the important factor because alveolar vapour concentration alters with changes in total barometric pressure at different altitudes, whereas minimum alveolar partial pressure remains constant. Therefore, MAC values are quoted under steady state conditions at 1 atmosphere pressure.

MAC has limited usefulness and the median anaesthetic dose to obtund reflex movement in 95% of subjects (AD_{95}) is more useful. The AD_{95} is about 1.5 times the MAC value.

When more than one agent is used their separate MAC fractions may be simply added together to estimate the total effect on the patient.

Other drugs that depress the CNS, such as opioids, sedatives and alcohol, reduce MAC values. MAC values are also reduced by hypothermia, hypoxaemia, hypotension and old age.

MAC values are higher in children, in states of excessive anxiety, hyperthermia, hyperthyroidism and in chronic ingestion of alcohol.

Two other derivatives of MAC are sometimes quoted:

● MAC-BAR refers to the blockade of the adrenergic response causing a rise in heart rate and blood pressure in 50% of subjects due to surgical stimulus.
● MAC-awake refers to the value at which 50% of subjects fail to respond to command during inhalational induction and may be related to the value required to prevent awareness.

Clinical Signs of Anaesthesia

Classic stages of anaesthesia are rarely seen now with the routine use of intravenous induction agents and inhalational agents with low blood/gas partition coefficients.

In 1937, Guedel described a series of physical signs describing the onset of anaesthesia and its subsequent depth. This was based on observations made on unpremedicated patients inhaling diethyl ether causing prolonged induction. The signs were classified into stages of progressive depth (Box 2.3.1).

Excitement is still seen in very light planes of anaesthesia, and ocular movements occur in light anaesthesia as does lacrimation. Autonomic responses can still occur in the presence of full muscular relaxation, and neuroendocrine responses occur in response to surgery or trauma.

General anaesthesia has three basic components:

● Narcosis
● Analgesia (with associated suppression of reflexes and the neuroendocrine stress response)
● Muscle relaxation

With appropriate selection of drugs, these three components can be varied individually.

BOX 2.3.1 Stages of Anaesthesia

Stage 1: Analgesia
Normal reflexes maintained until loss of consciousness
Abolition of the eyelash reflex

Stage 2: Excitement
Excitement
Breathing is irregular
Struggling and resisting
Regurgitation, coughing and laryngeal spasm
Pupillary dilatation

Stage 3: Surgical anaesthesia
Plane I
Eyes centrally placed, loss of conjunctival reflex
Swallowing, vomiting depressed
Pupils normal or small
Increased lacrimation

Plane II
Beginning of intercostal muscle paralysis
Regular deep breathing
Loss of corneal reflexes
Pupillary dilatation
Further increase in lacrimation

Plane III
Complete intercostal muscle paralysis
Shallow breathing
Depression of laryngeal reflexes
Depression of lacrimation

Plane IV
Complete diaphragmatic paralysis
Depression of cranial reflexes

Stage 4: Overdose
Apnoea
Pupils maximally dilated

Properties of an Ideal Inhalational Anaesthetic Agent

The desirable properties for an ideal inhalational anaesthetic agent would include the following:

- A stable molecule, not broken down by light or soda lime, not requiring preservatives and with a long shelf-life
- Nonflammable in air, O_2 or N_2O
- Potent enough to allow use with high concentrations of O_2
- Saturated vapour pressure (SVP) high enough to allow easy vaporization, but not so high as to boil at room temperature

- Low solubility in blood to allow rapid induction and recovery, and rapid response to changes in inhaled concentration
- Pleasant and nonirritating to inhale
- Devoid of organ-specific toxicity
- Lack of toxic effect when inhaled in low doses by theatre staff
- Should not undergo metabolism in the body
- Minimal cardiovascular and respiratory side-effects
- Should provide some analgesia
- No stimulant effects on the nervous system
- No sensitization of the heart to catecholamines
- No interactions with other drugs
- Cheap to manufacture

PHARMACOLOGY OF INHALATIONAL ANAESTHETIC AGENTS

The pharmacology of some of the more modern inhalational anaesthetic agents is reviewed here, together with diethyl ether, which is regarded as of historical importance (Table 2.3.2).

Desflurane

Desflurane (1-fluoro-2,2,2-trifluoroethyl difluoromethyl ether) was developed in the USA and introduced into clinical practice in 1994. The chemical structure is the same as that of isoflurane, but with fluorine substituted for chlorine.

Physical Properties

Desflurane is a colourless liquid with a pungent vapour and a molecular weight of 168 Da. Its SVP at 20°C is 88 kPa owing to its low boiling point of 23.5°C. Its blood/gas partition coefficient is 0.42 and oil/gas partition coefficient 19. MAC values range from 5% to 7% in adults to 10% in children.

No preservative is required, but desflurane can react with dry soda lime to produce carbon monoxide.

Because the boiling point of desflurane is so close to room temperature, standard vaporizers are unsatisfactory and electrically heated vaporizers are used to heat the liquid desflurane to 39°C (above its boiling point), thus vaporizing it completely. The internal vaporizer pressure at this temperature is about 200 kPa, and the vapour is then injected into the fresh gas flow, rather than the fresh gas flow passing over the surface of the vapour. Electronic sensors monitor the fresh gas flow and adjust the vapour output automatically.

Pharmacodynamic Effects

Cardiovascular System

Desflurane has similar effects on the cardiovascular system to isoflurane, with a reduction in systemic vascular resistance causing hypotension. However, some sympathetic stimulation has been reported, related partly to the absolute

TABLE 2.3.2 Physical Properties of Some Inhalation Anaesthetic Agents

Agent	Molecular Weight	Boiling Point (°C)	SVP (kPa) @ 20°C	Specific Gravity @ 20°C	Oil/Gas Partition Coefficient	Blood/Gas Partition Coefficient	MAC (%) (in Adults)	Metabolism (%)
Desflurane ($CF_2H–O–CHF.CF_3$)	168	23.5	88	–	19	0.42	6.0	0.2
Diethyl ether ($CH_3CH_2–O–CH_2CH_3$)	74	36.5	55	–	–	12	1.92	10–15
Enflurane ($CHF_2–O–CF_2.CHFCl$)	184.5	56.5	24	1.52	98.5	1.9	1.68	3
Halothane ($CF_3.CHClBr$)	197	50	32	1.87	220	2.3	0.75	20
Isoflurane ($CHF_2–O–CHCl.CF_3$)	184.5	48.5	33	1.5	98.5	1.4	1.15	0.2
Methoxyflurane ($CHCl_2.CF_2–O–CH_3$)	165	105	3.07	–	960	13	0.16	50–75
Nitrous oxide (N_2O)	44	–88.5	5200	1.2	1.4	0.47	104	0.004
Sevoflurane ($CFH_2–O–CH(CF_3)CF_3$)	200	58.5	21	1.52	53	0.69	2.0	3
Xenon (Xe)	131	–108	–	4.64	–	0.15	63–68	< 0.004

concentration of desflurane (>1.25 MAC) and also when the inspired concentration is increased rapidly, and tachycardia and hypertension can then result. The myocardium is not sensitized to catecholamines and there are no reports of coronary steal.

Respiratory System

Although desflurane vapour is not unpleasant to inhale, desflurane is much more irritant to the airways than sevoflurane, with a higher incidence of coughing and laryngeal spasm at induction in both adults and children, making its use unsuitable for inhalational induction. The threshold for irritation is 1–1.5 MAC. There is a dose-dependent reduction in tidal volume and a compensatory increase in breathing rate.

Nervous System

There is an increase in CBF and intracranial pressure with desflurane, together with a reduction in cerebral oxygen consumption. Cerebral autoregulation is abolished >1.5 MAC. EEG changes are similar to those produced by isoflurane, with anticonvulsive properties. Very little analgesia is produced. Muscle relaxation occurs and nondepolarizing neuromuscular blockers may be potentiated.

Other Systems

Desflurane has no effect on renal function.

It causes a dose-dependent relaxation of the pregnant uterus.

Desflurane has been reported to trigger malignant hyperthermia.

Pharmacokinetics

Only 0.02% of desflurane is metabolized, the rest being excreted unchanged by the lungs.

Toxicity

The minimal metabolism of desflurane means there is a very low risk of toxicity. However, very small amounts of trifluoroacetic acid are produced, which can interact with hepatic protein to trigger an immune response. Nevertheless, there are no reports of significant liver or kidney toxicity.

Desflurane is degraded by dessicated CO_2 absorbers to produce substantial amounts of carbon monoxide ($>14,000$ ppm).[1]

Clinical Use

Due to its extremely low blood/gas partition coefficient, desflurane provides the most rapid induction and recovery of all of the inhalational agents. It is therefore particularly suitable for day surgery and for bariatric surgery. Desflurane solubility in body tissues is also low, so that in a closed breathing system the concentration of vapour in the system will approach that in the basal flow more rapidly than in the case of other agents.

Diethyl Ether

Diethyl ether (ether; ethoxyethane) is now of historical interest only, although the majority of inhalational anaesthetic agents in current use are derivatives of ether. It was still being used up until 2012 in Indonesia.

Physical Properties

The SVP of diethyl ether at 20°C is 55 kPa, and the blood/gas partition coefficient 12 resulting in a very slow induction and recovery. The MAC is 1.92. It is flammable in air and explosive in O_2.

Pharmacodynamic Effects

Cardiovascular System

Diethyl ether causes sympathetic stimulation, which maintains blood pressure. There is little cardiac depression. Arrhythmias are rare. Epinephrine (adrenaline) is relatively safe with diethyl ether.

Respiratory System

Diethyl ether has an irritant vapour, which can readily induce laryngeal spasm and make induction even slower. It stimulates salivary and bronchial secretions. Bronchial smooth muscle is relaxed.

Toxicity

Although diethyl ether undergoes extensive metabolism, its metabolites (alcohol, acetaldehyde and acetic acid) are relatively nontoxic.

Enflurane

Enflurane (2-chloro-1,1,2-trifluoroethyl difluoromethyl ether) was developed in the USA and introduced into clinical practice in 1973.

Physical Properties

Enflurane is a colourless volatile liquid with a halogenated hydrocarbon-like smell. Its molecular weight is 184.5 Da and boiling point is 56.5°C, giving an SVP of 24 kPa at 20°C.

The MAC for enflurane is 1.68% in O_2 and 1.28% in 70% N_2O for adults, but up to 2.4% in children. Its blood/gas partition coefficient is 1.9 and oil/gas partition coefficient is 98.5.

Concentrations of enflurane above 4.25% are flammable in 20% O_2 with N_2O.

Enflurane is stable with soda lime and metals and does not require preservative.

Pharmacodynamic Effects

Cardiovascular System

As the depth of anaesthesia is increased, there is a reversible fall in arterial pressure with enflurane due to myocardial depression with some vasodilatation. Arrhythmias are uncommon and there is only slight sensitization of the myocardium to catecholamines. The safe dose of epinephrine (adrenaline) is up to three times that permitted with halothane.

Respiratory System

Minute volume is reduced more with enflurane than with halothane or isoflurane because of a reduction in tidal volume, often with a slight compensatory rise in respiratory rate. Airway reflexes are well maintained, and tracheal intubation is more difficult than with halothane. Salivary and bronchial secretions are not increased. Bronchodilatation occurs and there may be occasional deeper inspirations.

Nervous System

The main disadvantage of enflurane is that EEG changes of an epileptiform nature often occur. These are more common during hypocapnia and may persist for several weeks. Convulsions may occur at 2 MAC and enflurane should be used with extreme caution in patients who have a history of epilepsy. CBF is doubled at 1 MAC.

Muscle relaxation is greater with enflurane than with halothane or isoflurane, enhancing the action of nondepolarizing muscle relaxants.

Enflurane has weak analgesic properties.

Other Systems

Postoperative nausea and vomiting are uncommon with enflurane.

Enflurane causes a dose-dependent relaxation of the pregnant uterus but is suitable for caesarean section in a concentration of 1%.

There is a reduction in intraocular pressure.

Enflurane has been reported to trigger malignant hyperpyrexia.

Pharmacokinetics

Enflurane is eliminated mostly via the lungs, although about 3% is metabolized in the body and the resultant fluoride ions are excreted by the kidney.

Toxicity

Peak fluoride concentrations are similar to those seen after sevoflurane anaesthesia and are usually well below the possible toxic level of 50 µmol/L. Changes in renal function are not clinically significant, and enflurane seems to produce no further impairment of renal function, even when this is impaired preoperatively. However, caution should be exercised when potentially nephrotoxic drugs such as isoniazid are co-administered.

There have been reports of hepatitis following enflurane anaesthesia, and cross-sensitivity with halothane has been suggested.

Enflurane is degraded by dessicated CO_2 absorbers to produce substantial amounts of carbon monoxide ($>10,000$ ppm).[1]

Clinical Use

Enflurane is a more potent cardiac and respiratory depressant than more recently introduced agents. Emergence from anaesthesia is smooth and reasonably rapid, and shivering is infrequent.

It is unsuitable for neurosurgery.

Enflurane use is declining.

Halothane

Halothane (2-bromo-2-chloro-1,1,1-trifluoroethane) was developed in the UK and introduced into clinical practice in 1956.

Physical Properties

Halothane is a colourless liquid with a relatively nonpungent vapour. Its molecular weight is 197 Da, with a liquid density at 20°C of 1.87. The boiling point of halothane is 50°C, and its SVP at 20°C is 32 kPa.

The MAC for halothane is 0.75%, although up to 1.5% may be required in spontaneously breathing patients.

Partition coefficients for halothane are blood/gas 2.3, oil/gas 220, fat/blood 60.0 and brain/blood 2.6.

Halothane is decomposed by light and stabilized by 0.01% thymol but is stable when stored in amber-coloured bottles. It can be used safely with soda lime. The vapour is absorbed by rubber (rubber/gas partition coefficient at 20°C is 120). In the presence of moisture it attacks tin, brass and aluminium in vaporizers and circuits.

Halothane is nonflammable and nonexplosive when its vapour is mixed with O_2 in any concentration (including hyperbaric conditions) used clinically.

Halothane is decomposed by an open flame, liberating free bromine.

Pharmacodynamic Effects

Cardiovascular System

Arterial pressure falls with halothane owing to myocardial depression and significant vasodilatation. Sinus or nodal bradycardia is common due to increased vagal tone and can be reversed by atropine. Coronary arteries dilate, but there is an increase in myocardial oxygen demand.

Myocardial excitability is significantly increased, causing ventricular extrasystoles. These are more likely when there is CO_2 retention, sensory stimulation in light anaesthesia and with the use of β stimulant drugs and catecholamines. Ventricular fibrillation has occurred following epinephrine infiltration during halothane anaesthesia. Intravenous infusion of more than 10 µg/min of epinephrine (adrenaline) is likely to provoke an arrhythmia.

Respiratory System

Halothane depresses respiration by decreasing tidal volume and increasing respiratory rate. It causes bronchodilatation and has been used as an adjunct to ventilation in severe asthma in intensive care.

Halothane is not irritant to the airway, but depresses pharyngeal and laryngeal reflexes. Deep halothane anaesthesia allows relatively easy laryngoscopy and intubation where the airway is difficult and muscle relaxants are contraindicated.

Nervous System

Halothane produces a smooth and relatively rapid onset and emergence of anaesthesia. It increases CBF threefold at 1 MAC and abolishes autoregulation. It should only be introduced in neurosurgery if the PCO_2 has previously been lowered by hyperventilation to about 3.5 kPa. With halothane there is a moderate degree of muscle relaxation and a potentiation of nondepolarizing muscle relaxants.

Other Systems

Halothane causes a dose-dependent relaxation of the pregnant uterus. A concentration as low as 0.5% may increase blood loss during termination of pregnancy, even when oxytocin is administered.

Shivering (halothane shakes) and tremor are both common during the immediate postoperative period following halothane anaesthesia. They may be associated with a generalized increase in muscle tone, clonic or tonic. Although a fall in core temperature during anaesthesia may precipitate shivering, it has also been postulated that decreased descending inhibitory control of spinal reflexes may be important. Treatment with pethidine is sometimes helpful.

There is a reduction in intraocular pressure.

Halothane triggers malignant hyperpyrexia in susceptible individuals.

Pharmacokinetics

About 20% of the halothane taken up by the body is metabolized by the liver. This is mainly by oxidative pathways, but hypoxia may cause metabolism by alternative reductive pathways, leading to the possibility of liver damage. Metabolites include bromine, chlorine and trifluoroacetic acid, with very small numbers of fluoride ions.

Toxicity

Massive hepatic necrosis following halothane anaesthesia was first reported in 1958. Subclinical halothane hepatitis (a lesser degree of liver dysfunction, with a hepatocellular pattern of elevated transferases) may also occur in up to 20% of patients. The most susceptible patients are middle-aged women and the obese, and there may be a genetic predisposition. Conversely liver toxicity is extremely rare in children.

The incidence of halothane hepatitis is low, between 1 in 6000 and 1 in 30,000, making it difficult to study. The National Halothane Study in the USA (1969) reported on 850,000 cases of hepatitis within 6 weeks of anaesthesia, but less than 30% had received halothane.

Metabolites of halothane are slowly cleared from the body for up to 3 weeks. The pathways are complex, but the products of the reductive pathways appear more toxic and may cause direct damage to hepatocytes. There is also evidence, however, for an immune-mediated reaction, with the production of antibodies that react with liver cells altered by halothane.

Therefore, when considering using halothane:

- A careful history should be taken relating to previous halothane anaesthetics and any adverse effects.
- Halothane should not be used within 3 months of a previous halothane anaesthetic without overriding clinical circumstances.
- Unexplained jaundice or fever after a previous halothane anaesthetic is an absolute contraindication to further use of halothane.

Pre-existing liver disease unrelated to halothane is not a specific contraindication to the use of halothane. Severe liver damage is unlikely to follow a single administration of halothane. Hepatitis has been reported after the use of other inhalational anaesthetics, but repeat anaesthetics with these agents are thought to be safe.

Other causes of postoperative jaundice including side-effects of drugs (phenothiazines, monoamine oxidase inhibitors), blood transfusion, sepsis, hypotension and coincidental viral hepatitis should be excluded.

Halothane is not significantly degraded by dessicated CO_2 absorbers producing only small amounts of carbon monoxide.[1]

Clinical Use

Use of halothane is declining with the introduction of newer agents and it may soon disappear from clinical practice. It had a niche use in paediatrics for gaseous induction, but sevoflurane is now the agent of choice for this indication.

Isoflurane

Isoflurane (1-chloro-2,2,2-trifluoroethyl difluoromethyl ether) is the isomer of enflurane. It was developed in the USA but due to a misleading study, which showed hepatic carcinogenicity in mice, it was not introduced into clinical practice until 1980.

Physical Properties

Isoflurane is a colourless volatile liquid with a pungent vapour. Its molecular weight is 184.5 and its boiling point is 48.5°C. Its SVP is 33 kPa at 20°C which is similar to that of halothane, and it could theoretically be used in the same vaporizer as halothane, although this is not recommended.

Induction and recovery are rapid, partly because of the low blood/gas partition coefficient of 1.4, but also because of a fairly low fat solubility. The oil/gas partition coefficient is 98.5.

The MAC in O_2 ranges from 1.68% in children to 1.05% in patients over 60 years of age. The MAC falls to 0.66 in 70% N_2O.

Isoflurane is stable and no preservatives are necessary to prevent its decomposition. It does not react with metal in breathing systems, but can react with dry soda lime to produce carbon monoxide.

Pharmacodynamic Effects

Cardiovascular System

Isoflurane is a direct myocardial depressant, but less so than either halothane or enflurane. Isoflurane lowers arterial blood pressure less than halothane or enflurane, principally as a result of reduced systemic vascular resistance. The cardiac rhythm is stable, and the myocardium is not sensitized to catecholamines. Tachycardia is common, especially in young patients.

Isoflurane is a powerful coronary vasodilator at normal concentrations. Therefore, coronary steal may occur in patients with some types of coronary artery disease, where the healthy myocardium receives increased blood flow at the expense of myocardium supplied by the stenosed vessels. On the other hand, isoflurane with N_2O has improved the tolerance to pacing-induced myocardial ischaemia in patients with coronary artery disease. Animal work on this subject has yielded conflicting results.

Respiration

Isoflurane decreases tidal volume and increases respiratory rate. Isoflurane depresses respiration more than halothane but less than enflurane. It blunts the ventilatory response to hypercapnia, being 30% of the awake value at 1 MAC and 14% at 1.5 MAC. The ventilatory response to hypoxia is abolished at just 0.1 MAC (as with all volatile agents).

The incidence of coughing and laryngeal spasm during induction with isoflurane is greater than with halothane because the vapour is irritant, which limits its value for gaseous induction. Bronchodilatation and a reduction in hypoxic pulmonary vasoconstriction both occur.

Nervous System

Low concentrations up to 1 MAC do not increase CBF in normocapnia, so isoflurane is widely used in neurosurgical anaesthesia. Larger concentrations do increase CBF. At 2 MAC the electroencephalogram (EEG) may become isoelectric, and therefore afford some protection in cerebral hypoxia.

Isoflurane has anticonvulsive properties and does not affect the development of cerebral oedema after trauma. It has poor analgesic properties.

Muscle tone is reduced with isoflurane, as with other volatile agents, and isoflurane potentiates nondepolarizing muscle relaxants.

Other

Isoflurane decreases renal blood flow by 50% and glomerular filtration rate by 30%. Both return to normal when the drug is withdrawn.

Isoflurane causes a reduction in hepatic portal blood flow, but hepatic arterial blood flow is maintained. Repeated isoflurane administrations have failed to produce measurable changes in liver function.

Isoflurane causes a dose-dependent relaxation of the pregnant uterus but is suitable for caesarean section in a concentration of 0.75%.

There is a reduction in intraocular pressure.

Isoflurane has been reported to trigger malignant hyperpyrexia in susceptible patients.

Pharmacokinetics

About 0.2% of isoflurane is metabolized by cytochrome P450 2E1 in the liver and excreted by the kidneys. The rest is excreted unchanged by the lungs.

Toxicity

The likelihood of renal or hepatic toxicity following isoflurane anaesthesia is considered to be minimal. Serum fluoride concentrations after 3 MAC-h of exposure amount to 5% of the levels associated with renal toxicity.

Isolated cases of fatal hepatic necrosis have occurred after the use of isoflurane.

Isoflurane is degraded by dessicated CO_2 absorbers to produce significant amounts of carbon monoxide (>2500 ppm).

Clinical Use

Of the various inhalation agents available, isoflurane has the advantage of providing a stable cardiac rhythm and lack of sensitization of the heart to exogenous and endogenous epinephrine (adrenaline).

Rapid awakening is an advantage in the day-stay patient. Isoflurane is stable and is unlikely to be toxic. It produces hypotension with little cardiac depression. For maintenance with spontaneous breathing 1%–2% is usually required.

Methoxyflurane

Methoxyflurane (2,2-dichloro-1,1-2difluoroethyl methyl ether) was introduced into clinical practice in 1960, but in 2005 the Food and Drug Administration in the USA did not renew its licence due to safety concerns. However, it continued to be used in Australia as an inhalational analgesic. It was re-launched as an analgesic in the UK in 2015.

Physical Properties

Methoxyflurane is a clear, almost colourless volatile liquid with a halogenated hydrocarbon-like smell. Its molecular weight is 165 Da and boiling point is 105°C, giving an SVP of 3.07 kPa at 20°C.

The MAC for methoxyflurane is 0.16% in O_2 for adults. Its blood/gas partition coefficient is 13 and oil/gas partition coefficient is 960.

Recommended concentrations are nonflammable and nonexplosive in air and oxygen at room temperature. Concentrations of methoxyflurane above 5.4% and 7% are flammable in oxygen and air, respectively.

It is stable and does not decompose in contact with soda lime and metals and does not require preservative.

Pharmacodynamic Effects

Cardiovascular System

There is a reversible fall in arterial pressure with increasing concentration of methoxyflurane due to myocardial depression with some vasodilatation. Arrhythmias are uncommon and there is only slight sensitization of the myocardium to catecholamines.

Respiratory System

Airway reflexes are well maintained. Salivary and bronchial secretions are not increased. It relaxes bronchial muscle.

Nervous System

Unlike other inhalational agents methoxyflurane provides good analgesia at subanaesthetic concentrations.

Pharmacokinetics

Metabolism is the principal route of elimination of methoxyflurane accounting for 50%–75% of an administered dose. The metabolites formed (free fluoride ion, dichloroacetic acid and 2,2-difluoromethoxyacetic acid) are excreted in the urine.

Toxicity

Nephrotoxicity is greater with methoxyflurane than with other halogenated anaesthetic agents. Dose-dependent high output renal failure occurs following methoxyflurane anaesthesia. Exposure > 2 MAC-h is associated with serum fluoride ion induced renal tubular acidosis.

Methoxyflurane is metabolized by CYP450 2E1 and to some extent by CYP450 2A6. Enzyme inducers which increase its metabolism should be avoided.

Clinical Use

A hand-held device for methoxyflurane inhalation, the Penthrox® Inhaler, is available. Onset of pain relief occurs after about 4 min or 6–10 inhalations.

The maximum dose administered via the Penthrox® Inhaler is 6 mL of methoxyflurane which represents 0.59 MAC-h.

Analgesic use of methoxyflurane at subanaesthetic dose does not carry a risk of nephrotoxicity.

No significant adverse events have been associated with methoxyflurane at analgesic doses.

Nitrous Oxide

Nitrous oxide is a very useful agent that has been in use for over 150 years, although its undesirable properties may now outweigh its benefits. Although colloquially referred to as a gas, N_2O is actually a vapour at room temperature.

Physical Properties

Nitrous oxide is a sweet-smelling, nonirritating, colourless gas with a boiling point of $-88.5°C$, molecular weight 44 Da, critical pressure 72.5 bar, critical temperature 36.5°C, blood/gas partition coefficient 0.47 and oil/gas partition coefficient 1.4.

Nitrous oxide is a weak anaesthetic agent, with a MAC value between 100% and 105%.

The vapour pressure of N_2O at 15°C is 44 bar and 52 bar at room temperature. The vapour density at 15°C is 1.875 g/L (1.5 times that of air).

The velocity of sound in N_2O is 262 m/s (compared with 317 m/s for O_2) and a suitable whistle can be used to differentiate the two gases. Change from O_2 to N_2O causes the pitch to fall 1.5 tones.

Nitrous oxide is neither flammable nor explosive, but supports the combustion of other agents even in the absence of oxygen, if a high temperature (above 450°C) is supplied to initiate decomposition into nitrogen and oxygen.

Medical N_2O is made by heating ammonium nitrate to 240°C:

$$NH_4NO_3 \rightarrow 2H_2O + N_2O$$

At higher temperatures the percentage of impurities such as nitric oxide (NO) and nitrogen dioxide (NO_2) increases. The effects of contamination with NO has recently been reviewed and may be beneficial to the oxygenation of arterial blood.[2,3]

The issuing vapour is collected, purified and compressed into liquid at 5200 kPa.

N_2O cylinders are painted blue in the UK and USA, under the International Standard System for colour coding of medical gas cylinders (ISO 32).

The amount of N_2O present in the cylinder can only be ascertained by weighing to calculate the mass of the contents, which are in liquid form. The SVP above the liquid phase only varies with temperature. Up to four-fifths of the contents of a full cylinder is in the liquid state. Just before exhaustion of the cylinder, when all the liquid is vaporized, the pressure quickly drops to zero.

Cylinders are filled to a filling ratio (ratio of the mass of N_2O in the cylinder to the mass of water required to completely fill it) of 0.75 in temperate and 0.67 in tropical climates. The weight of the cylinder, full and empty (tare weight), is stamped on the side.

Pharmacodynamic Effects

Cardiovascular System

Nitrous oxide causes a small reduction in myocardial contractility, but this is more than compensated for by an increase in catecholamine release and is more marked under hyperbaric conditions.

Respiratory System

Nitrous oxide is nonirritant to the airway and causes a small reduction in minute volume.

Immediately following N_2O anaesthesia hypoxaemia may occur because N_2O diffuses into alveolar gas faster than nitrogen (from inspired room air) can diffuse into the blood, causing a reduction in alveolar O_2 tension. This phenomenon is called diffusional hypoxia and may be prevented by giving 100% O_2 for a few minutes at the end of anaesthesia, and continuing administration of O_2 in the recovery room.

Nervous System

Nitrous oxide is a weak anaesthetic agent. Unplanned awareness may occur if it is used as the sole anaesthetic. Tolerance to the analgesic effects has been demonstrated in volunteers, which can develop in 2 h, and may make awareness more likely (see Chapter 3.3).

Nitrous oxide is a potent analgesic. It may cause release of endorphins in the CNS. There is evidence of reversal of its analgesia by naloxone. Nitrous oxide 25%, has compared favourably with morphine for relief of postoperative pain despite having little general effect on consciousness.

Psychomotor performance is not affected at concentrations below 8%.

Other Systems

Postoperative nausea and vomiting is more likely with N_2O than when it is not used, possibly associated with its diffusion into the middle ear. Expansion of the gut and effects on opioid receptors have also been implicated.

In surgery for retinal detachment where sulphur hexafluoride is used, N_2O diffusion can cause a rise in intraocular pressure. Nitrous oxide should be discontinued up to 15 min before the bubble is injected.

Changes in middle ear pressure may cause postoperative hearing loss, and problems in otological surgery (e.g. myringoplasty) when tympanic grafts are used. It may be preferable to avoid N_2O in these cases.

Pharmacokinetics

Nitrous oxide is eliminated unchanged from the body, mostly via the lungs, but partly through the skin.

Toxicity and Adverse Effects

Nitrous oxide is an extremely safe nontoxic anaesthetic agent, provided it is administered with a sufficient concentration of O_2. It is unaffected by soda lime.

Poisoning as a result of contamination with NO and NO_2 resulting in methaemoglobinaemia and cardiorespiratory failure has been reported. Higher oxides of nitrogen can cause respiratory distress above 100 ppm, but clinical features may be delayed for several hours.

Diffusion into Gas-Containing Spaces

There is a 35-fold difference in the blood/gas partition coefficients of N_2O (0.47) and nitrogen (0.013), so for every molecule of nitrogen removed from gas-containing spaces, 35 molecules of N_2O will enter. The diffusion of N_2O between blood, tissue and gas is more rapid than that of nitrogen. This causes an increase in the volume of the gas space if the space can expand (pneumothorax, gut, air embolus) and an increase in pressure if the space cannot expand (sinuses, middle ear, pneumoencephalocoele).

Interaction with Vitamin B_{12}

Nitrous oxide inactivates the cobalt in vitamin B_{12} and so irreversibly inactivates the enzyme methionine synthetase. The time course of this interaction is much slower in humans than in rodents, in which it has been most extensively studied. A period of at least 8 h of N_2O anaesthesia is needed to demonstrate a significant fall in plasma methionine concentrations which interferes with the metabolism of folate and the synthesis of DNA and proteins. Megaloblastic anaemia and peripheral neuropathy have been reported after exposure of patients to N_2O for periods of 6–12 h. Pretreatment with folinic acid prevents these megaloblastic changes.

Very prolonged N_2O and O_2 anaesthesia could cause bone marrow aplasia.

Prolonged occupational exposure to N_2O may result in subacute combined degeneration of the cord.

Teratogenicity

Although teratogenic changes have been observed in pregnant rats exposed to N_2O for prolonged periods, there is no evidence of harm to the foetus in humans.

Clinical Use

Nitrous oxide has a number of advantages including its potent analgesic and nonirritant properties, its low solubility in blood and additive effects, allowing lower doses of inhalational agents. Nitrous oxide also speeds induction with volatile agents owing to the second gas effect.

Nitrous oxide is useful to supplement continuous or intermittent intravenous anaesthesia to reduce the chances of awareness.

Premixed Nitrous Oxide/Oxygen

Certain mixtures of N_2O and O_2 will remain in the gaseous phase at pressures and temperatures at which N_2O by itself would normally be a liquid (Poynting effect).

Entonox

Entonox is the trade name for a 50:50 mixture of gaseous N_2O and O_2. The cylinder shoulder is painted white and blue in quarters and the body is blue according to the ISO 32 classification.

If cylinders are exposed to temperatures of less than $-7°C$, the N_2O component can separate as a liquid (lamination) and may lead to delivery of uneven mixtures, too much O_2 at the beginning a ıd too much N_2O at the end of the cylinder life. Danger of lamination can be ɛ voided by immersing the cylinder in water at $52°C$ and inverting it three times, ɛ r by keeping it above a temperature of $10°C$ for 2 h before use.

Uses of Entonox include obstetric analgesia and analgesia for dressing wounds, chest physiotherapy, removal of chest drains, coronary infarction and dental surgery.

Entonox may be supplied by pipeline from large cylinders via a manifold and is usually delivered to patients through a demand valve.

Sevoflurane

Sevoflurane (1,1,1,3,3,3-hexafluoroisopropyl fluoromethyl ether) was developed in the USA but, as with isoflurane, its introduction was delayed because of fears about toxicity, in this case related to high levels of organic and inorganic fluoride, together with reports that breakdown products when used with CO_2 absorbents were nephrotoxic in rats. It was not introduced into clinical practice until 1990.

Physical Properties

Sevoflurane is a colourless liquid with a pleasant-smelling nonpungent vapour. It has a molecular weight of 200 Da, a boiling point $58.5°C$, and specific gravity of 1.52.

The SVP for sevoflurane is 21 kPa at $20°C$.

The blood/gas partition coefficient is 0.69 for sevoflurane (the second lowest of the volatile agents after desflurane, for which the blood/gas partition coefficient is 0.4) and the oil/gas partition coefficient is 53. The MAC ranges from 3.3% in neonates to 1.4% at 80 years of age.

Pharmacodynamic Effects

Cardiovascular System

Vasodilatation and hypotension may occur with sevoflurane, but blood pressure is better preserved than with isoflurane. There is no evidence of coronary steal, and coronary vasodilator properties are similar to those of isoflurane at equivalent MAC values. Sevoflurane is also less likely to cause tachycardia than isoflurane. Heart rhythm is stable and there is no myocardial sensitization to catecholamines.

Respiratory System

Sevoflurane vapour is sweet smelling and easy to breathe, making it ideal for gaseous induction in small children. Respiratory rate increases slightly, but tidal volume is reduced enough to decrease minute volume overall. Bronchodilatation and reduced hypoxic pulmonary vasoconstriction occur, as with isoflurane.

Nervous System

Sevoflurane produces a smooth and rapid onset of general anaesthesia at concentrations of between 4% and 8%. There is no increase in CBF or intracranial pressure below 1 MAC. It has anticonvulsant properties with no excitatory phenomena. Muscle tone is reduced, potentiating nondepolarizing muscle relaxants. Cerebral oxygen consumption is halved at 2 MAC. Analgesic properties are very poor.

Other Systems

The effects of sevoflurane on the uterus are similar to those of isoflurane, with a dose-dependent relaxation of the pregnant uterus. It may be used in caesarean section.

Sevoflurane may trigger malignant hyperpyrexia in susceptible individuals.

Pharmacokinetics

About 5% of sevoflurane is metabolized by cytochrome P450 2E1 in the liver with the production of hexafluoro-isopropanol and inorganic fluoride. The former is rapidly glucuronidated and excreted by the kidneys. The rest is excreted by the lungs.

Toxicity

There is no known hepatic or renal toxicity with sevoflurane, even after repeated administration.

Concentrations of inorganic fluoride are only likely to reach 50 μmol/L (the proposed threshold at which renal impairment may occur) after about 8 MAC-h of sevoflurane anaesthesia. In clinical practice sevoflurane does not cause renal damage, and the raised inorganic fluoride levels return to normal after the drug is withdrawn. However, some caution against its use if renal function is significantly impaired.

Isoflurane is degraded by CO_2 absorbers and five breakdown compounds have been identified: compounds A to E. This degradation is more marked at higher temperatures. Compound A (PIFE, pentafluoroisopropenyl fluoromethyl ether) is the only one likely to be produced in clinical use and is toxic to the liver, kidneys and CNS in rats. The concentrations of compound A found in patients have been generally less than 10 ppm, higher if baralyme is used. Concentrations over 30 ppm have been recorded after very prolonged exposure using low fresh gas flows. These values are substantially less than the 200 ppm that seems to be the minimum dose needed to cause renal damage in rats. Compound A is almost certainly of no clinical significance except when sevoflurane is used for a very long time with fresh gas flows under 2 L/min. Transient changes in renal function, attributed to compound A, have been noticed in volunteers after administration of 1.25 MAC of sevoflurane for 8 h with fresh gas flows of 2 L/min.

There is also evidence that production of compound A, fluoride, methanol and formaldehyde is more likely to occur if sevoflurane is passed over dessicated baralyme. This effect does not occur with dessicated soda lime, where the production of compound A actually decreases.

Only small amounts of carbon monoxide are produced when sevoflurane is passed over dessicated CO_2 absorbers.[1]

Clinical Use

Gaseous induction using sevoflurane is rapid, smooth and well tolerated in both children and adults.

Techniques include:

- Increasing the inspired concentration rapidly from 0.5% up to 4%–8%
- Taking a single vital capacity breath of 4.5% or higher
- Immediately breathing a high concentration (8%)

The incidence of coughing is extremely low.

The trachea may be intubated under deep sevoflurane anaesthesia. A supraglottic airway device can be inserted at about 1 MAC.

Emergence from anaesthesia is more rapid than with isoflurane and is comparable to that seen after continuous propofol anaesthesia. This makes it suitable for day surgery.

Xenon

Xenon is a weak anaesthetic agent which was first used clinically in 1951. It was approved for clinical use in Russia in 2000 and in Germany in 2005. Xenon compares favourably with N_2O in terms of haemodynamic, neuroendocrine and analgesic properties.[4,5]

Physical Properties

Xenon is a colourless, odourless gas with a boiling point of −108°C, molecular weight 131 Da, critical temperature 17°C and blood/gas partition coefficient 0.15.

Xenon is a weak anaesthetic agent, with a MAC in the range 63%–68%.
Xenon is nonflammable and nonexplosive.

Medical xenon is manufactured by fractional distillation of air, a by-product of oxygen production.

Pharmacodynamic Effects

Cardiovascular System

Xenon is highly cardiovascularly stable with no reduction in contractility, but a small reduction in heart rate may be seen. It does not sensitize the myocardium to catecholamines.

Respiratory System

In contrast to other inhaled anaesthetic agents, xenon slows the respiratory rate, while the tidal volume is increased so that the minute volume remains constant.

Compared with N_2O, xenon has a higher density ($\times 3$) and viscosity ($\times 1.5$), which may increase airway resistance at higher inspired concentrations and increase the need for higher driving pressures during ventilation.[4]

It does not cause respiratory irritation.

As the blood:gas solubility of xenon is close to that of nitrogen, diffusion hypoxia is less likely during recovery and diffusion into air-filled spaces is lower compared with N_2O.

Nervous System

Xenon inhibits plasma membrane Ca^{2+} pump and inhibits NMDA in dorsal horn neurones and may protect neural cells against ischaemic injury. In humans it appears to increase CBF in a variable manner and its use for neuroanaesthesia is not recommended.

Xenon has significant analgesic properties.

Clinical Use

Radioactive xenon[133] can be used to study regional CBF.

Currently there is no anaesthetic machine that is capable of delivering xenon.

ENVIRONMENTAL EFFECTS OF INHALATIONAL ANAESTHETIC AGENTS

There has been interest in the possible effects of inhalational anaesthetic agents on the environment. Modern halogenated inhalational agents undergo little metabolism and evaporate almost completely to the atmosphere. Chlorine-containing molecules are probably more destructive than those with fluorine.[6] Anaesthesia contributes at most 0.01% to the total atmospheric burden of chlorine-containing compounds.[6]

Over the 10 years to 2015, the abundances in the atmosphere of isoflurane, desflurane and sevoflurane have increased, while over the same period the abundance of halothane has declined, reflecting the change in pattern of their use. Desflurane now accounts for 80% of emissions of these long-lived greenhouse gases. The mean mole fractions in the global atmosphere in 2014 were:[7]

- Desflurane: 0.30 parts per trillion (10^{-12}) in dry air
- Sevoflurane: 0.13 parts per trillion (10^{-12}) in dry air
- Isoflurane: 0.097 parts per trillion (10^{-12}) in dry air
- Halothane: 9.2 parts per quadrillion (10^{-15}) in dry air

By comparison carbon dioxide currently makes up 400 parts per million (10^{-6}) in the atmosphere. However, on a kilogram-per-kilogram basis halogenated agents are much more potent than CO_2; 1 kg of desflurane produces the same greenhouse effect as 2500 kg of CO_2. Similarly, nitrous oxide is 230 times more potent as a greenhouse gas than CO_2, whereas xenon as a natural component of the atmosphere is not a greenhouse gas.

GASES USED IN ASSOCIATION WITH ANAESTHESIA

Oxygen

Oxygen has a molecular weight of 32 Da. Its solubility in water is 0.024 mL/mL at 37°C, 0.031 mL/mL at 20°C and 0.049 mL/mL at 0°C.

The boiling point of O_2 is −183°C, its critical temperature is −118.4°C and its critical pressure is 50.8 bar.

The specific gravity of O_2 is 1.1 (air is 1.0) and its density is 1.35 kg/m^3 at 15°C. Electric sparks convert O_2 into ozone (O_3).

It encourages fires, although it is not in itself flammable.

Medical O_2 is manufactured by the fractional distillation of liquid air; nitrogen boiling off first at −195°C followed by oxygen at −183°C.

Oxygen cylinders are painted black with white shoulders in the UK, blue in some European countries and green in the USA. The recommended ISO 32 colour code is white. However, within Europe it has been agreed that all medical gas cylinders shall be identified by the colour coding of the shoulder and have the body of the cylinders painted white. This change will be phased in by 2025 (Table 2.3.3). The cylinders contain gaseous O_2 compressed to 137 bar. When rapidly compressed, O_2 may ignite grease or oil, which should not therefore be used in cylinder pressure gauges. Oxygen is also supplied as a liquid at about −183°C in vacuum-insulated evaporators with a vapour pressure above the liquid of around 10.5 bar: 1 mL of liquid O_2 gives 842 mL of gas at 15°C. Hospital pipeline pressure is set at 4.1 bar.

The oxygen concentrator produces O_2 from ambient air by preferential absorption of nitrogen on zeolites (crystalline aluminosilicates). It behaves like a molecular sieve with a pore size of 0.5 nm. The resultant gas contains 6% of harmless impurities, mostly argon, and is suitable for use in hospitals and homes, remote areas, developing countries and in the military. Small machines producing about 2 L/min are cheaper than cylinders for domestic use.

TABLE 2.3.3 Colour Coding of Medical Gas Cylinders

Product	Current ISO Colour Code		New European Colour Code*	
	Shoulder	Body	Shoulder	Body
Oxygen	White	Black	White	White
Nitrous oxide	Dark blue	Dark blue	Dark blue	White
Medical air	Black/white	French grey	Black/white	White
Carbon dioxide	French grey	French grey	White	White
Helium	Brown	Brown	Brown	White
Nitrous oxide/ oxygen	Dark blue/ white	Dark blue	Dark blue/ white	White
Helium/oxygen	Brown/ white	Brown	Brown/ white	White

* From 2025 onwards

Medical Air

Atmospheric air contains 78.08% nitrogen, 20.95% O_2, 0.93% argon, 0.03% CO_2 and traces of neon, helium, krypton, hydrogen and xenon in descending order of abundance.

Medical air is supplied in the UK in grey cylinders with black and white shoulder quadrants, compressed to 137 bar. In hospitals, it is also supplied through two sets of pipelines at 4 bar and 7 bar.

Medical air is used as a respired gas and to drive ventilators at 4 bar, and drives surgical drills and saws at a pressure of 7 bar. Medical air has fewer impurities than industrial compressed air, contains no water and less than 0.5 mg/m^3 of oil mist.

Carbon Dioxide

Carbon dioxide is a colourless gas with a pungent odour in high concentration. It has a molecular weight of 44 Da, a boiling point of −78.5°C and a solubility in water of 0.88 mL/mL at 20°C. Its critical temperature is 31°C and critical pressure 73.8 bar.

The specific gravity of CO_2 is 1.52 and it has a density of 1.87 kg/m^3 at 15°C.

Carbon dioxide is stored in grey cylinders under the ISO 32 recommendation. Solid CO_2 is stored and transported in insulated containers. The filling ratio in cylinders is 0.75 in temperate climates and 0.67 in the tropics. The liquid phase disappears when about 83% of the gas by mass has been discharged.

Modern anaesthetic machines no longer have a yoke provided for it.

Effects

Inspired air contains 0.03% CO_2, mixed expired gas 3.5%–4% CO_2 and alveolar gas 5.3% CO_2 in health. Breathing 5% CO_2 in air or O_2 causes a tolerable rise in minute volume, but higher amounts cause dyspnoea, headache and increased sympathetic discharge. Above 10% CO_2 the narcotic effect becomes noticeable, and at 30% CO_2 the EEG becomes isoelectric as coma ensues. Muscle twitching, a flap of the hands and fits may occur before coma supervenes. At 40% CO_2 respiration is directly depressed.

The main medical use for CO_2 is to insufflate the abdomen for laparoscopy. It is also used as a cerebral vasodilator in studies of CBF.

Helium

Helium is an inert, colourless, odourless gas with a molecular weight of 4 Da, a boiling point of –269°C and solubility in water of 0.0088 mL/mL at 20°C. Its critical temperature is –268°C, specific gravity 0.14, critical pressure 2.3 bar and density 0.17 kg/m^3 at 15°C. Only hydrogen has a lower mass.

It is collected as a natural gas, from gas wells which contain air with 1% helium by volume (air contains 0.0005%). Huge reserves have been found in the Rift Valley in East Africa.

Helium cylinders are brown and helium–oxygen cylinders are brown with brown/white shoulder quadrants. The pressure in a full cylinder is 137 bar.

A mixture of 21% O_2 and 79% helium has a low density which enables flow through an orifice three times that air for the same pressure gradient. It may therefore be used for therapeutic benefit in patients with upper airway obstruction. Because its viscosity is very similar to that of O_2, it will make no difference to the laminar flow in smaller airways, but the lower Reynolds number for helium mixtures will encourage laminar flow in the larger airways.

Helium has a low solubility that enables it to be used in the measurement of lung volumes by gas dilution. High diffusibility and low solubility make helium less likely than nitrogen to be responsible for decompression sickness.

Its high thermal capacity encourages loss of body heat.

Water Vapour

Water has a high specific heat of 4.2 kJ/kg/°C or 10 times that of copper. Inspired air is warmed to body temperature and fully saturated with water vapour by the time it reaches the trachea. If the trachea is intubated and dry air is inspired, this important process is bypassed and has to take place in the tracheobronchial tree, with consequent drying of the mucosa. Air saturated with water vapour at 15°C, 20°C and 37°C has partial pressures of water vapour of 12, 18 and 47 mm Hg and water contents of 13, 19 and 50 mg/L, respectively.

REFERENCES

1. Keijzer C, Perez RSGM, De Lang JJ. Carbon monoxide production from five volatile anesthetics in dry sodalime in a patient model: halothane and sevoflurane do produce carbon monoxide; temperature is a poor predictor of carbon monoxide production. BMC Anesthesiol 2005;5:6. DOI:10.1186/1471-2253-5-6.
2. Hess WC, Kannmacher J, Kruse J. Contamination of anaesthetic gases with nitric oxide and its influence on oxygenation: study in patients undergoing open heart surgery. Br J Anaesth 2004;93:629–33.
3. Marczin N. Tiny wonders of tiny impurities of nitrous oxide during anaesthesia. Br J Anaesth 2004;93:619–23.
4. Harris PD, Barnes R. The use of helium and xenon in current clinical practice. Anaesthesia 2008;63:284–93.
5. Dickinson R, Franks NP. Bench-to-bedside review: Molecular pharmacology and clinical use of inert gases in anesthesia and neuroprotection. Crit Care 2010;14:229.
6. Brown AC, Canosa-Mas CE, Parr AD, Pierce JM, Wayne RP. Tropospheric lifetimes of halogenated anaesthetics. Nature 1989;341:635.
7. Vollmer MK, Siek Rhee T, Rigby M, Hofstetter D, Hill M, Schoenenberger F, et al. Modern inhalation anesthetics: Potent greenhouse gases in the global atmosphere. Geophys Res Lett 2015;42:1606–11.

FURTHER READING

Kety SS. The physiological and physical factors affecting the uptake of anesthetic agents by the body. Anesthesiology 1950;11:517–26.
Bunker JP, Forrest WH, Mostella F, editors. The National Halothane Study. A Study of the possible association between halothane anesthesia and post-operative hepatic necrosis. Washington: US Government Press Office: 1966.
McCaughey W. A summary of the National Halothane Study. Br J Anaesth 1972;44:918.

Chapter 2.4

Intravenous Anaesthesia

Susan Hill

This chapter describes those drugs given by the intravenous route for induction of anaesthesia. They may also be used for maintenance of anaesthesia, or at subanaesthetic doses as sedatives. Other intravenous drugs used as adjuvants to anaesthesia are discussed in Chapters 2.5 and 3.2.

The groups of drugs considered in this chapter are those with action(s) at:

- γ-Aminobutyric acid (GABA$_A$) receptors – barbiturates, benzodiazepines, etomidate and propofol
- N-methyl-D-aspartate (NMDA) receptor – ketamine
- α_2-Adrenergic receptor – dexmedetomidine

They differ physicochemically and in their pharmacodynamic and pharmacokinetic properties. The important common property is good lipid solubility, which enables them to penetrate the blood–brain barrier, particularly when largely unionized at pH 7.4 (Table 2.4.1).

TABLE 2.4.1 Physicochemical Properties of Induction Agents

Agent	Molecular Weight	Acid–Base Status	pKa	% Unionized at pH 7.4
Etomidate	342	Weak base	4.24	99.9
Ketamine	237.5	Weak base	7.5	44.3
Methohexital	284	Weak acid	7.9	75
Midazolam	326	Weak base	6.2	94.1
Propofol	178	Weak acid	11	99.97
Thiamylal	254	Weak acid	7.48	54.6
Thiopental	264	Weak acid	7.6	61.3

General anaesthesia may be maintained after intravenous induction either by converting to inhalation anaesthesia or by continuing intravenous administration of the induction agent using an infusion device.

There is an increasing number of microprocessor-controlled drug delivery systems for maintenance of the required effect site concentration either directly or indirectly through control of plasma concentration. Total intravenous anaesthesia (TIVA) and the more sophisticated target-controlled intravenous anaesthesia (TCI) are discussed later in this chapter.

PROPERTIES OF AN IDEAL INDUCTION AGENT

These include pharmaceutical, physicochemical, pharmacodynamic and pharmacokinetic properties (Box 2.4.1). Maintenance of anaesthesia, particularly with TIVA or TCI, also introduces cost as an important consideration.

None of the currently available induction agents is ideal, although propofol comes closest.

BOX 2.4.1 Properties of an Ideal Induction Agent

Pharmaceutical
Needs no mixing or diluting
Long shelf-life without refrigeration
pH close to plasma
No preservatives needed

Pharmacodynamic
Affects only CNS
No excitatory phenomena
No unwanted effects, particularly respiratory or cardiovascular
Good correlation between plasma concentration and clinical effects
High therapeutic index
Analgesic
No important drug interactions
No pain on injection
No histamine release or anaphylactic reactions

Pharmacokinetic
No organ-based metabolism
Rapid onset and offset of action
No active metabolites

Physicochemical
High lipid solubility
High proportion unionized at plasma pH

Economic
Cheap to produce
Sustainable supply at low cost

HISTORICAL PERSPECTIVE

Barbiturates were the first intravenous induction agents to be used in clinical anaesthesia. Hexobarbital was the first rapidly acting agent but was soon superseded by thiopental, which had fewer unwanted effects. Methohexital, an ultra-short-acting barbiturate, was popular because of its more rapid recovery than thiopental, but has largely been replaced by propofol.

Steroid-based intravenous induction agents have been used in clinical anaesthesia. Althesin, a 3:1 mix of alphaxalone and alphadolone, had several advantages compared to thiopental, but was withdrawn because its solvent polyethoxylated castor oil (Cremophor EL) was associated with severe allergic reactions. Another steroid-based induction agent, eltanolone (5-β-pregnanolone), which was solubilized in soybean oil, was withdrawn owing to a high incidence of urticaria. It had few advantages over propofol.

The eugenol derivative propanidid was also solubilized in Cremophor EL. It had a very short duration of action and minimal accumulation due to rapid metabolism by tissue and hepatic esterases. It too was withdrawn because of allergic reactions. A new intravenous induction agent, AZD3043 (previously named THRX-918661), a chemical analogue of propanidid, has reached the clinical trial stage of development.[1] AZD3043 is an ester that undergoes rapid hydrolysis. This results in a short constant context-sensitive half-time that may be advantageous for maintenance of anaesthesia or long-term sedation without accumulation. Like thiopental, propofol and etomidate, AZD3043 is a positive allosteric modulator at the $GABA_A$ receptor. However, clinical development has been slow because of problems with the formulation of the drug.

CURRENTLY AVAILABLE INTRAVENOUS INDUCTION AGENTS

The structures of the most commonly used intravenous induction agents currently available are shown in Fig. 2.4.1.

Anaesthetic barbiturates are derivatives of barbituric acid, formed by a condensation reaction between urea and malonic acid. They are weak acids and have pKa values above plasma pH, making them largely unionized and hence able to cross the blood–brain barrier. They differ in substitutions on the carbon at position 5 in the heterocyclic ring. Thiobarbiturates have oxygen replaced by sulphur on the urea-derived carbon at position 2 (Table 2.4.2; Fig. 2.4.2). A short duration of action is associated with the thio- substitution and a branched group on C5. Larger, unbranched groups prolong the duration of action and increase convulsant activity.

Barbiturates are almost water insoluble but are weak acids in the tautomeric enol form (–C(OH):N– rather than –CO.NH–). This allows formation of the sodium salt.

Thiopental is the sulphur derivative of pentobarbital, both of which have a single chiral carbon. Other barbiturates used as intravenous induction agents include methohexital and thiamylal.

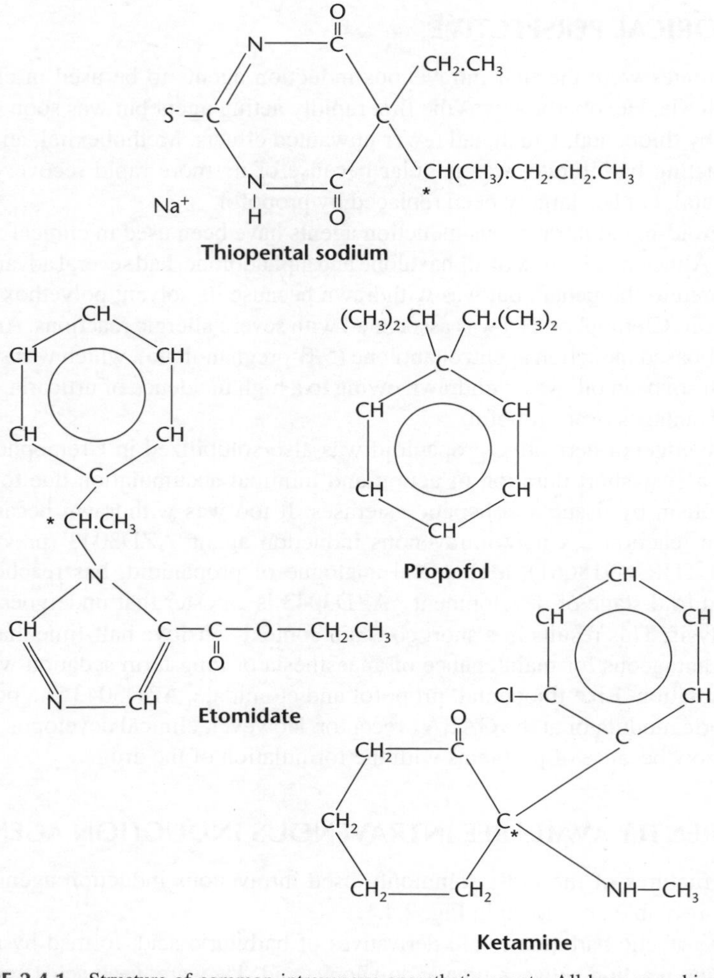

FIGURE 2.4.1 Structure of common intravenous anaesthetic agents. All have one chiral centre (indicated by *), except propofol, which is achiral.

Thiopental

Thiopental (sodium 5–ethyl–5′–(1–methylbutyl)–2–thiobarbiturate) is presented as a yellow powder containing 6% anhydrous sodium carbonate and is prepared and stored under nitrogen, which prevents release of free thiobarbituric acid in the presence of atmospheric carbon dioxide. It is dissolved in water for injection and usually diluted to give a 2.5% (25 mg/mL) alkaline solution, pH 11, which may be stored for up to 48 h if refrigerated. Injection into a vein may cause precipitation because the lower pH of blood increases the proportion in the union-ized form. Once in the blood, thiopental is highly protein bound.

TABLE 2.4.2 Structures of Barbiturate Induction Agents

Barbiturate	C2 (O or S)	N1	R1	R2
Methohexital	O	Methyl ($-CH_3$)	Propenyl (allyl) ($-CH_2.CH:CH_2$)	1–methyl pentene–2–yl ($-CH(CH_3).CH:CH.CH_2.CH_3$)
Thiamylal	S	H	Propenyl (allyl) ($-CH_2.CH:CH_2$)	1–methyl butyl ($-CH(CH_3).CH_2.CH_2.CH_3$)
Thiopental	S	H	Ethyl ($-CH_2.CH_3$)	1-methyl butyl ($-CH(CH_3).CH_2.CH_2.CH_3$)

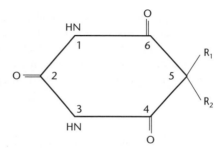

FIGURE 2.4.2   Barbituric acid nucleus.

Dose of Thiopental

The dose of thiopental varies between 3 and 5 mg/kg, with an effective plasma concentration of 15 μg/mL. Thiopental can also be given rectally, using a 5% or 10% solution at a dose of 50 mg/kg.

Pharmacodynamic Effects

Mechanism of Action

Barbiturates are positive allosteric modulators at $GABA_A$ and glycine receptors. They cause increased channel opening time for chloride, which increases inhibitory effects. Evidence of stereoselective differences between the enantiomers, *S*– more potent than *R*–thiopental, suggests specific binding sites. Other inhibitory activity can be demonstrated at central sodium and calcium channels, particularly neuronal nicotinic receptors.

Central Nervous System

Central effects of thiopental include sedation, anaesthesia, respiratory depression, anticonvulsant action, retrograde amnesia and depression of the vasomotor centre.

Thiopental has no analgesic action and may be antanalgesic in low dose.

Thiopental, like other intravenous general anaesthetic agents, is a cerebral vasoconstrictor, causing a reduction in cerebral blood flow and intracranial pressure and depression of cerebral metabolism. These are features of neuro-protection. Burst suppression of the EEG can be induced with high doses when used in the treatment of status epilepticus or intractable rises in intracranial pressure following head injury.

Respiratory System

Thiopental causes centrally mediated respiratory depression and reduced sensitivity to raised CO_2, which is dependent on dose and rate of injection. Transient apnoea is common and may require supportive manual ventilation. Laryngeal reflexes remain intact. Coughing, laryngeal spasm and mild bronchoconstriction can occur, particularly in asthmatics.

Cardiovascular System

Myocardial contractility is depressed in a dose-dependent manner with thiopental. Peripheral vascular resistance falls, leading to reduced preload and cardiac output. There is hypotension and tachycardia. Hypotension will be exaggerated if there is hypovolaemia and may be dramatic if the myocardium cannot compensate for abnormalities such as autonomic dysfunction, tight aortic stenosis and tamponade.

Other Actions

Pupils initially contract but then dilate with thiopental. Pupillary response is lost with surgical anaesthesia. Loss of the eyelash reflex is commonly used as a clinical endpoint for an adequate induction dose. Skeletal muscle tone falls more than that of smooth muscle. Uterine tone is unaffected. Lipid solubility allows passage across the placenta, with peak fetal plasma levels lower and delayed compared to maternal levels.

Pharmacokinetics

The pharmacokinetic parameters of thiopental are summarized in Table 2.4.3 for comparison with other induction agents.

The effect compartment equilibration half-life for thiopental is very short, 1.2 min, which is faster than for propofol.

Thiopental is highly protein bound depending on pH: binding falls as pH rises. Clearance is by hepatic metabolism, not renal excretion ($<1\%$). Plasma concentration falls rapidly after a bolus dose of thiopental owing to uptake by vessel-rich tissues, not metabolism. Hepatic extraction ratio is low (0.15), with saturable metabolism by oxidation to the carboxylic acid derivative, 5–ethyl–5′(4–carboxyl–1–methylbutyl) –2–thiobarbituric acid, which is inactive, and to a lesser extent by S–oxidation to pentobarbital, an hypnotic oxybarbiturate with slow elimination.

TABLE 2.4.3 Pharmacokinetic Parameters for Induction Agents

Agent	Protein Bound (%)	Clearance (mL/kg/min)	Vd$_{ss}$ (L/kg)	t$_{1/2}\beta$ (h)	Active Metabolites
Etomidate	76	18	2.5	3	None
Ketamine	60	19	3	3	Norketamine, dehydronorketamine
Methohexital	85	11	2.2	4	Hydroxymethohexital
Midazolam	98	7	1	2	1– and 4–Hydroxymidazolam
Propofol	98	30	2–3	6	None
Thiamylal	85	3	4	14	Quinalbarbital
Thiopental	85	4	2.5	10	Pentobarbital

Notes: Vd$_{ss}$, steady state volume of distribution; t$_{1/2}\beta$, elimination half-time.

After a single bolus dose or short infusion, pharmacodynamic decay curves follow typical first-order kinetics. With longer, high-dose infusions hepatic metabolic capacity may be exceeded and zero-order kinetics may be seen. Desulphurization may then become a significant metabolic pathway. Recovery will be prolonged as a result of both reduced metabolism and the presence of an active metabolite.

The elderly show reduced metabolism and a smaller volume of distribution, and a reduced dosage is needed.

Barbiturates are able to induce hepatic metabolism by several isoforms of the cytochrome P450 system. This is of importance only after repeated dosage or with prolonged infusion. CYP 1A2 (warfarin) and CYP 3A3/4 (midazolam, fentanyl, alfentanil, hydrocortisone) may be of importance to anaesthetists.

Adverse Effects

Inadvertent Intra-Arterial Injection

Inadvertent intra-arterial injection of thiopental requires prompt recognition and treatment. Surgery should be postponed if possible.

Immediate pain, blanching of the hand and loss of the radial pulse occur, followed by secondary thrombosis.

The cannula should be left in the artery to effect immediate sympathetic blockade using intra-arterial phentolamine or another vasodilator such as papaverine. This should be followed by brachial plexus or stellate ganglion block. A bolus of heparin should be given and long-term anticoagulation should be instituted as soon as possible.

Extravasation

Infiltration with lidocaine and hyaluronidase should reduce the pain caused by extravasation of thiopental.

Hypersensitivity

Anaphylactoid reactions are very rare with thiopental (1 in 15,000), but are severe.

Contraindications

Thiopental is contraindicated in porphyria, status asthmaticus, severe shock, pericardial tamponade and uncompensated myocardial disease.

Methohexital

Methohexital sodium (sodium 5–allyl–5′(1–methylpenten–2–yl)–N1–methyl–barbiturate) is presented as a white powder mixed with anhydrous sodium carbonate, as for thiopental. It is water soluble with pH of 10–11. The methyl group on the nitrogen in position 1 of the heterocyclic ring confers an ultra-short duration of action.

Unlike thiopental, methohexital has two chiral carbons and is presented as a racemic mix of just the two α-isomers. The β-isomers produce excitation.

Dose of Methohexital

The dose of methohexital is 1–2 mg/kg of a solution containing 10 mg/mL.

Pharmacodynamic Effects

Methohexital is more potent than thiopental and has a shorter onset and duration of action. Induction is often accompanied by pain on injection and involuntary myoclonic movements, particularly of the hands. Methohexital is proconvulsant.

Pharmacokinetics

Metabolism of methohexital is by oxidation at the N1 position to hydroxy-methohexital, which has some hypnotic activity. Intrinsic hepatic clearance of methohexital is far higher than for thiopental and saturation kinetics is not seen (see Table 2.4.3).

Adverse Effects

There is less risk of tissue damage than with thiopental following extravasation or inadvertent intra-arterial injection owing to its lower concentration.

Thiamylal

Thiamylal (5–allyl–5–(1–methylbutyl)–2–methyl–barbiturate) is presented as a white crystalline powder mixed with anhydrous sodium carbonate. It is dissolved in water for injection and usually diluted to give a 2% (20 mg/mL) alkaline solution. Its chemical structure is very similar to that of thiopental with an allyl group instead of ethyl group in position 5 of the heterocyclic ring.

Dose of Thiamylal

The dose of thiamylal is 3–4 mg/kg of a solution containing 20 mg/mL. A higher dose of 5–6 mg/kg has been reported for procedural sedation, particularly in children. Thiamylal can also be given rectally.

Pharmacodynamic Effects

Like thiopental, thiamylal is a positive allosteric modulator of the $GABA_A$ receptor. It is slightly more potent than thiopental and has properties very similar to those of thiopental.

Pharmacokinetics

Like thiopental, it is metabolized in the liver and has a short distribution half-life (see Table 2.4.3).

Etomidate

The sulphate of etomidate (R–1–(methylbenzyl)–imidazole–5–ethylcarboxylate sulphate) is water soluble and is presented as a 0.2% solution with pH 7 in 35% propylene glycol.

Etomidate has a single chiral carbon; the R– and S–isomers have very different potencies and the clinical preparation is just the R–enantiomer.

Dose of Etomidate

The dose of etomidate is 0.3 mg/kg. It may cause pain on injection. Etomidate does not release histamine.

Pharmacodynamic Effects

Mechanism of Action

Etomidate is a selective positive allosteric modulator at the $GABA_A$ receptor and, unlike thiopental, does not appear to affect other pentameric ion channels. A single point mutation on the β-subunit can alter the sensitivity of the $GABA_A$ receptor to etomidate.

Central Nervous System

As with thiopental, cerebral blood flow and metabolism, intracranial and intra-ocular pressure all fall with etomidate.

As with methohexital, excitatory phenomena may be seen on induction, which can be prevented by benzodiazepine premedication or concomitant use of opioids.

Central sympathetic outflow is stimulated, which maintains haemodynamics.

Respiratory System

Respiratory depression is increased with etomidate in the presence of opioids, but is less than with thiopental.

Cardiovascular System

Etomidate has no effect on mean blood pressure, cardiac output or coronary perfusion. Myocardial oxygen consumption may fall.

Pharmacokinetics

Etomidate has a rapid onset and offset of action owing to redistribution (see Table 2.4.3). Metabolism is mainly by ester hydrolysis in the liver, with a clearance that is flow limited, unlike thiopental. Metabolites undergo both renal (78%) and biliary excretion. None are active.

Due to its pharmacokinetics etomidate is suitable for maintenance of anaesthesia by continuous infusion, but adverse effects have restricted its use to bolus dose only.

Adverse Effects

Adrenocortical Suppression

A synthesis of both mineralo- and glucocorticoids is inhibited in the adrenal cortex following continuous infusion of etomidate, leading to higher than predicted mortality in the critically ill.

It has been suggested that a single dose of etomidate is sufficient to cause suppression in susceptible patients. The mitochondrial P450 enzymes inhibited are responsible for 11-β and 17-α hydroxylation of the steroid nucleus.

Nausea and Vomiting

Etomidate is more likely to be associated with nausea and vomiting than other induction agents.

Propofol

Propofol (2,6-di-isopropylphenol) has replaced thiopental as the most commonly used induction agent in many countries. It is highly lipid soluble but insoluble in water and is therefore presented as a 1% or 2% emulsion in 10% soybean oil with 1.2% egg phosphatide as the emulsifying agent.

Ampoules of 20 mL and 50 mL, and 100 mL bottles of 1% propofol are available, as well as 1% and 2% 50 mL prepackaged electronically tagged syringes for use in Diprifusor™ TCI devices. With the expiry of the patent on propofol the Diprifusor chip has been incorporated into other 'open label' TCI syringe drivers.

Propofol may be used as an induction agent alone or for both induction and maintenance of anaesthesia.

Dose of Propofol

The dose of propofol is 1–2.5 mg/kg for induction. The lower dose should be used in the elderly.

The effective blood concentration for anaesthesia (ED_{90}; the dose at which the effect is seen for 90% of patients) is 3.4 μg/mL when used with 67% nitrous oxide.

Sedation may be produced with a 0.2 mg/kg bolus dose intravenously or an infusion of 1 mg/kg/h, which produces a blood concentration of about 1.5 μg/mL.

Co-induction with either an opioid or midazolam enables the induction dose and initial target level for TCI to be reduced.

Myoclonic movements are common on induction, especially with slow injection. Emergence is more rapid than with thiopental, with less hangover.

Pharmacodynamic Effects

Mechanism of Action

Propofol is a positive allosteric modulator, binding to the β-subunit of the $GABA_A$ receptor, leading to an increased hyperpolarization owing to increased chloride channel opening time.

A point mutation resulting in replacement of methionine by tryptophan at position 286 on the β-subunit abolishes indirect receptor activation by propofol. This site is distant from that for benzodiazepines.

Other centrally located ion channels are depressed by propofol, particularly nicotinic cholinergic Na^+ and $5-HT_3$ channels, but often at higher doses than for the GABA effect.

Central Nervous System

Like thiopental, propofol is a cerebral vasoconstrictor. It reduces cerebral blood flow and metabolism, and intracranial pressure.

A central anticholinergic response may be responsible for bradycardia.

Propofol causes dose-dependent burst suppression of the EEG and is used to treat status epilepticus. Myoclonic movement is associated with increased δ-waves on the EEG during induction.

Respiratory System

Central respiratory depression occurs with propofol. Laryngeal tone is reduced more than with thiopental, making it easier to insert a laryngeal mask. There is less risk of coughing and laryngospasm than with thiopental.

Cardiovascular System

Myocardial depression is dose dependent with propofol and seen more commonly in ischaemic heart disease. Systemic vascular resistance is reduced by up to 30% without compensatory tachycardia. Associated arterial hypotension is more pronounced in the hypertensive patient. Centrally mediated bradycardia can lead to heart block. Prior administration of glycopyrrolate or atropine may be helpful. Slow, low-dose induction maintains cardiac output in hypertrophic obstructive cardiomyopathy.

Other Effects

Propofol has been used as a low-dose infusion (target 1 μg/mL) to reduce pruritus due to epidural morphine.

Nausea and vomiting are very uncommon after propofol-based anaesthesia.

Placental transfer of propofol is rapid and causes fetal depression.

Propofol is an antioxidant and may act as a free radical scavenger.

Pharmacokinetics

Propofol is lipophilic and a weak acid with a pKa of 11, existing in the unionized form, which allows fast onset of action (see Table 2.4.1). Effect compartment concentrations rise rapidly, but not quite as fast as for thiopental. The rapid distribution to tissues and high hepatic clearance account for rapid recovery after a bolus dose. Steady-state volume of distribution is large, but clearance is high (see Table 2.4.3).

Hepatic metabolism of propofol is by glucuronidation (40%) through the hydroxyl group and oxidation (60%) to 4–hydroxypropofol, a quinol derivative thought to be responsible for the green colour of urine. CYP 2B6 and, to a lesser extent, CYP 2C9, are the hepatic isoforms of the cytochrome P450 system involved in metabolism. The quinol undergoes 4-glucuronidation (85%) or sulphation. The metabolites are inactive and renally excreted. Hepatic metabolism is flow limited. Extrahepatic metabolism has been demonstrated.

After continuous infusion, terminal elimination half-life is long but context-sensitive half-time is short, being 20 min after a 12-h infusion. This is due to rapid metabolism and slow redistribution.

Adverse Effects

Unwanted Movements

There are reports of persistent epileptiform activity in myotonic dystrophy following propofol. Myoclonic movements are commonly seen. Fits have also been reported up to several hours postoperatively.

Pain on Injection

Pain on injection of propofol is often severe, may extend to the upper arm and shoulder, and most common when a rapid bolus is given into too small a vein. Addition of lidocaine may reduce pain. A new preparation of propofol in a 50:50 mixture of medium- and long-chain triglycerides (propofol-lipura) is associated with less pain on injection. Thrombophlebitis is rare.

Hypersensitivity

The incidence of hypersensitivity to propofol is low and less than for etomidate. Initial reports attributed the sensitivity to the preparation in the solvent

Cremophor EL. Few hypersensitivity reactions attributable to the emulsion have been reported.

Support of Bacterial Growth

Support of bacterial growth was demonstrated with earlier preparations of propofol. Newer formulations contain ethylenediaminetetraacetic acid (EDTA) or sodium metabisulphite as preservatives.

Propofol Infusion Syndrome

Propofol infusion syndrome is a very rare but potentially lethal syndrome of metabolic acidosis, acute cardiomyopathy and skeletal myopathy associated with prolonged (>48 h), high-dose (>5 mg/kg/h) infusion. It appears to be due to failure of free fatty acid (FFA) metabolism secondary to inhibition of both FFA entry into mitochondria and specific sites in the respiratory chain. It was first identified in paediatric intensive care.

Midazolam

Midazolam exists as two dynamic isomers; the open diazepine ring form is water soluble, but the closed-ring form is not. It is presented as a solution at pH 4, favouring the ionized, open-ring isomer. On intravenous injection, a rise in pH alters the equilibrium that favours ring closure and passage across the blood–brain barrier.

Dose of Midazolam

The dose of midazolam is 0.15–0.3 mg/kg for induction. The onset of anaesthesia is slower than for other agents and less predictable.

Co-induction with a small intravenous dose (1–3 mg of midazolam) allows a reduction in the dose of propofol required for induction and adds to the hypnotic and amnesic effect.

A combination of midazolam and opioids with nitrous oxide can also be used for intravenous anaesthesia.

Use as a Premedicant

Midazolam can be administered by the intranasal (0.2 mg/kg), oral (0.5 mg/kg) or rectal (0.3–0.5 mg/kg) routes. It has an unpleasant bitter taste that needs masking, particularly for children.

Use as a Sedative

Midazolam is more frequently used as a sedative agent by infusion (2–5 µg/kg/min) in intensive care.

Pharmacodynamic Effects

Mechanism of Action

Midazolam is a full agonist at the benzodiazepine site on the γ-subunit of the $GABA_A$ receptor complex. It augments hyperpolarization by increasing the frequency of channel opening (unlike thiopental, propofol and etomidate, which all increase the duration of channel opening). Its actions are reversed by the benzodiazepine antagonist flumazenil.

Central Nervous System

Midazolam produces sedation and hypnosis and is anticonvulsant. The amnesic effect is greater than that of diazepam. Intranasal midazolam (0.3 mg/kg) has been demonstrated to be more effective at terminating seizures in children than rectal diazepam.

Respiratory System

Respiratory depression occurs at a relatively low dose of midazolam, which is useful in intensive care. During induction, apnoea commonly occurs before anaesthesia is established.

Cardiovascular System

Midazolam is stable when used in combination with opioids for anaesthesia. Overdose in the elderly can cause hypotension, but in low doses blood pressure is relatively well maintained. Reflex tachycardia compensates for any fall.

Pharmacokinetics

Midazolam has a short terminal elimination half-life and a low steady-state volume of distribution, although its clearance is not high (see Table 2.4.3).

Effect compartment concentration rises more slowly than for other induction agents, accounting for a slower onset time for hypnosis.

Hepatic metabolism is by hydroxylation by CYP 3A4 and CYP 2A19 isoforms of cytochrome P450 to active compounds, 1– and 4–hydroxymidazolam. These are then glucuronidated for renal excretion.

Adverse Effects

Confusional State

A confusional state is commonly encountered in intensive care after stopping a prolonged infusion of midazolam.

Ketamine

Ketamine (2– (2–chlorophenyl) –2–methylaminocyclohexanone hydrochloride) is a phencyclidine derivative presented as a racemic mixture of R– and S–ketamine. The S-enantiomer is three times more potent and is associated with fewer unwanted effects. It is lipophilic but more water soluble than thiopental. It is available as a 1%, 5% or 10% solution (pH 4), with benzethonium chloride as a preservative. An enantiopure preparation of S–ketamine is available in some countries.

Dose of Ketamine

The dose of ketamine is 1–2 mg/kg intravenously for induction. Ketamine can also be used to induce anaesthesia using the intramuscular (4–6 mg/kg) or rectal (8–10 mg/kg) routes. Ketamine has become the induction agent of choice for major trauma patients due to its advantageous effects on the cardiovascular system. At lower doses there is little evidence for a rise in intracranial pressure sufficient to worsen primary traumatic brain insults.

Onset of anaesthesia is rapid, but recovery from a bolus dose is slower than for propofol and thiopentone.

An infusion of ketamine at 25–100 μg/kg/min may be used for maintenance of anaesthesia. Ketamine, unlike other induction agents, is an analgesic agent even at subanaesthetic dosage.

Ketamine produces a different form of anaesthesia from other agents, known as dissociative anaesthesia. Muscle tone is maintained, spontaneous respiration is preserved and there is profound analgesia and amnesia. Patients appear to keep their eyes open and involuntary movement is common. It is useful in the asthmatic patient and for children undergoing short, painful procedures.

Unpleasant emergence phenomena restrict the usefulness of ketamine.

Pharmacodynamic Effects

Mechanism of Action

Ketamine is a non-competitive inhibitor at the N–methyl–D–aspartate (NMDA) receptor. It is also a ligand at opioid receptors, both μ and κ, where S–ketamine is more potent than R–ketamine.

Central Nervous System

Unlike propofol and thiopental, ketamine increases cerebral blood flow and metabolism and intracranial pressure, making it unsuitable for neuroanaesthesia. Central sympathetic stimulation and inhibition of catecholamine (and serotonin) reuptake lead to increases in catecholamine levels. These can be prevented by premedication with 2 μg/kg clonidine intramuscularly. Movement of the eyes and limbs may occur spontaneously during anaesthesia.

Respiratory System

Respiratory depression is much less with ketamine than with other induction agents. Pharyngeal reflexes are preserved. Ketamine is a powerful bronchodilator owing to its indirect sympathomimetic activity.

Cardiovascular System

Heart rate, blood pressure, cardiac output and myocardial oxygen consumption all increase on induction with ketamine. Indirect sympathomimetic effects predominate over direct negative inotropic and vasodilatatory effects. Ketamine sensitizes the heart to small doses of epinephrine (adrenaline) and can precipitate arrhythmias in the anxious patient.

Pain

Ketamine reduces central sensitization after tissue injury and secondary hyperalgesia. It prevents growth of new pain pathways by inhibition of c-fos oncogene induction. Pre-emptive analgesic effects and opioid sparing are seen at low doses (0.15 mg/kg).

Reports suggest that ketamine is useful in the treatment of neuropathic pain. Ketamine appears to have found a useful role at low doses as part of a multimodal analgesic plan. A pure preparation of *S*-ketamine may replace the racemic mix for analgesic use.

Other Effects

Mood and memory disturbance may be seen.

Ketamine readily crosses the placenta and fetal levels exceed maternal within 1.5–2 min. Apgar scores may be lower.

Pharmacokinetics

Onset of action for ketamine is less rapid than for other agents. Recovery is slower than for propofol by infusion. Metabolism of the racemate is slower than for either enantiomer, suggesting mutual inhibitory effects. *S*–ketamine is metabolized more rapidly and recovery is faster than with *R*–ketamine. High-affinity, low-capacity N-demethylation is associated with the CYP 2B6 isoform and high-capacity, low-affinity demethylation with CYP 3A4 and CYP 2C9 isoforms. In vivo, CYP 3A4 is probably the most important route for N-demethylation. Elimination follows a three-compartment model, with clearance slower than for propofol but similar to that of etomidate (see Table 2.4.3).

Adverse Effects

Emergence Phenomena

Emergence phenomena can occur for up to 24 h with ketamine and include hallucinations and vivid dreams that are very unpleasant for the patient. Their incidence is less in children. These may be reduced by premedication with a benzodiazepine or clonidine, using propofol as the maintenance agent, and by allowing a slow wake-up with minimal disturbance.

Drug of Abuse

Ketamine may produce psychosis.

Contraindications

Ketamine should be avoided in patients with intracranial pathology, particularly raised intracranial pressure or penetrating eye injury. It should be used with caution in patients with hypertension.

Dexmedetomidine

Dexmedetomidine, the S–enantiomer of medetomidine, is a potent, selective α_2-adrenergic agonist (α_2 to α_1 ratio 1620:1). It is freely soluble in water and is available in a ready to use liquid formulation of dexmedetomidine 4 μg/mL in 0.9% saline.

Dexmedetomidine can be used as a premedicant, as an infusion for sedation in intensive care and for radiological imaging or in combination with remifentanil for more stimulating procedures such as awake craniotomy and insertion of spinal cord stimulators. It may also be used as sedation for fibre-optic intubation. As an adjunct to general anaesthesia it can reduce anaesthetic requirements and has been reported to reduce emergence phenomena in children.

Dosage

Dexmedetomidine is used commonly as an adjunctive agent in paediatric anaesthetic practice, although this is currently an off-label application. An intravenous bolus dose of 0.5 μg/kg or alternatively 0.1–0.5 μg/kg/min by infusion can be used to reduce postoperative adverse effects.[2]

Use as a Premedicant

For premedication in children, dexmedetomidine 1 μg/kg intranasally is superior to oral midazolam (0.5 mg/kg).

Use as a Sedative

For sedation in the intensive care unit, an initial bolus of 1 μg/kg over 10 min is given followed by 0.2–1.4 μg/kg/min intravenously by infusion. In the elderly, the loading dose should be halved and may be omitted altogether in patients who are already hypotensive.

For procedural sedation, a similar loading dose is suggested followed by a maintenance infusion rate of 0.2–1.0 μg/kg/min titrated to effect. When used in combination with remifentanil, the loading dose should be reduced and the maintenance rate is normally in the range 0.2–0.6 μg/kg/min.

Pharmacodynamics

Mechanism of Action

Dexmedetomidine has sedative and anxiolytic effects by acting on α_2-adrenergic receptors located in the pons, which inhibit the release of noradrenaline in a dose-dependent manner. This is part of the natural sleep pathway and patients sedated using dexmedetomidine maintain muscle tone and are more likely to move spontaneously and be more readily aroused than agents acting on the $GABA_A$ system.

Cardiovascular System

Its most common cardiovascular effects include hypotension and bradycardia, although hypertension and atrial fibrillation may occur less commonly; the QT interval can be prolonged so should be avoided in combination with other drugs with similar activity.

Other Effects

It reduces shivering and emergence phenomena in the postoperative period.

Pharmacokinetics

Dexmedetomidine has a distribution half-life of 6 min and a terminal elimination half-life of 2 h with a total body clearance of 39 L/h. It undergoes hepatic metabolism by CYP2A6 followed by glucuronidation to inactive metabolites, which are excreted in the urine. Tolerance and tachyphylaxis occur with prolonged infusion beyond 24 h.

TOTAL INTRAVENOUS ANAESTHESIA

Induction and maintenance of anaesthesia using the intravenous route is increasingly popular. Advantages are both clinical and environmental. Short-acting opioids and nitrous oxide may be used as adjuncts for analgesia and to reduce infusion requirements.

Suitable Drugs

A drug suitable for TIVA should ideally have the following pharmacokinetic profile:

- Rapid onset of action – short effect compartment half-life ($t_{1/2}k_{eo}$) (i.e. rapid equilibration between blood and brain)
- Rapid offset with a constant context-sensitive half-time (CSHT, the time taken for plasma concentration to fall to half its value when the infusion is stopped) – rapid elimination, not by organ metabolism and slow redistribution from tissues compared with metabolism
- Not accumulative – small steady-state volume of distribution

Propofol

The pharmacokinetic profile of propofol is suited to TIVA because the combination of high lipid solubility and rapid clearance ensures plasma levels fall rapidly, even after long infusions.

Context-sensitive half-time (CSHT) is not a fixed value but varies according to its context (i.e. the duration of the infusion). Although the CSHT for propofol does increase with the duration of infusion, it never exceeds about 20 min. The time to wake up is therefore dependent on both the duration of the infusion and the plasma concentration reached. A patient will wake up once plasma levels fall below about 1–1.2 μg/mL. Wake-up time is also affected by residual effects of any other hypnotic and analgesic drugs. There is variation between patients, which is to be expected when elimination depends on hepatic metabolism, although there do not appear to be major pharmacogenetic influences.

Propofol and Remifentanil

A combination of propofol and remifentanil infusions is ideally suited to TIVA.

Remifentanil is a very short-acting opioid with a CSHT that varies very little regardless of infusion duration. It undergoes rapid ester hydrolysis with a clearance in excess of 3 L/min. Its use reduces the plasma concentration of propofol required for adequate anaesthesia by about 50%.

Remifentanil is rapidly eliminated, so awakening is much faster than with other opioids. It is important to give longer acting analgesics before the patient awakens fully, or the analgesic effect of remifentanil will have disappeared, leaving the patient in severe pain.

Propofol and Alfentanil

Alfentanil has also been used in combination with propofol for TIVA. Alfentanil has a longer CSHT than remifentanil, with a maximum of 40 min after a 90-min infusion, longer than for propofol. The combination is useful for short procedures, but not for prolonged surgery.

Unsuitable Drugs

Fentanyl is unsuitable for use by continuous infusion during anaesthesia. Although it has a rapid clearance its intercompartmental clearance is such that the CSHT of fentanyl rapidly escalates with increasing duration of infusion (Fig. 2.4.3).

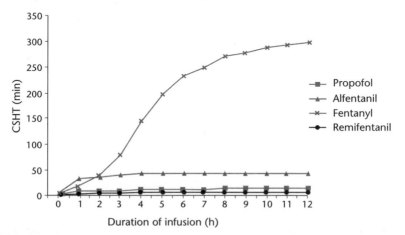

FIGURE 2.4.3 Context-sensitive half-times (CSHT) for propofol, remifentanil, alfentanil and fentanyl. Fentanyl is unsuitable for infusions of long duration but has a shorter CSHT than alfentanil for infusions of less than 2 h.

Clinical Application of TIVA

Manually Controlled Infusion of Propofol

The Bristol infusion regimen[3] for propofol ('10–8–6') based on lean body weight produces an approximate plasma concentration of 3.5 µg/mL, which is adequate for body surface surgery (Fig. 2.4.4). Higher infusion rates may be required for other surgery.

The technique involves premedication, induction with 3 µg/kg of fentanyl and a 1.0 mg/kg bolus of propofol. This is followed by an infusion of 10 mg/kg/h for 10 min then 8 mg/kg/h for the next 10 min with a final maintenance level of 6 mg/kg/h using 67% nitrous oxide in oxygen.

Recovery after procedures lasting up to 90 min is within 5–10 min, with minimal airway irritability and coughing.

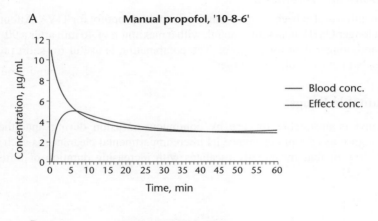

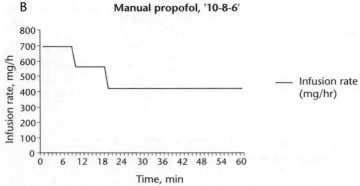

FIGURE 2.4.4 (A) Predicted plasma and effect concentrations using a manual infusion regimen ('10–8–6'). The initial plasma concentrations are high due to a bolus dose, with peak effect compartment concentration of 5 µg/mL. This is commonly compared with TCI propofol to a target of 6 µg/mL; (B) the corresponding infusion rates.

Target-Controlled Infusion of Propofol

The manual technique described above has some disadvantages, particularly for use in surgery with great variations in stimulus intensity and for long procedures. TCI devices have been available for propofol since 1996. These use microprocessor technology incorporating a pharmacokinetic model to control the rate of infusion to maintain a given target concentration. It is possible to target either plasma or site of action (effect compartment) concentration of propofol and remifentanil. Patient body weight and required target concentration are entered by the user. A visual display shows calculated concentrations for both plasma and effect compartment, together with actual infusion rate in mg/h. Often the decrement time is also displayed (i.e. time to reach predicted wake-up concentration) and there is a record of total dose infused.

The longer-established technique targets plasma concentration. The device first gives a bolus dose of propofol followed by a decreasing infusion rate according to the model. The effect compartment is in communication with plasma, but there is a rate constant for equilibration, k_{eo}, so the effect compartment concentration lags behind plasma. For a rapid onset of anaesthesia, the initial plasma target must be higher than that needed for intubation to take this lag-time into account and the target must then be reduced at around 2 min to avoid unnecessary hypotension.

Currently available devices also give the option of targeting the effect compartment concentration, which reflects pharmacodynamic activity more closely. Two pharmacokinetic models are available: the original model developed by Marsh et al.[4] and a newer one by Schneider et al.,[5] which uses a different value of k_{eo}. Unlike the Marsh model which needs just lean body mass, the Schneider model requires actual body weight, height, age and gender to be entered. In the Marsh model all compartmental volumes are weight-dependent whereas for Schneider the central and third compartment volumes are fixed and the second compartment volume and its intercompartmental clearance are both age-dependent; total body clearance is dependent on all factors (Table 2.4.4). These models differ predominantly

TABLE 2.4.4 Comparison of Factors Used to Calculate Parameters for Marsh and Schneider Models for TCI Propofol

	V_1	V_2	V_3	Cl_{10}	Cl_{12}	Cl_{13}
Marsh (modified)	LBM	LBM	LBM	LBM	Fixed	Fixed
Schneider	Fixed (4.27 L)	Age	Fixed	Weight, height, gender, age	Age	Fixed

Notes: V_1, central compartment volume; V_2, second compartment volume; V_3, third compartment volume; Cl_{10}, clearance out of model; Cl_{12}, intercompartmental clearance between compartments 1 and 2; Cl_{13}, intercompartmental clearance between compartments 1 and 3; LBM, lean body mass. In the Schneider model, LBM is calculated, so actual weight is required.

in the amount of propofol delivered for induction. The Schneider model predicts a more rapid rise in effect compartment concentration during induction (Fig. 2.4.5), with the Marsh model predicting plasma levels during recovery more accurately than Schneider.

None of the commercially available models for propofol are accurate for the morbidly obese. Both the Schneider and the Minto[6] (for remifentanil) models use the James' formulae to calculate lean body mass, which is not predicted appropriately in this group of patients. New models, such as the Eleveld model,[7] are currently being developed.

Two microprocessors with different algorithms calculate targeted concentrations. One acts as a monitor to check the accuracy of the control processor, which in turn determines the pump motor speed and rate of infusion. Performance therefore depends not only on the pharmacokinetic model but also on the algorithms used and the mechanics of the pump, syringe and infusion line.

The performance of such devices has been compared with actual plasma concentrations. There is a positive bias of about 16% (i.e. plasma concentrations tend to be a higher than calculated). Delivery must be within 5% to meet device regulations.

A suitable plasma target level for induction depends on premedication, opioid dose at induction, type of surgery, lean body mass and age.

The elderly need a lower target concentration than the young for induction and maintenance.

For a young day-case patient, without opioids, without intubation and for body surface surgery of short duration, a target of 6 μg/mL is suitable. For a premedicated patient requiring intracranial surgery also using a remifentanil infusion, this may be reduced to 3 μg/mL. The maintenance level is usually 4–6 μg/mL without opioids, but reduces to 2–3 μg/mL when using a remifentanil infusion.

TIVA using propofol is associated with a lower incidence of postoperative nausea and vomiting than volatile agent anaesthesia. The rapid awakening is particularly useful in day surgery and also for neurosurgery where early neurological assessment is required. Long periods of anaesthesia using manually controlled infusion pumps, as opposed to TCI, can lead to longer wake-up times. Recovery cannot be hastened, unlike a volatile technique where agents may be removed by ventilation.

Many anaesthetists are concerned that awareness during TIVA may be greater than for inhalation anaesthesia, although a common time for awareness is during the transition from induction agent to volatile, when intubation takes place. The end-tidal volatile agent concentration needed for adequate anaesthesia shows similar variation between patients to that for plasma levels of propofol measured during TIVA. But there is no similar indirect measure of plasma propofol concentration. End-tidal volatile concentration is measured, so is a surrogate for (indirect measure of) plasma concentration of volatile, but the TCI pump for propofol gives the calculated plasma concentration of propofol

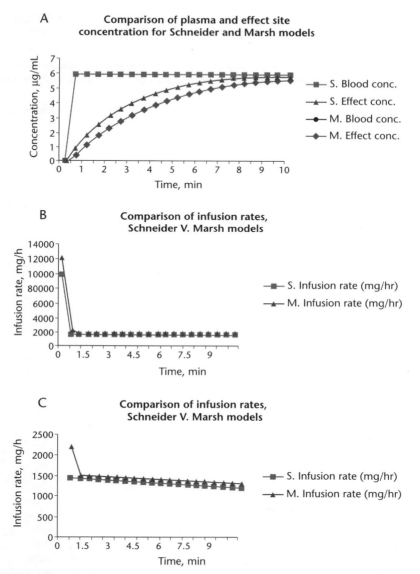

FIGURE 2.4.5 (A) Comparison of the Marsh and Schneider models for predicted rise in plasma and effect compartment concentration for the first 10 min during a TCI of propofol to 6 μg/mL. The Marsh model predicts a slower rise of effect compartment concentration because the effect compartment half-life ($t_{1/2}k_{eo}$) is longer (2.6 min) than in the Schneider model ($t_{1/2}k_{eo}$ 1.8 min); (B) comparison of the Marsh and Schneider model infusion rates. These are similar, but the Marsh model has a slightly faster initial infusion rate; (C) Comparison of the Marsh and Schneider model infusion rates. The Schneider model requires a slightly lower infusion rate over the entire 10-min period of induction.

according to the pharmacokinetic model. There is therefore a big difference in the confidence anaesthetists attribute to a measured against a calculated value for a plasma concentration. However, there is still a wide individual variation between end-tidal and actual plasma concentration of volatile agent. Monitoring depth of anaesthesia has therefore taken on a greater significance with the rise in popularity of TIVA.

Of the currently available monitors, bispectral analysis (BIS) is probably the most valuable.

Target-Controlled Infusion of Remifentanil

TCI remifentanil devices are available, with a pharmacokinetic model derived by Minto[6] which target both plasma and effect compartment concentration. As with the Schneider model for propofol, age is an essential parameter. Effect site concentrations are achieved more rapidly than with propofol (Fig. 2.4.6).

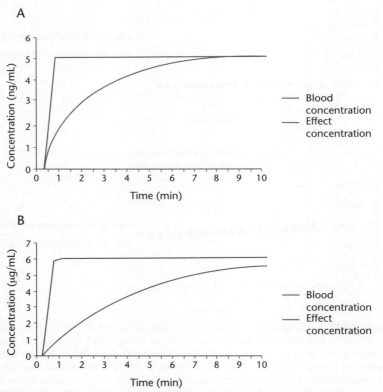

FIGURE 2.4.6   (A) Rate of rise of effect compartment concentration for remifentanil. Remifentanil reaches an effect compartment concentration of 90% of the targeted plasma concentration within 4 min; (B) rate of rise of effect compartment concentration for propofol. Propofol takes just under 9 min to reach an effect compartment concentration of 90% of the targeted plasma concentration (Marsh model).

For patients over 70 years of age, the infusion rate needs to be reduced to one-third of that for a fit young patient. Typical manually controlled remifentanil infusion rates are 2–2.5 µg/kg/min for induction and 1–2 µg/kg/min for maintenance, adjusted in anticipation of variation in surgical stimulation.

For TCI remifentanil, target levels are 4–10 ng/L depending on the nature of surgery. Offset of action is rapid and almost constant despite prolonged infusion because remifentanil has an almost constant and short CSHT of 3.5 min. This means remifentanil can be continued to the end of surgery, after propofol has been discontinued.

Provision of adequate postoperative analgesia is essential because the analgesic effects of remifentanil will dissipate soon after discontinuing the infusion. This may be provided by morphine 0.1–0.15 mg/kg intravenously or intramuscularly about 20–30 min before the completion of surgery.

Advantages of Propofol TIVA

Advantages of propofol TIVA are as follows:

- Predictable and extremely clear-headed awakening, which is especially useful after neurosurgery
- Rapid emergence, especially when used with remifentanil
- Reduced incidence of nausea and vomiting compared to volatile anaesthesia
- Reduced release of scavenged anaesthetic gases into the atmosphere
- Safe in patients susceptible to malignant hyperpyrexia
- Paralysis not always required when used with remifentanil, avoiding reversal agents
- Can be used when an anaesthetized patient needs to be transferred (e.g. between radiology and theatres)

Disadvantages of Propofol TIVA

Disadvantages of propofol TIVA are as follows:

- Propofol is more expensive than volatiles used in low-flow systems.
- It needs electrical power and infusion devices.
- It requires experience to run smoothly.
- There is a risk of awareness if intravenous access is not maintained (e.g. disconnection, blockage, dislodgement) – the infusion site must be visible at all times.
- There is no direct monitoring of plasma concentration, unlike end-tidal concentration of volatile agents – BIS or similar monitoring may be desirable to reduce the possibility of awareness.

SEDATION TECHNIQUES

Conscious sedation is a term used to describe a variety of techniques used to enable therapeutic and diagnostic procedures to be carried out without recourse to general anaesthesia. It is of particular importance in children, in the accident and emergency department and for imaging, dental and endoscopic procedures.

Premedication with or without intermittent bolus doses of intravenous anaesthetic agents can be used for short periods of sedation. The dose required is subanaesthetic and depends on the selected combination of agents.

Low-dose TCI propofol, setting a target of $1–1.5$ μg/mL, is appropriate for sedation and is particularly useful in conjunction with a regional anaesthetic technique.

Infusions of ketamine have been used successfully in children during dressing changes for burns, when analgesia requirements would otherwise be high.

Patient-controlled sedation, analogous to patient-controlled analgesia, is another technique of interest. Protocols exist for different drugs, doses and lock-out times.

Sedation in Intensive Care

Sedation in intensive care usually consists of a combination of agents tailored to the needs of individual patients and their underlying disease processes. In critically ill patients, changes in pharmacokinetics, protein binding and metabolism lead to much more variable plasma levels as well as responses. Tolerance can also become a problem, particularly in very long-term illness.

Commonly encountered drug combinations are morphine with midazolam for long periods, and propofol with alfentanil for shorter periods. Renal failure can prolong the effects of morphine due to accumulation of the active 6-glucuronide metabolite.

Thiopental is unsuitable for long-term sedation because of accumulation, except in status epilepticus and the management of intractable increases in intracranial pressure.

Etomidate is not licensed in the UK for infusion because of adrenal suppression.

REFERENCES

1. Norberg A, Koch P, Kanes SJ, Björnsson MA, Barassin S, Ahlén K, et al. A bolus and bolus followed by infusion study of AZD3043, an investigational intravenous drug for sedation and anesthesia: safety and pharmacodynamics in healthy male and female volunteers. Anesth Analg 2015;121:894–903.
2. Mahmoud M, Mason KP. Dexmedetomidine: review, update and future considerations of paediatric perioperative and procedural applications and limitations. Br J Anaesth 2015;115:171–82.
3. Spelina KR, Coates DP, Monk CR, Prys-Roberts C, Norley I, Turtle MJ. Dose requirements of propofol infusion during nitrous oxide anaesthesia in man. I: Patients premedicated with morphine sulphate. Br J Anaesth 1986;58:1080–4.
4. Marsh B, White M, Morton N, Kenny GN. Pharmacokinetic model driven infusion of propofol in children. Br J Anaesth 1991;67:41–8.
5. Schneider T, Minto C, Schaefer S, Gambus PL, Andresen C, Goodale DB, et al. The influence of age on propofol pharmacodynamics. Anesthesiology 2000;90:1502–16.

6. Minto CF, Schneider TW, Egan TD, Youngs E, Lemmens HJ, Gambus PL, et al. Influence of age and gender on the pharmacokinetics and pharmacodynamics of remifentanil. I. Model development. Anesthesiology 1997;86:10–23.
7. Eleveld DJ, Proost JH, Cortinez LI, Absalom AR, Struys MM. A general purpose pharmacokinetic model for propofol. Anesth Analg 2014;118:1221–37.

FURTHER READING

Vuyk J, Schraag S, editors. Advances in modelling and clinical applications of intravenous anaesthesia. Adv Exp Med Biol. vol. 523. New York: Springer; 2003.

Chapter 2.5

Neuromuscular Blocking Drugs

James Montague

Neuromuscular blocking drugs (NMBs; also referred to as muscle relaxants) provide skeletal muscle relaxation to facilitate tracheal intubation, control mechanical ventilation and optimize surgical operating conditions. These drugs principally interrupt the transmission of nerve impulses at the neuromuscular junction. This junction is the most thoroughly studied synapse of any type, and although some questions remain unanswered, it is a model for our understanding of synaptic transmission.

PHYSIOLOGY OF NEUROMUSCULAR TRANSMISSION

Motor Unit

The combination of a motor neuron and the muscle fibres it innervates is a motor unit. The number of muscle cells per motor unit varies, depending on the function of the muscle. The motor neurons that control skeletal muscle are long cells with bodies in the ventral horn of the spinal cord, and axons that are typically 10–20 microns in diameter and are myelinated.

The synapse is the area of the nerve lying closest to the muscle cell, situated opposite a specialized area of the muscle cell called the endplate (Fig. 2.5.1). The synaptic cleft is only 20 nm wide. A nerve impulse causes the release of acetylcholine into the cleft, activating the postsynaptic receptors and leading to depolarization and contraction of the muscle fibres.

Motor Endplate

The motor endplate is a small specialized area of muscle that is rich in acetylcholine receptors. The surface of the muscle at the endplate is deeply folded, with a high density of acetylcholine receptors of 10,000–20,000 per square micron. There are 1–10 million receptors at each endplate.

Acetylcholine Synthesis, Storage and Release

Acetylcholine is synthesized in the presynaptic terminal from the substrates choline and acetate, catalysed by choline acetyltransferase. About half the choline formed by the breakdown of acetylcholine at the neuromuscular junction is

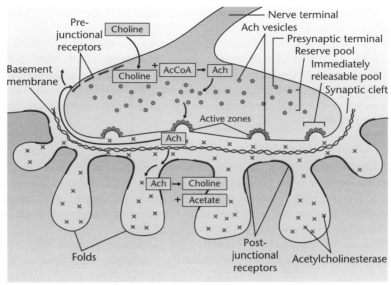

FIGURE 2.5.1   The neuromuscular junction. *Source:* Reproduced from Donati F. Physiology: nerve junction and muscle. In: Harper NJN, Pollard BJ, eds. Muscle Relaxants in Anaesthesia. London: Edward Arnold; 1995; 1–12.

taken up again into the nerve terminals by a carrier-facilitated transport mechanism before being converted back to acetylcholine.

Different pools or vesicles of acetylcholine in the nerve terminal have variable availability for release. About 1% of the vesicles are responsible for the maintenance of transmitter release under conditions of low nerve activity. Around 80% of acetylcholine is in a reserve pool, released in response to nerve impulses. Each vesicle contains approximately 12,000 molecules of acetylcholine. Acetylcholine is loaded into the vesicles by an active transport process in the vesicle membrane involving a magnesium-dependent proton-pumping ATPase.

The release of acetylcholine may be spontaneous or in response to a nerve impulse. Random miniature endplate potentials (MEPP) of 0.5–1 mV may be detected in the absence of an axon potential. When a nerve impulse reaches the nerve terminal, calcium channels in the terminal membrane are opened, calcium enters and there is a calcium-dependent synchronous release of the contents of 50–100 vesicles.

To enable the contents of the vesicle to be released, the vesicles must be docked at special release sites (active zones). Once the vesicle contents have been discharged, they are rapidly refilled from the reserve store.

Reserve vesicles are anchored to actin fibrils in the cytoskeleton by vesicular proteins called synapsins. Some of the calcium ions that enter the axoplasm on arrival of the nerve impulse bind to calmodulin. Calmodulin then activates protein kinase 2, which phosphorylates synapsin allowing the vesicle to move to and dock with the release site.

Acetylcholine release and receptor stimulation in response to a nerve action potential is far greater than that required to elicit a single muscle fibre contraction. This large safety margin means that up to 70%–80% of receptors can be occupied by a nondepolarizing muscle relaxant before surgical relaxation develops. Conversely, reversal can be clinically adequate even though many receptors are still blocked.

Acetylcholine Receptors

Acetylcholine receptors in the postjunctional membrane of the motor endplate are of the nicotinic type. They are made up of five protein subunits, designated α, β, γ, δ and ε joined to form a transmembrane ion channel that is narrower within the membrane than at the entrance. All receptors contain two α-subunits and one δ-, β- and ε-subunit. In the fetus, γ replaces ε.

When acetylcholine receptors bind to the pentameric complex, they induce a conformational change in the proteins of the α-subunits which open the channel. Potassium ions leak out from the cell, but there is a much greater movement of sodium ions into the cell.

The inside of the cell has a resting membrane potential of -80 mV with respect to the outside. Movement of sodium ions into the cell induces depolarization. Once a threshold of -50 mV is reached, voltage-gated sodium channels on the sarcolemma open, allowing the flow of sodium ions into the muscle. This increases the rate of depolarization resulting in an action potential that causes muscle contraction.

Only 6%–25% of acetylcholine normally released is required to reach the threshold potential. The activated acetylcholine receptor stays open for 1 ms. This receptor also acts as a switch, which is closed until the acetylcholine binds to the two α binding sites. The receptor then snaps open and passes current. When the acetylcholine leaves, the channel shuts and the current ceases.

Acetylcholinesterase

Acetylcholine molecules that do not react with a receptor or are released from the binding site are destroyed almost immediately by acetylcholinesterase in the junctional cleft. This protein enzyme is secreted from the muscle but remains attached to it by thin stalks of collagen attached to the basement membrane. Acetylcholine is destroyed in less than 1 ms after it has been released.

Other Acetylcholine Receptors

As well as the postjunctional receptors described above, there are also prejunctional and extrajunctional acetylcholine receptors.

Prejunctional Receptors

Prejunctional receptors are nicotinic receptors that control an ion channel specific for sodium, which is essential for the synthesis and mobilization of acetylcholine.

They are blocked by D-tubocurarine, resulting in 'fade' and exhaustion. They are also blocked by aminoglycosides and polymyxin antibiotics.

Extrajunctional Receptors

Extrajunctional receptors tend to be concentrated around the endplate, where they mix with postjunctional receptors, but may also be found anywhere on the muscle membrane. In the fetus, the ε unit is replaced by the γ unit.

Extrajunctional receptors are not found in normal active muscle, but appear very rapidly after injury or whenever muscle activity has ended. They can appear within 18 h of injury and an altered response to neuromuscular blocking drugs can be detected within 24 h of the insult.

There is a difference in the response to depolarizing and nondepolarizing muscle relaxants when large numbers of extrajunctional receptors are present. Resistance to nondepolarizing relaxants develops, yet there is an increased sensitivity to depolarizing relaxants such as suxamethonium. Suxamethonium depolarizes postjunctional and extrajunctional receptors with an exaggerated efflux of intracellular potassium, resulting in a potentially lethal hyperkalaemic response.

The longer opening time of the ion channel on the extrajunctional receptor also results in a larger efflux of ions from each receptor.

Physical Channel Blockade

Many different drugs, apart from muscle relaxants, are capable of blocking ion channels at the neuromuscular junction and preventing depolarization. This blockade can occur in two modes; blocked when open and blocked when closed.

Physical block by a molecule of an open channel (by cationic drugs only) relies on the channel being open in the first place, and the development of this is proportional to the frequency of channel opening. Provided its molecular size is small enough and concentration high enough, any drug may enter and occlude open ion channels. This mechanism may explain the synergy that occurs with certain drugs such as local anaesthetics, antibiotics and other muscle relaxants. In addition, the difficulty in antagonizing profound neuromuscular blockade may be due to open channel block by the muscle relaxant itself.

Tricyclic drugs and naloxone may cause physical blockade of a closed channel by impeding interaction of acetylcholine with the receptor.

CHARACTERISTICS OF NEUROMUSCULAR BLOCKERS

Muscle relaxants used in anaesthesia can be classified as:

- Nondepolarizing agents (tachycurares)
- Depolarizing agents (leptocurares)

Under certain circumstances depolarizing agents can exert a nondepolarizing effect: phase 2 block. Muscle relaxation can also be produced centrally by deep general anaesthesia or peripherally by nerve blockade.

Mechanisms of Neuromuscular Block

Cholinergic agonists (such as suxamethonium) and antagonists (such as rocuronium and cis-atracurium) compete at the α-subunit binding site on the nicotinic receptor. Neuromuscular blocking drugs are positively charged quaternary ammonium compounds (Fig. 2.5.2). The positive charge combines with the α-subunit in the same way as the quaternary nitrogen radical of acetylcholine.

All currently available blocking drugs contain one or more quaternary ammonium groups, which are separated by a lipophilic bridging structure of varying length. The lipophilic bridge may be a major determinant of potency.

With a depolarizing or noncompetitive block, the drug occupies the α-subunits of a receptor binding site to produce depolarization and remains attached for longer than acetylcholine, rendering the receptor insensitive to further stimulation. With a nondepolarizing or competitive block, the drug competes with acetylcholine to occupy the receptor-binding site but does not produce any initial stimulation or depolarization.

Depolarizing (Noncompetitive) Neuromuscular Block

Depolarizing drugs are structurally similar to acetylcholine. Suxamethonium chloride (succinylcholine) is comparable to two molecules of acetylcholine linked together. If the two quaternary ammonium radicals of suxamethonium interact with two α-subunits of a receptor, they open the ion channel in the same way as acetylcholine. Because suxamethonium is not metabolized by acetylcholinesterase in the synaptic cleft, depolarization of the endplate continues for longer than with acetylcholine, inactivating the voltage-gated sodium channels in the muscle membrane, which are immediately adjacent to the motor endplate. A zone is created around the endplate through which impulses temporarily cannot pass, preventing further action potentials. The muscle becomes flaccid and repolarization does not occur. Recovery only occurs as the drug diffuses away from the receptor down a concentration gradient as the plasma level falls.

Desensitization Block

Prolonged exposure of the neuromuscular junction to agonists (acetylcholine or depolarizing drugs) leads to receptor desensitization. This may represent a safety mechanism that prevents overexcitation. The membrane potential may return almost to its resting level despite the continued presence of the agonist, yet neuromuscular transmission remains blocked. The exact mechanism of desensitization block is not fully understood.

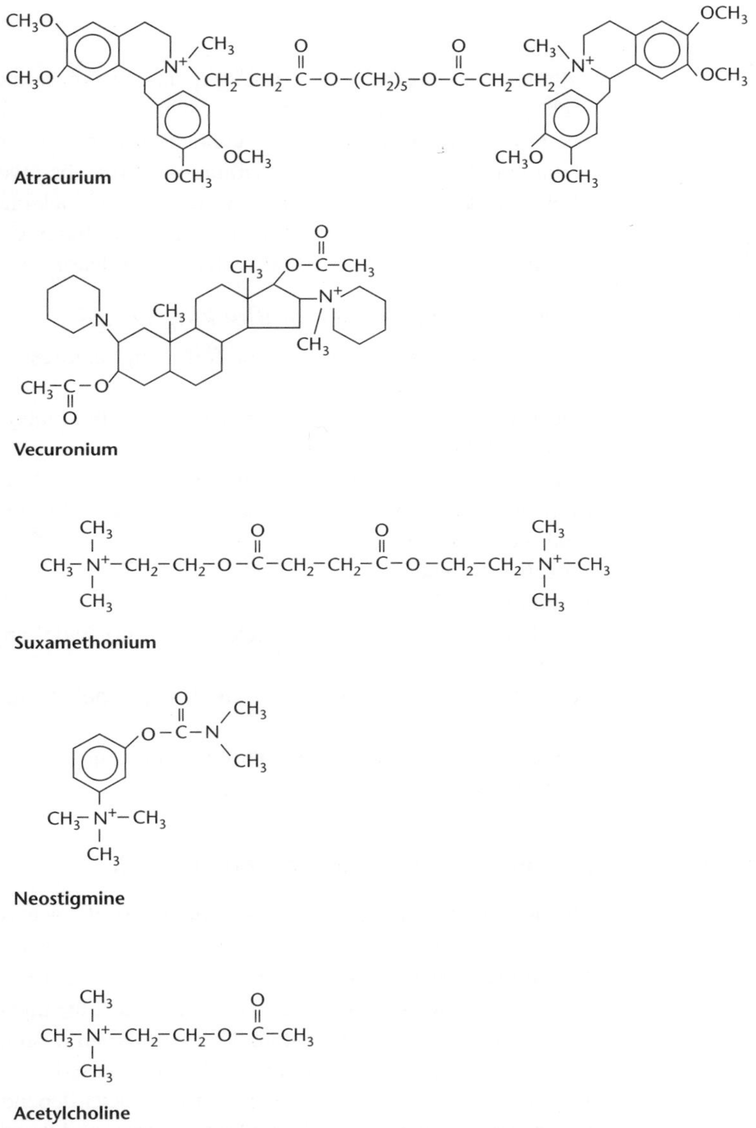

Atracurium

Vecuronium

Suxamethonium

Neostigmine

Acetylcholine

FIGURE 2.5.2 Chemical structures of atracurium, vecuronium, suxamethonium, neostigmine and acetylcholine.

Phase 2 Block

High doses of suxamethonium (between 3 and 17 mg/kg) generate a phenomenon known as phase 2 block (previously called dual block), when a short-lived depolarizing block changes into a nondepolarizing block, characterized by fade of the train of four (TOF), tetanic fade and post-tetanic facilitation. It may be reversed by low doses of anticholinesterase. Possible mechanisms of phase 2 block include postjunctional receptor desensitization, postjunctional ion channel block or presynaptic receptor blockade inhibiting acetylcholine synthesis or release.

Features of Depolarizing Neuromuscular Blocking Drugs

Depolarizing neuromuscular blocking drugs have the following features:

- They cause muscle fasciculation (but not in myasthenic individuals), and extraocular muscles exhibit a tonic response.
- Sodium channels are blocked open – muscle is unresponsive to mechanical or electrical stimuli, and repolarization does not happen until the resting membrane potential returns to –80 mV.
- There is fast dissociation at receptors.
- Block is not reversed by anticholinesterases.
- In partial paralysis there is depression of muscle twitch, no 'fade' and no post-tetanic facilitation.
- They are potentiated by isoflurane, respiratory alkalosis, hypothermia and magnesium.
- They are antagonized by acidosis and nondepolarizing relaxants.
- Repeated or continuous use leads to phase 2 block.

Nondepolarizing (Competitive) Neuromuscular Block

Nondepolarizing drugs do not alter the structural conformation of the acetylcholine receptor but prevent depolarization by combining reversibly with one or both of the α-subunits, preventing access by acetylcholine and opening of the ion channel. This results in a lower endplate potential, which does not reach the threshold necessary to fire off a propagating action potential. This is a dynamic situation with the various molecules repeatedly combining and being released from the receptor. The outcome (i.e. neuromuscular transmission or block) depends on the relative concentrations of acetylcholine and the blocking drug, and their relative affinities for the postsynaptic nicotinic receptor: 70%–80% of receptors have to be occupied by a nondepolarizing drug before the response to nerve stimulation is affected. Thus, during recovery from a nondepolarizing block, even when respiratory force and vital capacity are normal and head lift is sustainable for 5 s, 70% of the postsynaptic receptors may still be occupied by the drug.

The phenomena of fade and post-tetanic facilitation are thought to be due to block of the prejunctional nicotinic receptor. The blocking drug is thought to inhibit the positive acetylcholine feedback, which stimulates acetylcholine synthesis and mobilization in the presynaptic nerve endings.

Features of Nondepolarizing Neuromuscular Blocking Drugs

Nondepolarizing neuromuscular blocking drugs have the following features:

- No muscle fasciculation.
- They are mostly hydrophilic mono- or bisquaternary salts with interonium distances of 0.7–1.4 nm.
- They have a relatively slow onset (1–5 min) and slow dissociation at receptors.
- They are reversed by anticholinesterases.
- The relaxed muscle remains responsive to mechanical and electrical stimuli.
- In partial paralysis there is depression of muscle twitch, 'fade' and post-tetanic facilitation, followed by exhaustion (Fig. 2.5.3).
- The effects are reduced by suxamethonium (but not in myasthenic individuals).
- They are potentiated by volatile agents, acidosis, magnesium and hypo-kalaemia.
- Mild cooling antagonizes their effects, but further cooling below about 33°C potentiates them.

Pharmacokinetics

The concentration of drug at the receptor (biophase) is in equilibrium with the plasma concentration, which in turn depends on the dose administered and its individual pharmacokinetic behaviour. A relationship therefore exists

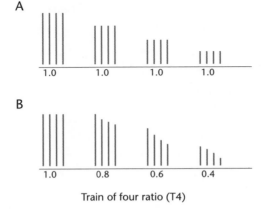

Train of four ratio (T4)

FIGURE 2.5.3 Representation of train of four (TOF) responses to a depolarizing (A) and a non-depolarizing (B) relaxant. Note that there is no fade with the depolarizing relaxant and progressive fade with the nondepolarizing relaxant as blockade develops.

between plasma concentration and the degree of paralysis, and the time course of action of nondepolarizing muscle relaxants is a reflection of the plasma concentration–elimination curve. Pharmacokinetic variables can be calculated from this curve (Table 2.5.1).

As a result of the positively charged quaternary ammonium groups all muscle relaxants are highly water soluble, relatively insoluble in fat and confined to the extracellular fluid. They are poorly absorbed from the gut and their onset is delayed when administered intramuscularly.

Protein binding of muscle relaxants varies between 30% and 85% and is influenced by changes in protein concentration in disease and protein binding of other drugs. This influences the volume of distribution, metabolism and excretion of the relaxants.

For most muscle relaxants a two-compartment model is suitable and thus two half-lives can be determined: the distribution half-life ($t_{1/2}\alpha$) and the elimination half-life ($t_{1/2}\beta$). The volume of distribution is limited owing to high water solubility.

Volume of distribution and clearance can be markedly affected by hepatic and renal disease, and cardiovascular disturbances.

Reduction in cardiac output usually leads to slower and lesser distribution, with lengthening of $t_{1/2}\alpha$, slower onset of action and eventually a stronger effect.

In hypovolaemia, the volume of distribution is smaller and peak concentration higher, with a stronger clinical drug effect.

TABLE 2.5.1 Pharmacokinetic Data of Muscle Relaxants

Drug	Vd$_{ss}$ (L/kg)	Clearance (mL/kg/min)	Excretion	
			Urinary (%)	*Biliary (%)*
Atracurium	0.09	6.6	10	–
Cis-atracurium	0.15	4.5–5.7	15	–
Doxacurium	0.22	2.7	25–30	–
Mivacurium	0.2–0.27	55	< 10	–
Gallamine	0.20	1.3	95	<1
Pancuronium	0.24	1.8	40	10
Pipecuronium	0.35	3.0	38	2
Rocuronium	0.21	2.9	9	54
D-Tubocurarine	0.30	2.3	45	–
Vecuronium	0.20	5.3	15	40

In patients with oedema, the volume of distribution increases and plasma concentrations are lower, with a weaker clinical effect.

Renal Function

Many relaxants are strongly dependent on renal excretion for their elimination. Only suxamethonium, mivacurium, atracurium and cis-atracurium are independent of renal function.

Plasma cholinesterase activity is frequently decreased in renal failure, prolonging the effects of suxamethonium and mivacurium.

Changes in renal function have a significant impact on clearance and elimination, but minimal effect on volume of distribution and $t_{1/2}\alpha$.

Liver Function

In comparison with renal function, liver function is a modest determinant of the pharmacokinetics of muscle relaxants:

- Decreased liver perfusion (e.g. in shock) – lower clearance and prolongation of paralysis.
- Increased extraction ratio (e.g. enzyme induction) – increased metabolism and a shorter effect for some muscle relaxants.
- Decreased protein binding (e.g. in hypoproteinaemia) – can increase liver extraction and shorten the duration of action.
- Cirrhosis – may increase the volume of distribution causing an apparent resistance to many nondepolarizing muscle relaxants.
- Plasma cholinesterase levels – may be depressed in hepatic failure, prolonging the effects of suxamethonium and mivacurium.

Age

Neonates and infants have a decreased plasma clearance, prolonged elimination and prolonged paralysis. In addition, the initial volume of distribution is increased, leading to a relative resistance to relaxants.

The elderly usually have a decrease in total body water, lean body mass and protein binding, resulting in an altered volume of distribution and plasma clearance of most relaxants. Increased sensitivity and prolonged effects are seen. A decrease in renal function and renal blood flow contributes to a decreased clearance with a more prolonged effect of muscle relaxants.

Pharmacodynamics

Muscle relaxants have neither anaesthetic nor analgesic properties. Therapeutic doses produce the following effects in sequence: ptosis, imbalance of extraocular muscles with diplopia (which rarely may last several days), relaxation of muscles of the face, jaw, neck and limbs, and finally relaxation of the abdominal wall and diaphragm.

Respiration

Paralysis of respiratory muscles causes apnoea. The diaphragm is less sensitive than other muscles and is usually the last to be paralysed.

Cardiovascular Effects

Cardiovascular effects include hypotension (D-tubocurarine), hypertension (pancuronium), tachycardia (gallamine, rocuronium and pancuronium), and skin flushing with hypotension (atracurium; Table 2.5.2).

Histamine Release

D-Tubocurarine is the most likely to cause histamine release and vecuronium is the least likely. True allergy with antibody formation is rare, but more frequent in females and atopic individuals. Often there is no obvious history of previous exposure.

Hypersensitivity Reactions

Robust data on muscle relaxant-related anaphylaxis is lacking. Geographical variation may reflect the different prevalence of Ig_e sensitizing agents consumed in different countries.

TABLE 2.5.2 Cardiovascular Side-effects of Muscle Relaxants

Drug	Histamine release[a]	Ganglionic effects	Vagolytic activity	Sympathetic stimulation
Suxamethonium	+	Stimulation	[b]	0
Atracurium	+	0	0	0
Cis-atracurium	0	0	0	0
Doxacurium	0	0	0	0
Gallamine	0	0	++	+
Mivacurium	+	0	0	0
Pancuronium	0	0	+	+
Pipecuronium	0	0	0	0
Rocuronium	0	0	±	0
D-Tubocurarine	++	Blockade	0	0
Vecuronium	0	0	0	0

[a]Histamine release is dose dependent and less pronounced if drugs are given slowly over 75 s.
[b]Suxamethonium may cause bradycardia by muscarinic stimulation at the sinoatrial node.

The incidences of anaphylaxis associated with nondepolarizing relaxants are as follows:

- Rocuronium – 8 in 100,000 doses
- Atracurium – 4 in 100,000 doses
- Vecuronium – 2.8 in 100,000 doses

Suxamethonium-related reactions are more complicated to quantify but it appears to cause anaphylaxis at least as frequently as rocuronium when measured per new patient exposure.

Registry data suggest that rocuronium accounts for 56% of anaphylaxis related to muscle relaxants, suxamethonium 21% and vecuronium 11%. Pancuronium and cis-atracurium appear less allergenic.

Cis-atracurium has the lowest cross-reactivity for those patients testing positive to rocuronium and vecuronium.

CLINICAL USE

Following induction of anaesthesia and intravenous administration of the muscle relaxant, tracheal intubation is possible after 1–3 min when the relaxant has taken its full effect.

The following suggest the need for more relaxant:

- Hiccough due to contraction of the periphery of the diaphragm, abdominal wall tightening, coughing on the tracheal tube or decreased compliance of the chest wall
- Irregular capnograph pattern
- Neuromuscular monitoring

These should be distinguished from signs of light anaesthesia or inadequate analgesia, such as muscle movement in the limbs, head or neck in response to surgical stimulation, or sympathetic activity (i.e. sweating, raised blood pressure and pulse).

Choice of Nondepolarizing Muscle Relaxant

The ideal muscle relaxant would have the following characteristics:

- Nondepolarizing – most side-effects of suxamethonium related to its depolarizing characteristics
- Rapid onset of action – enables intubation within 45 s of administration, necessary for a rapid sequence induction technique
- Predictable duration of action – no accumulation, same elimination rate regardless of dose given and antagonism by a suitable drug
- No histamine release – this has been a problem associated with the benzyl-isoquinolinium drugs particularly D-tubocurarine and atracurium

- No vagolytic or ganglion blocking action – avoids cardiovascular side-effects
- Potency – increased potency may give fewer side-effects, but lower potency seems necessary for a rapid onset of action
- Properties unaltered by renal or hepatic dysfunction – metabolites should have no pharmacological action

The duration of surgery will influence the choice of muscle relaxant:

- Ultra-short duration – suxamethonium
- Short duration – mivacurium
- Intermediate duration – atracurium, vecuronium, rocuronium, cis-atracurium
- Long duration – pancuronium, D-tubocurarine, doxacurium, pipecuronium

The following relaxants are suggested for:

- Rapid sequence intubation – suxamethonium, or if this is contraindicated, rocuronium
- Haemodynamic stability – vecuronium
- Renal or hepatic failure – atracurium, cis-atracurium or mivacurium
- Myasthenia gravis (if relaxants are essential) – atracurium, initially at one-tenth of the normal dose and then titrate against response from neuromuscular monitor

PHARMACOLOGY OF SPECIFIC NEUROMUSCULAR BLOCKING DRUGS

Suxamethonium is the archetypical depolarizing neuromuscular blocking drug although decamethonium is available in some countries. Nondepolarizing blocking drugs can be subdivided into two chemical groups: benzylisoquinolinium compounds and aminosteroids (Table 2.5.3).

Depolarizing Neuromuscular Blocking Drugs

Suxamethonium Chloride

Suxamethonium chloride is the dicholine ester of acetylcholine. It is presented as a clear colourless aqueous solution of pH 3.0–5.0 with a shelf-life of 2 years, and stored at 4°C. Spontaneous hydrolysis occurs in warm or alkaline conditions.

Dose

The dose of suxamethonium is 1 mg/kg as an intravenous bolus. It is effective within 30 s and lasts for several minutes, with complete recovery in 10–12 min. Its dose is increased to 2 mg/kg in paediatrics as a result of greater volume of distribution.

Suxamethonium is rapidly acting by virtue of rapid redistribution to the neuromuscular junction and its depolarizing mode of action. Its effect is terminated by diffusion away from the neuromuscular junction followed by rapid

TABLE 2.5.3 Pharmacodynamic Data of Muscle Relaxants

Drug	ED$_{95}$ (mg/kg)[a]	Intubating Dose (mg/kg)	Onsetv Time (s)[b]	Clinical Duration (min)[c]
Suxamethonium	0.3	1.0	60	10
Atracurium	0.23	0.5	110	43
Cis-atracurium	0.05	0.15	150	45
Doxacurium	0.025	0.05	250	83
Gallamine	3.0	3.5	240	80
Mivacurium	0.08	0.2	170	16
Pancuronium	0.07	0.1	220	75
Pipecuronium	0.045	0.08	300	95
Rocuronium	0.3	0.6	75	33
D-Tubocurarine	0.5	0.5	220	80
Vecuronium	0.05	0.1	180	33

[a]ED$_{95}$ is the mean dose that depresses twitch height by 95%.
[b]Onset time is the time to 95% depression of twitch height following an intubating dose.
[c]Clinical duration is time to 25% recovery of twitch height.

redistribution and hydrolysis. Elimination is by hydrolysis by plasma cholinesterase and its elimination half-life is 3.5 min.

Mechanism of Action

Suxamethonium acts by stimulation of the acetylcholine receptor and depolarization. Persistence of the agonist at the receptor prevents repolarization of the endplate, which is therefore refractory to further stimulation. As the suxamethonium diffuses away from the junctional cleft repolarization occurs and muscle action potentials are once more possible. The block may be enhanced by anticholinesterases.

Clinical Features

Suxamethonium has a rapid onset, where muscle fasciculation as groups of muscle fibres are depolarized. Neuromuscular monitoring shows reduced single twitch height, reduced TOF, all of equal amplitude, no tetanic fade and no post-tetanic facilitation.

Blood pressure increases, and bradycardia occurs, especially in children or after a second dose, when prior administration of atropine is advised. There may be a small increase in intracranial pressure, although rapid control of the airway and PCO_2 is of greater importance for brain protection. There is an increase in intraocular pressure. Although gastric pressure is increased, barrier pressure (upper and lower oesophageal sphincter pressure) is maintained, so there is no increased tendency for regurgitation.

Abnormalities of Suxamethonium Metabolism

Plasma cholinesterase seems to have no known physiological purpose. Its half-life is about 7–10 days. Abnormal inherited genetic variants of plasma cholinesterase were first identified by the extent to which the enzyme is inhibited by dibucaine, the percentage inhibition using benzylcholine as substrate being called the dibucaine number. The normal value is 75%–85%; heterozygotes for the atypical gene have numbers of about 50% and homozygotes about 30%. Different abnormal genetic variants have also been identified using inhibition by sodium fluoride. Other rarer variants have been identified, such as the 'silent' gene.

The atypical genes are autosomal, 1 in 3000 of the population is homozygous, when hydrolysis proceeds at only 5% per hour and there is 1–2 h of apnoea after suxamethonium, during which phase 2 block may develop. In the commoner heterozygote (about 1 in 25 of the population), apnoea lasts only 10–20 min.

Cholinesterase deficiency may also be acquired, as in liver disease, malnutrition, carcinomatosis (reduced production), pregnancy, uraemia, connective tissue disorders or hypothyroidism. The enzyme is antagonized by anticholinesterases such as neostigmine.

Mivacurium and ester local anaesthetics such as cocaine are also metabolized by plasma cholinesterase. Their actions are prolonged if this enzyme is deficient whereas esmolol and remifentanil are unaffected because they are metabolized by other esterases.

Adverse Effects

Hyperkalaemia: The serum potassium may rise transiently by up to 0.5 mmol/L with suxamethonium, even in the normal patient. This is exaggerated after burns, tetanus and spinal cord injuries, and also in patients with many other neurological and muscular disorders, such as stroke, cerebral palsy and muscular dystrophy. This is due to the proliferation of extrajunctional receptors, which cause a massive outpouring of potassium when stimulated by suxamethonium. It is probably safe to use suxamethonium within 24–48 h of an acute lesion such as burns or spinal cord injury, but the safe period after injury has not been accurately determined.

Intraocular pressure: Intraocular pressure increases by 7–8 mm Hg with suxamethonium, with a maximal effect 2 min after administration, and is due to tonic contraction of the extraocular muscles. Suxamethonium may still be used in a perforating eye injury if essential (see Chapter 5.9).

Muscle pains: Muscle pains with suxamethonium are more frequent in women, young to middle-aged adults and those who are ambulant shortly after surgery. They may be prevented by a small dose of a nondepolarizing agent 3 min before the suxamethonium, although a larger dose of the latter is then likely to be needed.

Malignant Hyperpyrexia

Suxamethonium is one of the drugs most commonly implicated in the development of malignant hyperpyrexia, which has an incidence of 1 in 100,000 general anaesthetics.

Allergy

Suxamethonium causes the highest incidence of anaphylaxis per new patient exposure of any muscle relaxant, but much more frequently causes histamine release from mast cells and circulating basophils, resulting in flushing or urticaria.

Dystrophia

Suxamethonium should not be given in dystrophia myotonica because it causes severe muscle rigidity, preventing respiration and intubation.

Nondepolarizing Neuromuscular Blocking Drugs: Benzylisoquinolinium Compounds

Atracurium Besylate

Atracurium is presented as a 10% solution with pH 3.5, stored at 4°C.

Atracurium is metabolized by Hofmann degradation and alkaline ester hydrolysis in the plasma and elsewhere in the body. Hofmann degradation is the spontaneous fragmentation of atracurium at the bond between the quaternary nitrogen and the central chain, which occurs at body temperature and pH, producing the tertiary metabolite laudanosine and a quaternary monoacrylate. Laudanosine has slow renal elimination and crosses the blood–brain barrier.

Atracurium is also metabolized by ester hydrolysis, producing a quaternary alcohol and quaternary acid.

Dose

The dose of atracurium besylate is 0.5 mg/kg. The speed of onset is 1–2 min, and duration of action is dose dependent, 20–40 min, even in anephric patients. The elimination half-life is 20 min.

Clinical Features

Atracurium is distributed throughout the extracellular fluid with no effective crossing of the placenta. It is a suitable drug for patients with impaired renal or hepatic function.

The effect of atracurium is prolonged in hypothermia.

Adverse Effects

Histamine release is observed in up to 40% of patients with doses over 0.5 mg/kg, giving transient hypotension and tachycardia associated with facial and truncal flushing. This effect can be prevented by injecting the drug slowly over 75 s, reducing the dose, or prior treatment with 0.1 mg/kg chlorpheniramine and 2 mg/kg cimetidine intravenously.

Laudanosine can cause convulsions but this has not been of significance in clinical practice.

Cis-atracurium Besylate

Cis-atracurium is the purified form of one of the 10 isomers of atracurium. It is stored at 4°C and is approximately three times more potent than atracurium.

Dose

The dose is 0.15 mg/kg, and the duration of action is about 30 min.

Clinical Features

The features of cis-atracurium are similar to those of atracurium, except that it does not release histamine within the clinical dose range. It is slightly slower in onset, consistent with the inverse relationship between potency and the speed of onset observed in nondepolarizing relaxants.

Cis-atracurium is haemodynamically stable, noncumulative and a suitable agent as an infusion in intensive care. It undergoes Hofmann degradation but not hydrolysis by plasma esterases.

Adverse Effects

Laudanosine levels are much lower than with atracurium.

Mivacurium Chloride

The structure of mivacurium resembles that of both atracurium and doxacurium, but in common with doxacurium the ether oxygen and the carboxyl group are reversed and so do not permit Hofmann degradation.

Mivacurium exhibits stereoisomerism, is a geometric isomer and is presented as a racemic mixture of *trans–trans* (58%), *cis–trans* (36%) and *cis–cis* (6%). Although the *trans–trans* and *cis–trans* isomers are hydrolysed by plasma cholinesterase, the *cis–cis* isomer may be metabolized in part by the liver.

Block is prolonged by atypical or reduced plasma cholinesterase, as with suxamethonium. Heterozygotes for the atypical enzyme show a prolongation of block by about 10 min.

Dose

The dose is up to 0.25 mg/kg. Mivacurium is ideal for use by continuous intravenous infusion at 0.24–0.48 mg/kg/h. The duration of action is 10–20 min (about twice that of suxamethonium and one-half to one-third that of atracurium or vecuronium).

Clinical Features

Mivacurium is a short-acting muscle relaxant metabolized by plasma cholinesterase.

Adverse Effects

Transient decreases in arterial pressure as a result of histamine release may be observed following doses greater than 0.15–0.2 mg/kg.

Doxacurium Chloride

Doxacurium chloride is the most potent neuromuscular blocking drug currently available. It has a slow onset and very long duration of action. Although it has diester groupings, it does not undergo significant hydrolysis by plasma cholinesterase and is largely eliminated by the kidney with some hepatic excretion unchanged in the bile.

Dose

The dose of doxacurium chloride is 0.03–0.05 mg/kg, and its duration of action is over 1 h.

Clinical Features

The cumulative potential is difficult to ascertain because repeat dosing is rarely needed. Antagonism by anticholinesterase is satisfactory provided considerable spontaneous recovery has already taken place.

Adverse Effects

Unlike other benzylisoquinolinium analogues doxacurium has no significant cardiovascular effects or histamine-releasing propensity within the clinical dose range.

D-Tubocurarine Chloride

Dose

The dose is 0.3–0.5 mg/kg and its duration of action is over 40 min. It shows cumulation.

Adverse Effects

D-Tubocurarine chloride may cause histamine release and blockade of sympathetic ganglia, resulting in significant hypotension. It was formerly used to assist controlled hypotension.

Nondepolarizing Blocking Drugs: Aminosteroids

The aminosteroids have a bulky steroidal nucleus which, when bound to the nicotinic receptor at the endplate, competitively impedes the interaction of acetylcholine with the α-subunits.

Vecuronium Bromide

Ring D of the steroidal nucleus has a quaternary ammonium similar to that of pancuronium and is probably the area that interacts with the endplate nicotinic receptor. Ring A has been modified by a tertiary nitrogen, giving greater vascular stability and less stability in solution, and encouraging elimination in the bile as well as in the urine. The duration of action of vecuronium is therefore shorter than that of pancuronium.

Vecuronium is eliminated by spontaneous deacetylation and hepatic metabolism. Of the total dose, 10%–25% is excreted in urine and the rest in bile. Most is excreted unchanged. Hepatic failure may prolong the clinical effect. Phenytoin and other anticonvulsant therapies reduce the efficacy of vecuronium by enzyme induction. There are three potential active metabolites, 3–OH, 17–OH and 3,17–OH. The 3–OH metabolite is the only one found in any significant quantity and it has 50% of the neuromuscular blocking potency of vecuronium. This may cause prolonged block if used by infusion in intensive care.

Dose

The dose of vecuronium is 0.1 mg/kg and its onset of action is 1–2 min, but this can be shortened by priming with one-tenth of the intubating dose 6 min before the main dose.

Clinical Features

Vecuronium has the best haemodynamic stability of all muscle relaxants.

Adverse Effects

There is minimal vagolytic activity.

Rocuronium Bromide

Rocuronium bromide is a monoquaternary aminosteroid. It is a rapid-onset deacetoxy analogue of vecuronium and is slightly vagolytic, resulting in a tachycardia at higher doses (more than 0.9 mg/kg). It is presented as a clear colourless to pale brown solution with pH 3.8–4.2, stored at 4°C and protected from light. It can cause pain on injection. Rocuronium exhibits predominantly biliary excretion with 10% excreted in urine. Clearance is decreased in renal failure and the elimination half-life is significantly increased in hepatic disease. The main metabolite, 17–deacetyl rocuronium, has weak neuromuscular blocking action.

Dose

For routine use the dose of rocuronium is 0.6 mg/kg allowing intubating conditions in 60–90 s. Although the time to 80% block (for intubation) is more rapid than with other nondepolarizing relaxants, the overall time to 100% block is similar to that for vecuronium. Even at high doses, the onset of block is still slower than for suxamethonium. In rapid sequence induction the dose is increased to 1.2 mg/kg. Ongoing paralysis can be provided with an infusion of 0.3–0.4 mg/kg/h under inhalational anaesthesia and 0.3–0.6 mg/kg/h under intravenous anaesthesia. This is titrated to a TOF count of 1–2.

In obesity, the dose is calculated using lean body mass.

Pancuronium Bromide

Pancuronium bromide is a long-acting bisquaternary aminosteroid, devoid of hormonal activity. The additional quaternary ammonium group on ring A of the steroidal nucleus enhances vagolytic activity by blocking cardiac muscarinic M_2 receptors and neuronal norepinephrine (noradrenaline) reuptake. It can also cause norepinephrine release.

Pancuronium becomes strongly bound to gamma globulin and moderately bound to albumin. Less than 13% of the dose is unbound and active; 50% is excreted unchanged, of which 80% appears in the urine, 40% is deacetylated in the liver to 3–OH, 17–OH and 3,17–OH derivatives, which are eliminated in the bile. The 3–OH metabolite has some neuromuscular antagonist activity.

Dose

The dose of pancuronium is 0.05–0.15 mg/kg, and the initial dose lasts 45–60 min.

Adverse Effects

There is no histamine release. It tends to cause tachycardia and hypertension and complements induction with high dose opioids. It is safe in patients susceptible to malignant hyperpyrexia.

Pipecuronium Bromide

Pipecuronium bromide is a quaternary aminosteroid. It is 25% more potent than pancuronium, but clinically and pharmacodynamically very similar, but without pancuronium's vagolytic side-effects. As 85% is excreted by the kidneys it has a prolonged effect in renal failure, 4% is metabolized by the liver to 3-desacetyl pipecuronium and only 2% is excreted in the bile. Cumulation may occur, particularly with impaired renal function.

Dose

The dose of pipecuronium is 0.05 mg/kg.

Clinical Features

It has a slow onset, over 3 min, and a long duration of 1–2 h.

Adverse Effects

Like other aminosteroids used clinically, it does not produce histamine.

PHARMACOLOGY OF SPECIFIC ANTAGONISTS

Anticholinesterase Drugs

Acetylcholinesterase has an esteratic site and an anionic site in close proximity. Physiologically, the positively charged quaternary amine of acetylcholine binds to the anionic site, the acetyl ester combines with the esteratic site and the acetylcholine is hydrolysed. Anticholinesterases competitively occupy these sites and prevent acetylcholine access.

Anticholinesterases have a quaternary amine group that is attracted to the anionic site and a carbamyl ester that binds covalently to the serine amino acid of the esteratic site. The quaternary amine group conveys enhanced potency and stability and results in poor absorption following oral administration with minimal transfer of the drug across the blood–brain barrier. When neostigmine is used for the treatment of myasthenia gravis large oral doses are therefore necessary. Anticholinesterases also have some direct cholinergic agonist activity.

Anticholinesterases have widespread effects subsequent to the increased cholinergic, muscarinic and nicotinic activity. Heart rate, vasomotor tone and blood pressure are reduced. At high doses sympathetic ganglion stimulation may predominate.

Excess acetylcholine causes bronchoconstriction, increased bronchial secretion, increased gastrointestinal tone with severe colic and increased secretion of saliva, sweat and tears. These problems are prevented by the concomitant use of muscarinic anticholinergic drugs such as atropine or glycopyrronium.

Anticholinesterases can also cause a depolarizing neuromuscular blockade when used in excess or in the absence of nondepolarizing blockade.

Neuromuscular blockade terminates either by endogenous elimination of the muscle relaxant drug and diffusion of the blocking agent away from the neuromuscular junction, or in the case of the nondepolarizing agents the effects can be overcome in part by inhibiting the metabolism of acetylcholine.

In administering anticholinesterase drugs, the clearance of relaxants is not accelerated but the dose–response curve for neuromuscular blockade shifts to the right. The pharmacodynamic recovery is therefore accelerated. This process of reversal is superimposed upon the mechanisms responsible for relaxant clearance.

Neostigmine

Neostigmine binds to the esteratic subsite of acetylcholinesterase with its carbonate group. It is the only anticholinesterase routinely used to reverse neuromuscular blockade in anaesthesia. It can cause a depolarizing block in its own right owing to build-up of acetylcholine. Phase 2 block can eventually result. The amount of neostigmine needed to cause paralysis by persistent depolarization is much greater than that required to antagonize a clinical dose of nondepolarizing relaxant.

Dose

The dose of neostigmine is 2.5 mg to a maximum of 5 mg, with atropine 1 mg or glycopyrronium 0.5 mg. Its duration of action is 40 min.

Neostigmine is eliminated via hydrolysis by the acetylcholinesterase that it antagonizes, and by plasma cholinesterase to a quaternary alcohol. Renal excretion accounts for 50% of its clearance. Some hepatic metabolism occurs with biliary excretion.

Edrophonium

Edrophonium forms an ionic bond to the anionic subsite of acetylcholinesterase. It is quicker in onset; however, small doses are rapidly metabolized and are not as long-lasting. It is used for the assessment of myasthenia gravis, to distinguish between a myasthenic or a cholinergic crisis.

Dose

The dose of edrophonium is 1 mg/kg, repeated if necessary, with atropine or glycopyrronium.

Pyridostigmine

Pyridostigmine is used in the treatment of myasthenia gravis in total daily doses up to 720 mg (sometimes more). Its duration of action is 6 h.

Physostigmine

Physostigmine is an anticholinesterase derived from the West African calabar bean and has a tertiary amine structure that can cross the blood–brain barrier. It does not adequately antagonize neuromuscular block but may be used in the treatment of anticholinergic syndrome produced by atropine, hyoscine and other related alkaloids.

Selective Muscle Relaxant Encapsulating Agents

Sugammadex

Sugammadex is a synthetic γ-cyclodextrin. It is presented as a clear and colourless to slightly yellow solution for injection with pH 7–8 and concentration of 100 mg/mL. It is licensed for the reversal of muscle relaxation from rocuronium and vecuronium for patients aged 2 years and upwards.

Mechanism of Action

Cyclodextrins are ring-shaped oligosaccharides composed of α–D–glucopyranoside units attached in a circular fashion via α-1–4 linkages. Sugammadex is a γ–cyclodextrin with polar hydroxyl moieties attached to each α–D–glucopyranoside unit. These hydroxyl groups form its rim. The periphery of the molecule is hydrophobic ensuring solubility while the centre, or toroid, is lipophilic and allows the encapsulation of aminosteroids in a 1:1 ratio. Rocuronium bromide is sequestered most avidly, but there is also affinity for vecuronium and, to a lesser extent, pancuronium. It has no effect on nonaminosteroid molecules. Binding of the muscle relaxant prevents it antagonizing the acetylcholine receptor and it encourages its diffusion down a concentration gradient, away from the nicotinic acetylcholine receptor. Sugammadex possesses no cholinergic side effects.

Dose

Routine reversal: If two twitches of the TOF have returned after rocuronium or vecuronium administration a dose of 2 mg/kg is used, returning the T_4/T_1 ratio to 0.9 in a median time of 2 min. In deeper levels of muscle relaxation where post-tetanic count has reached 1–2 a dose of 4 mg/kg returns a T_4/T_1 ratio of 0.9 in 3 min.

Immediate reversal: For immediate reversal of neuromuscular blockade after rapid sequence induction with 1.2 mg/kg of rocuronium a dose of 16 mg/kg is recommended and returns the T_4/T_1 ratio to 0.9 in a median time of 1.5 min.

Use in Special Situations

- In exceptional circumstances postoperative residual curarization can occur and a repeat dose of 4 mg/kg is recommended.
- In the obese patient actual body weight should be used when calculating doses.
- Use of sugammadex is not recommended in renal failure with creatinine clearance < 30 mL/min or in dialysis-dependent patients.

Although sugammadex can be used routinely for reversal of rocuronium in children over 2 years, in a dose of 2 mg/kg, currently it is not recommended for immediate reversal of a rapid sequence intubation dose of rocuronium. It is not recommended for routine use in neonates and infants.

Readministration

If the original dose of rocuronium was 1.2 mg/kg, sugammadex may be re-administered after waiting a minimum of 5 min. If the original dose of rocuronium was 0.6 mg/kg (or vecuronium 0.1 mg/kg), sugammadex may be readministered after waiting a minimum of 4 min.

Other Encapsulating Agents

The cucurbit[n]uril (CB[n]) family of molecular containers have a similar action to the cyclodextrins, in that they form host-guest complexes with a specific target drug and thus modify the characteristics of drug bound within the interior of the complex.

An acyclic glycoluril tetramer CB[n] based molecular container, is undergoing evaluation as a reversal agent. Unlike sugammadex, it binds to both aminosteroidal and benzylisoquinolinium neuromuscular blocking agents.

NEUROMUSCULAR MONITORING

Monitoring of neuromuscular function involves pulsed electrical stimulation of a peripheral motor nerve and assessment of the muscular response.

Stimulus

Needle or surface electrodes are located over or close to a peripheral motor nerve. The stimulator pulse should be a square wave with an appropriate amplitude (i.e. low amplitude [0.5–5.0 mA] for needle electrodes and higher amplitude for skin electrodes [10–40 mA]).

The optimal duration of the pulse is 0.2 ms for various patterns of pulses including single, trains of pulses at 1–2 Hz and tetanic bursts at 50–100 Hz. This provides supramaximal stimulation that ensures maximum recruitment of muscle fibres and provides a baseline control twitch for comparison with that obtained when using muscle relaxants.

Single Twitch

A single twitch results from application of a single supramaximal stimulus every 10 s. The twitch height falls steadily to zero as the nicotinic postsynaptic receptor occupancy increases from 75% or 80% to 100%. It has limited application owing to the narrow range of receptor occupancy detected (75%–95%) and the requirement for a means of measuring twitch height.

Train of Four

TOF stimulation is the application of four successive stimuli, each of which is similar to the single twitch, administered at 2 Hz every 10 s. The degree of neuromuscular blockade can be more objectively assessed by calculating the ratio of the fourth (T_4) and the first (T_1) measured twitch heights (T_4/T_1). When the T_4/T_1 ratio is > 0.9 muscle relaxation is considered reversed.

Tetanic Stimulation

Tetanic stimulation results from application of an electrical current identical to the single twitch, but repeated at a higher frequency, usually 50 Hz, applied for 5 s. The frequency of 50 Hz is similar to the stimulation of a voluntary maximal muscle movement. The test is painful and should only be performed under anaesthesia.

Tetanic stimulation causes mobilization of acetylcholine from the reserve pools to the readily available store. The depletion of acetylcholine changes the intensity of the basic response and therefore it is necessary to wait 15–20 min before the next tetanic stimulus can be given.

Post-tetanic Count

Post-tetanic count (PTC) describes the counting of responses to single twitch stimulation following a tetanic stimulation of 50 Hz for 5 s. This method can produce a response at relatively high levels of receptor occupancy, and a PTC less than 5 indicates profound neuromuscular blockade. A PTC greater than 15 is at least equivalent to two twitches of a TOF, and at this level reversal of remaining muscle blockade is possible.

Double Burst Stimulation

Double burst stimulation was introduced to improve manual assessment of fade. This consists of two tetanic bursts at 50 Hz. Each burst is separated by 750 ms. The user sees two contractions (T_1 and T_2). The ratio of T_2 to T_1 is more sensitive in detecting fade than the TOF ratio.

Sensitivities of the Different Modes of Stimulation

The different modes of stimulation have different sensitivities. The amplitude of a single twitch does not start to diminish until about 80% of receptors are occupied by muscle relaxants. For normal neuromuscular transmission, only 20% of receptors of the motor endplate are required. Neuromuscular blockade is not complete until 90%–95% of receptors are occupied. This percentage varies from muscle to muscle. Paralysis of the diaphragm does not become apparent until 90%–95% of the receptors are blocked. Tetanic stimulation is the most sensitive test. The response to stimulation at 50 Hz starts to diminish when 65% of receptors are occupied.

Assessment of Muscular Response

A variety of methods providing an indirect measure of contractile force have been employed during neuromuscular stimulation.

Vision and Touch

Vision and touch provide a simple and convenient method but are less accurate than other methods and provide only a gross assessment of muscle response.

Mechanomyography

With mechanomyography the muscle contracts against a preload, generating a tension that is proportional to the force of contraction. This is converted to an electrical signal for measurement. Mechanomyography is more accurate than vision and touch but does require correct positioning of the transducer, selection of the preload and immobilization of the hand.

Acceleromyography

In acceleromyography, a piezo-electrode wafer is fixed to the distal part of the digit. Acceleration is converted into an electrical signal for measurement. This technique is more objective than vision and touch, but problems exist with joint positioning creating inconsistencies.

Electromyography

Electromyography measures muscle activity by recording the magnitude of the evoked compound potentials from either skin or needle electrodes overlying a particular muscle. This technique avoids the mechanical problems of using and calibrating transducers attached to joints, but simple alteration in hand position can alter electrode geometry enough to change the measured response.

Interpretation

A normal response to different stimulation patterns demonstrates different percentages of unoccupied or free receptors (Table 2.5.4). Clinically, depression of at least 95% of a twitch is needed to obtain absence of glottic movements, and depression of at least 90% is desirable for surgery when opening and closing the abdominal wall. The respiratory vital capacity will be diminished at more than 25% paralysis, but it is possible to maintain a tidal volume until about 75% paralysis. The most sensitive clinical test to evaluate residual paralysis is the 5 s head lift test.

Full recovery of the diaphragm corresponds with 25% recovery of the adductor pollicis muscle. A much higher degree of receptor occupation is necessary in the respiratory muscles than in the peripheral muscles to obtain the same intensity of neuromuscular blockade. Monitoring ulnar nerve function is recommended over facial nerve where possible.

Standards of Monitoring

To minimize the incidence of postoperative residual curarization (PORC), routine neuromuscular monitoring must be used as even routine sugammadex use without monitoring is still associated with a 10% incidence of PORC.

TABLE 2.5.4 Different Stimulation Patterns Demonstrate the Following Percentage of Unoccupied or Free Receptors

Normal Response to Stimulation	Percentage of Free Receptors
Single twitch	>20–25
Train of four	>25–30
30 Hz tetanic	>30
50 Hz tetanic	>40
100 Hz tetanic	>50
200 Hz tetanic	>60

It has been suggested that neuromuscular monitoring should be mandatory for those patients receiving a muscle relaxant under anaesthesia. A recovery to $T_4/T_1 > 0.9$ is suggested as a minimum criterion of motor function and reflects adequate ventilation and the ability to protect the upper airway and hence reduce aspiration risk.

FURTHER READING

Srivastava A, Hunter JM. Reversal of neuromuscular block. Br J Anaesth 2009;103:115–29.

Sadleir PH, Clarke RC, Bunning DL, Platt PR. Anaphylaxis to neuromuscular blocking drugs: Incidence and cross-reactivity in Western Australia from 2002 to 2011. Br J Anaesth 2013;110: 981–87.

Chapter 2.6

Airway Management

Patrick Wong

The primary goal of airway management is to safely provide adequate oxygenation to patients. Techniques commonly used to achieve this include the use of a facemask, supraglottic airway device (SAD) and tracheal intubation.

ANATOMY OF THE LARYNX

The larynx extends from the root of the tongue to the trachea and lies opposite C3–C6 vertebrae, higher in children and females. It is covered by the depressor muscles of the hyoid bone, thyroid gland and the cricothyroid muscles and is composed of the following cartilages, joined together by ligaments – thyroid, cricoid, two arytenoids, two corniculate (Santorini), two cuneiform (Wrisberg) and the epiglottis.

The cavity of the larynx extends from the superior laryngeal aperture to the lower border of the cricoid cartilage. The piriform fossa is a recess on each side, bounded by the aryepiglottic fold medially and the thyroid cartilage and thyrohyoid membrane laterally. The depression between the dorsum of the tongue and the epiglottis is divided into two valleculae by the glossoepiglottic fold.

The superior laryngeal aperture is wider in front than behind, sloping downwards and backwards. It is bounded anteriorly by the epiglottis, laterally by the aryepiglottic folds with two small nodules on each side, the cuneiform anteriorly and the corniculate posteriorly, and posteriorly by the arytenoids. This view (Fig. 2.6.1) is seen at laryngoscopy.

The vestibule of the larynx is the superior part of the cavity of the larynx and extends from the aryepiglottic folds to the vestibular (ventricular) folds. Each of the latter is a ridge formed by the vestibular ligament and extends from the angle of the thyroid cartilage anteriorly, backwards along the side cavity of the larynx to the cuneiform cartilage. The vestibular folds are the false cords and the space between them is the rima vestibuli, while a depression on the sidewall of the larynx between the vestibular fold and the vocal folds (false and true cords) is the saccule of the larynx.

The vocal folds (cords) stretch from the thyroid cartilage anteriorly to the arytenoid cartilage of the corresponding side posteriorly. The space between the

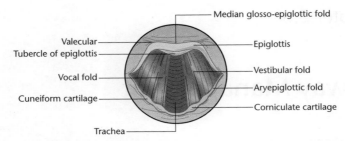

Median glosso-epiglottic fold
Valecular
Tubercle of epiglottis
Vocal fold
Cuneiform cartilage
Trachea
Epiglottis
Vestibular fold
Aryepiglottic fold
Corniculate cartilage

FIGURE 2.6.1   A laryngoscopic view of the interior of the larynx.

cords is the glottis, bounded anteriorly by the intermembranous part of the cords and posteriorly by the intercartilaginous part.

In adults the narrowest part of the larynx is the glottis, measuring about 2.3 cm from front to back in males, and 1.7 cm in females. In children it was thought that the narrowest part was at the cricoid ring. More recently, measurements using bronchoscopic images and magnetic resonance imaging have consistently found children to have glottic openings smaller than at the cricoid. The shape and width of the glottis vary with phonation and respiration and the tone of the muscles controlling it. When these are in spasm, the glottis is obliterated.

Extrinsic Muscles

The extrinsic muscles comprise the suprahyoid group attached to the hyoid (thyrohyoid, mylohyoid, stylohyoid, geniohyoid), the infrahyoid or strap muscles (sternothyroid, omohyoid, sternohyoid) and the inferior constrictor of the pharynx.

Intrinsic Muscles

The vocal folds abduct during inspiration and return nearly to the midline on expiration, and on phonation they actually touch. Intrinsic muscles that open and close the glottis are as follows:

● Cricoarytenoids – the posterior (open) and lateral (close)
● Interarytenoid (close)

Intrinsic muscles that control the tension of the cords are as follows:

● The cricothyroids – tense the cords
● Posterior cricoarytenoids – abduct the cords
● Thyroarytenoids – relax the cords
● Vocales – relax the cords

Intrinsic muscles that control the inlet of the larynx are as follows:

● The aryepiglottics
● Thyroepiglottics – in laryngeal spasm, both the true and the false cords are adducted

Nerve Supply

The superior laryngeal branch of the vagus arises near the base of the skull and divides into the internal laryngeal nerve (sensory supply to both surfaces of the epiglottis and to the larynx down to the vocal cords) and the external laryngeal nerve (motor supply to the cricothyroid muscle and the inferior constrictor of the pharynx).

The external laryngeal nerve may be injured during ligation of the superior thyroid vessels at thyroidectomy, causing temporary huskiness of voice.

The recurrent laryngeal nerve branch of the vagus supplies the remaining intrinsic muscles and is sensory to the mucosa below the cords.

The recurrent laryngeal nerve carries abductor and adductor fibres but, if injured, abductor paralysis is greater than adductor paralysis. Bilateral injury results in respiratory difficulty because the cords lie together. Speech is also difficult, with valvular obstruction and inspiratory stridor. Complete paralysis of both recurrent nerves inactivates both abductor and adductor muscles, but the tensing action of cricothyroid maintains cords in adduction. Paralysis of one cord may be symptomless, but paralysis of both is serious and may require surgery.

Paralysis of both recurrent and superior laryngeal nerves together (or full muscle relaxation) produces the cadaveric position with the cords relaxed midway between abduction and adduction.

Topical analgesia of the larynx may, by paralysing branches of the external laryngeal nerves going to the cricothyroids, cause a temporary alteration in both the appearance of the cords and the voice.

All sensory nerve impulses from the larynx reach the nucleus solitarius in the medulla.

Arterial Supply

The larynx is supplied by laryngeal branches of the superior and inferior thyroid arteries, which accompany the nerves.

AIRWAY ASSESSMENT AND DEFINITIONS

Many definitions exist for the difficult airway and the techniques used for its management. Definitions from the American Society of Anesthesiologists (ASA) are given in Table 2.6.1.[1] Han's classification of difficulty in facemask ventilation (FMV) is given in Table 2.6.2.[2]

The laryngeal view obtained during laryngoscopy is commonly graded using the modified Cormack and Lehane classification (Table 2.6.3). Subdivision into Grades 2a, 2b, 3a and 3b are based on the anatomical structures seen on direct laryngoscopy. However, a Grade 1 or 2a view at laryngoscopy may not equate to easy intubation, which can still be difficult, e.g. awkward dentition. T.M. Cook reclassified the laryngeal view based on the practical techniques required

TABLE 2.6.1 Difficult Airway Definitions from the American Society of Anesthesiologists[1]

Clinical Scenario	Definition
Difficult airway	The clinical situation in which a conventionally trained anaesthetist experiences difficulty with facemask (or SAD) ventilation of the upper airway, difficulty with tracheal intubation, or both
Difficult face mask or SAD ventilation	It is not possible for the anaesthetist to provide adequate ventilation because of one or more of the following problems: inadequate mask or SAD seal, excessive gas leak or excessive resistance to the ingress or egress of gas
Difficult SAD placement	SAD placement requires multiple attempts, in the presence or absence of tracheal pathology
Difficult laryngoscopy	It is not possible to visualize any portion of the vocal cords after multiple attempts at conventional laryngoscopy
Difficult tracheal intubation	Tracheal intubation requires multiple attempts, in the presence or absence of tracheal pathology

TABLE 2.6.2 Han's Classification of Facemask Ventilation[2]

Classification (Grade)	Definition
0	Ventilation by mask not attempted
1	Ventilated by mask
2	Ventilated by mask with oral airway or other adjunct
3	Difficult mask ventilation (inadequate, unstable or requiring two practitioners)
4	Unable to mask ventilate

to achieve intubation: easy, restricted or difficult. The latter two may require the use of adjuncts such as the bougie or indirect laryngoscopy, respectively. The intubation difficulty scale (IDS) incorporates seven factors linked to difficult intubation: number of attempts, number of operators, number of alternative techniques used, glottic exposure, lifting force applied during laryngoscopy, necessity to apply external laryngeal pressure and position of vocal cords.[3] The resulting composite score is used to compare difficult intubation under varying circumstances.

TABLE 2.6.3 Various Classifications of Laryngeal View Obtained on Direct Laryngoscopy[4]

Cook's Modification of the Cormack and Lehane Classification		Cook's Classification	Anatomical Relevance (Laryngeal Inlet View)	Clinical Relevance for Tracheal Intubation
1	Most of the vocal cords visible	Easy	Visible	Usually easy under direct vision without need for adjuncts
2a	Posterior vocal cords visible			
2b	Only arytenoids visible	Restricted	Not visible	Requires use of a bougie
3a	Epiglottis visible and liftable			
3b	Epiglottis adherent to posterior pharyngeal wall	Difficult	Not visible	Requires advanced airway techniques (e.g. indirect laryngoscopy)
4	No laryngeal structures seen			

Prediction of the Difficult Airway

The incidences of the various types of difficult airways are given in Table 2.6.4. These patients are at increased risk of complications including dental damage, hypoxia, awareness and brain damage. It is important to predict who these patients are and manage them appropriately. This involves a full assessment based on history, examination and investigations. However, airway tests are not reliable and many difficult airways remain unanticipated.

Independent predictors for impossible FMV are neck radiation changes, male sex, sleep apnoea, Mallampati III or IV (see Chapter 1.1) and presence of beard.[5]

Predictors for Difficult Laryngoscopy and Intubation

General Predictors

- Weight (obese patients)
- Head and neck anatomical/mechanical abnormalities, e.g. rheumatoid arthritis, ankylosing spondylitis and acromegaly
- Previous head and neck surgery, trauma, infection and burns, and radiotherapy.
- Congenital disorders, e.g. Down's, Marfan's, Pierre-Robin, Treacher Collins and Goldenhar syndromes
- History of previous difficult airway

TABLE 2.6.4 Incidences of Difficult Airway

Clinical Scenario	Incidence	Aide Memoire ('rule of 5s')	Incidence of Unanticipated Cases
Difficult face mask ventilation	0.9%–5%	<5%	Up to 94%
Failed face mask ventilation	0.2%	<<0.5%	
Difficult laryngos-copy	1.0%–5.8%	<5%	50%–93%
Failed intubation	0.005%–0.43%	<<0.5%	
'Cannot intubate, cannot oxygenate'	1 in 5000 to 1 in 1,000,000	1 in 5000	

Specific Predictors

Specific predictors include symptoms such as shortness of breath, hoarse voice, stridor, 'hot potato' voice, postural symptoms (worsening of symptoms when lying down, or unable to lie down).

Specific 'Airway Tests'

Teeth:
- Top teeth – presence of an overbite
- Between the teeth – mouth opening (interdental distance) < 2.5–5.0 cm
- Behind the teeth – Mallampati Grade III or IV
- Lower teeth – underbite (micro-/retrognathism), jaw protrusion – unable to protrude lower incisors beyond upper incisors

Neck:
- Thyromental distance < 6.5 cm
- Long thyromental distances also associated with difficult intubation; a caudal larynx and a hypopharyngeal tongue ('anterior larynx')
- Sternomental distance <12.5 cm
- Neck movement – a difficult airway is indicated by Delikan sign – a patient is asked to look up to the ceiling and the level of the tip of the jaw cannot be raised higher than the level of the occipital tuberosity

The degree of mouth opening serves two functions, as a predictor of difficult laryngoscopy/intubation but also determines the ability to insert an oral airway or SAD. Mouth opening > 2 cm is required for comfortable insertion of an SAD.

Airway tests alone have poor to moderate predictive value; 50%–90% of difficult airways remain unpredictable (Table 2.6.5).

TABLE 2.6.5 Predictive Value of Airway Tests (%)

Airway Tests	Sensitivity	Specificity	PPV
Neck movement	10–21	92–98	6–30
Modified Mallampati score	35–81	66–91	8–9
Mouth opening (inter-dental distance)	26–47	93–95	7–25
Retrognathism	14	98	15
Jaw protrusion	17–26	95–96	5–21
Thyromental distance	21–62	25–92	6–16

Note: PPV, positive predictive value.

Multivariate models (combinations of airway tests and physiological parameters) have better accuracy than individual tests. They can be constructed using different weighting and cut-off values for each airway test to give an optimal sensitivity and specificity ratio. Multivariate logistic regression allows (otherwise independently predictive) covariates to be excluded.

There are numerous reasons for the varied ranges in predictive values:

● Nonstandard definitions (e.g. ASA, Cormack and Lehane, or IDS)
● Nonstandard values for individual tests (e.g. mouth opening from <2.5 to <4.0 cm, thyromental distance from <4.0 to < 7.0 cm)
● Intra- and interobserver variation
● Heterogeneous study populations
● Varied levels experience of operator and techniques/adjuncts used to achieve intubation

Other Investigations

In addition to clinical tests, other investigations include:

● Flexible nasendoscopy – It is valuable in cases of actual or potentially obstructed upper airway to decide on whether awake or asleep intubation is the safest technique. As it is performed in an awake patient, a difficult airway may still occur after induction of anaesthesia and loss of airway tone.
● Radiological – Neck, chest X-ray, CT scan and MRI; to determine the location and extent of obstruction and presence of local tissue invasion (only if there is time and the patient is stable). For facial or neck trauma or disease – identification of fractures, cervical instability, soft tissue damage or oedema. 3D CT scans are helpful in cases of airway distortion and can reconstruct a virtual endoscopy.
● Ultrasound of the neck – Location of anatomical landmarks for percutaneous tracheostomy/cricothyroidotomy; it has been used to measure pretracheal fat as a predictor of difficult airway.

- Flow volume loops – These may differentiate small or large airway, intra- or extrathoracic, fixed or variable obstruction. These are of little clinical benefit in the acute setting.

FORMULATING AN AIRWAY STRATEGY – PLAN ABC APPROACH

Difficult airway guidelines are written by working parties of airway experts who gather the best available evidence and opinion to obtain a consensus for airway management. They are not intended to constitute a minimum standard of practice or absolute requirements, as each difficult airway scenario requires an individually tailored airway strategy.

The ASA algorithm can be applied to both anticipated and unanticipated difficult airway cases. In anticipated cases, it encourages proactive formulation of an ABC plan before induction of anaesthesia. Various 'complexity factors' are first considered to help determine which of the 'four basic management choices' (BMC) are chosen to make a final airway strategy. The UK Difficult Airway Society (DAS) algorithm applies to unanticipated difficult airway cases; this is a reactive algorithm containing guidelines on what to do after induction of anaesthesia.[6]

With regard to intubation, there are four main groups of patients (Table 2.6.6):

1. Can intubate, can oxygenate
2. Difficult to intubate, can oxygenate
3. Cannot intubate, can oxygenate
4. Cannot intubate, cannot oxygenate (CICO)

The majority of patients belong to the first group 'can intubate, can oxygenate' with easy FMV, easy SAD ventilation and easy tracheal intubation. They can be safely managed by the 'basic techniques' chosen from the four BMC (left side column of Table 2.6.6): intravenous induction of anaesthesia, ablation of spontaneous ventilation, conventional direct laryngoscopy and standard tracheal tube to achieve intubation. Alternatively, an SAD may be used, with or without muscle relaxants.

Full pre-oxygenation should be performed. After induction of anaesthesia, 'chin lift, head tilt' or 'jaw thrust', and use of airway adjuncts (e.g. oropharyngeal airways) open up the airway to facilitate FMV. The 'sniffing the morning air' position aligns the oral–pharyngeal–laryngeal axes for laryngoscopy (Fig. 2.6.2).

Anticipated Difficult Airway

Patients predicted or known to be in any of the other three groups require careful consideration of the 'DO ASK complexity factors' (see page 220) and an ABC airway strategy planned. These patients may require more 'advance techniques' to secure the airway (right side column of Tables 2.6.6 and 2.6.7).

TABLE 2.6.6 With Increasing Predicted Difficulty in Airway Management (from 'Can Intubate, Can Oxygenate' to CICO), the Basic Management Choices Will Shift towards the Right Side Column of 'Advanced Techniques'[1]

Airway Type (Predicted or Known)	Can Intubate, Can Oxygenate	Difficult to Intubate, Can Oxygenate	Cannot Intubate, Can Oxygenate	CICO
	Basic Techniques		*Advanced Techniques*	
Four basic management choices (ASA)[1]	Asleep intubation		Awake intubation	
	Ablate spontaneous ventilation		Preserve spontaneous ventilation	
	Direct laryngoscopy		Indirect laryngoscopy (e.g. videolaryngoscopy or fibreoptic intubation)	
	Noninvasive airway (e.g. SAD or TT)		Invasive airway (e.g. tracheostomy)	

Notes: TT, tracheal tube.
See text for full details.

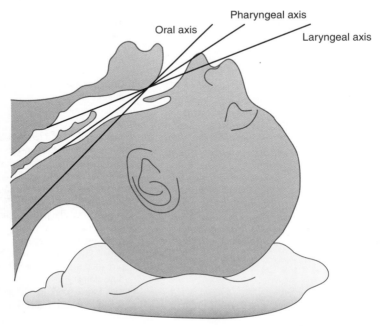

FIGURE 2.6.2 Alignment of oral, pharyngeal and laryngeal axis for laryngoscopy.

TABLE 2.6.7 Advantages and Disadvantages of the 'Advance Techniques' from the Four 'Basic Management Choices'[1]

	Advantages	Disadvantages
Awake intubation (e.g. awake fibreoptic intubation, awake videolaryngoscopy or awake tracheostomy)	• Maintain protective airway reflexes and ability to swallow secretions • Maintain airway tone and functional lung capacity • Minimize risk of regurgitation • Neurological assessment possible after intubation and positioning • Opportunity to consider alternative option if failed plan A intubation	• More complex procedure • Potentially unpleasant for the patient • Cooperative patient is required • Requires local anaesthesia topicalization or infiltration +/− supplementation with sedation, if safe • Airway collapse may occur during these interventions
Preserving spontaneous ventilation (e.g. gas induction and avoiding muscle relaxants)	• Spontaneous ventilation maintains inspiratory negative intrathoracic pressure – beneficial in airway obstruction (e.g. ball-valve, pedunculated lesions and central airway obstruction) • Cessation of volatile if airway obstruction occurs, allowing the patient to wake up	• Slow induction • Laryngospasm possible • Increased work of breathing • Poor conditions for laryngoscopy and intubation • Difficult to achieve correct depth of anaesthesia for airway manipulation • 2x MAC required for direct laryngoscopy/intubation
Indirect laryngoscopy (e.g. videolaryngoscopy or fibreoptic intubation)	• Videolaryngoscopy – better glottic view than direct laryngoscopy • Nasal flexible fibreoptic intubation • Bypass oropharyngeal lesions • Rescue intubation following failed attempts using direct laryngoscopy • Less head and neck movement	• Complex (with steep learning curve) • Videolaryngoscopes • Bulky • May require bougie/stylet to guide tracheal tube insertion • Airway trauma possible • Flexible fibreoptic intubation • Passage of FOB requires an airspace to reach the glottis – easiest in awake patient who can maintain airway tone. In anaesthetized patients (when safe to do so) – may be provided by a suitable SAD (low-skill FOI) • May cause 'cork in a bottle' scenario if severe airway obstruction

TABLE 2.6.7 Advantages and Disadvantages of the 'Advance Techniques' from the Four 'Basic Management Choices'—cont'd

	Advantages	Disadvantages
Invasive airway device/technique (e.g. tracheostomy)	• Bypass obstructive lesions of the upper airway (e.g. oropharyngeal or laryngeal lesions)	• Complex • Complications (e.g. bleeding) • May not be possible due to large or distal lesions (e.g. retrosternal goitre or tracheobronchial lesions)

Notes: MAC, minimum alveolar concentration. FOB, fibreoptic bronchoscope. FOI, fibreoptic intubation.

For patients deemed safe to have asleep intubation, a pre-induction check should be performed:

● A – Assistance (skilled) available.
● B – Brief (team) between anaesthetists, surgeons and theatre staff communicating the anticipated difficult airway and explaining the airway strategy. ENT surgeons scrubbed and ready to perform an emergency tracheostomy may be indicated.
● C – Consent checked and valid.
● D – Drugs checked.
● E – Equipment checked, intubating aids, e.g. bougie or stylet, alternative laryngoscopes, and a difficult airway trolley.
● Standard patient monitoring.

Alternative laryngoscopes include:

● Short handle – This is for patients with short necks, barrel chest and large breasts.
● McCoy – This has a lever-operated hinged tip blade that lifts the epiglottis to improve glottic view.
● Miller straight blade – This is used via a paraglossal approach to reduce tongue compression and backwards displacement of the tongue and epiglottis. However, there is reduced space to manipulate the tracheal tube, so a bougie or stylet may be needed.
● Videolaryngoscopes.

Unanticipated Difficult Airway

The basic sequence for the provision of oxygenation in the anaesthetized patient is:

● FMV (single person, two hands)
● Insertion of an oropharyngeal airway (less often a nasopharyngeal airway)
● Two person (four hands) FMV

- SAD insertion and ventilation (and/or step 5)
- Laryngoscopy and intubation
- Front of neck access (FONA) for CICO (see page 233)

The 2015 DAS algorithm for the unanticipated difficult airway consists of a plan ABCD approach, where subsequent plans are enacted if the preceding plan fails:

- Plan A – FMV, laryngoscopy and intubation
- Plan B – Maintain oxygenation using SAD
- Plan C – FMV
- Plan D – FONA

Whenever difficulties are encountered, a 'call for help' should be made early. Timely progression from plan A to B helps avoid task fixation such as the need to intubate, when the priority is to oxygenate. Moreover, repeated intubation attempts are associated with airway complications such as oedema, trauma and bleeding, and delay attempting alternative, possibly more appropriate airway plans.

If plan B is successful, then a brief 'stop and think' juncture allows the team to consider the merits of the following four options:

- Wake up the patient.
- Proceed with surgery using the SAD for ventilation.
- Intubate via the SAD (see page 230).
- FONA.

Decision-making during successful plan B is based on patient, anaesthetic and surgical factors. Note that the option of an elective FONA during plan B (successful oxygenation via SAD) is different from an emergency FONA during plan D following failed plan B and C.

If plan C is successful, then the patient should be woken up since arrival at this stage was preceded by failure of plans A and B. Surgery should only proceed for exceptional circumstances. If plan C fails, then a CICO should be declared and FONA should be obtained expeditiously.

Consider 'DO ASK' Complexity Factors

Time sensitive 'complexity factors' should be considered when constructing an airway strategy. Unfavourable factors may indicate more 'advance techniques' from the BMC (right side column of Table 2.6.6).

These factors can be summed up by the mnemonic 'DO ASK':

- Desaturation – Healthy patients have apnoea times (5–6 min) after full pre-oxygenation allowing other treatment options to be implemented; others such as obese, children, obstetric and septic patients desaturate more quickly.

- Obstruction – This depends upon the location (can it be reached and bypassed), size and type (e.g. stenosis or pedunculated, ball-valve).
- Aspiration risk – Patients at increased risk of aspiration should have regional anaesthesia, if possible. Alternatively, their airway secured with a second-generation SAD or ideally a tracheal tube (including the use of rapid sequence induction [RSI]); aspiration of gastric contents is a common cause of anaesthesia-related deaths (~50%).[7] Antacid prophylaxis should be administered as per local guidelines.
- Skills and kit – The skill set of personnel (anaesthetic or ENT surgeon) and equipment available, e.g. to perform low-skill fibreoptic intubation or FONA.

Four Basic Management Choices (BMC)

The ASA difficult airway algorithm offers four BMC for securing the airway (Table 2.6.6):

1. Asleep versus awake intubation.
2. Ablate versus preserve spontaneous ventilation.
3. Direct versus indirect laryngoscopy.
4. Noninvasive versus invasive airway device/technique for intubation.

After 'consideration of the relative clinical merits and feasibility' of these choices, the anaesthetist can construct a logical plan A, B, C airway strategy. The primary goal is to use airway devices and techniques that provide and maintain oxygenation of the patient. Plan A should be the best and safest method of achieving this. The advantages and disadvantages of the various advance airway techniques from the BMC are described in Table 2.6.7. Subsequent plans should be chosen such that they can be implemented in a timely and effective manner should there be failure in the preceding plan. Again, task fixation must be avoided; if a certain plan is not working, then one needs to change drug, device, technique or operator.

OXYGENATION

Maintenance of oxygenation is the priority in all patients and can be achieved by:

- Pre-oxygenation in the awake patient
- FMV in the anaesthetized patient
- Apnoeic insufflation during attempts at securing the airway in the anaesthetized patient
- Extracorporeal oxygenation (rarely used, and as a last resort)

The first two methods use a tight sealing mask to help deliver 100% oxygen. A high fresh gas flow (>10 L/min) and reservoir bag are required to prevent rebreathing exhaled gases when the patient's peak inspiratory flow (30 L/min) is greater than fresh gas flow.

Difficult airways are not always predictable and pre-oxygenation is recommended for all patients to increase apnoea time (defined as the time taken for haemoglobin to desaturate to given limit, usually 93%–95%). Methods to achieve pre-oxygenation include:

● Tidal volume breathing for 3 min (TVB)
● Four vital capacity breaths in 30 s (4DB)
● Eight vital capacity breaths in 60 s (8DB)

Optimal pre-oxygenation requires delivery of 100% oxygen from the anaesthetic machine, absence of leak from the anaesthetic circuit and maximum lung denitrogenation. It is indicated by three signs:

1. Emptying and refilling of the anaesthetic circuit reservoir bag.
2. Adequate capnography tracing.
3. End tidal oxygen (EtO_2) of at least 85%. However, if there is a circuit leak (indicated by a lack of the above two signs), the EtO_2 may over read due to supplementation by the anaesthetic machine delivery of 100% oxygen.

More recently, apnoeic oxygenation during laryngoscopy has been shown to considerably increase apnoea time. Oxygen delivered to an apnoeic patient can be delivered in a variety of ways:

● Low flow (up to 6 L/min) nasal cannula
● High flow (6–70 L/min) nasal cannula (HFNC) via a heated humidification system; this allows the paralysed patient with a patent airway to remain oxygenated for up to a median (range) time of 14 (5–65) min

In certain situations (e.g. patients with large tracheal or bronchial tumours or mediastinal masses), attempts at securing the airway may be hazardous or impossible. Extracorporeal oxygenation, by providing systemic oxygenation and carbon dioxide clearance without the need to intubate or provide pulmonary ventilation, may be the only remaining option.

NEUROMUSCULAR BLOCKING DRUGS

Anaesthetists are traditionally taught to administer neuromuscular blocking drugs (NMBs) after confirmation of adequate FMV as muscle paralysis may prevent resumption of spontaneous ventilation and/or the 'waking up' of the patient with impossible FMV. However, this has now been questioned. The incidence of impossible FMV in the general population is very low, 0.2% and the majority (97%) of these patients can be intubated. Even if FMV fails, there are alternative methods for oxygenation, e.g. SAD or tracheal tube. In most cases of difficult or impossible FMV, anaesthetists tend not to wake up patients and often give NMBs, as these can relieve laryngospasm and chest wall rigidity and make airway management easier (including FMV, SAD insertion and ventilation). In addition, direct laryngoscopy and intubation may resolve some causes of difficult FMV and NMBs may improve ventilation in patients with fixed, annular subglottic/tracheal stenosis. If rocuronium is used and failed FMV is then encountered, sugammadex provides quick and effective reversal.

However, in certain circumstances of airway obstruction, the use of NMBs may be contraindicated. Positive pressure ventilation in cases of large pedunculated airway lesions may cause a ball-valve obstruction. In large central airway obstruction, preservation of spontaneous ventilation (and therefore negative intrathoracic inspiratory pressure) maintains airway patency.

NONINVASIVE AIRWAY TECHNIQUES

Tracheal intubation provides the most secure airway and also protects the lower airway against aspiration. However, complications include failure, dental damage, sore throat, oesophageal or endobronchial intubation, and cervical injury in patients with cervical spine disease or injury.

SAD can be safely used in selected patients for appropriate types of surgery. The first generation SAD, the classic laryngeal mask airway (cLMA, Laryngeal Mask Company Ltd, Henley-on-Thames, UK), was invented by Archie Brain and introduced into clinical use in 1988. It consists of an airway tube with a distal elliptical silicone cuff (soft for atraumatic insertion). The airway tube has a proximal 15 mm connector that fits standard anaesthetic circuits. The cuff is designed to sit snugly in the oropharynx. The proximal, anterior part of the cuff abuts the posterior tongue. The distal part sits in, and plugs, the upper oesophageal sphincter (composed primarily of the cricopharyngeus). The bowl of the cuff aligns with the glottis and has epiglottic bars to prevent the epiglottis obstructing the airway. It is made in eight sizes.

Cuff pressure should be less than 60 cm H_2O to reduce sore throat and nerve injury. The recommended manufacturer's cuff inflation volumes = (cuff size − 1) × 10 mL. However, inflating a size 4 LMA with 30 mL air may produce inflation pressure of 100–200 cm H_2O. Cuff manometry is therefore recommended.

Oropharyngeal leak pressure (OLP) is a marker of performance between the various SADs. It is measured by fully closing the expiratory value of the circle system at a fixed gas flow of 3 L/min. The OLP is the airway pressure at which gas leak occurs in the mouth or is the value at which the airway pressure gauge reaches equilibrium (limited to a maximum of 40 cm H_2O). OLP is optimal when using less than recommended cuff volumes (e.g. 15–20 mL for size 4). Inflation with higher volumes decrease OLP, as it displaces the tip of the SAD, moves the epiglottis into the bowl and exposes the oesophageal inlet. It also worsens fibreoptic view of the glottis.

There are many advantages of SAD over the tracheal tube[8]:

- Speed and ease of insertion, even by novices
- High success rates for insertion and ventilation (up to 99%)

- During insertion – more haemodynamic stability, minimal increase in intra-ocular pressure
- Lower anaesthetic requirements
- Emergence – smoother and higher oxygen saturation
- Lower incidence of sore throat

The disadvantages over the tracheal tube:

- Lower OLP.
- Gastric insufflation – minimized by use of maximum ventilatory pressures of 15–20 cm H_2O.
- Contraindicated in patients at risk of aspiration as protection is less than with a cuffed tracheal tube. However, the risk of aspiration is still low with cLMA (1 in 5–10,000). The tip acts as a physical block to regurgitation and careful patient selection (starved and excluding those with aspiration risk factors).

There are now many 'second-generation' SAD designed to reduce the risk of aspiration. Features (not shared by all) include:

- Oesophageal drainage tube – common to all second-generation SAD; functionally separating the respiratory and gastric tracts, allowing escape of regurgitated gastric contents. A nasogastric tube may also be inserted to suction out stomach contents.
- Respiratory port – sufficiently large enough to act as a conduit for fibreoptic intubation.
- Posterior inflatable cuff – the ProSeal LMA™ has an additional cuff, producing higher OLP than the cLMA (30 versus 20 cmH₂O, respectively).
- Noninflatable cuff – a feature of the i-gel™ (OLP of 27–30 cmH₂O) and the streamlined liner of the pharyngeal airway (SLIPA™).
- Integral bite block – prevents biting and complete obstruction of the SAD, which may cause negative pressure pulmonary oedema.
- Epiglottic fins – found in the bowl of the LMA supreme™ to prevent epiglottic obstruction.

INDIRECT LARYNGOSCOPY

These can be broadly divided into videolaryngoscopes (VL) and optical stylets. They allow the anaesthetist to 'look around the corner' to visualize the glottis, not relying on the conventional alignment of the oral, pharyngeal and laryngeal (OPL) axes for intubation.

VL devices are based on the traditional Macintosh laryngoscope. They have a camera/video chip mounted in the distal part of the blade, which allows the transmission (usually by fibreoptics) of images to a monitor. Optical laryngoscopes have prisms and lenses to obtain an indirect view, but images can also be relayed to a monitor. For simplicity, this latter group is grouped with VL devices. They provide a better view of the glottis compared with direct laryngoscopy devices.

VL devices can be channelled or nonchannelled. The latter have either a similar Macintosh-style blade or an extra-curved blade. The 'channelled' blades have an integrated tube that guides the tracheal tube to the visualized glottis. Most have disposable blades, and there is also a single-use fibreoptic flexible intubating bronchoscope. Differences between the various devices are described in Table 2.6.8.

VL devices are used to manage anticipated and unanticipated difficult airways and all anaesthetists should be trained in their use. There is little evidence that VL is superior to DL in the general population. However, they have a 67%–100% intubation success rate for predicted or known difficult airways and have been used as a rescue technique after failed direct laryngoscopy.

TABLE 2.6.8 Comparison of Different Types of Indirect Laryngoscopy Devices

	Nonchannelled	Channelled	Stylet

Examples	• AP Advance™
	• C-MAC®
	• Glidescope®
	• McGrath®
		• Airtraq®
		• AP
		  Advance™
		• CTrach™
		• Pentax
		  AWS®
			• Flexible FOB
			• Rigid
			  bronchoscope
			• Bonfils
			• Shikani

Device creates airspace for laryngoscopy and intubation	Y	Y	N (airspace created by awake patient, or by anaesthetist, e.g. inserted thumb, performing laryngoscopy or inserting SAD)
Can 'look around the corner'?	Y	Y	Y
Able to manipulate device inside oropharynx?	N (bulky +)	N (bulky ++)	Y (slim)
Guides tube to glottis?	N (may require stylet or bougie)	Y (via channel)	Y (railroad tube over stylet)
Awake and asleep intubation?	Y	Y	Y
Both oral and nasal intubation?	N (but may assist in nasal intubation)	N (but may assist in nasal intubation)	Y
Difficulty to learn	+	+	+++

Novice anaesthetists have a higher intubation success rate using VL devices than the Macintosh laryngoscope. This is in part due to the indirect view obtained, but also the shared view on the monitor allows teaching and correction of technique. As the first attempt at intubation should be the best attempt, some authors recommend (and some institutions have implemented) the use of VL devices as a first line technique for intubation. Some are portable, battery operated, with a mounted screen (e.g. McGrath™ VL) making them ideal as a 'scoop and go' device when an unexpected difficult airway is encountered. VL devices have also been used in difficult airways in 'awake' (or sedated) patients in combination with airway topicalization. There is less head and neck manipulation, making them more suitable for patients with cervical spine disease or trauma. The video capability allows recording of the intubation. This 'digital airway footprint' can be used for documentation (for clinical and medicolegal reasons) and for teaching.

Intubation using VL devices may still fail due to the following:

- Mouth opening of about 2 cm and 2.5 cm is required for insertion of non-channelled and channelled VL devices, respectively.
- Impaired view, e.g. fogging, secretions, and blood.
- A good glottic view may not equate with easy intubation. The tracheal tube still has to pass along a potentially nonaligned OPL axis. An intubating stylet or bougie may be needed but does not guarantee success. The discordance between glottic view and the ability to intubate makes the Cormack and Lehane scoring less appropriate for indirect laryngoscopy.
- The oropharyngeal space may be small due to less forceful tongue retraction or the bulkiness of the VL device.

Using VL devices is associated with the creation of a 'blind spot'. Passage of the tracheal tube alongside the blade, but before coming into view of the camera/lens, can produce airway trauma.

FIBREOPTIC INTUBATION

Awake Flexible Fibreoptic Intubation (FOI)

Indications for awake FOI include:

- Difficult airway – history or predicted difficult airway (intubation and FMV)
- Airway protection – severe risk of gastric aspiration
- Avoidance of trauma – unstable cervical spine (allowing neurological assessment post intubation in the awake patient), risk of dental damage, e.g. loose teeth

Contraindications include:

- Patient refusal or uncooperative patient
- Local anaesthetic allergy
- Severe acute upper airway obstruction

- Grossly distorted upper airway anatomy or unable to see the glottis on flexible nasendoscopy
- Coagulopathy
- Penetrating eye injury
- Basal skull fracture (relative contraindication)
- Lack of FOI skills

FOI allows visualization of almost the entire airway (from nose or mouth down to the bronchioles). However, devices are expensive, fragile and have a steep learning curve. Although considered the gold standard for the management of certain difficult airways and a core skill in training curriculums, opportunities to train and maintain FOI skills are often inadequate, in part due to increasing use of alternatives such as SAD and VL devices.

Where FOI is considered the optimal method of securing the airway, an awake technique should be considered unless contraindicated.[7] FOI is best avoided in anaesthetized patients with a predicted difficult airway. The awake patient has preserved airway tone and is able to perform manoeuvres such as tongue protrusion. In addition, the flexible bronchoscope is too flimsy to create the airspace needed to allow visualization and passage of the tracheal tube through the glottis in an anaesthetized patient (unlike rigid VL devices). An alternative is the insertion of a SAD allowing FOI to be performed through this (low-skill FOI, see page 230).

Awake FOI should be avoided in cases of severe airway obstruction for several reasons:

- Patients may be agitated or distressed due to hypoxia, hypercarbia and dyspnoea.
- Sedation and topicalization may result in the loss of critical airway tone or laryngospasm.
- FOI may be difficult and, for friable airway tumours, cause bleeding and airway obstruction.
- Inserting the fibreoptic bronchoscope (FOB) through an obstructed airway may cause a 'cork in a bottle' scenario, resulting in complete airway obstruction.
- Railroading the preloaded tracheal tube over the FOB may be difficult, traumatic or impossible.

Patient preparation includes airway topicalization and sedation (unless contraindicated, e.g. aspiration risk). Although sedation reduces anxiety and may help intubation conditions (Table 2.6.9), oversedation may cause loss of airway patency and cooperation. Topicalization decreases discomfort and attenuates or abolishes airway reflexes. It may be achieved by various methods (Table 2.6.10). Mucosal topicalization is used more commonly than specific airway nerve blocks. The maximum dose of lidocaine is 8.2 mg/kg.

Additional laryngeal and tracheal analgesia can be provided by spraying lignocaine down the channel of the FOB, perhaps via an epidural catheter, or

TABLE 2.6.9 Sedation Techniques for Awake Fibreoptic Intubation

	Bolus or Loading Dose	Advantages	Disadvantages
Midazolam	• 1–2 mg bolus	• Amnesic	
Propofol	• 1% 10 mL/h • 0.7 mg/kg bolus then 1 mg/kg/h • Ce 1–5 µg/mL	• Amnesic • Anti-emetic	• Sedative • Desaturation • Airway obstruction
Fentanyl	25–50 µg boluses		• Bradycardia • Respiratory depression • Pruritus
Remifentanil	• 50 µg/mL solution (1 mg in 20 mL) at 5–10 mL/h • 0.75 µg/kg bolus then 0.075 µg/kg/min • Ce 2 ng/mL	• Analgesic • Antitussive • Better patient cooperation and intubating conditions than propofol • Reversed by naloxone	• Higher recall than propofol • Bradycardia • Respiratory depression • Chest wall rigidity
Dexmedetomidine	• 0.4–1 µg/kg over 10 min then 0.7–1.0 µg/kg/h	• Less cardiovascular instability • Less respiratory sedation • Antisialogogue • Antitussive • Amnesic	• Slower offset than propofol • Hypertension during initial loading bolus

TABLE 2.6.10 Airway Anaesthesia for Awake Fibreoptic Intubation

Nerve Block	Anatomical Supply	Technique
Anterior ethmoidal	Anterior and lateral nasal cavity	LA soaked pledgets on a long applicator; this is inserted into the nasal cavity, upwards and parallel to its anterior border, and stopping at its cribriform plate and posterior nasopharyngeal wall
Sphenopalatine	Roof of the nasal cavity and septum	Applicator as above, but inserted 20° to the floor of the nasal cavity until bone felt (sphenopalatine foramen) behind the middle turbinate

TABLE 2.6.10 Airway Anaesthesia for Awake Fibreoptic Intubation—cont'd

Nerve Block	Anatomical Supply	Technique
Glossopharyngeal	Soft palate, pharynx, tonsil, posterior one-third tongue, vallecular and anterior epiglottis	LA injected (via 22G spinal needle) into the base of either the anterior or posterior tonsillar fold (palatoglossal and palatopharyngeal arches, respectively)
Superior laryngeal	Posterior epiglottis, arytenoids and vocal cords	External approach • Injection of LA after piercing the thyrohyoid membrane by walking off inferiorly from greater cornu of the hyoid bone, or superiorly from superior cornu of the thyroid cartilage Internal approach • LA soaked gauze inserted lateral to each side of the tongue into the piriform fossae via Jackson forceps
Mucosal topicalization	Respective areas where topicalization is applied	• Nebulizer – entire airway from nasal/oral mucosa to lower airways • Lidocaine gel • Mucosal atomizer devices (MAD) – nasal and oropharynx • 'Spray as you go' (SAYGO) – via epidural catheter inserted into the working channel of the fibreoptic intubating bronchoscope • Translaryngeal injection (see text)

Notes: LA, local anaesthetic solution. The nerve blocks are performed bilaterally.

by a translaryngeal block. The skin over the cricothyroid membrane is anaesthetized with lignocaine and an intravenous cannula, connected to a 5 mL syringe containing 2%–4% lidocaine, inserted. The cannula is advanced until air is freely aspirated indicating needle entry into the trachea. Advancing a further 2 mm ensures that the plastic cannula has also entered the trachea. Lidocaine injection is timed at the end of deep inspiration or expiration. The former causes coughing (forced expiration against a closed glottis) spreading lignocaine above and below the vocal cords although the distal trachea may not be fully anaesthetized. With the latter technique, there is mainly distal spread. Translaryngeal block should be avoided when there is local infection or malignancy.

Additional considerations include:

● For nasal FOI, the nose is sprayed with co-phenylcaine (phenylephrine for vasoconstriction and 5% lidocaine). Each metered spray is approximately

0.1 mL and therefore contains 5 mg (convert % straight into mg). Other nasal decongestants such as 0.05% oxymetazoline or 0.1% xylometazoline can be used.

● An antisialogogue may be given (glycopyrrolate 200 μg i.v.);
● For those at risk of aspiration (e.g. obstetric patients), antacid prophylaxis should be administered.

Airway adjuncts for awake oral FOI include Berman and Ovassapian intubating airways. These create an airspace, prevent biting, and guide the FOB to the larynx.

Proficient use of the FOB requires the development and practice of complex cognitive and psychomotor skills. Confusion and frustration from the learner may arise from not being aware that the direction of tip (up or down deflection) of the FOB determines how rotational movement of the body of the FOB will translate to that of the tip (Fig. 2.6.3). This body-to-tip relationship is dependent on the position of the operator relative to (i.e. standing in front or from behind) the patient and on the relative location of the FOB in the airway.

Failure of FOI may occur due to impingement of the tracheal tube during railroading, typically against the right arytenoid, epiglottis and tongue. This can be minimized by use of a narrower tracheal tube or one specially designed to promote smooth passage through the larynx, e.g. the intubating LMA tube or the Parker Flex-Tip™ tube.

Low-Skill Fibreoptic Intubation (LSFOI)

All anaesthetists should be trained in intubation through a SAD, often termed 'low-skill fibreoptic intubation'. This is usually performed in anaesthetized, paralysed patients; a SAD creates an airspace and guides the FOB to the glottis, often with minimal manipulation. It has been used successfully in patients with difficult airways as a first line technique and also as a rescue technique after failed intubation by other methods. It is one of the options in plan B of the DAS unanticipated difficult airway algorithm. If difficult ventilation after induction of anaesthesia is anticipated, an awake intubation technique should be considered rather than LSFOI.

There are two LSFOI methods after insertion of a SAD (Table 2.6.11): direct and indirect. The FOB is preloaded with a 5.0 or 6.0 mm microlaryngeal tube (MLT) (direct method) or an Aintree Intubating Catheter (AIC, indirect method).

Direct Method

1. FOB-MLT combination inserted through SAD – until carina viewed.
2. Railroad MLT over FOB – fully insert MLT through the SAD.
3. Remove FOB – leaving both SAD and MLT in situ.

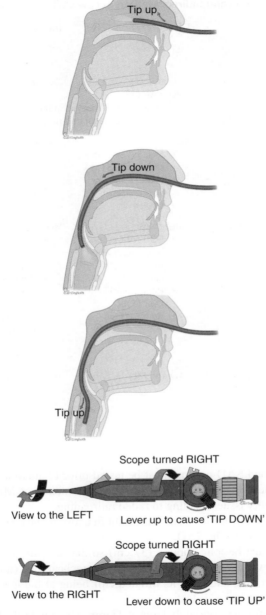

FIGURE 2.6.3 Demonstration of how tip orientation (up or down) alters the direction of rotation of the body of the fibreoptic bronchoscope in order to view a given direction. (See text for full description.)

TABLE 2.6.11 Direct and Indirect Method of Low Skill Fibreoptic Intubation

	Direct	Indirect
Fibreoptic bronchoscope preloading	MLT	AIC
Supraglottic airway device	• Most SAD, e.g. classic LMA, ProSeal™ LMA, i-gel™ and Air-Q® • LMA Supreme™ not recommended (due to its acutely curved shaft and presence of epiglottic fins)	
Tracheal tube	MLT • Size 5.0 mm for size 3 classic LMA • Size 6.0 mm for size 4 classic LMA 4	Tracheal tube • Internal diameter ≥7.0 mm (since AIC outer diameter is 6.5 mm)
Sequence of events after SAD insertion	Three steps: • FOB-MLT combination inserted into SAD to carina • Railroad MLT over FOB • Remove FOB	Five steps: • FOB-AIC combination inserted into SAD to carina • Remove SAD (ensuring AIC still deep in trachea) • Remove FOB • Railroad tracheal tube over AIC • Remove AIC
Devices left in the patient's airway after intubation completed	SAD and MLT	Tracheal tube

Precautions

- Each MLT and SAD pairing must be tested prior to attempting intubation. Varying inner diameters of SAD and outer diameters of MLT may cause incompatibility issues, leading to failed railroading.
- The MLT is left inside the SAD – the tight fit between the two devices makes it unsafe to remove the SAD.
- The MLT must be long enough (37 cm) so that its cuff, when inflated, is distal to the vocal cords. A standard 6.0 mm tracheal tube (for small adults) is 28–32 cm long and risks its inflated cuff being at the level of the vocal cords, resulting in an air leak.
- The MLT cuff is appropriately large at 27 mm. The standard 6.0 mm tracheal tube has a 22 mm cuff diameter, which may be too narrow for the adult trachea (range of internal tracheal diameter 10–25 mm).
- The SAD must be secured to the patient, and the MLT to the SAD.

Indirect Method

1. FOB-AIC combination inserted through SAD – until carina viewed
2. Remove SAD carefully – hold AIC in situ inside trachea
3. Remove FOB carefully – hold AIC in situ inside trachea
4. Railroad tracheal tube over AIC
5. Remove AIC – leaving tracheal tube inside trachea

The AIC is a 56-cm-long hollow tube exchanger with a 4.7 mm internal diameter (fits onto a 4.1 mm FOB) and a 6.5 mm outer diameter (only allowing $\geq$7.0 mm tracheal tubes to be railroaded over it). It comes with two Rapi-Fit® adaptors, one has a Luer lock connector to allow high pressure jet ventilation and the other a 15 mm standard connector to allow conventional low pressure ventilation. However, ventilating down the AIC is associated with barotrauma.

Precautions

- There are more steps involved than the direct method.
- Removal of the SAD also removes the ability to ventilate that patient.
- The AIC can be flipped out of the trachea and into the oesophagus.
- Railroading of the tracheal tube may fail due to impingement of the bevel onto airway structures.

FRONT OF NECK ACCESS (FONA)

Following failed plan ABC of the DAS difficult algorithm, plan D (emergency FONA) should be implemented without delay. Administration of NMBs is recommended in cases of CICO as this may potentially reverse contributory factors and to optimize conditions for airway management.[6,7]

FONA includes cricothyroidotomy and surgical tracheostomy. There are three types of cricothyroidotomy: needle, large bore and surgical techniques (Tables 2.6.12 and 2.6.13). The cricothyroid membrane lies between the thyroid and cricoid membrane. Its height and width in an adult are 10 mm and 25 mm, respectively. The cricothyroid artery lies superiorly, and there are large veins lateral to the midline. Therefore, cricothyroid puncture should be made midline and in the inferior half of the membrane.

Oxygen supply comes from either low or high-pressure sources, and each can produce low or high flows depending on the regulator or flowmeter settings. Inspiration requires high flow or high pressure to overcome the resistance of a small diameter cricothyroidotomy catheter (Table 2.6.13). Expiration requires an adequate expiratory pathway to prevent barotrauma. This pathway can be via a patent upper airway (proximal to the cricothyroidotomy), or via the cricothyroidotomy device itself. Adequate passive expiration is possible in devices with diameter $\geq$4 mm (large bore cannula or surgical, but not needle, cricothyroidotomy). Active expiration can be achieved via a needle cricothyroidotomy using the Ventrain® system (Table 2.6.13).

TABLE 2.6.12 Types of Cricothyroidotomy

	Needle	Large Bore	Surgical
Internal diameter of cricothyroid airway	2 mm	4 mm	6 mm
Complexity of technique	Easy, quicker	Moderate difficulty	Complex (DAS 'stab, twist, bougie, tube' technique)
Success rate	37%–79%	57%–100%	
Connectors	Luer	Fits standard connectors (15 mm ID/22 mm OD)	
Ventilator	• Manujet™ • Monsoon jet ventilator™ • Ventrain® • Rapid-O2™	• Anaesthetic machine • Self-inflating bag valve device	
Pressure for ventilation	High (1–4 bar)[a]	Low (10–20 cmH$_2$O)	
Patient with patent airway	• Safe if patent airway allows adequate exhalation to prevent barotrauma	• Requires cuff inflation (not present on all devices) to prevent air leak and ineffective ventilation	
Patient with total obstructed upper airway	• Exhalation of 500 mL tidal volume via 14G needle takes >30 s • Risk of barotrauma due to high pressure source	• Exhalation occurs through cricothyroidotomy device and takes less than 5 s	

[a]Jet ventilation scenario

For surgical cricothyroidotomy, a 6.0 mm tracheal tube is used for two reasons. First, its outer diameter of 8 mm fits the height of the cricothyroid membrane. Second, if used in the DAS-recommended 'stab, twist, bougie, tube' technique, the internal diameter snugly fits the bougie and decreases the chance of catching on soft tissues during railroading. The DAS technique involves:

1. Stab – transverse stab incision through the cricothyroid membrane.
2. Twist – turn scalpel so sharp edge faces caudally.
3. Bougie – pull scalpel laterally and insert bougie into the trachea.
4. Tube – railroad the tracheal tube over the bougie, remove bougie and inflate cuff.

Complications associated with emergency cricothyroidotomy are given in Table 2.6.14.

TABLE 2.6.13 Oxygen Source for Cricothyroidotomy Devices

Classification	Types
High flow	• High flow oxygen at 15 L/min from the anaesthetic machine, oxygen cylinder or wall-mounted oxygen flowmeter. • The Rapid-O2™ device is a low-compliance oxygen tubing circuit that connects to standard oxygen flowmeter at one end and Luer connector at the other. It has a large bore exhaust hole; occluding this causes lung inflation and subsequent release allows partial exhalation. Instructions for use: http://rhce-cico.edwise.edu.au/documents/session4-facilitator.pdf • Ventrain® is a single use portable, flow-controlled ventilator using a driving gas flow rate of up to 15 L/min. Active expiration is achieved and augmented by subatmospheric pressure created within the device. In healthy lungs, a minute volume of 7 L/min is possible via a 2 mm internal diameter catheter. In a pig and sheep studies, the Ventrain® performed better than the Manujet™ in CICO scenario (partially and completely obstructed airways). Its use resulted in rapid re-oxygenation, lower airway pressures, lower PCO_2, higher minute volume and near normal blood pH.
High pressure jet ventilation	• High-pressure jet ventilation (low or high frequency). • Low frequency jet ventilation results in normal tidal volume. High frequency (between 100–1600 breaths/min) results in small tidal volumes (in some cases less than dead space). • The Manujet™ is a lightweight, portable, pressure-controlled injector system consisting of an adjustable pressure regulator (0.5–4 bar), toggle switch, pressure hose and connecting tubing with a Luer connector (to allow connection to a needle cricothyroidotomy). This is manually operated, used at low frequency and delivers 100% oxygen. • The Monsoon™ jet ventilator has an air-oxygen blender (delivering 2 L, 100% oxygen) with heat/humidification functions. It delivers gas at a driving pressure of 0–3.5 bar. The main safety features are the pause pressure (pressure between jet streams) and peak inspiratory pressure alarms. If these are breached, the jet ventilator automatically stops, thereby minimizing barotrauma. Jet frequency is between 1 and 1600/min. Pause pressure only works when the jet ventilator is connected to catheters inside the trachea, e.g. subglottic catheter and cricothyroidotomy needles.

CRISIS MANAGEMENT

Many factors lead to major airway complications[7]:

1. Poor airway assessment
2. Poor plan or failure to plan
3. Wrong choice of airway technique (e.g. not performing awake FOI when indicated, or SAD used inappropriately)

TABLE 2.6.14 Complications of Cricothyroidotomy

Technique related	• Failure/misplacement • Kinking/obstruction of device (kinking of guidewire) • Displacement • Bleeding
Barotrauma	• Subcutaneous emphysema • Pneumothorax • Pneumomediastinum • Embolus from insufflation into a vessel • Cardio-respiratory arrest
Airway	• Voice changes • Laryngeal fracture • Subglottic stenosis • Persistent stoma • Tracheo-oesophageal fistula • Tracheomalacia
Others	• Infection • Aspiration

4. Multiple repeat attempts at intubation
5. Failure to correctly interpret a capnograph trace (unrecognized oesophageal intubation)
6. Poor judgement

RAPID SEQUENCE INDUCTION

This is used for rapid tracheal intubation in patients at high risk of aspiration. Introduced by WJ Stept and P Safar in 1970 it has since evolved, with many variants (Table 2.6.15). Cricoid pressure, described by BA Sellick in 1961, is performed by applying backward pressure on the ring-shaped cricoid cartilage to occlude the oesophagus, theoretically reducing the risk of aspiration. However, its use is not without controversy:

● There is no evidence that it decreases the incidence of aspiration.
● It may cause airway distortion and obstruction and worsen laryngoscopy view.
● The oesophagus is laterally displaced with or without cricoid pressure (50% and 95%, respectively); complete occlusion is not guaranteed.
● It may cause patient discomfort and increase the risk of regurgitation.
● Oesophageal rupture may occur if there is active vomiting.

Classically, suxamethonium is used for RSI due to its fast onset time (60 s) and relatively short duration time (8–10 min). Theoretically, in

TABLE 2.6.15 Components of Rapid Sequence Induction (RSI) before Tracheal Intubation

Steps	Component	Original or Traditional Methods	Modern Alternatives
1	Pre-oxygenation	• 3 min tidal volume	• 4 deep breaths (30 s) • 8 deep breaths (60 s)
2	Application of cricoid pressure	• 40 N	• 10 N in awake patient and then 30 N after loss of consciousness
3	Intravenous anaesthetic induction agent	• Thiopental	• Propofol mainly, but other induction agents have been used • Coinduction drugs to attenuate the pressor response of intubation (e.g. fentanyl)
4	Rapid onset muscle paralysis	• Suxamethonium	• Rocuronium 1–1.2 mg/kg
5	FMV	• Not performed (to avoid gastric insufflation and decrease risk of aspiration)	• Performed if risk of hypoxia (but using <20 cm H_2O)

cases of failed intubation, allowing recovery of spontaneous ventilation before critical oxygen desaturation (8 min in healthy patients after full pre-oxygenation) occurs. However, studies have shown that 10%–33% of patients will desaturate before spontaneous recovery. In addition, critical desaturation occurs much earlier in those with high oxygen consumption (e.g. morbidly obese, pregnancy or sepsis). This may be countered by the use of HFNC oxygenation.

Rocuronium and Sugammadex Reversal

An alternative NMB for RSI is high dose rocuronium (1–1.2 mg/kg), which has an onset time of 60–90 s. Duration of action is prolonged at this dose (70–120 min), but it can be effectively reversed by sugammadex (16 mg/kg) within 2 min. The option of 'waking up' the patient in case of a failed airway plan is more feasible with this rocuronium/sugammadex combination compared with the slower spontaneous recovery from suxamethonium (5–10 min).

EXTUBATION

Tracheal extubation is usually a smooth, incident-free process however occasionally, problems may occur including the following:

- Residual effects of anaesthetic agents, opioids, sedatives and muscle relaxants prevent the full return of airway tone and reflexes and effective ventilation.
- Physiological function and reserve may be decreased in sick patients.
- During light planes of anaesthesia, airway stimulation may cause breath holding, coughing and laryngospasm.
- Effects of surgery – there may be impaired ventilation due to pain, splinting of the diaphragm, decreased functional residual capacity, atelectasis and ventilation/perfusion mismatch.
- Trauma, bleeding and oedema of the airway may result in a difficult and/or unsafe airway.
- Human factors – there may be time pressure, lack of personnel, fatigue and distraction.

The aim of extubation is 'to ensure uninterrupted oxygen delivery to the patient's lungs, avoid airway stimulation, and have a back-up plan, that would permit ventilation and re-intubation with minimum difficulty and delay should extubation fail'.[9] Patients may be considered 'low risk' – fasted patients with uncomplicated airways – or 'at risk' – reintubation potentially difficult, ability to oxygenate uncertain or general risk factors (including aspiration) present.

Basic Principles

- Assess airway and physiological/pathological risk factors.
- Optimize patient and other task-related factors.
- Decide whether to perform 'awake' extubation or 'deep' extubation.

Awake extubation is considered the safest option as there is a return of airway tone (for patency), airway reflexes (to prevent aspiration) and ventilation.

Deep extubation is performed at a level of anaesthesia such that airway manipulation does not lead to unwanted airway responses, e.g. breath-holding, coughing, bucking or laryngospasm. As airway reflexes are obtunded and ventilation is suboptimal, this should only be performed on 'low-risk' patients and by experienced anaesthetists. There are several prerequisites to performing deep extubation:

- FiO_2 should be 100%.
- Neuromuscular paralysis fully reversed and spontaneous ventilation resumed.
- Oropharyngeal secretions suctioned (to clear the airway and to test adequate depth of anaesthesia).
- Oral or nasal pharyngeal airways inserted to keep the airway patent.
- Tracheal tube 'cuff deflation test' negative –after deflating the cuff, the capnograph remains unaltered and there is no bucking, cough or any signs of laryngospasm.

Other techniques to consider for 'at-risk' patients include laryngeal mask exchange, remifentanil technique and using an airway exchange catheter. If removing the tracheal tube is not safe, then consider postponing extubation or performing a tracheostomy.

REFERENCES

1. Apfelbaum JL, Hagberg CA, Caplan RA, Blitt CD, Connis RT, Nickinovich DG, et al. Practice guidelines for management of the difficult airway: an updated report by the American Society of Anesthesiologists Task Force on Management of the Difficult Airway. Anesthesiology 2013;118:251–70.
2. Han R, Tremper KK, Kheterpal S, O'Reilly M. Grading scale for mask ventilation. Anesthesiology 2004;101:267.
3. Adnet F, Borron SW, Racine SX, Clemessy JL, Fournier JL, Plaisance P, et al. The intubation difficulty scale (IDS): proposal and evaluation of a new score characterizing the complexity of endotracheal intubation. Anesthesiology 1997;87:1290–7.
4. Cook TM. A new practical classification of laryngeal view. Anaesthesia 2000;55:274–9.
5. Kheterpal S, Martin L, Shanks AM, Tremper KK. Prediction and outcomes of impossible mask ventilation: a review of 50,000 anesthetics. Anesthesiology 2009;110:891–7.
6. Frerk C, Mitchell VS, McNarry AF, Mendonca C, Bhagrath R, Patel A, et al. Difficult Airway Society 2015 guidelines for management of unanticipated difficult intubation in adults. Br J Anaesth 2015;115:827–48.
7. Royal College of Anaesthetists. 4th National Audit Project: Major Complications of Airway Management in the UK. London: 2011.
8. Brimacombe J. The advantages of the LMA over the tracheal tube or facemask: a meta-analysis. Ca J Anaesth.
9. Difficult Airway Society Extubation Guidelines G, Popat M, Mitchell V, Dravid R, Patel A, Swampillai C, et al. Difficult Airway Society Guidelines for the management of tracheal extubation. Anaesthesia 2012;67:318–40.

Chapter 2.7

Intravascular Techniques, Fluid Administration and Blood Transfusion

Andrew A. Klein, Anna Butcher

INTRAVENOUS TECHNIQUES

Peripheral Venous Cannulation

The most suitable veins for routine use for peripheral venous cannulation in adults include those on the forearm or dorsum of the hand. Veins in the leg should be avoided if possible.

A cold or frightened patient is likely to have constricted veins that are difficult to cannulate. If this is the case, or if the patient is hypovolaemic, an antecubital fossa or central vein may be preferred.

Prior application of EMLA cream (60 min) or AnGel® (45 min) is effective at reducing the pain of venepuncture, especially in children. Consider nitrous oxide for anxious children. In infants, the volar aspect of the forearm, the dorsum of the foot and the great saphenous vein at the ankle is often used. Consider practicalities of splinting, e.g. elbow, foot in a mobile child. Scalp veins should only be used by more experienced doctors.

Intra-osseous access is useful in emergencies when intravenous access is difficult by using the medullary space to provide access to the systemic venous system. Intra-osseous needles are typically placed in the epiphyses of long bones such as the tibia or humerus using either manual or drill-assisted devices. All acute care clinicians should be familiar with techniques and have ready access to devices.

Complications

Damage to a superficial cutaneous nerve caused by the needle or cannula has been reported after peripheral venous cannulation and may result in chronic neuropathic pain.

Thrombophlebitis is common if a cannula remains in place for more than a day or two, and it should be removed at the first sign of pain, redness or swelling developing at the cannulation site.

Minor extravasation of fluids is common and does not usually cause harm, but if the solution is irritant or hypertonic (e.g. sodium bicarbonate, calcium and some chemotherapeutic agents) this may cause extensive necrosis of skin, muscle and tendons, with permanent disability.

Central Venous Cannulation

The most common approach to a central (i.e. intrathoracic) vein is via the internal jugular vein. The right side is preferred. On the left side, the thoracic duct joins the venous system at the lower end of the left internal jugular vein and can be damaged. Also, a cannula passed from the left internal jugular vein is more likely to pass across into the right internal jugular or subclavian vein.

With the patient tilted head down and the head rotated to the left, the right internal jugular vein is often visible or palpable. The needle punctures the skin midway between the mastoid process and the sternoclavicular joint and is advanced towards the right nipple to enter the vein. A guidewire is inserted, over which the cannula is then passed. This method of percutaneous cannulation is known as the Seldinger technique and is thought to be associated with fewer complications than the cannula over needle technique. It can also be used for peripheral cannulation techniques.

Many guidelines have been produced recommending the routine use of ultrasound for internal jugular central venous catheter insertion and consideration for all other central venous access sites.[1]

The subclavian vein is often preferred for long-term use because it is more amenable to subcutaneous tunnelling.

Other approaches that have been used include the axillary, femoral or external jugular veins.

Alternatively, a long catheter may be passed from an antecubital vein, preferably on the medial side of the arm to avoid the pectoral fascia obstructing the passage of the catheter (peripherally inserted central catheter, PICC), using ultrasound and X-ray screening.

The choice of device depends on diagnosis, intended use and patient choice. The number of lumens required should be planned in advance to reduce the risk of having to insert further lines. The risk of a larger sized device needs to be weighed against the need for further lumens. The position of the cannula should usually be checked by radiography to ensure its tip lies above the pericardial reflection (i.e. above the level of the carina). This will avoid pericardial tamponade in the rare case where the tip penetrates the wall of the superior vena cava or right atrium. It is also valuable to exclude a pneumothorax.

Central venous cannulae should be removed when no longer required or if they are causing problems. The patient should lie flat with the exit site below the heart to reduce risks of air embolus. Firm pressure should be applied for at least 5 min after removal, followed by an occlusive dressing. Routine culture of tips is not considered necessary. Persistent bleeding may require a skin stitch.

Complications

Complications of central venous cannulation include haemorrhage, haematoma, air embolism, pneumothorax, damage to or compression of other structures in the neck such as the carotid artery, perforation of the vein or right atrium, thromboembolism and infection.

Arterial Cannulation

Any artery that can be compressed after cannulation may be used for arterial cannulation. The radial artery is normally preferred. Alternative sites are the dorsalis pedis, brachial or femoral arteries. The only sure confirmation of arterial, rather than venous, cannulation is to observe the pulse waveform or to measure a sufficiently high PO_2. It can be misleading to rely only on the colour of the blood. The cannula and any connecting lines should be clearly marked as arterial and kept as separate as possible from intravenous lines, to avoid the possibility of accidental arterial injection of drugs. Extreme care is also taken to avoid entry of air into an artery.

Before radial artery cannulation, some anaesthetists perform Allen's test – press on the radial and ulnar arteries while a fist is made, extend the patient's fingers and release the pressure on the ulnar artery only. Reflushing of the hand indicates an adequate alternative blood supply to the radial artery. The colour of the palm usually takes less than 5–10 s to return. Greater than 15 s is considered abnormal. However, many consider that the significant incidence of false positives and negatives makes this test misleading and therefore unnecessary.

The use of ultrasound should be considered early if arterial or peripheral venous cannulation proves difficult.

INTRAVASCULAR FLUID ADMINISTRATION

Crystalloids and Colloids

Constituents of some common crystalloid and colloid intravenous fluids are shown in Table 2.7.1 (all are essentially isotonic with plasma). There is a small but significant incidence of anaphylaxis with all colloids, and this is least common with albumin solutions.

Gelatins

Gelatins are produced by hydrolysis of collagen. The average molecular weight for both succinylated gelatin 4% and polygeline 3.5% is 30,000. They are widely used for temporary blood volume replacement. Gelatins lead to 70%–80% volume expansion. Duration of action is shorter than in comparison to albumin and starches.

Human Albumin Solution

Human albumin solution (HAS) is the serum albumin found in blood, the most abundant protein found. It is derived from plasma, serum or normal placentas.

TABLE 2.7.1 Constituents of Some Common Crystalloid and Colloid Intravenous Fluids

Fluid	Na⁺ (mmol/L)	K⁺ (mmol/L)	Cl⁻ (mmol/L)	HCO3⁻ (mmol/L)	Ca⁺⁺ (mmol/L)	pH
Normal saline (0.9% or 9 g/L)	154	–	154	–	0	5
Hartmann's	131	5	111	29	2	6.5
Dextrose (4%) with saline (0.18%)	30	–	30	–	–	4
Dextrose (5%)	–	–	–	–	–	4
Succinylated gelatin 4% (Gelofusine®)	154	0.4	120	–	0.4	7.4
Polygeline 3.5% (Haemaccel®)	145	5.1	145	–	6.25	7.3

The solution may be isotonic (containing 3.5%–5% protein) or concentrated (containing 15.25% protein). HAS is contraindicated in setting of severe anaemia and cardiac failure.

Dextrans

Dextrans are available as dextran 40 and 70 with average molecular weights of 40,000 and 70,000, respectively. Both are available either in 0.9% sodium chloride or in 5% dextrose. Dextran 40 is sometimes used to improve blood flow to ischaemic limbs. Both dextrans have some prophylactic value against deep venous thrombosis, but have been replaced for this purpose by heparin preparations. Dextrans interfere with blood grouping and cross-matching.

Starches

Starches are mainly amylopectin etherified with hydroxyethyl groups. Pentastarch is 50% etherified (i.e. 50 hydroxyethyl groups for every 100 glucose units). Tetrastarch and hexastarch are 40% and 60% etherified, respectively. Average molecular weights are generally high (130,000 for tetrastarch; 200,000 for pentastarch and hexastarch). They are usually presented as a 6% solution in normal saline.

They are considerably longer lasting as plasma expanders than the gelatins or dextrans. However, their use is associated with some controversy. In June 2013, the use of starches to treat critically ill patients and those undergoing surgery was suspended in the UK following the publication of two trials; 6S (Scandinavian Starch for Severe Sepsis/Septic Shock) and CHEST (Crystalloid

TABLE 2.7.2 Approximate Volume and Electrolyte Composition of Gut Secretions

	Na$^+$ (mmol/L)	K$^+$ (mmol/L)	Cl$^-$ (mmol/L)	HCO$_3^-$ (mmol/L)	Volume (mL/day)
Stomach	30–80	5–15	110–140	a	2000
Pancreas	130	10	60	90	1000–1500
Bile	130	10	100	35	500
Small bowel	130	10	110	30	1500+

^{a}pH is about 1.0.

versus Hydroxyethyl Starch Trial), which suggested an increased risk of renal injury and death.

Gastrointestinal Fluid Losses

For adult patients who need to be nil by mouth for significant periods, daily water requirements of 30–40 mL/kg/day, plus daily electrolyte requirements of Na$^+$, K$^+$ (1–1.5 mmol/kg/day) and Cl$^-$ (0.07–0.22 mmol/kg/day) should be replaced. For replacement of additional gastrointestinal fluid losses, it is helpful to compare the composition of the fluids given in Table 2.7.1 with the approximate volume and electrolyte composition of gut secretions (Table 2.7.2).

BLOOD TRANSFUSION

Allogeneic red cell transfusion is a commonly used treatment to correct anaemia and improve the oxygen carrying capacity of blood. Approximately, 85 million red cell units are transfused worldwide annually. New and emerging infections continually pose threats to the safety surrounding blood transfusion. Since 2009, governing bodies have identified 68 potential agents that are considered to be a threat to allogenic blood components.[2] Among these, the prions causing variant Creutzfeldt–Jakob disease (vCJD) and dengue virus have been of the greatest concern. Governments have strongly encouraged hospitals to continuously re-evaluate their practices, in particular, the measures put in place to reduce the need for perioperative transfusion.

It is fundamental to the use of any therapeutic agent to understand its contents and potential physiological effects, both beneficial and harmful. Transfusion of blood and blood products is potentially lifesaving in acute severe haemorrhage.

Our understanding of the effects of transfusion, the period of blood storage and when or why to transfuse red cells is still in its infancy. Until such questions are answered, we should be cautious with a product used so widely but with so little proven efficacy.

Recently, there has been a reduction in the number of units transfused yearly, both in the UK and Europe-wide. There are many reasons for this fall, including national and local initiatives, education about patient blood management, reduced Hb triggers for transfusion and awareness of the risks of allogeneic transfusion.

Blood and Blood Products

A transfusion can consist of blood or its related constituents (blood products). Blood is collected from the donor into polyvinyl chloride bags partly prefilled with one of several anticoagulants. It is then subjected to centrifugation, leucodepletion and separation into red blood cells (RBCs) and the haemostatic components. In the UK RBCs are resuspended in saline, adenine (to preserve cellular ATP stores), mannitol and glucose (to preserve the 2,3-diphosphoglycerate [DPG] as much as possible). They are then stored at 4°C.

Temporal, chemical and physical changes result from these mechanical processes and cold storage. These changes are well documented and result clinically in the infusion of hyperkalaemic, acidotic fluids containing RBCs that are much less deformable than normal and sometimes collected in aggregates or clumps. The mark of efficacy of a transfusion is defined by the US Food and Drugs Administration as survival of 70% or more of RBCs 24 h after a transfusion. By this time, therefore, up to 30% of the transfused cells may be dead.

Fresh Frozen Plasma

Fresh frozen plasma (FFP) is separated from whole blood at the time of collection, flash frozen and the cryoprecipitate withdrawn. A unit of FFP should contain:

- 400 mg of fibrinogen in 200 mL of plasma
- 1 unit of activity per mL for each clotting factor
- Na^+ 170 mmol/L, K^+ 4 mmol/L, glucose 22 mmol/L and lactate 3 mmol/L, with a pH between 7.2 and 7.4
- Labile clotting factors V and VIII – may decrease to less than 40% 4 h after thawing

Most guidelines for use after thawing recommend use up to 24 h but can extend up to 120 h to enable rapid provision of FFP for the management of unexpected major haemorrhage without excessive wastage. Plasma should be stored at 4 ± 2°C after thawing. Solvent detergents and treatment with methylene blue are used as additional measures to reduce viral loads in FFP.

Transfusion-related acute lung injury (TRALI) is recognized as a complication of the transfusion of FFP. It occurs if leuco-agglutinating specific antibodies are present in donor plasma. If this is the case, the donor is usually a woman who has become immunized against leucocyte antigens during pregnancy.

Traditionally, laboratory tests have been used to guide the administration of FFP, mainly prothrombin time (PT), international normalized ratio (INR) and activated partial thromboplastin time (APTT). However, there is increasing use of point-of-care tests to guide transfusion of FFP and other blood products, such as thromboelastography (TEG®) or rotational thromboelastometry (ROTEM®).

Cryoprecipitate

Cryoprecipitate is mainly administered as a source of fibrinogen replacement; however, fibrinogen concentrate is now also commercially available, although much more expensive. Cryoprecipitate is derived from controlled thawing of FFP at 1–6°C and contains between 9 and 15 mg/mL of fibrinogen compared with FFP, which contains only 2 mg/mL.

Guidelines recommend transfusion of cryoprecipitate if the fibrinogen level is <1.5 g/dL with clinical evidence of bleeding; there is some controversy about the trigger for administration of cryoprecipitate as the evidence is currently limited. Approximately 10 single bags of cryoprecipitate derived from whole blood are needed to raise the plasma fibrinogen level by 1 g/dL in an adult.

Platelets

Normal platelet count ranges between 150 and 450×10^9/L. Thrombocytopenia is commonly defined as a platelet count $< 150 \times 10^9$/L with mild thrombocytopenia being between 70 and 150×10^9/L and severe thrombocytopenia being $< 50 \times 10^9$/L. Thrombocytopaenia may be caused by:

- Bleeding and replacement of blood loss without replacing platelets
- Haemodilution
- Sepsis
- Chronic hepatic and/or renal dysfunction
- Myeloproliferative disorders

As well as measuring platelet count to guide transfusion of platelet concentrate, consideration should be given to impairment of platelet function. Causes of impaired platelet function include:

- Drugs (aspirin, clopidogrel, heparin, Glycoprotein IIb/IIIa antagonists, e.g. abciximab, tirofiban, – reduced adhesion and aggregation)
- Chronic hepatic and/or renal dysfunction
- Cardiopulmonary bypass
- Sepsis

- Hypothermia
- Acidosis

Platelets for transfusion are prepared by centrifugation of whole blood. One pooled unit contains 55×10^9 platelets in 50 mL (normal blood contains this number of platelets in about 200 mL, or 250×10^9/L). A single unit should raise the platelet count by between 5 and 10×10^9/L. An apheresis unit, often from a single donor, contains 30×10^{10} platelets and is the equivalent of six pooled platelet units.

Platelets are subject to rapid deterioration during storage, and only 40%–60% of platelets are active in any infusion. Cytokine levels in platelet infusions are higher than for any other blood product and may account for many of their adverse effects.

Therapeutic use of platelets has been increasing worldwide. Platelets are given prophylactically (patients with thrombocytopenia or in those with risk factors for bleeding, e.g. sepsis) to prevent bleeding during invasive procedures, as well as for the treatment of active bleeding.

Is Blood Transfusion Necessary?

It is clear from the above discussion that transfusion is not an exact science, and not without risk of considerable complications (Table 2.7.3).

Inappropriate transfusion of patients during surgery has often been criticized, but it is of interest to put these patients in the context of all those receiving blood transfusions. Table 2.7.4, published in 2016, shows that in England and Wales 67% of all transfused blood is used for medical (i.e. nonsurgical and nonobstetric) reasons, often with little scientific justification.[3]

A number of recent studies suggest that patients receiving red cell transfusion are at increased risk of death, ischaemic complications, delayed wound

TABLE 2.7.3 Complications of Blood Transfusion (Adapted from Reference 5)

	Complications of Blood Transfusion
Early	Haemolytic reactions – immediate or delayed Nonhaemolytic febrile reactions Transfusion-associated circulatory overload (TACO) Transfusion-associated acute lung injury (TRALI) Citrate toxicity Electrolyte disturbances – hyperkalaemia Hypothermia Post-transfusion purpura
Late	Infection Graft vs host disease Transfusion-related iron overload Immunomodulation

TABLE 2.7.4 Indications for Red Cell Transfusion; (n = 46,111)

No. (% of All Transfused)	
Medicine	
Anaemia	12,636 (27%)
Haematology	12,516 (27%)
Gastrointestinal bleed	5377 (12%)
Neonatal top-up/exchange transfusion	554 (1%)
Surgery	12,318 (27%)
Obstetrics and gynaecology	
All uses	2690 (6%)
No clinical details	20 (<1%)

healing and prolonged hospital stay. These studies, being observational, are controversial, and transfusion may only be associated with these complications (as opposed to being the cause). The results of ongoing randomized controlled trials are awaited.

Red cell transfusion is used to improve the oxygen carrying capacity of blood; however, increasing arterial oxygen content by increasing haemoglobin does not necessarily increase tissue oxygen delivery or uptake. To understand the aim of a perioperative blood transfusion, it is necessary to consider the relationship between oxygen delivery to the tissues (DO_2) and consumption ($\dot{V}O_2$).

Oxygen delivery (DO_2) is

$$\text{Cardiac output} \times \text{arterial oxygen content}$$

Arterial oxygen content depends mainly on the haemoglobin concentration and arterial oxygen saturation.

Oxygen consumption $\dot{V}O_2$ is often calculated by the Fick equation as:

$$\text{Cardiac output} \times \text{the arteriovenous oxygen content difference.}$$

The two terms are related by the graph shown in Fig. 2.7.1.

It can be seen that, as oxygen delivery is potentially reduced, whether by haemorrhage, myocardial dysfunction or hypoxic hypoxaemia, oxygen consumption is maintained by increasing oxygen extraction. However, as oxygen delivery is reduced further, the critical DO_2 is reached. $\dot{V}O_2$ then moves from being independent of supply to becoming dependent on supply, with resultant ischaemic injury and cell death. The aim of blood transfusion is to ensure that this point is never reached and forms the basis for the term 'transfusion trigger'.

The majority of the evidence published to date has shown that a restrictive strategy for red cell transfusion is not inferior to a liberal strategy. As a restrictive

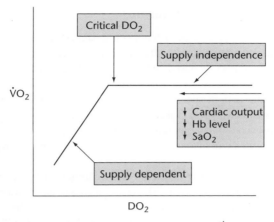

FIGURE 2.7.1. The relationship between oxygen consumption ($\dot{V}O_2$) and delivery (DO_2). As oxygen delivery to the tissues falls, whether due to reduced cardiac output, haemoglobin concentration or arterial oxygen saturation (SaO_2), $\dot{V}O_2$ is unaltered (i.e. is independent of supply) until delivery reaches a critical value, below which $\dot{V}O_2$ starts to drop (i.e. is dependent on supply).

strategy requires less resources and exposes the patient to less allogeneic blood, this is currently recommended. Therefore, most hospitals have agreed on Hb transfusion triggers around 7 g/dL in patients who do not have ongoing coronary ischaemia.

A meta-analysis performed by Holst and colleagues aimed to compare the benefit versus harm of restrictive versus liberal transfusion strategies to guide the prescribing and practices of red blood cells transfusion.[4] They showed that not only were restrictive transfusion strategies associated with a reduction in the number of red cell transfusions, but mortality, overall morbidity and risk of myocardial infarction were no different to liberal transfusion practice.

To Transfuse or Not to Transfuse?

In summary, there is now sufficient evidence to assume that transfusion would not be beneficial when the haemoglobin is greater than 10 g/dL in the absence of acute blood loss.[5] Furthermore, adopting more restrictive transfusion practices does not appear to impact on patient outcome. The individual patient's physiological requirements should be taken into account rather than adopting a slavish adherence to protocols.

Most units in the UK have now adopted a restrictive policy, with locally agreed triggers for transfusion, commonly Hb < 7 g/dL. In patients with ischaemic heart disease, especially if symptomatic, or after cardiac surgery, this is commonly revised to transfusion if Hb < 8 g/dL. However, these suggested thresholds are still controversial and should be agreed locally.

Reducing the Need for Transfusion

Patient blood management (PBM) has been designed to shift focus to patient-centred care and decisions regarding transfusion practices in the perioperative setting. The principle of PBM is based on three pillars of care: detection and treatment of preoperative anaemia, reduction of perioperative blood loss, and harnessing and optimizing the patient-specific physiological reserve of anaemia (including restrictive transfusion triggers) (Table 2.7.5).[6] The practice of PBM has been associated with improved clinical outcome and reduced transfusion requirements.

Similar principles will also apply to those who refuse blood transfusion such as Jehovah Witnesses.

PBM emphasizes the early detection and treatment of preoperative anaemia in surgical patients, which even in mild cases has been independently associated with increased morbidity and mortality. Functional iron deficiency, the most common cause of preoperative anaemia, should be treated with iron supplementation. Antifibrinolytic drugs such as tranexamic acid should be administered on induction of anaesthesia whenever moderate or major blood loss is expected, and cell salvage should also be used in these circumstances. As discussed above, a restrictive transfusion practice is recommended as the standard of care perioperatively.[6]

Mechanical Methods

Mechanical methods to reduce the need for transfusion include acute perioperative normovolaemic haemodilution (APNH) and cell salvage.

Acute Preoperative Normovolaemic Haemodilution

APNH is the withdrawal of a certain amount of blood and its replacement with an equivalent volume of crystalloid or colloid. It is used for surgery associated with major but controlled blood loss. Its aim is to reduce the red cell mass of blood loss due to surgical bleeding followed by the retransfusion of the previously withdrawn blood at the end of surgery.

Its ability as a blood conservation therapy is directly related to the amount of blood that can be collected from the patient, i.e. the greater the amount, the greater its efficacy. It can be considered if potential surgical blood loss is expected to exceed 20% of blood volume and with a starting haemoglobin of greater than 100 g/L. However, blood must be reinfused within 6 h. APNH is not commonly practiced as removal of blood may be associated with haemodynamic instability and there may be local barriers to the temporary storage of blood collected in this way intra-operatively. It is contraindicated in patients with severe cardiovascular disease.

Cell Salvage

Cell salvage consists of suction of red cells from the operative field using a purpose-designed double-lumen suction device, with anticoagulants (usually

TABLE 2.7.5 Components of a Patient Blood Management Programme (Adapted from Reference 6)

	Pillar 1 Optimize erythropoiesis	Pillar 2 Minimize blood loss	Pillar 3 Manage anaemia
Preoperative	Identify, evaluate and treat anaemia Refer for further evaluation as necessary	Review/stop medications (antiplatelet, anticoagulation therapy)	Assess and optimize patient's physiological reserve, e.g. pulmonary and cardiac function Formulate patient-specific management plan using appropriate blood conservation modalities
Intraoperative	Schedule surgery after anaemia has been corrected	Meticulous haemostasis and surgical techniques (consider minimally invasive surgery) Anaesthetic blood-sparing strategies (e.g. hypotension if appropriate) Acute normovolaemic haemodilution in select patients Cell salvage Pharmacological agents (tranexamic acid, ε aminocaproic acid)	Optimize cardiac output Optimize oxygenation and ventilation Evidence-based transfusion thresholds (restrictive transfusion unless ischaemic heart disease or after cardiac surgery)
Postoperative	Beware of drug interactions that can worsen anaemia	Monitor and manage bleeding Avoid secondary haemorrhage Maintain normothermia (unless indicated specifically) Autologous blood salvage Minimize iatrogenic blood sampling loss Haemostasis/anticoagulation management Awareness of adverse effects of medicines Prophylaxis of upper gastrointestinal haemorrhage	Maximize oxygen delivery Minimize oxygen consumption Avoid/treat infections promptly Evidence-based transfusion thresholds

heparin) added. The blood and anticoagulant are stored in a reservoir after suctioning, and when a sufficient amount has been collected this is centrifuged to separate out the components. The red cells are washed and filtered, removing debris (such as fat), free haemoglobin, white blood cells and plasma. The red cells are then stored in a bag, suspended in normal saline and are ready for transfusion. This entire process takes from 5 to 15 min, depending on the manufacturer, the design of the cell salvage machine and the volume of blood being processed. The red cells for autotransfusion are more concentrated than allogeneic (bank) blood, with a haematocrit of 50%–70%. This means that 200 mL of cell-salvaged red cells equates to one unit of bank blood, which is usually around 300–350 mL in volume.

The use of cell salvage has been shown to be cost-effective compared with transfusion and should be considered for operations with an anticipated blood loss greater than 500 mL. If blood loss is uncertain, the cell salvage system can be set up for collection only, and if sufficient blood is collected, the full set of disposables can be opened to permit processing.

Studies comparing cell salvaged with allogeneic blood show that salvaged blood has increased mean erythrocyte viability and increased 2,3-DPG and adenosine triphosphate (ATP) levels. Salvaged blood red cells maintain their normal biconcave disk shape, whereas allogeneic blood assumes an echinocyte shape (after 14 days), which is thought to impair its ability to cross the capillary beds. Therefore, patients who have had autologous transfusion following cell salvage should have improved oxygen carrying capacity and tissue oxygen delivery.

Although the use of cell salvage is generally accepted to be safe, there are a number of potential complications that should be considered. These include haemolysis, coagulopathy (especially when large volumes of blood are processed and autotransfused) and incomplete washing leading to contamination with activated white cells and cytokines. Suctioning of blood may cause sheer stress injury, which can result in haemolysis and therefore reduction in yield from blood salvage. One method of reducing red blood cell haemolysis is minimizing the pressure in the suction device.

Cell salvage is most commonly used in cardiac surgery, obstetrics, trauma, orthopaedics and other major surgery. It is also usually accepted by Jehovah's Witnesses, who generally refuse allogeneic blood or blood product transfusions on religious grounds.

Pharmacological Methods

Bleeding in surgery is multifactorial and impacted by a number of factors including patient comorbidities, medications, type of surgery and acquired defects in coagulation such as those seen in coronary bypass surgery. There are two classes of pharmacological agents known as antifibrinolytics that attempt to achieve haemostasis:

- Serine protease inhibitors (e.g. aprotinin), which prevent fibrinolysis by direct inhibition of plasmin

- Lysine analogues (e.g. tranexamic acid [TXA], ε-aminocaproic acid [EACA]), which prevent the conversion of plasminogen to plasmin

Multiple meta-analyses have demonstrated the superiority of aprotinin to TXA or EACA in reducing postoperative blood loss and rates of transfusion, and need for redo sternotomy in cardiac surgery.[7] However, observational studies have disputed the safety of aprotinin, resulting in the withdrawal of the agent from the worldwide market in 2008, due to its increased associated risk of death in high-risk cardiac surgical patients. Lysine analogues have now become the mainstay in prevention of hyperfibrinolysis, despite inconclusive outcomes with regards to blood loss, transfusion rates or overall complication rates. In the UK, tranexamic acid is most commonly used, with evidence for benefit in cardiac, orthopaedic, urological, gynaecological and obstetric surgery. In the USA, ε-aminocaproic acid is commonly used. Both have been shown to significantly reduce postoperative or traumatic bleeding. There is also some evidence for a reduction of perioperative blood transfusion.[7]

REFERENCES

1. Bodenham A, Babu S, Bennett J, Binks R, Fee P, Fox B, et al. Association of Anaesthetists of Great Britain and Ireland. Anaesthesia: Safe Vascular Access. Anaesthesia 2016;71:573–85.
2. Shander A, Lobel GP, Javidroozi M. Transfusion practices and infectious risks. Expert Review of Hematology 2016;9:597–05.
3. Tinegate H, Pendry K, Murphy M, Babra P, Grant-Casey J, Hopkinson C, et al. Where do all the red blood cells (RBCs) go? Results of a survey of RBC use in England and North Wales in 2014. Transfusion 2014;56:139–45.
4. Holst LB, Petersen MB, Haase N, Perner A, Wetterslev J. Restrictive versus liberal transfusion strategy for red blood cell transfusion: systematic review of randomized trials with meta-analysis and trial sequential analysis. BMJ 2013;350:h1354.
5. Shah A, Stanworth SJ, McKechnie S. Evidence and triggers for the transfusion of blood and blood products. Anaesthesia 2015;70:10–e3.
6. Clevenger B, Mallett SV, Klein AA, Richards T. Patient blood management to reduce surgical risk. Br J Surg 2015;102:1325–37.
7. Ortmann E, Besser MW, Klein AA. Antifibrinolytic agents in current anaesthetic practice. Br J Anaesth 2013;111:549–63.

Chapter 2.8

Acid–Base and Electrolyte Balance

Adel Badr, Peter Nightingale

ACID–BASE BALANCE

Internal acid–base homeostasis is fundamental for maintaining life. The hydrogen ion concentration $[H^+]$ is tightly regulated as any change in $[H^+]$ alters virtually all protein and membrane function. Consequently, an understanding of acid–base physiology is important for both clinical anaesthesia and critical care medicine.

The following definitions are used in acid–base physiology:

- Acid – A proton donor.
- Base – A proton acceptor (can be a cation, neutral or anion).
- pH – The negative logarithm to the base 10 of $[H^+]$. Normal $[H^+]$ in body fluids is 40 nmol/L. The normal range for arterial blood pH is 7.36–7.44 and the pH range compatible with life is 6.8–7.8.
- Acidosis – Excess H^+ in the body, as opposed to acidaemia which means low blood pH. Although pH is clinically measurable, acidosis is not a readily measurable parameter. The two terms are frequently associated but acidosis does not always lead to acidaemia.
- Alkalosis – Excess HCO_3^- in the body, as opposed to alkalaemia which means high blood pH.

An arterial blood gas (ABG) sample typically has a pH of 7.4 ± 0.04, PCO_2 of 5.3 ± 0.7 kPa (40 ± 5 mm Hg) and $[HCO_3^-]$ of 24 ± 2 mmol/L. The blood gas electrodes measure $[H^+]$ and PCO_2 directly, whereas $[HCO_3^-]$ is calculated using Hasselbach's modification of the Henderson equation. A chemical (calorimetric) method can be used to measure CO_2 generated from HCO_3^- plus dissolved CO_2, which is typically only 1 mmol/L.

ACID–BASE PHYSIOLOGY

The difference between the pool of total free H^+ in total body water (1.6×10^{-3} mol/L) and the very much larger continuous flux of H^+ from volatile acid

254

(CO_2) and nonvolatile acids (organic and inorganic) necessitate a tight system to regulate pH. The first step is the buffering system that acts immediately to sequester excess H^+; this is followed by excretion of H^+ by lungs and kidneys.

Buffer Systems

Buffers act to minimize change in pH in the blood that would otherwise occur when an acid or alkali is added. There are a number of buffer systems in the blood:

- Extracellular buffers
  - Bicarbonate
  - Albumin
  - Haemoglobin
  - Phosphate
- Intracellular buffers
  - Protein
  - Phosphate

The bicarbonate buffer system is the most important buffer in the body, whereas other buffers become more relevant with progression of acidosis.

Bicarbonate Buffer System

The bicarbonate buffer system is a very efficient buffer system with enormous power to deal with an acid load. The continuous respiratory elimination of CO_2 prevents accumulation of carbonic acid and allows HCO_3^- to be a very effective H^+ acceptor. The relationship between H^+, HCO_3^- and CO_2 is described by the Henderson equation. Thus,

$$CO_2 + H_2O \leftrightharpoons H_2CO_3 \leftrightharpoons HCO_3^- + H^+ \leftrightharpoons CO_3^{2-} + 2H^+$$

Simplified:

$$CO_2 + H_2O \leftrightharpoons HCO_3^- + H^+$$

This can be expressed as:

$$[H^+] = \kappa \times \alpha PCO_2/[HCO_3^-]$$

Where κ is a constant and α is the solubility coefficient for CO_2

Add measuring units:

$$[H^+] \text{ nmol/L} = 180 \times (PCO_2 \text{ kPa}/[HCO_3^-] \text{ mmol/L})$$

Hasselbach's transformation converts it to the more clinically friendly pH units:

$$pH = 6.1 + \log_{10} ([HCO_3^-]/\alpha PCO_2)$$

The final form of the equation known as the Henderson–Hasselbach (H–H) equation clearly illustrates the relative roles of the lung (CO_2) and kidney (HCO_3^-) in regulating plasma pH.

Urinary Buffers

The liver can metabolize organic acids, e.g. lactic and keto acids, into CO_2 + H_2O that can replace used HCO_3^-, but its main contribution is through production of glutamine from the metabolism of nitrogen-containing compounds. Glutamine is converted to ammonia (NH_3) in the kidney.

Ammonia is the most important urinary buffer. NH_3 provides a very high capacity buffer system that is protonated to ammonium (NH_4^+) and excreted as acid in the urine. The other major task of the kidney is to reabsorb very large amounts of filtered HCO_3^-.

As in CO_2 elimination by the lung, continuous renal excretion of ammonium massively increases the capacity of the ammonia buffer system to deal with very large acid loads.

Acid–Base Disorders

Assessment of acid–base disorders may be based on:

- HCO_3^-/CO_2 buffering (physiologic approach)
- Base excess
- Strong ion difference (physicochemical [Stewart] approach)

When interpreting arterial lood gas (ABG) results, the most common approach to quantifying acid–base disorders combines the physiologic approach with assessment of base excess. This approach is adequate for managing most everyday acid–base disorders.

The complexity of Stewart's equations has limited the clinical use of this approach but simplifying the equations has resulted in a resurgence of interest in the physicochemical approach. This approach is recommended for managing complex mixed acid–base disorders in critically ill patients.

Traditional Approach

Primary Acid–Base Disorder

Measuring $[H^+]$, PCO_2 and $[HCO_3^-]$ will indicate whether there is a primary metabolic or respiratory acidosis or alkalosis. Examining the change in PCO_2 in relation to $[HCO_3^-]$ will indicate whether there is a secondary (compensatory) change (Table 2.8.1).

Base Excess (BE)

BE is used to quantify the metabolic component of an acid–base disorder. It is defined as the amount of strong acid or base required to titrate 1 L of blood back to a pH of 7.4, while the PCO_2 is kept at 5.33kPa. BE is measured in mmol/L and is considered negative if base must be added (acidosis) and positive if acid is required. Base deficit has the opposite sign.

Standard BE (SBE) gives a better indication of the base excess of the entire extracellular fluid and is calculated assuming haemoglobin (Hb) of 50 g/L to reflect the average Hb across the extracellular space. SBE is a useful clinical

TABLE 2.8.1 Changes in PCO_2 and $[HCO_3^-]$ in Response to Acute and Chronic Acid–Base Disturbances[1]

Disorder	$[HCO_3^-]$ vs $PaCO_2$
Acute respiratory acidosis	$\Delta[HCO_3^-] = 0.2\ \Delta PaCO_2$
Chronic respiratory acidosis	$\Delta[HCO_3^-] = 0.5\ \Delta PaCO_2$
Acute respiratory alkalosis	$\Delta[HCO_3^-] = 0.2\ \Delta PaCO_2$
Chronic respiratory alkalosis	$\Delta[HCO_3^-] = 0.5\ \Delta PaCO_2$
Metabolic acidosis	$\Delta PaCO_2 = 1.3\ \Delta[HCO_3^-]$
Metabolic alkalosis	$\Delta PaCO_2 = 0.75\ \Delta[HCO_3^-]$

Notes: Δ, change in value; $[HCO_3^-]$, concentration of bicarbonate.

measure of metabolic acid–base status but it does not reveal anything about the underlying cause of the acid–base disorder.

Anion Gap (AG)

AG is a derived variable calculated from the difference between the primary measured cations (Na^+ and K^+) and the primary measured anions (Cl^- and HCO_3^-), but because $[K^+]$ is low usually it has little effect and AG is expressed as:

$$AG = [Na^+] - ([Cl^-] + [HCO_3^-])$$

The normal range for AG is 3–12 mmol/L.

Because a decrease in albumin of 1 g/dL results in a decrease in AG by 3, an albumin-corrected AG may be necessary:

$$\text{Albumin corrected AG} = AG + (0.25 \times [40\text{-measured albumin}])$$

Plasma electroneutrality means that any gap is the result of not measuring all plasma electrolytes. Unmeasured cations include Ca^{2+}, Mg^{2+} and immunoglobulins, whereas unmeasured anions include proteins, SO_4^{2-}, PO_4^{2-} and organic anions such as lactate and ketoacetate.

The most common cause of an increased AG is an increase in the unmeasured anions of non–chloride-containing acids, e.g. lactic acid, keto acids or decreased unmeasured cations. A decreased AG can result from hypercalcaemia, lithium administration or hypoalbuminaemia.[2]

Examining the degree of change of $[HCO_3^-]$ and AG is useful in classifying mixed acid–base disorders (Table 2.8.2).

Simplified Stewart's Approach

Combining BE with simplified equations from the physicochemical approach significantly improves the understanding and management of

TABLE 2.8.2 Changes in $[HCO_3^-]$ and AG as a Tool to Classify Metabolic Acidosis Disorders

Disorder	$[HCO_3^-]$ vs AG
Pure AG metabolic acidosis	$\Delta[HCO_3^-] = \Delta AG$
Mixed AG and non-AG acidosis	$\Delta[HCO_3^-] > \Delta AG$
Mixed metabolic acidosis and metabolic alkalosis	$\Delta[HCO_3^-] < \Delta AG$

Notes: Δ, change in value; $[HCO_3^-]$, concentration of bicarbonate; AG, anion gap.

the underlying pathophysiology of acid–base disorders in critically ill patients.[3]

The basic concept of Stewart's approach is that the main independent factors, which affect the acid–base status of water-based body fluids are not $[H^+]$ or $[HCO_3^-]$ but:

- Electrolytes (strong ions and the Na–Cl effect)
- CO_2
- Weak acids (mostly proteins, mainly albumin)

Strong ions are the completely dissociated plasma cations and anions that are routinely measured (Na^+, K^+, Mg^{2+}, Ca^{2+} and Cl^-, lactate$^-$). Normally there is an excess of measured cations over measured anions (strong ion difference; SID). This gap is filled by negatively charged CO_2 and weak acids to achieve electroneutrality of body fluids:

$$SID = (Na^+ + K^+ + Ca^{2+} \ 1 \ Mg^{2+}) - (Cl^- + lactate^-)$$

This gap is filled by negatively charged CO_2 and weak acids to achieve electroneutrality of body fluids:

$$SID - (CO_2 + A^-) = 0$$

Strong Ion Difference

As SID decreases (i.e. becomes less positive) more water dissociates releasing more H^+ to maintain electroneutrality. Another way of interpreting SID is to think of it as squeezing out HCO_3^-, so reduced SID suggest lower $[HCO_3^-]$ and the presence of an acid.

Na–Cl Effect

Chloride and sodium handling by the liver, kidney and gastrointestinal tract plays a predominant role in SID. The normal Na–Cl difference is 35 mmol/L (measured Na^+ – measured Cl^-) which translates to a Na–Cl base excess effect of −35.

Lactate

Lactate is the other strong ion that is important in clinical acid–base changes:

$$\text{Lactate base excess effect} = 1 - \text{measured lactate}$$

Albumin

Albumin is the main weak acid, and hypoalbuminaemia is a common cause of metabolic alkalosis in surgical and critical care patients. As the effect of albumin is based on its electric charge, its base excess effect is measured by the equation:

$$\text{Albumin base excess effect (mmol/L)} = 0.25 \times (42 - \text{measured albumin})$$

Table 2.8.3 lists the acidifying or alkalinizing effects of Stewart's independent variables.

Clinical Approach to Acid–Base Disorders

Proper interpretation of an ABG sample requires a good clinical history and complete physical examination and should be reviewed in conjunction with other laboratory investigations.

The following scheme may be helpful:

- pH: What is the dominant acid–base disturbance, acidosis or alkalosis?
- HCO_3^-/CO_2: Is it a primary metabolic or respiratory disorder with/without secondary compensatory changes?
- SBE: Quantify metabolic component.

AG is adequate for diagnosing most simple metabolic acid–base disorders but for mixed acid–base disorders the components of SBE should be quantified,

$$\text{SBE} = \text{Na–Cl effect} + \text{lactate effect} + \text{albumin effect} + \text{other ions (OI) effect}$$

where OI reflects the effects of other cations (K^+, Ca^{2+}), anions (protein, phosphate, lithium) and drugs.

TABLE 2.8.3 The Acidifying or Alkalinizing Effect of Stewart's Independent Variables

	Acidifying Effect	Alkalinizing Effect
CO_2	⇧	⇩
SID	⇩	⇧
Albumin	⇧	⇩
Phosphate	⇧	⇩

Metabolic Acidosis

Metabolic acidosis results in a negative base excess (i.e. a base deficit) and low standard bicarbonate.

Causes

Metabolic acidosis may occur due to an excess acid production, administration/ ingestion or under excretion. They are classified as normal AG acidosis (less common) and increased AG acidosis.

Normal AG Acidosis

- Acid under excretion – renal tubular acidosis, acetazolamide treatment
- Intestinal alkali loss – chronic diarrhoea, ileal conduit, ileostomy, colostomy, enteric fistula
- Hyperchloraemic acidosis – excessive normal saline administration

Increased AG Acidosis

Most commonly metabolic acidosis is secondary to acid overproduction:

- Lactic acidosis
  - Type A due to tissue hypoperfusion/hypoxia – shock, severe anaemia, hypoxaemia
  - Type B due to increase lactate production or decrease uptake and metabolism – liver failure, metformin, acute thiamine deficiency, large solid tumours, lymphoma or toxin related (ethanol, salicylate, ethylene glycol, methanol)
- Ketoacidosis – diabetic ketoacidosis, starvation and ethanol-induced

Keto acids do not elevate AG if kidney function is preserved. Functioning kidneys excrete the organic anion with Na^+, which results in a normal AG, hyperchloraemic acidosis.

Effects

- Increased respiration (stimulated via the peripheral chemoreceptors) – hyperventilation reduces PCO_2, which partially compensates for the acidosis
- Palpitations
- Nausea and vomiting
- Hyperkalaemia

Acute acidaemia suppresses cardiac contractility with decreased myocardial response to circulating catecholamines. Peripheral venous congestion shifts plasma volume to the pulmonary circulation and increases susceptibility to pulmonary congestion.

Right shift of the oxyhaemoglobin dissociation curve (OHD) facilitates oxygen offloading in the tissues.

Treatment

Treatment of metabolic acidosis is mainly of the primary cause.

Intravenous sodium bicarbonate to treat metabolic acidosis is controversial. Most studies suggest either no benefits or worse haemodynamics with bicarbonate. Occasionally, treatment with intravenous sodium bicarbonate is necessary, e.g. following reperfusion and cardiac arrest secondary to hyperkalaemia, tricyclic antidepressant overdose and pre-existing metabolic acidosis.

One common formula for the dose of bicarbonate is:

$$(\text{Base excess} \times \text{weight in kg})/3$$

The disadvantages of giving bicarbonate include:

- Increased CO_2 production causing intracellular acidosis and hyperventilation
- Hypocalcaemia
- Hypertonic hypernatraemia and fluid overload
- Hyperosmolarity
- Left shift of OHD curve with decreased oxygen availability in the tissues
- No evidence of improved outcome

Although giving bicarbonate improves blood pH and plasma $[HCO_3^-]$, the underlying process of increased lactate production continues.

Metabolic Alkalosis

Metabolic alkalosis results in positive base excess and high standard bicarbonate. It is the most common clinical acid–base disorder.

Causes

Chloride depletion leads to alkalosis by increasing renal bicarbonate reabsorption.

Potassium depletion leads to alkalosis by increasing renal H^+ secretion. Although alkalosis itself causes hypokalaemia as it favours intracellular movement of K^+, hypokalaemia can lead to hypochloraemia by reducing renal Cl^- reabsorption.

Contraction of extracellular volume is common with metabolic alkalosis as hypovolaemia is associated with reduced glomerular filtration rate (GFR) and in turn reduced bicarbonate filtration and excretion.

Metabolic alkalosis may occur following:

- Chloride depletion
- Gastrointestinal or other nonrenal losses – pyloric stenosis, vomiting, nasogastric drainage, cystic fibrosis
- Renal loss – diuretics (loop, thiazide), genetic disorders, e.g. Bartter syndrome
- Isolated potassium depletion – laxative abuse

- Ingestion of large amounts of bicarbonate or its precursors – citrate drinks, milk–alkali syndrome
- Mineralocorticoid excess
  - Cushing syndrome
  - Primary aldosteronism
  - Renin-secreting tumours
  - Fludrocortisone, prednisolone

Effects

In metabolic alkalosis the body compensates by hypoventilation and increased renal bicarbonate excretion. The consequences of metabolic alkalosis on organ systems depend on the severity of the alkalaemia and the degree of respiratory compensation and include:

- Reduced oxygen delivery due to alkalaemia may be worsened by a compensatory hypoventilation to elevate PCO_2
- Arrhythmias
- Muscle weakness
- Renal potassium and magnesium loss that may be symptomatic
- Reduced ionized calcium
- Stimulating phosphofructokinase, so increasing lactate production

With moderate alkalosis, symptoms are due to intravascular volume depletion or hypokalaemia.

Rarely, severe alkalaemia can lead to agitation, stupor and coma.

Treatment

Treatment of metabolic alkalosis is mainly of the primary cause, but potassium and magnesium will need to be replaced and serum levels closely monitored. Dilute hydrochloric acid can be given orally or intravenously. Acetazolamide may be considered.

Respiratory Acidosis

Respiratory acidosis is caused by inadequate alveolar ventilation with a consequent increase in PCO_2.

Causes

Hypercarbia is common in anaesthesia and intensive care practice and is usually well tolerated. Common causes of respiratory acidosis include:

- Increased CO_2 production – strenuous physical activity, shivering, fever, hyperthyroidism, prolonged seizure
- Inhibition of medullary respiratory centre
  - Drugs – sedatives, narcotics, anaesthetics
  - Central sleep apnoea

- Extreme obesity
- Metabolic alkalosis
- Patients with chronic hypercapnia when given high flow oxygen in whom hypoxia serves as an important stimulant of respiratory drive
- Disorders in respiratory muscles and chest wall– myasthenia gravis, Guillain–Barré syndrome, extreme obesity, kyphoscoliosis
- Upper airway obstruction – foreign body, laryngospasm, obstructive sleep apnoea
- Abnormal gas exchange across the pulmonary capillaries, either acute, e.g. acute pulmonary oedema, severe asthma, or chronic, e.g. chronic obstructive pulmonary disease, extreme obesity

Effects

Acute respiratory acidosis is typically more symptomatic than acute metabolic acidosis due to the ease with which CO_2 diffuse across the blood–brain barrier. Acute changes produce far more manifestations than chronic carbon dioxide retention, as follows:

- Central nervous system (hypercapnic encephalopathy) – cerebral vasodilatation and increased intracranial pressure; headache. As the PCO_2 rises towards 25 kPa, narcosis deepens into coma, and over 25 kPa there is a profound narcosis and respiratory failure resembling curarization. If the hypercapnia is chronic the cerebrospinal fluid (CSF) bicarbonate rises, restores the CSF pH and so sets a new baseline for cerebral vascular resistance.
- Autonomic nervous system – sympathetic activation, with a rise of circulating catecholamines and sweating. Any parasympathetic activation is overshadowed by the sympathetic effect.
- Respiratory system – carbon dioxide stimulates the respiratory centre. There is right shift of the oxyhaemoglobin dissociation curve, the Bohr effect, via an increase in hydrogen ions, which facilitates oxygen release in the tissues.
- Cardiovascular system – increased rate and force of contraction, and vasodilatation due to direct effect of carbon dioxide on the blood vessels, increases cardiac output. There is sympathetic stimulation and increased circulating catecholamine; blood pressure often rises. Arrhythmias may occur, particularly during halothane anaesthesia. Severe hypercapnia can suppress myocardial contractility. A direct peripheral effect leads to vasodilatation, with flushed skin and distended veins.

Treatment

Respiratory acidosis is treated by increasing alveolar ventilation with or without reducing carbon dioxide production.

In cases of severe hypercapnia and severe acidosis, assisted ventilation should be initiated promptly.

Recovery from severe respiratory acidosis may be associated with hypophosphataemia, so this should be monitored carefully.

If the PCO_2 is reduced too rapidly after a long period of hypercapnia there may be:

- Sudden hypotension
- A left shift of the haemoglobin dissociation curve
- A rapid rise in CSF pH leading to cerebral vasoconstriction and convulsions

For patients with chronic respiratory acidosis in whom hypoxaemia is important in driving ventilation, so long as PO_2 does not exceed 8 kPa, the hypoxic drive remains functional. In these patients, care should be taken to carefully lower the PCO_2 as there is a risk of overshoot. This process of posthypercapnoeic metabolic alkalosis can be corrected with normal saline, discontinuation of loop diuretics. Acetazolamide may be required in oedematous patients with heart failure.

Respiratory Alkalosis

Respiratory alkalosis is caused by hyperventilation, producing hypocapnia and a rise in pH.

Causes

Increase in alveolar ventilation relative to CO_2 production:

- Hypoxaemia – high altitude, pulmonary disease
- Pulmonary disorders – pneumonia, interstitial pneumonitis, pulmonary oedema, pulmonary embolism, pneumothorax, bronchial asthma
- Cardiovascular – congestive heart failure, hypotension
- Metabolic – acidosis, liver failure
- Central nervous system – anxiety, psychogenic hyperventilation, CNS infection, CNS tumours, severe head injury
- Drugs – salicylates, β-adrenergic agonists, methylxanthines
- Miscellaneous – fever, sepsis, pain and pregnancy

Effects

Effects of respiratory alkalosis are as follows:

- Nervous system – cerebral vasoconstriction and reduced cerebral blood flow, clouding of consciousness and analgesia, voluntary hyperventilation lessens, tetany due to the fall in ionized calcium
- Cardiovascular system – peripheral vasoconstriction, but fall of blood pressure and cardiac output; coronary vasoconstriction
- Respiratory system – lack of stimulation of the respiratory centre may lead to hypoventilation; left shift of the haemoglobin dissociation curve

- Pregnancy – hyperventilation causes a reduction in uteroplacental blood flow that, with the left-shifted haemoglobin dissociation curve, causes a fall in fetal oxygen supply and acidosis

Treatment

Respiratory alkalosis is managed by treating the underlying cause and by a decrease in alveolar ventilation.

ELECTROLYTE BALANCE

Sodium

Normal serum level is 138–142 mmol/L, and the daily maintenance requirement is 1.0 mmol/kg. Most sodium is extracellular; normal intracellular concentration is 10 mmol/L.

Hyponatraemia

A relative excess of water to plasma electrolytes is usually noted by the presence of hyponatraemia and a fall in plasma osmolality. The incidence of postoperative hyponatraemia is reported to be approximately 1% and when severe (Na < 125 mmol/L with neurological symptoms) is a medical emergency.

The endocrine stress response to surgery or trauma increases plasma antidiuretic hormone (ADH) and impairs free water excretion (also seen with administration of oxytocin), which leads to an inappropriately high urine osmolality in the face of a low plasma osmolality. Osmolality (normal 280–290 mOsmol/L) is calculated as:

$$2 \times [Na^+] + [urea] + [glucose]$$

Causes

An assessment of volume status and total body water should be attempted and the urine sodium concentration, and plasma osmolality (calculated and measured), should be determined. An increase in the plasma calculated to measured osmolar gap suggests the presence of unmeasured substances such as alcohol or mannitol. Pseudohyponatraemia may be seen with severe hyperlipidaemia/hyperproteinaemia.

The causes of hyponatraemia in hypovolaemic, euvolaemic and hypervolaemic patients are given in Box 2.8.1.

Effects

The effects of hyponatraemia relate to the speed at which it develops, as well as the absolute degree. Anorexia and vomiting occur first, but then neuropsychiatric effects predominate when sodium is below 125 mmol/L. There is brain swelling with lassitude, apathy, confusion, weakness and eventually peripheral circulatory failure. In chronic hyponatraemia, compensatory mechanisms such as loss of solutes from the brain lead to a decrease in brain swelling.

BOX 2.8.1 Causes of Hyponatraemia in Hypovolaemic, Euvolaemic and Hypervolaemic Patients

Hypovolaemic patient
Extrarenal salt loss
Vomiting, diarrhoea, intestinal fistulae
Unrecognized losses in burns, pancreatitis or bowel obstruction (third space)
Renal salt loss
Diuretics including osmotic effect
Mineralocorticoid deficiency
Salt-losing nephropathy

Euvolaemic patient
Water excess
Intravenous hypotonic solutions
Primary polydipsia
Fluid absorption during transurethral resection of prostate (TURP) or endometrial surgery
Associated factors
Glucocorticoid deficiency
Syndrome of inappropriate antidiuretic hormone secretion (SIADH)
Hypothyroidism
Drugs (e.g. antipsychotics)

Hypervolaemic patient
Nephrotic syndrome
Cirrhosis
Heart failure
Acute or chronic renal failure

Treatment

Rapid correction of hyponatraemia, especially if chronic, may lead to central pontine myelinolysis (osmotic demyelination syndrome), which is a life-threatening neurologic emergency.

The management of acute severe symptomatic hyponatraemia should be in an environment that allows careful monitoring and measurement of electrolytes every hour.

In hypovolaemic patients ADH will be high, so first resuscitate with isotonic fluids.

Treatment of hyponatraemia is as follows:

● Treat the primary cause
● Stop any implicated drug therapy
● Water restriction
● For acute symptomatic hyponatraemia, hypertonic saline (1.8%) is given to raise the sodium by 1–2 mmol/L/h

- Loop diuretic to increase free water clearance
- In chronic and asymptomatic hyponatraemia, the rate of increase should be no more than 1 mmol/L/h

Hypernatraemia

Hypernatraemia results from increased total body Na^+ or decreased total body water.

An assessment of volume status and total body water should be attempted and the urine sodium concentration, and plasma osmolality (calculated and measured), should be determined.

Causes

The causes of hypernatraemia in hypovolaemic, euvolaemic and hypervolaemic patients are given in Box 2.8.2.

Effects

Intense thirst is prominent in hypernatraemia, but there is unlikely to be any oedema. Central nervous system symptoms predominate, with confusion, apathy, hyperreflexia and eventually coma.

BOX 2.8.2 Causes of Hypernatraemia in Hypovolaemic, Euvolaemic and Hypervolaemic Patients

Hypovolaemic patient
Extrarenal losses of more water than salt
Excessive sweating
Burns, diarrhoea, intestinal fistulae
Renal loss of more water than salt
Diuretics including osmotic effect
Renal disease
Postobstruction diuresis

Euvolaemic patient
Excess water loss
Diabetes insipidus
    Neurogenic (e.g. head injury)
    Nephrogenic (e.g. congenital or acquired [e.g. severe hypokalaemia])
    Drug induced (e.g. amphotericin B, demeclocycline or lithium)

Hypervolaemic patient
Excess sodium administration
High sodium-containing fluids (e.g. hypertonic saline, sodium bicarbonate)
Inappropriate replacement of daily insensible losses with high-sodium fluids
Inability to excrete sodium
Primary hyperaldosteronism
Cushing syndrome or high-dose corticosteroid therapy

Treatment

As with hyponatraemia, the speed of correction of the high sodium depends on the degree and acuity of the hypernatraemia. The generation of 'idiogenic osmoles' in the brain in chronic hypernatraemia increases the risk of acute brain swelling if the plasma osmolality is decreased too quickly. In hypovolaemic patients, water deficit should be restored first. Treatment of hypernatraemia is as follows:

- Treat the primary cause – consider desmopressin for diabetes insipidus, and review drug therapy, especially diuretics
- Withhold sodium-containing fluids
- Administer water by the enteral route or hypotonic fluids intravenously
- Furosemide (frusemide) or dialysis may be needed if hypervolaemic
- The rate of decrease in plasma sodium should be no more than 1 mmol/L/h

Potassium

Normal serum potassium level is 3.5–5.0 mmol/L. The daily maintenance requirement is 1.0 mmol/kg or 5–7 mmol/g nitrogen, with a higher requirement if severely malnourished. Most potassium is intracellular, with about 2% in the extracellular compartment, and only 0.4% in the serum. Normal intracellular concentration is 150 mmol/L. Maintenance of the normal ratio of ECF $[K^+]$ to ICF $[K^+]$ is vital for proper function of all excitable tissue.

Hypokalaemia

Causes

Causes of hypokalaemia are as follows:

- Inadequate intake, especially when reliant on intravenous therapy
- Excessive loss from the gastrointestinal tract – vomiting, diarrhoea, fistulae, etc.
- Excessive loss in the urine – diuretics, aminophylline overdose, renal tubular acidosis, etc.
- Hyperadrenal states or intensive steroid therapy
- Catecholamine-induced shift of potassium into cells, e.g. intravenous salbutamol
- Alkalosis – causes potassium to move into cells
- Insulinoma – drives potassium into cells
- Familial periodic paralysis
- Hypomagnesaemia

Effects

Hypokalaemia results in a clinical picture of lethargy, apathy, anorexia and nausea related to disordered function of the three types of muscles:

- Smooth muscle – resulting in constipation, distension and ileus.
- Skeletal muscle – resulting in hypotonia, weakness and paralysis.

- Cardiac muscle – resulting in hypotension, arrhythmias and cardiac arrest, in which case the ECG shows ST segment depression, lowering, widening or inversion of T waves, prolongation of PR and QT intervals and the appearance of U waves. Hypokalaemia increases the risk of digoxin toxicity.
- Hypokalaemia leads to metabolic alkalosis that can only be treated with K^+ repletion.

Treatment

- If there are life-threatening arrhythmias, a small slow intravenous bolus dose of potassium may be needed, 5 mmol over 60 s with ECG monitoring and repeated as necessary.
- Replace the expected deficit, either orally or intravenously; the deficit may be in the order of 200 mmol or more. Only dilute solutions are given peripherally, no more than 40 mmol/L because of pain and thrombosis.
- The recommended maximum replacement rate of 20 mmol/h can be exceeded under close monitoring, if clinically indicated.
- Potassium administration may not increase intracellular potassium concentration in the presence of magnesium deficiency, treat any coexisting magnesium deficiency.
- The correction of hypokalaemia with potassium chloride will correct any concurrent metabolic alkalosis.
- In renal tubular acidosis potassium hydroxide will ameliorate the metabolic acidosis.
- Surgery may have to be delayed if the serum potassium is below 3.0 mmol/L because of the risk of cardiac arrhythmias, muscle weakness, inability to reverse muscle relaxants, myopathy and renal failure.

Hyperkalaemia

Hyperkalaemia is dangerous, chiefly because of its effects on the heart. Acute changes are more dangerous than chronic changes. Severe hyperkalaemia ($K^+ > 6.5$ mmol/L) requires urgent treatment.

Causes

Causes of hyperkalaemia are as follows:

- Excessive administration – usually intravenously, but may occur with commercial salt substitutes.
- Renal failure.
- Trans-cellular shift of K^+ from cells to ECF:
  - Administration of suxamethonium – the hyperkalaemia occurs within minutes and may be up to 1.0 mmol/L in normal patients but is often much higher in patients with trauma and burns, muscle injury or diseases such as myopathies, motor neurone disease, muscular dystrophy, denervation and spinal cord transection and tetanus. The hyperkalaemia may be ameliorated by pretreatment with a nondepolarizing agent.

- Cell lysis, e.g. rhabdomyolysis, massive haemolysis.
- Hyperkalaemic periodic paralysis.
- Metabolic acidosis, including diabetic ketosis.
- Massive blood transfusion − stored blood may contain 25 mmol/L potassium.
- Drugs − potassium-sparing diuretics, angiotensin-converting enzyme (ACE) inhibitors, angiotensin receptor blockers and nonsteroidal anti-inflammatory drugs (NSAIDs), β blockers, heparin, digoxin.
- Hypoaldosteronism decreases K^+ renal secretion, e.g. Addison disease, spironolactone, NSAIDs.

Effects

Toxic manifestations of hyperkalaemia may occur at concentrations above 7.0 mmol/L, when the ECG shows peaking of the T wave, ST depression, absence of the P wave, widening of the QRS and finally a biphasic QRST. Ventricular fibrillation may supervene.

Treatment

Treatment of hyperkalaemia is as follows:

- Stop further administration or precipitating factors
- Protect the heart by administering calcium 5 mmol intravenously
- Decrease extracellular K^+:
  - Increase ECF volume with fluids
  - Increase cellular uptake of potassium by administering 5–15 units of insulin plus 25 g of dextrose (50 mL of 50%; glucose and insulin), as appropriate for the patient, with sodium bicarbonate 1 mmol/kg over 15 min; β_2-agonists such as salbutamol (albuterol) by inhalation (avoid in patients with ischaemic heart disease) may also be effective
- Remove K^+ from the body:
  - Loop diuretic
  - Cation exchange resin − give 15 g 6-hourly orally or 30 g as a retention enema
  - Dialysis

Calcium

The normal serum level of calcium is 2.1–2.6 mmol/L; the daily maintenance requirement is 0.2 mmol/kg. Calcium binding to albumin is pH dependent and the ionized level is the active fraction, so it is more appropriate to measure this fraction, which is normally 1.15–1.25 mmol/L.

Serum calcium plays a major role in biologic processes like bone mineralization, blood clotting and neuromuscular excitability. Intracellular calcium is important in physiologic processes like muscle contraction, nerve conduction, hormone secretion, cell proliferation and mobility.

Hypocalcaemia

Total calcium corrected for albumin is > 2.5 mmol/L and ionized calcium > 1.4 mmol/L.

Causes

Causes of hypocalcaemia are as follows:

● Postoperative hypoparathyroidism
● Alkalosis – usually due to acute hyperventilation
● Acute pancreatitis – associated with fat necrosis
● Acute hyperphosphataemia – tumour lysis syndrome, crush injury
● Transfusion with citrated blood – rarely requires treatment
● Vitamin D deficiency/resistance
● Chronic renal failure due to chronic hyperphosphataemia and reduced renal mass

Effects

The symptoms of hypocalcaemia correlate with the rate and magnitude of the fall in serum calcium. Neuromuscular irritability leads to circumoral and distal paraesthesia, muscle cramps, laryngospasm, tetany and seizures. Hypocalcaemia results in a long QT interval, bradycardia, hypotension and congestive cardiac failure.

Treatment

Treatment of hypocalcaemia is as follows:

● Oral or intravenous calcium and correction of any concurrent hypomagnesaemia. Patients with hypoparathyroidism do not respond to vitamin D till hypomagnesaemia is corrected. Calcium is irritant to veins and can cause tissue damage if extravasation occurs.
● Treating any acidosis will cause the ionized calcium to fall further, so defer this until the hypocalcaemia is corrected.
● Dialysis against high calcium and bicarbonate dialysate will correct both hypocalcaemia and acidosis.
● Further treatment will depend on the underlying cause, but may include vitamin D analogues, phosphate binders and parathyroidectomy.

Note that calcium and bicarbonate solutions must not mix in the giving set.

Hypercalcaemia

Causes

Hypercalcaemia may be genetic or associated with malignancy, primary hyperparathyroidism, secondary hyperparathyroidism associated with chronic renal failure, thiazide diuretics, immobilization, sarcoid, excessive vitamin D and the milk–alkali syndrome.

Effects

Symptoms of hypercalcaemia correlate with the rate and magnitude of increase in serum calcium. Above 3.0 mmol/L nausea, vomiting, constipation, polyuria and polydipsia are common; peptic ulcers may occur. Higher levels lead to confusion, coma and death. The ECG shows a short QT interval; the toxicity of digoxin is enhanced.

Treatment

Treatment of hypercalcaemia is as follows:

- Treat or remove any obvious cause.
- Those with symptomatic, moderate or severe hypercalcaemia should be well hydrated.
- Consider furosemide (frusemide) to enhance urinary calcium loss (the opposite occurs with thiazide diuretics).
- Those with primary hyperparathyroidism may need urgent surgery when stabilized.
- Further treatment involves bisphosphonates to reduce bone resorption, although precipitated calcium biphosphate may lead to renal insufficiency.
- In very severe cases calcitonin may be considered.
- Corticosteroids may be useful in malignancy or sarcoidosis.
- Haemodialysis against a low-calcium dialysate can be used for dialysis-dependent patients.

Magnesium

The normal serum level of magnesium is 0.8–1.0 mmol/L; the daily maintenance requirement is 0.2 mmol/kg or 1 mmol/g nitrogen.

Hypomagnesaemia

Causes

Causes of hypomagnesaemia are as follows:

- Serum magnesium levels frequently fall in ill patients.
- Gastrointestinal losses – gastric aspiration, diarrhoea, malabsorption.
- Renal losses – vigorous fluid therapy, diuretics, alcohol, aminoglycosides, cardiac glycosides, amphotericin and cisplatin, phosphate depletion and cardiopulmonary bypass.

Effects

Effects of hypomagnesaemia are as follows:

- Magnesium is a cofactor in various cellular enzymes – insufficient activation of Na^+/K^+-ATPase reduces intracellular potassium concentration.

- Chronic hypomagnesaemia leads to hypocalcaemia by inhibiting parathyroid hormone.
- Neuromuscular – paraesthesia, muscle twitching, tremor, cramps, tetany.
- Neuropsychiatric – apathy, depression, hallucinations and coma.
- Cardiovascular – arrhythmias, prolonged QT interval, hypertension.

Treatment

Treatment of hypomagnesaemia is routine replacement of 40 mmol/day, preferably by the oral route, although magnesium sulphate is cathartic. Therapeutic infusions may be larger and more rapid, but hypotension may occur because magnesium is a direct-acting vasodilator.

Hypermagnesaemia

Causes

Hypermagnesaemia results from excessive administration, either intravenously or by mouth, especially in those with renal impairment.

Hypermagnesaemia may be associated with a reduced inability to excrete magnesium and calcium via the kidney and a hypokalaemic alkalosis.

High levels of magnesium (1.5–4.0 mmol/L) have been used therapeutically in many conditions including pre-eclampsia, cardiac arrhythmias and asthma.

Effects

Above 2 mmol/L hypermagnesaemia causes nausea, flushing and reduced deep tendon reflexes. When levels are over 3 mmol/L there is drowsiness, decreased muscle tone, hypotension and bradycardia. Levels over 5 mmol/L lead to paralysis of voluntary muscle and respiratory depression; eventually there is cardiopulmonary arrest.

Treatment

To treat hypermagnesaemia, stop administration of magnesium. In severe cases, 5 mmol of intravenous calcium is given as necessary. Haemodialysis may be needed.

Phosphate

The normal serum level of phosphate is 0.9–1.4 mmol/L. The maintenance requirement is 0.3 mmol/kg (less if in renal failure and more if very catabolic).

Hypophosphataemia

A low serum phosphate is common in critically ill patients.

Causes

Causes of hypophosphataemia are as follows:

- Poor nutrition – chronic alcoholism, poor feeding in hospital
- Malabsorption – chelating antacids, diarrhoea, vitamin D deficiency

- Uptake of phosphate into cells – β_2 agonists, insulin and alkalosis
- Excessive renal loss – acetazolamide, acidosis, hyperparathyroidism and loss during haemodialysis

Effects

Hypophosphataemia results in paraesthesia, confusion and eventual metabolic encephalopathy with coma. Muscle weakness may lead to respiratory failure or failure to wean from mechanical ventilation. Dysphagia and ileus may occur. The oxygen dissociation curve shifts to the left, which may hinder offloading of oxygen in the tissues.

Treatment

To treat hypophosphataemia phosphate is best administered orally as effervescent tablets containing 16 mmol. Rapid or large infusions are dangerous, but in severe cases regimens have been described as high as 20 mmol over 12 h; it should not be mixed with calcium or magnesium for injection. Phosphate levels should be monitored at least daily.

Hyperphosphataemia

Causes

Causes of hyperphosphataemia are as follows:

- Excessive administration – oral or intravenous supplements, vitamin D poisoning
- Increased endogenous load – tumour lysis syndrome, rhabdomyolysis
- Reduced excretion – renal failure, hypoparathyroidism, sickle cell disease

Effects

Hyperphosphataemia results in hypocalcaemia and tetany if the increase is acute. Metastatic calcification occurs if the product of the serum Ca^{2+} and PO_4^{3-} exceeds 70.

Treatment

To treat hyperphosphataemia stop administration, reduce absorption with phosphate-binding salts (not aluminium based in renal failure) and increase renal excretion of phosphate with volume expansion and acetazolamide.

REFERENCES

1. Badr A, Nightingale P. An alternative approach to acid-base abnormalities in critically ill patients. Continuing Education in Anaesthesia. Critical Care & Pain 2007;7:107–11.
2. Berend K, de Vries A, Grans R. Physiologic approach to assessment of acid-base disturbances. N Engl J Med 2014;371:1434–45.
3. Story D. Stewart acid-base: a simplified bedside approach. Anesth Analg 2016;123:511–15.

FURTHER READING

Severinghaus J, Astrup P. History of blood gas analysis. II. pH and acid-base balance measurements. J Clin Monit 1985;1:259–77.

Michael R, Moe W, Moe O. Core concepts and treatment of metabolic acidosis. In: Mount DB, Sayegh MH, Singh AK, editors. Core concepts in the disorders of fluid, electrolytes and acid-base balance. New York: Springer; 2013.

Chapter 2.9

Nutrition

Matthew Jackson

ASSESSMENT OF NUTRITIONAL STATUS

Malnutrition is common in hospitalized patients and occurs when there is a negative balance between nutritional supply and demand. It is poorly recognized and inadequately treated. Malnutrition is associated with an increased morbidity and mortality during hospital admission. A clinical assessment of nutritional status is outlined in Box 2.9.1. Many hospitals use a formal standardized assessment, such as the malnutrition universal screening tool (MUST).[1]

NUTRITIONAL REQUIREMENTS

Nutritional requirement varies according to clinical condition. Typical energy requirements fall within the range of 105–147 kJ/kg/day (25–35 kcal/kg/day). Approximate nutritional requirements are given in Table 2.9.1.

A number of formulae and tables can be used to calculate patient energy requirement under specific clinical conditions (Fig. 2.9.1). Energy requirements can be more accurately assessed using bedside indirect calorimetry, which determines $\dot{V}O_2$, $\dot{V}CO_2$ and respiratory quotient (RQ). Direct measurement is the gold standard, but rarely performed in clinical practice.

NUTRITIONAL SUPPORT AND ARTIFICIAL FEEDING

Nutritional support includes any dietetic formulation intended to meet predicted nutritional requirements; it can be given orally or via an enteral tube or venous catheter.

Indications

Indications for nutritional support include:[2]

- Body mass index (BMI) less than 18.5 kg/m^2
- Unintentional weight loss of over 10% body weight over 3–6 months
- Poor nutritional intake for over 5 days
- Predicted poor nutritional intake over next 5 days

BOX 2.9.1 Clinical Assessment of Nutritional Status

History of associated disease, e.g. alcoholism, inflammatory bowel disease
Dietary history
Present problem, e.g. burns, trauma, sepsis
Recent severe weight loss – body mass index (BMI) < 20 kg/m^2
Signs of malnutrition, e.g. muscle wasting
Simple measurements of body composition such as:

- Mid-triceps skinfold thickness – indicates fat stores
- Mid-arm muscle circumference – indicates muscle mass
- Muscle ultrasound and bioelectrical impedance analysis. But limited usefulness in seriously ill patients due to the presence of oedema, etc

Biochemical markers:

- Albumin – a poor marker because of its long half-life
- Proteins with a rapid turnover, e.g. transferrin, retinol-binding protein fibronectin – there is normally a turnover of some 100 g of protein per day

---

Source: Adapted from 'Malnutrition Universal Screening Tool' ('MUST') for adults. Available at http://www.bapen.org.uk/pdfs/must/must_full.pdf

TABLE 2.9.1 Daily Nutritional Requirements

	Requirement per kg Body Weight	Requirement for 70 kg Man
Water	30–35 mL	2100–2500 mL (lower range in the elderly)
Sodium	1.0 mmol	60–100 mmol
Potassium	1.0 mmol	50–100 mmol
Phosphate	0.3 mmol	25 mmol
Calcium	0.2 mmol	20 mmol
Magnesium	0.2 mmol	12 mmol
Protein	1 g	70 g
Nitrogen	0.15–0.2 g	10–14 g
Carbohydrate	2 g	140 g
Fat	1–2 g	140 g
Calories	125 kJ (25–35 kcal)	8750 kJ (2100 kcal)

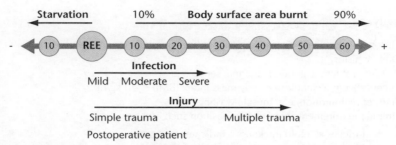

FIGURE 2.9.1   Nomogram for metabolic rate adjustment. REE, resting energy expenditure.

Clinical indications for artificial feeding include:

● Gastrointestinal failure – paralytic ileus, multiple fistulae or blind loops
● Catabolic state – major surgery, trauma, burns, sepsis
● Inability to feed – coma

Aims

Feeding aims to provide:

● Calories in the form of carbohydrate and fat because this is optimal for protein anabolism and provision of essential fatty acids
● Protein to provide essential amino acids and nitrogen so reducing muscle breakdown
● Water and electrolytes
● Trace elements and vitamins

Daily Requirements

Carbohydrate

Body stores of carbohydrate are limited, the average adult having only 5 g of blood glucose and 100 g of liver glycogen. Adequate carbohydrate is needed to allow fat utilization without ketosis, the minimum for this being 1.7 MJ (400 kcal) of carbohydrate energy per day, although normally at least 50% of the administered calories are from glucose.

Glucose provides 17 kJ (4.0 kcal)/g; 1 L of isotonic (5%) solution provides only 840 kJ (200 kcal), so concentrated solutions are needed to give enough calories without overhydration. In parenteral nutrition (PN) and separate infusions, 25% and 50% glucose are commonly used, respectively, and these solutions require a central vein for administration.

The metabolic response to surgery, sepsis or trauma includes an increase in energy expenditure and impaired glucose tolerance, but insulin does not often need to be given if less than 500 g glucose is given per day. If needed it may be given intravenously by infusion, normally about 1 unit per 4 g glucose infused, ideally to keep the blood sugar normal. There is good evidence of improved outcome from intensive care when blood glucose is kept at less than 10.0 mmol/L.[3]

Fat

Fat provides 38 kJ (9.0 kcal)/g. Advantages include iso-osmolarity and neutral pH (it can be given into a peripheral vein). No losses occur in the faeces or urine in health.

Fat is provided as a 10% or 20% soya oil emulsion, with particle diameters 0.2–1.0 microns, as similar size as a chylomicron. The surfactant is egg phospholipid, glycerol is added to make the solution isotonic and 500 mL of 20% emulsion provides 4.2 MJ (1000 kcal). This also provides essential fatty acids.

Excessive milkiness of serum calls for a reduction in fat intake. This is more likely in liver insufficiency, acute pancreatitis, uraemia and septicaemia. Occasional side-effects are shivering, flushing and fever.

Patients receiving infusions of propofol for sedation may receive a considerable proportion of their daily fat requirements by this route (4.6 kJ/mL; 1.1 kcal/mL). This should be considered when planning a parenteral feeding regimen; serum lipids should be checked periodically.

There is a theoretical benefit from a high fat, low carbohydrate feeds in patients with a severe limitation of ventilatory reserve as less carbon dioxide is produced than with carbohydrate (RQ 0.71 vs. 1.0).

Protein

Protein can theoretically supply 17 kJ/g (4 kcal/g). It is convention when calculating energy content of artificial nutrition to count only nonprotein calories. Protein is administered to provide the body with nitrogen.

Protein intake should be 0.8–1.5 g/kg/day (0.13–0.24 g nitrogen/kg/day). Nitrogen excretion in critical illness can exceed 20 g/day, which represents the breakdown of 125 g of protein or 600 g of muscle. This can be estimated from urea and protein loss in the urine and any rise in total body urea plus an estimate of losses from skin and stool. In practice, these calculations are rarely done.

For enteral feeding standard polymeric solutions are used that do not contain gluten or lactose. These solutions contain long-chain triglycerides and may also contain fibre. Elemental and semi-elemental feeds are also available that contain amino acids or peptides, glucose or oligosaccharides, and medium-chain triglycerides.

For parenteral feeding, a mixture of essential and nonessential crystalline amino acids is given in the physiological laevorotatory form. Solutions with higher proportions of branched-chain amino acids have no real advantage. Most solutions are hyperosmolar and acidic and must be given in central veins. Less irritant solutions designed for peripheral are only suitable for short-term use.

Micronutrients

Many micronutrients are conveniently provided by commercial additive preparations, although others are given individually (e.g. vitamin B_{12}) or in much higher doses according to the clinical circumstances (e.g. folate). The B vitamins and vitamins A and C degrade when exposed to light (Table 2.9.2).

Introducing Nutritional Support

Patients who have had minimal nutritional intake for over 5 days have a caloric deficit, but are at risk refeeding syndrome if feeding is started at full caloric load. The syndrome is characterized by electrolyte and fluid shifts; it can be life threatening. To avoid these risks, nutrition should be started at no more than

TABLE 2.9.2 Parenteral Daily Requirements of Vitamins and Minerals

Nutrient	Parenteral Daily Requirement
Biotin	60 µg
Folate	0.2–0.4 mg
Niacin	40 mg
Pantothenic acid	10–20 mg
Vitamin A	1–2.5 mg
Vitamin B_1 (Thiamine)	3–20 mg
Vitamin B_2 (Riboflavin)	3–8 mg
Vitamin B_6 (Pyridoxine)	4–6 mg
Vitamin B_{12}	5–15 µg
Vitamin C	100 mg
Vitamin D	5 µg
Vitamin E	10 mg
Vitamin K	1.0 µg/kg
Chromium	0.2–0.4 µmol
Copper	20 µmol
Fluoride	50 µmol
Iodine	1 µmol
Iron	20–70 µmol
Manganese	5–10 µmol
Molybdenum	0.2–1.2 µmol
Selenium	0.25–0.5 µmol
Zinc	100 µmol

half of the estimated requirement and slowly titrated to target over 1–2 days, as tolerated. High dose vitamins should be given and serum electrolytes, including phosphate and magnesium, monitored regularly.

Critically ill patients are catabolic. Paradoxically they are less able to absorb and use artificially delivered nutrition.

Choice of Feeding Route

The choice of feeding route is dependent upon the clinical situation. When available, the oral route is preferred to enteral feeding; parenteral feeding is the third choice. An alternative route should be considered when the chosen route is not meeting the patient's nutritional requirements. Current international guidance and clinical trials offer subtlety conflicting frameworks as to how quickly feeding routes should be changed to achieve these goals.[2,4]

Oral Supplements

Oral supplements are used in patients who can tolerate oral feeding, but are unable to meet their nutritional requirements with ordinary food. Supplements are presented as high calorie drinks or powders which are mixed into food. To achieve their aim, supplements should be pleasant to consume. Steroids are occasionally used to stimulate a poor appetite.

Enteral Feeding

Most enteral feeds provide 4.2 kJ/mL (1 kcal/mL). They are used when the patient has a viable alimentary tract but the oral route is either insufficient or unsafe. Contraindications to enteral feeding include severe gut pathology (e.g. generalized peritonitis, ischaemia and severe shock), but in general enteral feeding is the preferred route if the gut is functioning at all because it is less costly, more effective and less hazardous than intravenous nutrition. Also, gut integrity and function are enhanced.

Some nutrients, such as glutamine, short-chain fatty acids and polyunsaturated fatty acids, may be trophic to the gut and be of particular benefit to septic patients. Glutamine is central to protein synthesis and the function of enterocytes and the immune system. During critical illness, glutamine becomes a conditionally essential amino acid and the demand has to be met by skeletal muscle breakdown. There is some evidence in a number of critical illnesses that glutamine supplementation may improve outcome, but universal use is not recommended.[5] There is continued interest in immunomodulating feeds.

Confirmation that a tube is in the stomach is achieved by detecting a pH of 5.5 or below using indicator strips; use of proton-pump inhibitor medication can cause aspirates to be less acidic. Insufflating air down the nasogastric tube (NGT) and listening for borborygmi is not recommended. Aspiration is difficult through such small-lumen tubes, so to rule out misplacement into the lungs their position must be checked by radiography or endoscopy. Feeding through a misplaced tube is considered a 'Never Event' in many health care systems.

For longer term feeding, small-bore feeding tubes are placed in the stomach or duodenum. These need a wire stylet insertion, but are less traumatic and better tolerated, although blockage is more common. Percutaneous gastrostomy and jejunostomy tubes may also be used postoperatively and for longer term feeding.

Numerous protocols are available for starting and maintaining enteral feeding. Feeding continuously at a constant rate over 24 h makes glycaemic control easier. Early feeding, even after complex bowel surgery, has become common place and is supported by high quality trials and international guidance.[4,6]

A number of complications may arise during enteral feeding:

- Tube related – trauma and ulceration of the nose, pharynx and gut mucosa, sinusitis (if nasal), misplacement in the lungs, regurgitation and aspiration (reflux can be reduced by nursing the patient head up – aim for 45°).
- Gastrointestinal – change of gut flora, vomiting, regurgitation, large residue on aspiration of the nasogastric tube and diarrhoea. Large gastric aspirates can be managed pharmacologically with erythromycin, neostigmine and metoclopramide. Diarrhoea is common and may have a number of causes (e.g. antibiotics, lactose intolerance or high osmolality feed) and loperamide or codeine phosphate can be useful.
- Metabolic – water and electrolyte abnormalities, hyperglycaemia, deficiencies of essential nutrients.

Parenteral Feeding

Parenteral nutrition (PN) is used when full feeding via the gut is either not possible or not meeting the patient's total nutritional requirements. The aim with PN is to maintain nutrition until the gut failure is corrected, so it is usually started when prolonged feeding difficulties are expected, e.g. major abdominal surgery. In some conditions where PN was formerly used extensively, e.g. acute pancreatitis, the evidence now suggests that enteral feeding is better.[7]

A central venous catheter is necessary for most parenteral solutions, except those designed for peripheral veins. Catheters must be inserted under aseptic conditions and scrupulous care is needed in use. For long-term feeding, the line should be tunnelled and not used for other infusions or blood sampling, but if a multi-lumen catheter is used, one lumen should be reserved exclusively for parenteral nutrition.

Best practice is to have the desired mixture made up aseptically in pharmacy, presented in a 'big-bag' and infused over 24 h with a controlled volumetric pump. The electrolyte composition can be varied based on daily blood results by the pharmacy.

Total parenteral nutrition is best managed by a dedicated multidisciplinary team and can be successfully carried out at home. Complications may occur related to catheter insertion and use, e.g. pneumothorax, haemorrhage, infection and thrombophlebitis.

Other complications can be minimized by adequate biochemical monitoring and include the following:

- Glucose related – hyperglycaemia, ketoacidosis, hypercapnia.
- Amino acid metabolism – patients in acute renal failure will have to be dialysed or have haemofiltration more frequently due to prerenal uraemia. Hyperchloraemic metabolic acidosis.
- Fats – sicker patients are less able to metabolize fat so fatty liver and cholestasis may occur. Essential fatty acid deficiency may occur with predominantly glucose-based feeds.
- Water and electrolytes – circulatory overload, electrolyte imbalance, e.g. hypophosphataemia, pseudohyponatraemia.
- Vitamin and trace element deficiencies – thiamine, vitamin K, vitamin B_{12}, folate, zinc and copper deficiency should be considered and rectified.

REFERENCES

1. 'Malnutrition Universal Screening Tool' ('MUST') for adults. Available at http://www.bapen. org.uk/pdfs/must/must_full.pdf.
2. National Institute for Health and Care Excellence. Nutrition support in adults. NICE quality standard 24. Manchester: NICE; 2012. Available at https://www.nice.org.uk/guidance/qs24.
3. The NICE-SUGARS study investigators. Intensive versus conventional glucose control in critically ill patients. N Engl J Med 2009;360:1283–97.
4. McClave S, Martindale R, Vanek VW, McCarthy M, Roberts P, Taylor B, et al. Guidelines for the provision and assessment of nutrition support therapy in the adult critically ill patient: Society of Critical Care Medicine (SCCM) and American Society for Parenteral and Enteral Nutrition (A.S.P.E.N.). J Parent Ent Nutr 2009;33:277–316.
5. Oldani M, Sandini M, Nespoli L, Coppola S, Bernasconi DP, Gianotti L. Glutamine supplementation in intensive care patients: A meta-analysis of randomized clinical trials. Medicine 2015;94:e1319.
6. Soop M, Carlso GL, Hopkinson J, Clarke S, Thorell A, Nygren J, et al. Randomized clinical trial of the effects of immediate enteral nutrition on metabolic responses to major colorectal surgery in an enhanced recovery protocol. Br J Surg 2004;91:1138–45.
7. Marik PE, Zaloga GP. Meta-analysis of parenteral nutrition versus enteral nutrition in patients with acute pancreatitis. Br Med J 2004;328:1407.

Chapter 2.10

Resuscitation

Charles Deakin

The current resuscitation guidelines were developed by the International Liaison Committee on Resuscitation (ILCOR), of which the European Resuscitation Council is a member, and were published in 2015.[1]

Guidelines are continually updated and links are provided thropughout the text for access to the most up to date guidelines.

Successful resuscitation relies on a chain of survival that begins with calling for help, progresses to basic life support (BLS) and early defibrillation, and concludes with the postresuscitation care. Delivery of this chain of survival (Fig. 2.10.1) is equally important for cardiac arrest both outside and inside the hospital. The earlier links in this chain of survival have a far greater impact on survival than the latter.

ADULT RESUSCITATION

Cardiac arrest is diagnosed if someone shows no signs of life and is not breathing normally. It is important not to mistake agonal respiration that occurs transiently in 40% of patients following cardiac arrest, for normal respiratory effort.

Basic Life Support[2]

Basic life support must be initiated immediately. Bystander CPR will treble survival from cardiac arrest but in the UK it is only given to 30% of those

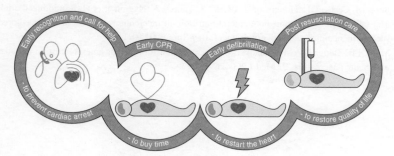

FIGURE 2.10.1   Chain of survival.

suffering cardiac arrest prior to ambulance arrival. Ambulance instructions encourage bystanders to give CPR and instruct how to do so.

Approximately 30% of adult cardiac arrests are secondary to shockable arrhythmias, primarily ventricular fibrillation. Every minute's delay in defibrillation increases mortality by approximately 10%. With the increasing availability and simplicity of use of automated external defibrillators, defibrillation is now considered part of BLS and the use of public access defibrillation (PAD) will further improve survival. PAD schemes aim to place defibrillators in public areas (e.g. airports, shopping centres) to enable early defibrillation before the arrival of the emergency services.

BLS follows the sequence of ABC – opening the Airway, supporting Breathing and assisting the Circulation (Fig. 2.10.2). Compression-only CPR is acceptable for those unable or unwilling to perform rescue breaths, but survival is greater in hypoxic-related arrests when rescue breaths are also given (paediatric arrests, drowning, hanging, etc.). Aim for a compression depth of 5–6 cm and a compression rate of 100–120/min, allowing the chest to completely recoil after each compression.

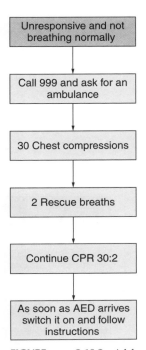

FIGURE 2.10.2 Adult basic life support algorithm. *Source:* Reproduced from algorithms published in the 2015 Resuscitation Guidelines (available at www.resus.org. uk) with permission from the Resuscitation Council UK.

Advanced Life Support[3]

Advanced life support (ALS) secures the airway and supports the circulation with pharmacological adjuncts, aiming to restore sinus rhythm and a spontaneous cardiac output. The ALS algorithm is shown in Fig. 2.10.3. The treatment pathway follows the route of either a shockable (VF/VT) or nonshockable (asystole/pulseless electrical activity) rhythm.

Tracheal intubation secures the airway from aspiration, allows ventilation while chest compression is performed and enables delivery of drugs via the endotracheal tube. Although it has been considered to be the gold standard in airway management, there is no firm evidence that outcome is better when compared with a supraglottic airway or bag and mask. Supraglottic airways are effective in delivering early ventilation and are easier to insert after relatively little training.

Early establishment of intravenous access is necessary for the administration of resuscitation drugs and fluids. A large forearm vein or the external jugular vein is ideal for initial access, but both require a saline infusion to flush the drugs through to the central circulation. In hospital, central venous access is

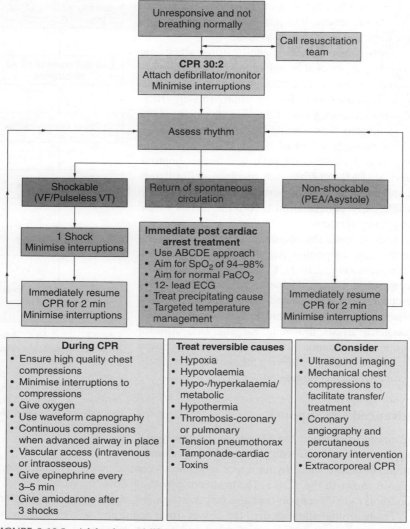

FIGURE 2.10.3 Adult advanced life support algorithm. *Source:* Reproduced from algorithms published in the 2015 Resuscitation Guidelines (available on www.resus.org.uk) with permission from the Resuscitation Council UK.

optimal. Intraosseous access (humeral head, sternum and tibia) is a suitable alternative to IV access if this cannot be gained quickly.

The evidence base for the effectiveness of ALS drugs is limited. The initial drug indicated for both VF/VT and non-VF/VT is epinephrine 1 mg intravenously. Epinephrine has been shown to increase the chances of return of spontaneous circulation (ROSC), but there is no evidence that it improves neurologically intact survival. Some studies have suggested that survival may be worse if epinephrine is administered, particularly if late in the cardiac arrest. Epinephrine should be administered with caution following ROSC, as excessive doses are liable to re-induce VT/VF. Epinephrine should be administered every 3–5 min when indicated (every second cycle).

Atropine is no longer indicated for asystole because vagal tone is not thought to be the cause of this arrhythmia. It remains indicated for bradyarrhythmias. Amiodarone 300 mg i.v. is indicated after three shocks have been given, followed by a further 150 mg amiodarone i.v. after a total of five shocks.

Causes of pulseless electrical activity should be actively sought and treated, and include:

- Hypoxia
- Hypovolaemia
- Hyper/hypokalaemia
- Hypothermia
- Tension pneumothorax
- Tamponade
- Toxic/therapeutic disturbance
- Thromboembolism

Defibrillation

Defibrillation aims to deliver sufficient transmyocardial current to depolarize a critical mass of myocardium, allowing restoration of synchronized electrical activity. Inadequate energy fails to defibrillate, but excessive energy may cause myocardial damage and risks the resumption of fibrillation.

Defibrillation should be performed through self-adhesive pads, placed with the sternal pad to the right of the sternum below the clavicle and the apical pad in line with the nipple in the left mid-axillary line. Antero-posterior and bi-axillary pad positions are also acceptable.

For biphasic waveforms (rectilinear biphasic or biphasic truncated exponential), use an initial shock energy of at least 150 J. For pulsed biphasic waveforms, begin at 120–150 J. With manual defibrillators, consider escalating the shock energy if feasible, after a failed shock and for patients where refibrillation occurs.

Minimize the delay between stopping chest compressions and delivery of the shock (the preshock pause); even a 5–10 s delay will reduce the chances of the shock being successful. Without pausing to reassess the rhythm or feel for a pulse, resume CPR immediately after the shock, starting with chest compressions to limit the postshock pause and the total perishock pause. Even if the defibrillation attempt is successful in restoring a perfusing rhythm, it takes time to establish a postshock circulation and a pulse is not usually palpable immediately after defibrillation.

Defibrillation of supraventricular arrhythmias should be synchronized to avoid delivering a shock on the T-wave of the ECG, which may induce VF.

Other Therapy

Thrombolysis should be considered for cardiac arrest patients when the presumed aetiology is pulmonary embolus. Cardiopulmonary resuscitation (CPR) is not a contraindication to thrombolytic therapy but may need to be continued for up to 90 min to ensure clot dissolution in these patients.

The routine use of mechanical chest compression devices is not recommended, but they are a reasonable alternative in situations where sustained high-quality manual chest compressions are impractical or compromise provider safety such as prolonged CPR (thrombolysis, hypothermia, etc.) and situations where effective CPR is difficult (cardiac arrest in the cath lab, ambulance transport, etc.).

Once ROSC is achieved, reduce the FiO_2 to a level that achieves SaO_2 94%–98%.

Resuscitation during Pregnancy[4]

The main causes of cardiovascular collapse during pregnancy are amniotic fluid embolus, pulmonary embolus, eclampsia, congestive cardiomyopathy, drug toxicity (e.g. hypermagnesaemia, total spinal anaesthetic) and haemorrhage:

- Below 25 weeks of gestation, treatment is as for a nonpregnant adult.
- Above 25 weeks of gestation, aortocaval compression significantly impedes venous return; a wedge is required to tilt the body to the left, together with manual uterine displacement in order to reduce aortocaval compression.
- Above 32 weeks of gestation, the extent of aortocaval compression precludes effective CPR and immediate caesarean section is indicated while CPR is continued.

In the third trimester, the mediastinum is pushed cranially by the gravid uterus and external chest compressions should be performed higher on the sternum than usual.

Traumatic Cardiac Arrest[4]

The management of traumatic cardiac arrest follows the principles discussed above, but aims to identify and treat any reversible causes, most commonly hypoxia, hypovolaemia, tension pneumothorax and cardiac tamponade. The recommended treatment pathways for traumatic cardiac arrest are shown in Fig. 2.10.4.

POST ARREST MANAGEMENT[5]

Following ROSC, those patients with evidence of ST-elevation should undergo urgent coronary artery catheterization and percutaneous coronary intervention (PCI) after out-of-hospital cardiac arrest of likely cardiac cause. This should also be considered in patients with non-ST elevation ROSC.

Targeted temperature management (TTM) is recommended for adults following out-of-hospital cardiac arrest (consider for in-hospital cardiac arrest) with

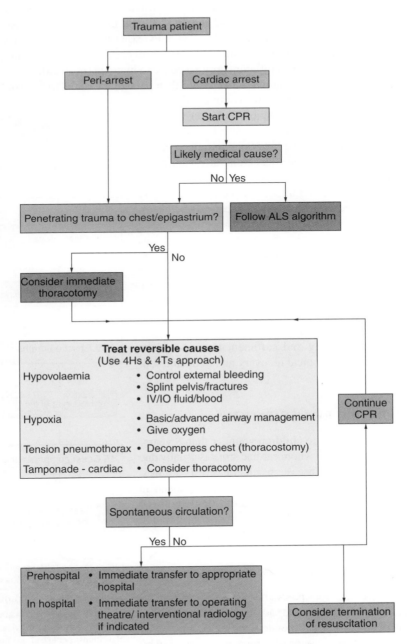

FIGURE 2.10.4 Algorithm showing the management of traumatic cardiac arrest.
Source: Reproduced from algorithms published in the 2015 Resuscitation Guidelines (available on www.resus.org.uk) with permission from the Resuscitation Council UK.

an initial shockable rhythm who remain unresponsive after ROSC. A constant, target core temperature between 32°C and 36°C should be used. It is suggested that the duration of TTM should be at least 24 h. Pyrexia (>37.5°C) is disastrous for neurological recovery and should be avoided at all costs. It occurs commonly following ROSC due to an inflammatory response to hypoxia (postcardiac arrest syndrome) and usually requires active rather than passive measures to control.

In the critically ill adult survivor of cardiac arrest who requires mechanical ventilation after return of spontaneous circulation, strict control of blood glucose with insulin may be beneficial to outcome.

Seizures are common after cardiac arrest and occur in approximately 30% patients who remain comatose after ROSC. Use intermittent electroencephalography (EEG) to detect epileptic activity in patients with clinical seizure manifestations. Consider continuous EEG to monitor patients with a diagnosed status epilepticus and effects of treatment. Propofol, clonazepam and sodium valproate are suitable therapies. Maintenance therapy should be started after the first seizure, once potential precipitating causes (e.g. intracranial haemorrhage, electrolyte imbalance) are excluded.

Prognostication should be undertaken using a multimodal strategy and sufficient time should be allowed for neurological recovery and to enable sedatives to be cleared.

PAEDIATRIC RESUSCITATION[6]

This section refers to children younger than 8 years.

Unlike adults, in whom cardiac arrest is usually due to ischaemic heart disease, paediatric arrests are usually secondary to hypoxia. Resuscitation of patients in this age group therefore emphasizes the importance of securing the airway and delivering high-concentration oxygen as a priority in the resuscitation sequence.

Basic Life Support

The algorithm for paediatric BLS is shown in Fig. 2.10.5 and, as with adults, follows the ABC sequence. For trained responders, the 30:2 compression ventilation ratio recommended for adults is replaced by a 15:2 ratio. Rescue breaths should be given before the first chest compression. For all children, compress the lower half of the sternum. The compression should

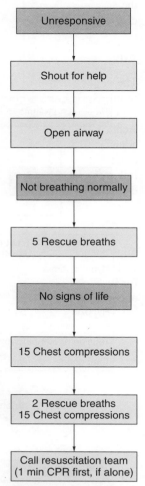

FIGURE 2.10.5 Paediatric basic life support algorithm. *Source:* Reproduced from algorithms published in the 2015 Resuscitation Guidelines (available on www.resus.org.uk) with permission from the Resuscitation Council UK.

be sufficient to depress the sternum by at least one-third the anterior–posterior diameter of the chest, given at a rate 100–120/min.

Choking is more common in infants than adults. Conscious infants should be encouraged to cough. Never perform a finger sweep that may impact the foreign body further. Unconscious infants should be given five back blows in the prone position, alternating with five chest thrusts. In children, abdominal thrusts replace chest thrusts (when they are less likely to damage abdominal viscera) after the second round of back blows. Subsequently, back blows are alternated with chest thrusts/abdominal thrusts until the airway is cleared (Fig. 2.10.6).

Advanced Life Support

The algorithm for paediatric ALS is shown in Fig. 2.10.7. As with adults, the sequence should follow an A, B, C, D, E approach.

Open the airway and ensure adequate oxygenation, starting with 100% oxygen. Achieving adequate ventilation and oxygenation may require the use of airway adjuncts ± bag-mask ventilation (BMV), the use of a supraglottic airway, securing a definitive airway by tracheal intubation and positive pressure ventilation. The following formula is useful in estimating the appropriate endotracheal tube internal diameter:

$$\text{Internal diameter (mm)} = (\text{age in years}/4) + 4$$

Having secured the airway, breathing must be assessed. It is particularly important to exclude a tension pneumothorax in both trauma patients and those with acute asthma. In the latter, a high index of suspicion must be maintained for a bilateral tension pneumothorax. If there is any doubt, decompress the chest once the child is intubated.

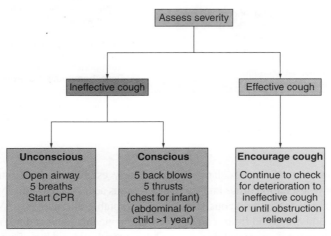

FIGURE 2.10.6 Paediatric choking algorithm. *Source:* Reproduced from algorithms published in the 2015 Resuscitation Guidelines (available on www.resus.org.uk) with permission from the Resuscitation Council UK.

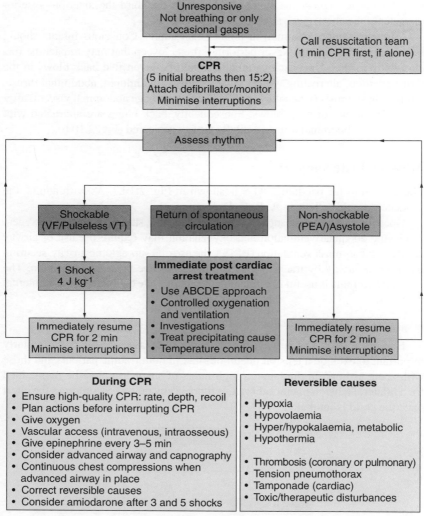

FIGURE 2.10.7 Paediatric advanced life support algorithm. *Source:* Reproduced from algorithms published in the 2015 Resuscitation Guidelines (available on www.resus.org.uk) with permission from the Resuscitation Council UK.

Management of the circulation requires early establishment of intravenous access for resuscitation drugs and fluid. Intravenous access is particularly difficult in infants, and the intraosseous route is an acceptable alternative to IV access. Resuscitation drugs and fluids can be given safely via this route and marrow aspirate used to estimate haemoglobin, electrolytes, venous pH and blood group. Drug doses are based on patient weight. An annotated tape measure (Broselow tape) or a length–weight–age nomogram (Oakley chart) both give specific drug doses according to the length or weight of the child and reduce the chances of error. The weight of infants and children can be estimated from the following formula:

$$\text{Weight (kg)} = (\text{age} + 4) \times 2$$

For CPR, the recommended i.v./i.o. dose of epinephrine in children for the first and for subsequent doses is 10 μg/kg. If indicated, give further doses of epinephrine every 3–5 min, i.e. every two cycles. Higher doses of epinephrine (>10 μg/kg) are not recommended because they do not improve survival or neurological outcome after cardiopulmonary arrest.

Atropine 20 μg/kg intravenously is only indicated as a treatment for brady-cardia once any hypoxia has been reversed.

Ventricular fibrillation in children is uncommon. If present, the following diagnoses should be actively excluded:

- Tricyclic overdose
- Hypothermia
- Hyperkalaemia
- Congenital heart disease

Energy levels of 4 J/kg are recommended for initial and all subsequent shocks. If paediatric self-adhesive pads are not available, adult pads are accept-able. Give amiodarone after the third shock as a 5 mg/kg bolus, repeated if nec-essary after a fifth shock.

Although acidosis is known to depress myocardial contractility, reduce tis-sue oxygen delivery and increase susceptibility to VF, there is no good evidence that correction of pH improves the outcome of CPR. Sodium bicarbonate may be considered during prolonged CPR or for severe metabolic acidosis, ideally titrated against arterial blood gases. Sodium bicarbonate may also be consid-ered in case of haemodynamic instability and co-existing hyperkalaemia, or in the management of tricyclic antidepressant drug overdose. When given without knowledge of acid–base status, a dose of 1 mmol/kg is recommended. Excessive quantities of sodium bicarbonate may impair tissue oxygen delivery and cause hypokalaemia, hypernatraemia, hyperosmolality and cerebral acidosis.

When circulatory collapse results from hypovolaemia (e.g. blood loss, acute gastroenteritis) or sepsis and fluid resuscitation is required, give a 20 mL/kg bolus of isotonic crystalloid. Repeat three times and then give 10 mL/kg of blood if shock persists.

Hypoglycaemia is common in infants and blood sugar should be checked and treated appropriately.

ETHICAL ASPECTS OF RESUSCITATION AND END OF LIFE CARE[7]

All establishments that face decisions about attempting CPR, including hospi-tals, general practices, care homes, hospices and ambulance services, should have a policy about CPR decisions. Ethical aspects of resuscitation have recently been addressed in a joint statement from the British Medical Association, Royal College of Nursing and Resuscitation Council.[8] Literature on CPR should be available to patients, who should be involved in decision-making, and these decisions should be reviewed regularly. In emergencies, CPR should be performed unless:

- The patient has refused CPR
- The patient is in the terminal phase of an illness
- The burdens of treatment outweigh the benefits

Each decision about CPR should be subject to review based on the person's individual circumstances and involve the patient in the decision-making process. If the patient lacks capacity, those close to them must be involved in discussions to reach a 'best interests' decision. It is not necessary to obtain the consent of a patient to decide not to attempt CPR if there is no realistic prospect of success. The patient and those close to them do not have a right to demand treatment that is clinically inappropriate and healthcare professionals have no obligation to offer or deliver such treatment.

FURTHER READING

Detailed guidelines for adult and paediatric resuscitation can be found on the websites of the Resuscitation Council (UK) at www.resus.org.uk and the European Resuscitation Council at www.erc.edu.

REFERENCES

1. Monsieurs KG, Nolan JP, Bossaert LL, Greif R, Maconochie IK, Nikolaou NI, et al. European Resuscitation Council Guidelines for Resuscitation 2015: Section 1. Executive summary. Resuscitation 2015;95:1–80.
2. Perkins GD, Handley AJ, Koster RW, Castrén M, Smyth MA, Olasveengen T, et al. European Resuscitation Council Guidelines for Resuscitation 2015: Section 2. Adult basic life support and automated external defibrillation. Resuscitation 2015;95:81–99.
3. Soar J, Nolan JP, Bottiger BW, Perkins GD, Lott C, Carli P, et al. European Resuscitation Council Guidelines for Resuscitation 2015: Section 3. Adult advanced life support. Resuscitation 2015;95:100–47.
4. Truhlar A, Deakin CD, Soar J, Khalifa GE, Alfonzo A, Bierens JJ, et al. European Resuscitation Council Guidelines for Resuscitation 2015: Section 4. Cardiac arrest in special circumstances. Resuscitation 2015;95:148–201.
5. Nolan JP, Soar J, Cariou A, Cronberg T, Moulaert VR, Deakin CD, et al. European Resuscitation Council and European Society of Intensive Care Medicine 2015 guidelines for post-resuscitation care. Intensive Care Med 2015;41(12):2039–56.
6. Maconochie IK, Bingham R, Eich C, López-Herce J, Rodríguez-Núñez A, Rajka T, et al. European Resuscitation Council Guidelines for Resuscitation 2015: Section 6. Paediatric life support. Resuscitation 2015;95:223–48.
7. Bossaert LL, Perkins GD, Askitopoulou H, Raffay VI, Greif R, Haywood KL, et al. European Resuscitation Council Guidelines for Resuscitation 2015: Section 11. The ethics of resuscitation and end-of-life decisions. Resuscitation 2015;95:302–11.
8. Decisions relating to cardiopulmonary resuscitation. Guidance from the British Medical Association, the Resuscitation Council (UK) and the Royal College of Nursing. 3rd ed. (1st revision). 2016. https://www.resus.org.uk/dnacpr/decisions-relating-to-cpr/.

Section 3

Care of the Patient after Surgery

Chapter 3.1

Care in the Recovery Area

Sock Koh

THE POSTOPERATIVE RECOVERY WARD

Location

The recovery ward (postanaesthesia care unit; PACU) should occupy a central area within the operating suite, as far as possible equidistant from all the operating theatres, but with separate access for patients to and from the wards. As well as minimizing transfer times this also means that the recovery staff will have more ready access to expert anaesthetic help should it be required.

Ideally, the recovery area should also be located close to the critical care units. Typically, these comprise the intensive therapy unit (ITU; level 3 critical care) and high-dependency unit (HDU; level 2 critical care) but may include a specific step-down postoperative critical care unit (POCCU) also referred to as a surgical intermediate care unit.[1] These different units will admit, as appropriate, patients who are too sick or too unstable to be cared for safely in a general ward, who require invasive monitoring, or who require the organ support offered by full intensive care. They may also be appropriate for those for whom specialized pain regimens have been prescribed, such as those delivered by patient-controlled epidural analgesia (PCEA) devices with which ward staff may not be familiar. This generalization will not apply to all hospitals, many of whose general nursing staff may well have received specific training in some of these areas.

Design

Recommendations for the ratio of recovery bays to operating theatres vary from 1.5:1 to not less than 2:1. The final number will depend on clinical specialities, patient numbers and casemix.[2,3,4]

Recommendations for the total floor space, which includes the bed space, open space, nurses' station, etc., range from 14 m^2 (150 square feet) to 20 m^2 (220 square feet) per recovery bay. A patient entering recovery after prolonged major surgery requires more space and equipment than a young fit adult who has undergone knee arthroscopy as a day case. A quarter of the total number of recovery bays should be suitably sized and equipped to care for level 2 critical care patients.

There should be curtains or screens to allow privacy. These should ideally be lead-lined to facilitate compliance with radiation protection requirements. Where possible there should be separation of the sexes although this is rarely done.

There should be a dedicated recovery unit for children. In smaller hospitals where this may not be practical, there should be a designated area in the general recovery unit dedicated to the care of children. Such an area should be decorated appropriately and should allow access to parents who wish to be reunited with their children.

Each bay should have sufficient electrical sockets, pipeline outlets for oxygen, air and suction, and a push button emergency call system. It is increasingly common for each bay to require a computer terminal.

There should be adequate storage, a dirty utility area, washing facilities and a communications base.

Adequate air exchange is important, because exhaled anaesthetic gases in a busy recovery will otherwise accumulate in the working area.

Equipment

Potential postanaesthetic and surgical problems mean that there must be immediate access to the same drugs and equipment, both standard and emergency, as are available in the anaesthetic room and operating theatre.

Airway Equipment

Airway adjuncts such as oropharyngeal and nasopharyngeal airways, laryngoscopes and a range of tracheal tubes should be available. There should also be readily available an effective (and familiar) cricothyroidotomy puncture kit with a means of attachment, after insertion, to the fresh gas supply.

A breathing system (circuit) must be present in every bay. Typically this is a Mapleson C system (also known as a Waters' circuit), which although convenient does require a high gas flow of two to three times minute volume to avoid rebreathing. Some units prefer to use self-inflating bags, particularly during resuscitation, although these tend to be less popular with anaesthetists.

Continuous capnography should be used if patients remain intubated or their airways are maintained with a supraglottic airway device.

Suction

Powerful and effective suction must be present in every bay, together with a range of suction catheters.

Monitoring

Minimum monitoring equipment in each bay comprises pulse oximeter, non-invasive blood pressure monitor, ECG, capnography as mentioned above and infrared tympanic thermometer. More complex cases may require more sophisticated monitoring such as invasive monitoring.

Emergency Equipment

Drugs, fluids and equipment (including a defibrillator) for resuscitation and management of complications should be immediately available. These may be located on dedicated trolleys in the recovery area.

Beds or patient trolleys that can be rapidly tipped head-down should be standard. There must also be sufficient room round the bed or trolley to allow whatever resuscitative or emergency manoeuvres may be necessary.

Warming Devices

Forced air warming devices should be available to actively warm patients who are hypothermic (<36.0°C) postoperatively.

Staffing

There should be sufficient trained staff to allow continuous one-to-one care of every patient passing through the recovery unit. An anaesthetist must also be immediately available. Ideally this would be a named individual with responsibilities only to the patients in recovery, but at the least they should be supernumerary to requirements in the operating theatre.

The particular skills of the staff will vary according to the case mix of the surgical unit, but their core skills should include basic airway management, immediate life support and the ability to assess accurately a patient's cardiac, respiratory and volaemic status.

Whether the staff feels competent to manage patients in whom a supraglottic airway device or tracheal tube remains in place usually depends on local policies and training. Supraglottic airway devices (SAD) tend to be very forgiving and much of their inherent safety lies in the fact that patients will tolerate them as consciousness returns and airway reflexes are restored. The same is not true of a tracheal tube. Yet although the uneventful removal of an endotracheal tube can be more difficult to achieve, there is no reason why this task cannot also be undertaken by properly trained recovery personnel, given appropriate anaesthetic supervision and support.

Staff should be able to assess and deliver appropriate treatments for common problems such as postoperative pain, nausea and vomiting. Hence, they should be trained to administer intravenous drugs, in particular opioid analgesics, set up intravenous fluids and drug infusions. Ideally they should be allowed by local protocols to set up and initiate patient-controlled analgesia (PCA), PCEA devices and increasingly local anaesthetic infusion devices for wound or nerve infiltration.

TRANSFER OF CARE TO RECOVERY

The imperative of maintaining surgical throughput means that the anaesthetist rarely has the luxury of transferring a patient who is fully conscious and whose protective reflexes are completely intact. More commonly the patient is in the inherently unstable state of emergence from anaesthesia. Transfer from the operating theatre to the recovery area should therefore be as swift as possible, but with supplemental oxygen provided as a routine.

Handover

When continued care of the postoperative patient is delegated to a member of the recovery team, pertinent details should be provided. It is standard practice for a member of the theatre team to convey operative information such as details of the surgical procedure and the presence of any drains or other devices.

The anaesthetist should supplement this with a brief verbal summary detailing any other relevant information (Table 3.1.1). In less straightforward cases, such information may be crucial to the continuing quality of care.

The anaesthetist should ensure that the anaesthetic record is legible and that prescriptions for fluid therapy, oxygen therapy, analgesia and antiemesis are clear and comprehensive.

Recovery Plan

The plan for recovery from anaesthesia should in effect begin at the stage of the preoperative assessment, because even though the effects of anaesthesia on the major systems are usually only temporary, they are nevertheless almost uniformly deleterious.

Cardiovascular function may often worsen, renal function may be compromised, CNS function is by definition impaired and respiratory function can deteriorate.

TABLE 3.1.1 Handover Information

Preoperative	Anaesthetic/ Intraoperative Events	Postoperative
Existing diseases, e.g. asthma, ischaemic heart disease, diabetes, dementia	Type of anaesthetic (GA, regional anaesthesia if used, sedation)	Instructions for monitoring, analgesia, fluids, discharge criteria
Allergies	Anaesthetic or surgical complications or interventions	For complex cases, extra requirements may include: blood tests, arterial blood gas sampling, radiological investigations, e.g. chest X-ray
Severe preoperative anxiety		
Previous complications of anaesthesia		
Significant abnormalities of patient's physiological parameters, e.g. hypotension, tachy/brady arrhythmias, low oxygen saturations	Drugs and fluids administered relevant to postoperative care, e.g. analgesics, antiemetics	Potential complications
Significant dentition concerns, e.g. loose teeth		
Airway concerns		

Even nonanaesthetic agents may have significant adverse effects, e.g. aminoglycoside antibiotics may potentiate neuromuscular blockade.

At the preoperative assessment therefore, the anaesthetist should be planning a technique that will mitigate these effects in any given patient and will facilitate rapid and safe recovery from anaesthesia. However, a large number of potential complications can still occur despite careful anaesthetic planning.

PROBLEMS ENCOUNTERED IN THE IMMEDIATE POSTOPERATIVE PERIOD

There are a number of ways of viewing the various clinical problems that may occur in recovery. One is to apply the typical airway, breathing, circulation, disability (ABCD) algorithm and to list the critical events with which each may be associated.

A different, and arguably more practical, method of dealing with these events is to incorporate the ABCD algorithm within a problem-based approach, because recovery staff will ask an anaesthetist to review a patient not because they have 'upper airways obstruction' or 'cardiogenic shock', but because they have low oxygen saturations or are hypotensive (Box 3.1.1).

Presentations of important problems that may require the urgent attention of an anaesthetist during the immediate postoperative period are outlined below.

Low Oxygen Saturation

Airway

Upper Airway Obstruction

Decreasing oxygen saturations may reflect the fact that the airway is obstructed, either partially or totally. There are no exceptions to the rule that noisy breathing is always partially obstructed breathing.

Airway obstruction may occur at any part of the respiratory tract.

Upper airway obstruction may be due to common and well-recognized causes such as the position of the tongue, persistent loss of tone in the pharyngeal

---

BOX 3.1.1 Common Problems in Recovery

Low oxygen saturation
Hypotension
Hypertension
Delayed awakening
Confusion and agitation
Pain
Nausea
Temperature disturbance
Shivering
High, low or irregular pulse

muscles and inappropriate positioning of the neck and jaw. It may also be due to foreign bodies in the oropharynx (such as a pack that has not been removed) or to blood clot or debris. These latter causes are all likely to be difficulties associated with intraoral and maxillofacial surgery.

A more general and common problem is laryngeal spasm, in which there is reflex closure of the vocal cords, precipitated often by stimulation during a light stage of anaesthesia.

The definitive management of laryngeal spasm comprises tracheal intubation following a full dose of neuromuscular blocking agent. Laryngeal spasm may respond to a small dose of suxamethonium (10 mg in an adult), to a subhypnotic bolus dose of propofol and to low-dose midazolam (0.5–1.0 mg increments). Incomplete laryngeal spasm may be managed by delivering 100% oxygen by facemask with a tight seal in order to overcome the spasm.

Doxapram has been advocated for partial spasm (dose of 1 mg/kg) but there is a risk of inducing negative pressure pulmonary oedema.

With upper airway obstruction, the patient will desaturate at a rate proportional to the oxygen that remains within the functional residual capacity, which in an adult is about 2000–2500 mL. The basal requirement for oxygen is around 250 mL/min, and so if a patient has been breathing 50% oxygen the alveolar oxygen reserve of 1000–1250 mL will be exhausted within 5 min.

If upper airway obstruction is total then there will be pronounced ventilatory efforts, but the airway will be silent. These extreme respiratory efforts, particularly if the patient is young and fit, can generate negative intrathoracic pressures as great as -100 cm H_2O. This is more than sufficient to cause negative-pressure pulmonary oedema. Onset can be rapid (within a few minutes) or delayed (up to 2–3 h) and will usually resolve within 12–24 h. Treatment is supportive with oxygen therapy, continuous positive airways pressure (CPAP) and occasionally intermittent positive pressure ventilation (IPPV).

Lower Airway Obstruction

Bronchoconstriction in the lower airways may occur in patients with a history of asthma, in individuals who are atopic, *de novo* in response to airway irritants, to the presence of inhaled gastric contents and as part of an allergic drug response. Wheeze is often transient, but if it persists to the detriment of gas exchange it can be treated with nebulized β sympathomimetics (such as salbutamol, 2.5–5.0 mg) or with intravenous salbutamol (250 μg slowly), aminophylline (5 mg/kg over 20 min) or magnesium sulphate (1.2–2 g over 20 min).

Breathing

Apnoea

A patient may be apnoeic because of drug-induced respiratory depression. Opioids are the most potent agents in this respect, but most anaesthetic agents, including nitrous oxide, also depress respiration and may exert a synergistic effect. Oxygen desaturation may occur relatively late in this situation.

If the airway remains patent ambient gas is drawn into the lungs by mass movement down the trachea. If room air is the ambient gas then hypoxia will occur almost as swiftly as it does in obstructed apnoea. If, however, the ambient gas is 100% oxygen then (in theory) it will take about 100 min before hypoxia supervenes.

Other causes of apnoea include residual neuromuscular paralysis, and hypocapnia associated with mechanical hyperventilation. Rarely, patients may fail to breathe because of an intracranial catastrophe.

Hypoventilation

Hypoventilation results in the failure of the patient to generate minute ventilation sufficient to supply tissue oxygen needs. This may be due to drug-induced respiratory depression and residual neuromuscular block, although inadequate ventilation may also be associated with poor pain control.

Low oxygen saturation may be reversed by supplemental oxygen, but if the cause of hypoventilation is not treated, the high inspired oxygen concentration may mask respiratory failure due to failure of carbon dioxide elimination.

An oxygen saturation of 95% in the presence of high inspired oxygen concentrations is not normal, but low.

Patients who remain partly paralysed by the effects of residual neuromuscular blocking agents may exhibit characteristic jerky and athetoid movements. The diagnosis is supported if a patient has weak grip strength or is unable to support head lift off the pillow for 5 s.

A peripheral nerve stimulator can be used to confirm the diagnosis. Tetanic stimulation (50 or 100 Hz for 5 s) is more sensitive for demonstrating residual block than double burst or train-of-four stimulation. Tetanic stimulation is painful and should not be used in the conscious patient.

For patients who exhibit residual neuromuscular blockade, check if an adequate dose of neostigmine (0.05 mg/kg) had been administered at the end of anaesthesia.

Sugammadex is very effective in reversing residual paralysis in patients who were paralysed using rocuronium. It can also be used for vecuronium and pancuronium-induced residual paralysis. The dose of sugammadex will be determined by the depth of residual neuromuscular blockade.

Circulation

Low oxygen saturation may also reflect impaired cardiac output (CO).

Cardiac output may be reduced by severe bradycardia and by an abnormally fast heart rate which can compromise diastolic filling and coronary artery perfusion. It may also be reduced by hypovolaemia, and by acute left ventricular dysfunction.

Hypotension

Hypotension has numerous causes, and although the immediate reason may be very obvious, such as excessive blood loss via a wound drain, it is better to follow a systematic diagnostic path that is based on first physiological principles. This may lead to a quicker diagnosis in a difficult case and may help unravel situations in which causation is multifactorial.

It is important to recognize that normal cerebration indicates adequate cerebral perfusion irrespective of the absolute blood pressure.

Hypovolaemia is a common cause of hypotension in the recovery area. Hypovolaemia may be actual (following blood and/or fluid loss), or effective (with insufficient volume effectively to fill the capacity of the venous system). Effective hypovolaemia may be associated with neuraxial (and hence sympathetic) block, with peripheral vasodilatation due to pyrexia or sepsis, and with severe drug reactions.

Stroke volume may also be diminished by myocardial depression, injury and ischaemia.

Causes of bradycardia include vagal reflexes, e.g. due to visceral distension, and the persistent effects of preoperative cardiac medication (such as β-adrenergic receptor blockers and angiotensin converting enzyme (ACE) inhibitors).

Most anaesthetic agents decrease in systemic vascular resistance (SVR) and their effects may persist into the recovery period. SVR may also be decreased by pyrexia, hypercapnia and sepsis.

Hypertension

Hypertension occurs less frequently in recovery than hypotension, and its most common cause is unrelieved pain. It can be due to distension of viscera, particularly of the urinary bladder, and it may also be associated with pre-existing essential hypertension. Rarely, it may be a rebound phenomenon secondary to the preoperative withdrawal of antihypertensive drugs (typically clonidine and β-adrenergic receptor blockers). Volume overload can be a contributory factor, as can hypercapnia and the perioperative use of ketamine.

Severe postoperative hypertension may be associated with coronary ischaemia, particularly if it is accompanied by a tachycardia, and so it should be treated. In addition to managing the cause, it may be necessary to treat with intravenous vasodilators such as glyceryl trinitrate (start infusion at 3 mg/h and titrate to response), magnesium sulphate (2–4 g over 10 min) or β-adrenergic receptor blockers such as labetalol (5–10 mg).

Delayed Awakening

The most common cause of delayed awakening is persistent CNS depression by anaesthetic and analgesic drugs. If the clinical context suggests that opioids or benzodiazepines are implicated, then their effects can be reversed by the cautious intravenous administration respectively of naloxone (1–3 μg/kg) or flumazenil (3 μg/kg followed by 1.5 μg/kg at 60 s intervals).

High inspired oxygen concentrations may disguise CO_2 retention. In nonhabituated patients, CO_2 narcosis will supervene at $PCO_2 \sim 12$ kPa.

Persistent coma may rarely be due to a hypoxic or ischaemic insult during surgery and anaesthesia. A number of metabolic derangements may also be responsible. The most important of these is hypoglycaemia.

Other abnormalities include hyponatraemia associated with the irrigation of large volumes of glycine-containing solutions during transurethral procedures, and rare endocrine disorders such as undiagnosed myxoedema coma associated with hypothyroidism.

If a patient has received a neuraxial or major plexus block in addition to a general anaesthetic, consideration must be given to the possibility of extensive central spread.

Confusion and Agitation

Confusion, agitation, disorientation and aggression may complicate immediate postanaesthetic recovery, and such psychological upsets may be relatively common in elderly patients.

The most important cause is hypoxaemia (which can be both cause and effect).

Confusion may be a nonspecific manifestation of persistent anaesthetic drug actions. It may be a direct adverse effect of an anaesthetic agent (e.g. racemic ketamine).

Confusion can be a sign of alcohol withdrawal.

More commonly confusion results from the residual hypnotic effects of drugs, which may prevent a patient being able to communicate effectively that they are in pain or have urinary retention.

Other causes of immediate postoperative confusion include pyrexia and sepsis as well as hyponatraemia and hypoglycaemia, as above.

In some patients, especially the elderly, postoperative cognitive deficit may persist for days or longer. It may be associated with pre-existing mental infirmity in which dementias and mild confusional states are exaggerated by the effects of anaesthetic drugs on memory processing. It is also associated with procedures in which there is a risk of embolism, such as joint replacement surgery and carotid endarterectomy.

Pain

Pain is a common problem as patients' experience of pain from the same surgical stimulus varies widely. The recovery area provides a safe environment in which to manage acute pain properly, and there should be no arbitrary limit on the dose of opioid that can be given.

Simple pain scoring scales are adequate for grading the response to analgesic drugs.

In addition to opioid medication, adjuvant analgesics may be helpful. Clonidine (up to 3 μg/kg) is useful, particularly when significant anxiety is present. Intravenous ketamine (up to 1 mg/kg) and magnesium sulphate

(40 mg/kg over 30 min) may be beneficial, particularly when large doses of opioids have already been used. Ketamine is associated with increased psychotomimetic effects with increasing doses.

Patient should be discharged from recovery only when they themselves are satisfied that their pain is tolerable.

Nausea and Vomiting

Immediate postoperative nausea and vomiting (PONV) is common and affects > 15% of all patients with multifactorial causes. Consequently administration of an antiemetic has become routine. Nevertheless an attempt should be made to identify the most likely cause.

Antiemetics should not be the first-line treatment for nausea and vomiting caused by hypoxia, hypotension or pain.

In the absence of an obvious cause for PONV which is amenable to treatment a range of antiemetics acting at different sites are available. These include antihistaminic/antimuscarinic agents such as cyclizine (50 mg; i.m., i.v.), serotonin (5-HT$_3$) antagonists such as ondansetron (4 mg; p.o., i.m., i.v.) and dopamine D$_2$-antagonists such as prochlorperazine (6.25–12.5 mg; i.m.).

Combination therapy may be necessary for intractable postoperative nausea with or without vomiting.

Temperature Disturbance

A high temperature may herald malignant hyperpyrexia (see Chapter 3.3). More common causes include sepsis, transfusion reactions and reactions to medication. The overefficient use of a warm air blanket perioperatively can also lead to a rise in core temperature. The use of anticholinergic drugs in the presence of any of these factors may cause pyrexia by preventing effective heat loss through the inhibition of sweating.

A fall in core temperature is more common, especially in the elderly and the very young, and is associated with factors such as intraoperative exposure, prolonged surgery and the intravenous infusion of cool fluids.

Shivering

Shivering that is not associated with a drop in body temperature may accompany the use of volatile anaesthetic agents. Not only is it a distressing symptom, but by increasing metabolic oxygen consumption by 300%–500% it may also impose an unacceptably high metabolic burden on susceptible individuals (such as those with ischaemic coronary or cerebrovascular disease).

Shivering may be aborted by a small dose of intravenous pethidine (25 mg) or clonidine (1 μg/kg).

High-flow oxygen should be given continuously.

High, Low or Irregular Pulse

Sinus tachycardia is a response to unrelieved pain, hypoxia, hypercapnia and hypovolaemia. It may also be caused by sympathomimetic drugs and by agents with anticholinergic actions.

Sinus bradycardia at worst may be a pre-agonal rhythm due to hypoxia. More usual causes include treatment with β-adrenoceptor antagonists, overdose of neostigmine, vagal stimulation and the higher vagal tone that may accompany physical fitness. Bradycardia needs treating only if it is causing symptoms.

Any tachyarrhythmia that is accompanied by inadequate cardiac output needs urgent treatment, if necessary by DC cardioversion.

Pharmacological treatment of supraventricular tachycardia (SVT) is with intravenous adenosine (6 mg initially, increasing to 12 mg). Amiodarone (5 mg/kg) is useful both for SVT and for ventricular arrhythmias.

Atrial fibrillation is usually chronic. Acute AF may be provoked by relatively trivial stimuli, but is also associated with sepsis.

PAEDIATRIC RECOVERY

The same principles that govern the care of adults following anaesthesia also apply to children, but there are some important additional aspects. The smaller paediatric airway may be more vulnerable to the complications already described in adults, and the higher metabolic rate and enhanced oxygen consumption in children mean that airway or breathing problems will lead to a more rapid fall in oxygen saturation. The younger the child, the more pronounced these factors become, and this applies also to the maintenance of body temperature.

Postoperative distress in children can be difficult to interpret. It may be due to pain, which should be managed just as energetically as it is in adults, but it may also be due to disorientation, hunger or separation (from parent, dummy or other comforter). This means that it is important that children should be cared for by recovery staff who, as well as being trained in the general aspects of paediatric postoperative care, are experienced enough to be familiar with these particular considerations.

PROTOCOLS AND DISCHARGE CRITERIA

Various scoring systems have been described, based on physical signs, but none holds universal currency. Their main advantage lies in the fact that they encourage a systematic approach to patient assessment before discharge from the recovery area.

The criteria are neither complex nor ambiguous. Patients must be able to maintain their airway unassisted and protective reflexes should be intact. Respiratory and cardiovascular indices should be within the anticipated range for that particular patient. Patients should be able to demonstrate recovery from neuromuscular blockade by sustaining a head lift off the pillow for at least 5 s, and symptoms such as pain and nausea should be under control to the patient's own satisfaction.

In routine practice, much of the care during the immediate period of postoperative recovery is delegated to recovery room staff. It remains good professional practice for the anaesthetist to leave the theatre and recovery suite only when the patient is awake and comfortable, with airway reflexes restored and with a circulation that is stable. If the anaesthetist wishes to delegate discharge to the ward to another individual, he or she is free to do so but must not lose sight of the uncomfortable reality that the final legal responsibility for ensuring that patients are safe when they leave the recovery area is going to be theirs.

HIGH DEPENDENCY CARE

Some patients benefit from critical care monitoring and input postoperatively. This may be due to type of surgery (e.g. cardiac surgery, oesophagectomy), patient comorbidities that may require organ support or significant intraoperative events such as anaphylaxis and major blood loss. Risk stratification using different strategies such as POSSUM (Physiological and Operative Severity Scoring for the enUmeration of Mortality & Morbidity) scoring or cardiopulmonary exercise testing (CPET or CPEX) may guide referrals to criteria care.

There are occasions when critical care units are full, necessitating prolonged stays in recovery to enable appropriate management of high-risk postoperative patients. In such an event, the staff should be trained and the area equipped to the standard of an intensive care unit to allow the monitoring and treatment of patients. Such patients remain the responsibility of the intensive care team.

NONSTANDARD AREAS

A subset of patients undergoes anaesthesia and is recovered in areas of the hospital outside the operating theatre suite. Nonstandard areas include radiology suites, mental health units and cardiology intervention units. Standards and guidelines for staffing, equipment and management of patients should be followed as if they are in the operating theatre suite.

INTERNATIONAL STANDARDS OF CARE

It is recognized that not all countries have resources to implement the above. The World Federation of Societies of Anaesthesiologists have proposed standards that pertain to different health care settings (such as small hospital, district/provincial hospital, referral hospital).[5] These guide organizational, personnel and equipment resource allocation. Of importance is the presence of an anaesthetically trained professional at all times during each patient's anaesthetic. A skilled and vigilant anaesthesia professional provides continuous clinical monitoring of patients, aided by continuous pulse oximetry which should be used until consciousness has recovered.

Patients who have had an anaesthetic should remain where anaesthetized or be transferred to a dedicated postanaesthetic recovery area. If care is delegated in the postanaesthetic phase, it should be to appropriately trained personnel who are given relevant information about the patient. The anaesthesia professional still retains overall responsibility for the patient. Clinical, and ideally quantitative, monitoring of patients should ensure that they have adequate oxygenation, ventilation, circulation and temperature. They should also receive appropriate medications to manage postoperative pain.

REFERENCES

1. Whitaker DK, Booth H, Clyburn P, Harrop-Griffiths W, Hosie H, Kilvington B, et al. Immediate post-anaesthesia recovery 2013. London: Association of Anaesthetists of Great Britain and Ireland. 2013. Available at http://onlinelibrary.wiley.com/doi/10.1111/anae.12146/abstract
2. Guidance on the provision of anaesthesia services for postoperative care 2017. In: GPAS editorial board. Guidelines for the provision of anaesthesia services. London: Royal College of Anaesthetists; 2017. Available at http://www.rcoa.ac.uk/gpas2016
3. Recommendations for the post-anaesthesia recovery room. Melbourne: Australian and New Zealand College of Anaesthetists; 2006. Available at http://www.anzca.edu.au/documents/ps04-2006-recommendations-for-the-post-anaesthesia.pdf
4. Haret D, Kneeland M, Ho E. 2012 Postanesthesia care units. In: Block FE, Helfmn S, editors. Operating room design manual. Schaumberg: American Society of Anesthesiologists; 2012. Available at https://www.asahq.org/resources/resources-from-asa-committees/operating-room-design-manual
5. Merry AF, Cooper JB, Soyannwo O, Wilson IH, Eichhorn JH. International standards for a safe practice of anesthesia 2010. Can J Anesth 2010;57:1027–34.

Chapter 3.2

Acute Pain Management

Lenny Ng, Jeremy Cashman

Pain is defined as 'an unpleasant sensory and emotional experience associated with actual or potential tissue damage, or described in terms of such damage' (www.iasp-pain.org/taxonomy).

Acute pain is defined as 'pain of recent onset and probable limited duration. It usually has an identifiable temporal and causal relationship to injury or disease'.[1]

PATHOPHYSIOLOGY OF ACUTE PAIN

A number of theoretical frameworks have been proposed to explain the physiological basis of pain, none of which completely account for all aspects of pain perception. The Gate Control Theory of Pain, which provides a neural basis for pain, is the most popular of the theories but is now recognized as an over simplification of pain perception.

The Periphery

Tissue damage results in the release of cell contents into the interstitial space. This initiates an inflammatory response which draws in white cells and mast cells that release histamine. The resulting mixture has been referred to as the 'sensitizing soup' and the contents bind to receptors on the primary afferent nociceptors.[2]

Primary afferent nociceptors (PAN) consist of:

- Aδ fibres – medium diameter lightly myelinated fibres that project into laminae I, III and IV of the dorsal horn. These conduct so-called 'fast pain', described as pricking or sharp pain.
- C fibres – slow conducting unmyelinated fibres, with their cell bodies in the dorsal root ganglia (DRG) and dendrites extending into lamina I, II and V of the dorsal horn. These conduct more slowly than Aδ fibres and pain is described as burning and aching pain.

The phenotypes of the nociceptors change in response repeated to nerve injury and inflammation. This dynamic neural plasticity lowers the transduction threshold

309

of nociceptors and contributes to primary hyperalgesia, which is defined as abnormal intensity of pain relative to stimulus.[2]

The Dorsal Horn and Spinal Cord

The cell bodies of nociceptive afferents that innervate the trunk, limbs and viscera are found in the DRG, while those innervating the head, oral cavity and neck are in the trigeminal ganglia and project to the brainstem trigeminal nucleus.[1]

Primary afferent nociceptors activate dorsal horn neurons by releasing two major classes of neurotransmitters:

- Glutamate as the primary neurotransmitter
- Neuropeptides such as substance P, calcitonin gene-related peptide (CGRP), galanin and somatostatins

Glutamate binds to two receptors on the secondary afferent, N-methyl-D-aspartate (NMDA) and α-amino-3-hydroxy-5-methyl-4-isoxazoleproprionic acid (AMPA) (Table 3.2.1). During the initial phase, glutamate binds to AMPA receptors, and the incoming traffic in the PAN matches traffic in the secondary nerve. When a threshold of AMPA receptors is reached due to repetitive stimuli, conformational changes occur which allow binding of glutamate to NMDA receptors, which causes traffic in the secondary afferent to rise dramatically and is known as 'wind-up'.[2]

TABLE 3.2.1 Examples of Primary Afferent and Dorsal Horn Pain-Related Receptors and Ligands

Receptor	Subtype	Ligand
Serotonin (5-HT)	$5\text{-}HT_3$	5-Hydroxytryptamine
Nicotinic acetylcholine (nAch)	Nn	Acetylcholine
Glutamate (Glu)	NMDA ($GluN_{1\text{-}2}$), AMPA ($GluA_{1\text{-}4}$), kainate ($GluK_{1\text{-}5}$)	Glutamate
Histamine (HA)	H_1	Histamine
Bradykinin (BK)	B_1, B_2	Bradykinin
Cannabinoid	CB_1, CB_2	Anandamide, 2-arachidonylglycerol (2-AG)
Opioid	μ, δ, κ, NOP	Dynorphin, endorphin, enkephalin, endomorphin, nociceptin

Central Projections of Nociceptive Pathways

Different qualities of overall pain experience are subserved by five major ascending spinal cord projection pathways: the spinothalamic, spinoreticular, spinomesencephalic, cervicothalamic and spinohypothalamic pathways.[1]

The spinothalamic tract originates from lamina V and predominantly distributes nociceptive information to the somatosensory cortex associated with sensory-discriminative aspects of pain.

The spinoparabrachial pathway originates from the dorsal horn and influences areas of the brain concerned with affect.

Descending Pathways

Descending pathways from higher centres project to the dorsal horn and inhibit pain transmission. The activation of these pathways releases the neurotransmitters noradrenaline and serotonin.

Other inhibitory systems in the dorsal horn include the cannabinoid receptor type 1 (CB1) and $\alpha_4\beta_2$ nicotinic acetylcholine receptor.[2]

ACUTE POSTOPERATIVE PAIN

Pain Assessment

The assessment of acute pain should include a general medical history, relevant physical examination, a specific 'pain history' and an evaluation of associated functional impairment.[1] Pain is also affected by behavioural, environmental, social and cultural factors which may influence the patient's response to therapy. In the postoperative period, preoperative anxiety, depression and catastrophizing have been shown to correlate with higher pain intensity and opioid requirements.

Pain can be broadly classified into two types: nociceptive and neuropathic pain.

Nociceptive Pain

Nociceptive pain (somatic and visceral pain) has the following characteristics:

- Somatic pain – may be described as sharp, hot or stinging, generally well localized and is associated with local and surrounding tenderness
- Visceral pain – may be dull, cramping or colicky, is often poorly localized and may be associated with symptoms such as nausea, sweating and cardiovascular changes

Neuropathic Pain

Neuropathic pain is defined as 'pain caused by a lesion or disease of the somatosensory system' (www.iasp-pain.org/taxonomy). It has the following characteristics:

- History of injury or disease leading to damage of peripheral or central nervous system

- Described as burning, shooting or stabbing
- May be paroxysmal
- Associated with surgery that has a risk of nerve injury, e.g. amputations and hernia repairs
- May have the presence of dysaesthesias, hyperalgesia, allodynia or areas of hypoaesthesia
- May have regional autonomic features and phantom phenomena

Pain Measurement

Regular and repeated pain measurements enable the assessment of the patient's response to treatment. This is done at both rest and when undertaking appropriate functional activity such as on movement or with coughing. A reduction in pain intensity of 30%–35% has been rated as clinically meaningful by patients with acute pain from a variety of sources (e.g. after surgery, trauma and acute cancer pain).[1] Self-reporting of pain should be done whenever appropriate due to the subjective nature of pain.

Unidimensional Pain Measurement

Unidimensional pain scales include:

- Visual analogue scale – a 100-mm horizontal line with 'no pain' at the left end and 'worst pain imaginable' at the right end. The patient is asked to mark a score to represent their pain, a rating of > 70 is indicative of severe pain.
- Verbal numerical rating scale – the patient is asked to give their pain a numerical score out of 10, where 0 is no pain and 10 is worst pain imaginable.
- Verbal rating scale – four-descriptor; none, mild, moderate and severe pain.
- Pictorial scales – useful for measuring pain in children with a series of faces, usually five or six depicting a range of expression from tearfulness to happiness. The child can point to the face which mirrors how they feel.

Multidimensional Pain Measurement

Multidimensional tools aim to provide further information about the characteristics of pain and its impact on the individual. Examples used in assessing acute pain include:

- Abbey Pain Scale – for patients with dementia or communication difficulties
- Neuropathic Pain Questionnaire – comprises 12 items and can be self-reported
- Critical Care Pain Observation Tool (CPOT) – for patients in critical care units

Other Measures of Pain

These include:

● Patient surveys – patient experience and satisfaction data
● Requirement for analgesics, e.g. morphine consumption as recorded by patient-controlled analgesia (PCA) machines

Outcomes

Treatment of acute pain is important not only for the humanitarian reasons of patient comfort and satisfaction, but it also leads to better outcomes in both the short and long term.

Short-Term Adverse Effects

Adverse sequelae of uncontrolled postoperative pain include delayed postoperative recovery, increased postoperative morbidity, delayed return of normal physiological functions, restriction of mobility with increased risk of thromboembolism and heightened catecholamine response leading to increased oxygen consumption.

Uncontrolled pain is recognized as the primary cause of pulmonary dysfunction after surgery, with reduced sputum clearance, atelectasis, regional under ventilation, perfusion inequality, shunting of venous blood and reduced functional residual capacity all contributing to hypoxia.

Psychologically, failure to relieve acute pain may result in increased anxiety, inability to sleep, a feeling of helplessness, loss of control and autonomy.

Long-Term Adverse Effects

Poorly controlled acute pain may lead to the development of persistent postsurgical pain (PPSP), which is pain that develops after surgery and lasts at least 2 months. PPSP appears to be higher in operations with the risk of nerve injury such as thoracotomy, mastectomy, limb amputation and hernia repair.

It is also possible that ongoing treatment of acute pain with opioids after discharge from hospital may lead to inadvertent long-term opioid use and the risk of diversion and abuse.[3]

DRUGS USED IN ACUTE POSTOPERATIVE PAIN MANAGEMENT

Pharmacological interventions may be administered before the surgical event (pre-emptive analgesia), before pain onset (preventive analgesia) or by repeat administration over the postoperative period.

Pre-emptive analgesia is treatment that is more effective than the same treatment administered after surgical incision. Pre-emptive analgesia prevents the development of altered processing of afferent input that would otherwise amplify postoperative pain (central sensitization).

Preventive analgesia is demonstrated when treatment is effective beyond the duration of action of the target drug. Preventive analgesia aims to minimize peripheral and central sensitization arising pre-operatively, intra-operatively and postoperatively.

Preventive analgesia encompasses multimodal analgesia.

Multimodal Analgesia

Multimodal analgesia compared to mainly opioid-based analgesia improves pain control and reduces opioid consumption and adverse effects.[1]

A multimodal analgesia approach is achieved by combining different analgesics that act by different mechanisms at different sites in the nervous system, resulting in additive or synergistic analgesia with lowered adverse effects of sole administration of individual analgesics.[4] For example, nonsteroidal anti-inflammatory (NSAIDs) drugs consistently reduce opioid consumption, and gabapentin has opioid sparing affects in the perioperative period.[4]

The knowledge of pain pathways enables different sites of pharmacological intervention and is represented in Fig. 3.2.1.

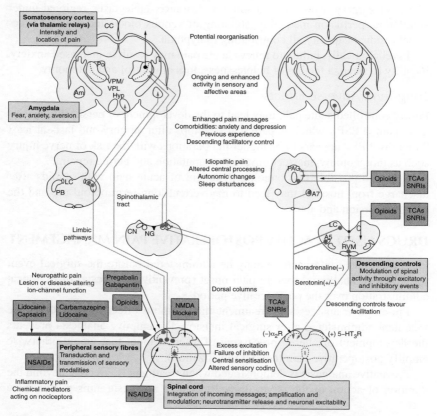

FIGURE 3.2.1 Pain pathways. *Source:* With permission from Elsevier: *The Lancet Neurology* 2013;12(11):1084–95.

Nonsteroidal Anti-inflammatory Drugs

The term nonsteroidal anti-inflammatory drugs refers to both nonselective NSAIDs and selective COX-2 inhibitors (Coxibs). Coxibs can be classified on the basis of their chemical structure (Table 3.2.2). NSAIDs are reversible cyclooxygenase (COX) inhibitors with the exception of aspirin, which binds covalently and acetylates the enzyme irreversibly. Nonselective NSAIDs block both COX-1 and COX-2, whereas the COX-2 inhibitors selectively block COX-2.

The enzymes exist in several isoforms; COX-1 is the constitutive isoform that takes part in the regulation of platelet and renal function, COX-2 is the inducible form which is upregulated in inflammatory processes and COX-3 is a variant of COX-1 and has a key role in the CNS.

Mechanism of Action

The main action of NSAIDs is inhibition of prostaglandin synthesis in peripheral tissues, nerves and the CNS. They have other actions independent of effects on prostaglandins, including basic cellular and neuronal processes.

TABLE 3.2.2 Chemical Classification of NSAIDs

Chemical Classification	NSAID
Acetic acids	
Indoleacetic acids	Acemetacin, indomethacin, sulindac
Naphthylacetic acid	Nabumetone
Phenylacetic acids	Aceclofenac, diclofenac
Pyrroleacetic acids	Ketorolac, tolmetin
Coxibs	Celecoxib, etoricoxib, valdecoxib
Fenamates	Mefenamic acid
Oxicams	Piroxicam, tenoxicam, meloxicam
Propionic acids	
Phenyl propionic acids	Ibuprofen, fenbufen, fenoprofen, flurbiprofen, ketoprofen, tiaprofenic acid
Naphthyl propionic acids	Naproxen
Pyrazolones	Azapropazone, phenylbutazone
Salicylic acids	
Acetylated	Aspirin
Nonacetylated	Diflunisal, salicyl salicylate
Others	Licofelone, paracetamol (acetaminophen)

Efficacy

NSAIDs have the following properties:

- Analgesic, anti-inflammatory and antipyretic
- Multiple routes of administration – oral, intravenous, intramuscular, rectal and topical
- Similar efficacy of nonselective NSAIDs and Coxibs for postoperative pain
- Provide better pain relief in combination with paracetamol than either drug alone
- Effective as sole analgesics after minor to intermediate surgery
- Opioid sparing effect $\cong 30\%$ – useful after major surgery

The time to peak plasma concentration with standard oral formulations of NSAIDs is >1 h. This time is halved using soluble formulations. Rectal administration is associated with slower and more varied response.

Adverse Effects

NSAIDs have a number of adverse effects affecting the gastrointestinal, respiratory, renal, haematological and cardiovascular systems. They should be used with caution in the elderly.

Gastrointestinal System

Reductions in prostaglandin levels by inhibition of COX-1 may lead to erosions of the gastrointestinal mucosa. This is not a local problem and erosions will not be avoided by using parenteral or rectal routes of administration. Acute damage can occur with short-term use. All long-term nonselective NSAIDs increase the risk of upper gastrointestinal (GI) complications. Ibuprofen and diclofenac appear to have the lowest rates of side effects while piroxicam and ketorolac are associated with the highest rates. Limited prophylaxis against gastric, but not small intestine ulceration is possible with prostaglandin analogues (e.g. misoprostol) and proton pump inhibitors (e.g. omeprazole), which are far more effective than H_2 antagonists (e.g. ranitidine)

There is a reduced risk of GI complications with Coxibs compared to nonselective NSAIDs.

Anastomotic Leak after Bowel Surgery

The evidence for this is conflicting with studies showing both no difference and an increase in anastomotic leakage for nonselective NSAIDs. There is no increased risk with Coxibs.[1]

Respiratory System and Allergic Reactions

Nonselective NSAID-exacerbated respiratory disease affects 10%–15% of people with asthma and precipitation of bronchospasm by aspirin and other NSAIDs is a recognized phenomenon in individuals with moderate asthma, chronic rhinosinusitis or nasal polyps.

Nonselective NSAIDs also cause drug-induced hypersensitivity reactions which include rhinitis, asthma, urticaria, angioedema, anaphylaxis, toxic epidermal necrolysis, maculopapular reactions, pneumonitis, nephritis or aseptic meningitis.[1]

Coxibs do not induce bronchospasm in patients with NSAID-exacerbated respiratory disease.

Renal System

Renal prostaglandins regulate and maintain renal blood flow and glomerular filtration rate in the presence of circulating vasoconstrictors. The risk factors for renal toxicity are as follows:

- Pre-existing renal impairment
- Where the circulating blood volume is decreased such as hypovolaemia, hypotension, dehydration and sepsis
- Use of other nephrotoxic agents including angiotensin-converting enzyme inhibitors, aminoglycosides, methotrexate and IV contrast media

Long-term use may cause sodium and water retention, which may exacerbate hypertension and even induce cardiac failure.

The risk of kidney injury increased with a decrease in COX-2 selectivity although the same renal precautions should apply for both nonselective and selective NSAIDs.

Haematological System

Nonselective NSAIDs impair platelet function and increase surgery-related bleeding.

COX-2 is not expressed by platelets; hence, COX-2 inhibitors do not impair platelet function. The use of COX-2 inhibitors is associated with less surgical blood loss in comparison to nonselective NSAIDs.

Bone Healing

The evidence for the effect on bone healing is conflicting and a structured review of over 300 papers has concluded that there is not enough clinical evidence to deny patients with simple fractures the analgesic benefits of these compounds.[1]

There is no good evidence of clinically significant inhibitory effect of Coxibs on bone healing.

Cardiovascular System

All NSAIDs approximately double the risk of congestive heart failure.[1]

Individual drugs have specific risk profiles of their pro-thrombotic effect irrespective of their COX selectivity. For example, the risk of cardiovascular events appears to be lowest with naproxen and highest with diclofenac and the Coxibs.

In noncardiac surgery, the short-term use of NSAIDs does not increase the risk of postoperative cardiovascular adverse effects. However, these concerns remain with cardiac surgery and the US FDA does not support the use of all NSAIDs in the immediate postoperative period following cardiac surgery.

Co-administration of an NSAID with various opioids including codeine, oxycodone and tramadol provides better pain relief than either drug alone.

Paracetamol (Acetaminophen)

Mechanism of Action

The mechanism of action of paracetamol is not well understood as there are no known endogenous binding sites. Paracetamol causes weak inhibition of COX and it has a central antinociceptive effect. It also appears to activate the endocannabinoid system and spinal serotorgenic pathways.

Efficacy

Paracetamol has the following properties:

- Analgesic and antipyretic, but not anti-inflammatory
- Oral and intravenous routes – good oral bioavailability 63%–89%
- Effective postoperative intravenous analgesic – Number needed to treat (NNT) 4.0 over 4 h
- Reduces opioid requirements by 30% over 4 h after a single dose

A limit of 4 g/day is recommended, with a maximum of 60 mg/kg/day in patients weighing less than 50 kg. A higher dose, 1 g 4-hourly up to a maximum dose of 6 g/day, has been suggested in adults with normal body weight and no contraindications.

The time to peak plasma concentration with standard oral formulations of paracetamol is <1 h, whereas onset of analgesia is faster with intravenous paracetamol. Rectal administration is associated with slower and more varied response with a time to peak plasma concentration of 2–4 h.

Adverse Effects

Paracetamol is generally well tolerated. Hepatic damage occurs in overdose but is very rare at therapeutic doses.

Paracetamol use in pregnancy and infancy is associated with an increase in the incidence of childhood asthma and there is a potential association between paracetamol and acute liver failure in children with myopathies.

Long-term use of paracetamol in adults, particularly at higher doses, may be linked with a small increased risk of adverse cardiovascular events, gastrointestinal bleeding and impaired kidney function. In newly diagnosed chronic kidney disease patients, paracetamol use is associated with an increased risk of end stage renal failure.[1]

Opioid Analgesic Drugs

Opioids are very effective as postoperative analgesics and are the main drugs used for the treatment of moderate to severe pain. Doses have to be titrated for each patient, because of considerable interpatient variation in requirements. In adults, age is a better determinant of dose than weight in opioid naïve patients.

Opioids influence the emotional aspects of pain, such as anxiety and fear, as well as reducing the actual pain threshold, so making intolerable pain tolerable.

In the absence of any contraindications, the oral route is the route of choice for opioid administration, unless a patient has severe acute pain. In treating acute pain, one opioid is not superior to others but some opioids are better in some patients.

Opioids can be categorized according to their affinities for opioid receptors present in the brain and spinal cord. This ranges from pure agonists, through partial agonists and partial antagonists to pure antagonists (Table 3.2.3).

TABLE 3.2.3 Opioid Drugs

Agonists	Mixed Agonist/ Antagonist	Antagonist
Phenanthrene alkaloids of opium		
Codeine		Methylnaltrexone
Morphine		
Papaveretum		
Thebaine	Buprenorphine	
Semisynthetic alkaloids		
Diamorphine		
Dihydrocodeine		
Dihydromorphinone		
Oxycodone		
Oxymorphone	Nalbuphine	Naloxone
Synthetic agents		
Morphinans		
Levorphanol	Butorphanol	
	Dezocine	
Benzomorphinans	Meptazinol	
	Pentazocine	

TABLE 3.2.3 Opioid Drugs—cont'd

Agonists	Mixed Agonist/ Antagonist	Antagonist
Phenylpiperidine derivatives		
Alfentanil		
Fentanyl		
Pethidine		
Phenoperidine		
Remifentanil		
Sufentanil		
Tapentadol		
Tramadol		
Diphenylheptane derivatives		
Dipipanone		
Dextromoramide		
Methadone		
Piritramide		
Propoxyphene		

Mechanism of Action

Opioids act on opioid receptors, which are found in the brain, spinal cord, gastrointestinal and urinary tracts, lungs and peripheral nerve endings.[3] There are four types of opioid receptors: δ-receptor (OP1), κ-receptor(OP2), μ(OP3) and orphan receptor (ORL1).[2] Opioid analgesic drugs act at the μ-receptor to produce analgesia.

Actions of Opioids

Central Nervous System

- Depress – awareness, anxiety, pain sensation, respiration
- Stimulate – vomiting centre, secretion of antidiuretic hormone, Edinger–Westphal nucleus (causing small pupils), hallucinations (rarely)

Smooth Muscle

- Depress – vascular tone, peristalsis
- Stimulate – bronchoconstriction, bowel sphincters, biliary sphincter, fallopian spasm, arrectores pilorum

Psychological and Physical Addiction

Patients may develop both tolerance (tachyphylaxis) and dependence (or addiction). In addicts, withdrawal results in agitation, severe abdominal cramps, diarrhoea and lacrimation (so-called 'cold turkey'). It is relieved by further doses of opioid.

Other

- Stimulate secretion of catecholamines
- Depress metabolism
- Release histamine
- Induce vagally mediated bradycardia (short-acting opioids)

Routes of Administration of Opioids

Oral

Oral opioids can give good analgesia and should be used in preference to parenteral injection when possible. There are several oral formulations of oral morphine; morphine in solution and immediate-release and modified-release tablets. Peak plasma concentrations occur within 1 h of morphine in solution and immediate-release tablets, with analgesia lasting 4 h. Modified-release tablets produce delayed peak plasma concentrations and long-lasting analgesia (12 h MST Continus®; 24 h MXL®). The potency ratio of oral:parenteral morphine is 1:6 for acute pain, but 1:2 to 1:3 for nonacute pain. An antiemetic may be needed.

Oral oxycodone is an effective analgesic and is available in immediate-release (Oxynorm® 5–10 mg 4-hourly) and sustained-release (Oxycontin® 12-hourly) preparations. Oxycontin may have a more rapid onset than other sustained-release opioid preparations.

Oral Transmucosal (Sublingual and Buccal)

Fentanyl is equally well absorbed after both buccal and sublingual administration. Sublingual buprenorphine is used as an analgesic and as an alternative to methadone in opioid addiction.

Sublingual sufentanil administration using a portable electronic dispenser is being investigated for the treatment of postoperative pain as an alternative to PCA.

Rectal

Morphine suppositories have similar bioavailability and duration to oral morphine. The potency ratio to oral morphine is 1:1.

Parenteral

Traditionally opioids have been given intramuscularly or subcutaneously. Neonates, infants, the elderly and the unfit are more susceptible to respiratory depression. Children and young adults are often quite resistant.

Continuous intravenous infusions of opioid analgesic can be given until pain is relieved, and then the dose titrated against the pain. Continuous infusions should only be used in an appropriately monitored clinical environment. Opioid infusions are not necessarily followed by either psychological dependence or physical sequelae. Intravenous PCA gives good pain relief at a lower dosage than intramuscular injection.

PCA commonly refers to a method of pain relief which uses electronic or disposable infusion devices and allows patients to self-administer an opioid as required. Many opioids, including morphine, fentanyl, oxycodone and tramadol have been used with PCA and there is no good evidence to suggest any major differences in either efficacy or the incidence of side effects.

Transdermal

The high lipophilicity of fentanyl makes it ideal for transdermal delivery. Fentanyl patches provide sustained delivery of 25–100 µg/h, and although these are not recommended for routine acute pain management, they can be of use for patients who have high or prolonged opioid requirements.

Once the fentanyl patch is placed on the skin, it may take 24 h or longer before peak blood concentrations are reached, and if the patch is removed, the depot of fentanyl in the skin reservoir means blood levels will decrease slowly with the elimination half-life around 17 h after patch removal.

An ionotophoretic patient-controlled transdermal delivery system for fentanyl is also available.

Extradural

Lipophilic opioids are no more potent by this route than when given systemically, unless they are mixed with local anaesthetics.

An extended release (ER) suspension of morphine (Depodur™) has been developed for epidural use consisting of morphine molecules suspended in liposome complexes (lipofoam). Studies have shown it to give better pain relief compared to standard epidural morphine; however, respiratory depression is more likely with extended release epidural morphine than with PCA opioids.[1]

Intradural

Intrathecal morphine improves analgesia and is opioid-sparing for up to 24 h. After major surgery, the incidence of opioid-induced ventilatory impairment and pruritus is higher with intrathecal morphine compared with intravenous PCA opioids.[1]

Adverse Effects

Opioids have a number of adverse effects affecting the gastrointestinal, respiratory and cardiovascular systems. Adverse gastrointestinal effects include nausea and vomiting in up to 50% of patients. Respiratory depression and hypotension may be troublesome. Bradycardia can also occur with short-acting opioids.

Opioids have a relatively slow onset of analgesia. Intravenous remifentanil and alfentanil are fastest (1–2 min), whereas fentanyl may take 15–20 min to produce analgesia; unfortunately, respiratory depression has a faster onset. However, because of the considerable variation of individual response (up to tenfold) it is difficult to predict the correct dose.

In susceptible individuals addiction may be a problem, and tachyphylaxis and occasional hallucinations may occur with prolonged administration.

Opioid Agonists

Naturally Occurring Alkaloids of Opium

Morphine

Morphine (Morpheus, Greek God of dreams, son of Somnus, God of sleep) has been in use for over 2000 years. Morphine remains the standard against which other opioids are compared.

Opium comes from the dried latex of unripe capsules of the poppy head (*Papaver somniferum*). Morphine is one of over 25 alkaloids contained in opium, but only morphine, codeine and papaverine have wide clinical use. The concentration of morphine in opium is 9%–17%. Morphine was isolated from opium in 1806, its chemical structure determined in 1925 and synthesized in 1952. Morphine salts are not destroyed by boiling.

Morphine is a good analgesic and a poor relaxer of smooth muscle. There is large interpatient variability with morphine.

Pharmacodynamics

Central nervous system: Morphine is analgesic, sedative, anxiolytic, euphoric, addictive, a respiratory depressant, and causes nausea and vomiting. It is more effective against dull, continuous, visceral than against sharp, intermittent pain. Very rarely, restlessness and delirium follow its injection and dysphoria follows. Intracranial pressure increases because of the raised PCO_2.

Effect on the eye: Morphine causes miosis by a central action, via the oculomotor nerve, stimulating the Edinger–Westphal nucleus. Intraocular tension is reduced in both normal and glaucomatous eyes.

Cardiovascular system: Morphine causes mild vasodilation in clinical doses, and sometimes bradycardia. Patients in shock should be given morphine intravenously so that it does not accumulate unabsorbed in the ischaemic tissues only to produce a massive effect when absorption occurs with improvement in the circulation. Only small doses are needed.

Respiratory system: Morphine reduces the response of the respiratory centre to PCO_2 with 50% depression of the PCO_2 response curve at plasma levels of 100 μg/L (postoperative analgesia occurs at 12–25 μg/L). Respiratory rate, rather than tidal volume, is decreased.

The risk of respiratory depression is increased in patients with a history of obstructive sleep apnoea or on concurrent central nervous system depressant drugs.[3]

Respiratory depression is difficult to define or measure clinically, and the respiratory rate is often used, by default. However, sedation scores are a better indicator of morphine toxicity.

Breathing may become periodic (Cheyne–Stokes) or irregular.

Bronchoconstriction can occur and is worse in asthmatic patients.

Maximal respiratory depression comes on 30 min after intramuscular injection, and sooner after intravenous injection. Morphine also depresses the cough reflex.

Gastrointestinal tract: Morphine constricts the sphincters of the gut and reduces peristalsis, more so when given intramuscularly than when given orally. Constipation is a significant adverse effect of prolonged morphine administration.

Nausea and vomiting are due to central stimulation. This is seen most strongly with the allied drug apomorphine. Vomiting after morphine depends partly on the movements of the body and the position of the patient; it sensitizes the vomiting centre to vestibular movements. Early ambulation after morphine will cause more nausea than quiet bed rest. Antiemetics can control this nausea, some more effectively than others. About one-third of postoperative patients feel nauseous after opioids, females much more so than males.

Morphine contracts the sphincter of Oddi, raising the pressure in the bile ducts, which rarely causes severe pain. Atropine does not fully antagonize this action, but glyceryl trinitrate, nalorphine, levallorphan, epinephrine (adrenaline), aminophylline and amyl nitrite do.

Genitourinary tract: The tone and peristalsis of the ureters and other smooth muscles (e.g. of the hollow viscera, bladder sphincter and fallopian tubes) are increased with morphine, an action antagonized by atropine.

The tone of the vesical sphincter is increased and may hinder micturition – a common postoperative problem. Urinary output is decreased owing to stimulation of secretion of antidiuretic hormone. There is little relaxation of the uterus during labour. Morphine crosses the placental barrier and depresses fetal respiration.

Endocrine system: The posterior pituitary and adrenal medulla are stimulated by morphine, so antidiuretic hormone and blood catecholamine levels increase. Blood glucose may rise.

Other: Morphine sometimes causes itching, especially of the nose, face, neck and trunk. It is thought that pruritus is due to the activation of μ-opioid receptors, and possible dopamine and $5\text{-}HT_3$ activation.[3] If it needs to be treated, the following options may be considered; a change in the opioid, low-dose naloxone or ondansetron.[3]

Pharmacokinetics

Routes of administration of morphine are many; oral, buccal, intramuscular, intravenous, subcutaneous, rectal, transcutaneous and intra-articular.

Morphine has a pKa of 7.9, is poorly lipid soluble, is 40% bound to plasma albumin (30% in neonates) and exhibits triexponential elimination kinetics. The elimination half-life varies with age; neonate 629 min, infant 233 min, child 120 min adult 180 min.

Oral morphine undergoes significant first-pass metabolism. Biotransformation is by conjugation with glucuronic acid in the liver, followed by excretion in the bile and by the kidneys. Both active (morphine-6-glucuronide [M6G]) and inactive (morphine-3-glucuronide [M3G]) metabolites depend on the kidneys for excretion. Deficient renal excretion may cause accumulation and respiratory depression.

Morphine appears in breast milk, saliva and sweat. Special care is necessary in infants under 6 months of age, elderly or debilitated patients, and in patients with a raised PCO_2, suprarenal insufficiency, myasthenia, myotonia, hypothyroidism, asthma, raised intracranial pressure, respiratory depression, hepatic failure, renal failure, acute alcoholism and diverticulitis and in labour.

The dose of morphine is 0.15 mg/kg intramuscularly, although in adults age rather than weight is a better determinant of dose. The intravenous bolus dose is 0.03 mg/kg, repeated as necessary. A dose of 0.1–1 mg/kg intravenously prevents the 'stress response'.

Onset of analgesia with morphine is 3–10 min (intravenously) and 10–20 min (intramuscularly). The duration is 3–4 h.

Codeine

The name is from the Greek for poppy-head. Codeine phosphate is classed as a weak opioid, and metabolic conversion of about 10% of the dose to morphine accounts for most of the analgesic effect. The enzyme responsible for this conversion is the CYP-2D6 cytochrome P450 isoenzyme. In the Caucasian population, 8%–10% of people are poor metabolizers, whereas 3%–5% are ultrarapid metabolizers. Those who are ultrarapid metabolizers have significantly higher levels of morphine and morphine metabolites after the same dose of codeine. Codeine is contraindicated in postpartum women as there may be a higher level of morphine in the breast milk of ultrarapid metabolizers.[1]

Semi-synthetic Alkaloids of Opium

Diamorphine

Diamorphine hydrochloride (heroin) is the diacetyl ester of morphine. It is a prodrug and is hydrolysed to 6-monoacetyl morphine and morphine. It is a drug of addiction, because of the euphoria it creates, and was introduced into medicine in 1898. Diamorphine is not licensed for medical use in many countries including the USA and Australia.

Diamorphine hydrochloride depresses the respiratory centre and the cough reflex more than morphine and is twice as efficient as an analgesic.

Diamorphine 5 mg has a faster onset of activity and fewer emetic sequelae than morphine 10 mg. It is an excellent postoperative analgesic, although its effect does not last as long as that of morphine. In coronary occlusion, 5 mg intravenously causes little cardiovascular depression or vomiting if given slowly.

Epidurally administered diamorphine resulted in a longer time to first PCA use and lower 24-h total morphine requirements compared to the same dose given as an intramuscular injection.[1]

Excretion of diamorphine hydrochloride is chiefly by the kidneys after conversion to morphine in the body.

Dihydrocodeine

Dihydrocodeine tartrate is a semisynthetic derivative of codeine with inherent analgesic activity. It is metabolized to dihydromorphine and is an analgesic and antitussive. It may cause nausea, constipation, dysphoria and vertigo, and it releases histamine.

Oxycodone

Oxycodone is a potent opioid agonist that is useful for the treatment of severe pain. It produces predictable and reliable analgesia after oral administration because of its higher, and less variable, bioavailability than morphine (50%–75%). Intravenous oxycodone produces similar analgesia to the same doses of morphine and can be given by PCA. It is metabolized in the liver to noroxycodone and oxymorphone (the latter is weakly active).

The dose of immediate release oral oxycodone is 5–10 mg 2–3-hourly.

Hydromorphone

Hydromorphone is five times as potent as morphine, from which it is derived. It has a similar efficacy and side effect profile to morphine and is metabolized to hydromorphone-3-glucuronide, which is dependent on renal excretion.

Synthetic Alkaloids of Opium

Pethidine (Meperidine)

Pethidine hydrochloride is the hydrochloride of the ethyl ester of 1-methyl-4-phenyl-piperidine-4-carboxylic acid.

Pethidine use is diminishing because of multiple disadvantages, of which the accumulation of norpethidine is the most significant. Norpethidine toxicity is associated with a variety of neuroexcitatory effects, ranging from nervousness to convulsions.

In clinical practice there is no evidence that pethidine is better than morphine for the relief of renal or biliary colic.

Pharmacodynamics

Analgesia: Pethidine relieves most types of pain, especially those associated with plain muscle spasm. It depresses the respiratory centre and cough reflex and is also a local analgesic. It has no effect on the ciliary body or iris. It raises the cerebrospinal fluid pressure and can cause addiction.

Smooth muscle: Pethidine has a direct papaverine-like effect on the smooth muscle of the bronchioles, intestine, ureters and arteries. It will often relieve bronchospasm. Vasodilation may be unwelcome in trauma patients and uncontrolled hypertensives.

Cholinergic effects: Pethidine has an atropine-like effect on cholinergic nerve endings.

Histamine release: Pethidine may release histamine from tissues.

Side effects: Side effects of pethidine include sweating, hypotension, vertigo and limb tingling.

Postoperative nausea is similar to that following morphine but comes on earlier. It is worse after intravenous than after intramuscular injection.

Like morphine, pethidine may cause hypotension if the head of the patient is raised, or with sudden movement. Because of its circulatory depressant effects, it is probably not the ideal drug for the relief of pain in myocardial infarction.

Norpethidine can produce nervousness, tremors, twitches, myoclonus and seizures.

Precautions: The administration of pethidine to patients receiving monoamine oxidase inhibitors may cause severe reactions and even death. There is restlessness, hypertension, convulsions and coma, with absent tendon jerks and an extensor plantar response. Hypotension may also be seen. The reaction is said to be due to serotonin reuptake inhibition.

Pharmacokinetics

The routes of administration of pethidine are the same as for morphine. Oral bioavailability is 45%–75% and 64% is bound to plasma protein.

Pethidine is metabolized at the rate of 17%/h. The biological half-life is 3–4 h in man and 80% is hydrolysed in liver. About 5%–10% is excreted unchanged by the kidneys. One metabolite, norpethidine, may cause convulsions or hallucinations if pethidine is given in large doses, for prolonged periods or with monoamine oxidase inhibitors. Patients in renal failure are at increased risk of norpethidine toxicity.

The dose of pethidine is 0.5 mg/kg intravenously and 1.5 mg/kg intramuscularly. Its onset of action is 2–5 min and its duration 2 h.

Fentanyl

Fentanyl, a 4-anilidopiperidine compound, is a pure opioid agonist with a high affinity for the μ-receptor. It is 75–125 times more potent than morphine as an analgesic. Unlike morphine, it has high lipid solubility and as a result is rapidly and extensively distributed in the tissues. Its metabolites are inactive and hence it is useful in patients with renal disease.

Fentanyl can be used for PCA, with a 5–10-min lockout interval.

Because of its high lipid solubility fentanyl can also be administered transdermally, but the fixed delivery rate of the patches is a major disadvantage in postoperative pain control.

The dose of fentanyl is a 10–20 μg as an intravenous bolus using PCA, and from 25 μg/h up to 100 μg/h using a transdermal patch.

Tramadol

Tramadol is a synthetic 4-phenyl-piperidine analogue of codeine. It has a weak central action on opioid receptors and also acts on descending monoaminergic pathways, whereby it acts as a serotonin and noradrenaline-reuptake inhibitor, and thus is commonly referred to as an atypical centrally acting analgesic.

Tramadol is an effective treatment for neuropathic pain with a NNT of 3.8.

The risk of respiratory depression is significantly lower with tramadol than with other opioids given at equianalgesic doses. Tramadol also causes less constipation. However, nausea and vomiting are common side effects.

There is a risk of inducing serotonin toxicity when tramadol is combined with other serotonergic medicines, in particular SSRIs. Administration of tramadol to elderly patients in the postoperative period is a risk factor for delirium.[1]

Tapentadol

Tapentadol is a combined μ-agonist and noradrenaline-reuptake inhibitor. Tapentadol is eliminated by glucuronidation and the dose may need to be adjusted in liver impairment.

Tapentadol is effective in treating nociceptive and neuropathic pain.[1] It has a similar efficacy to opioids with a reduced rate of gastrointestinal effects such as nausea, vomiting and constipation.

Tapentadol shows a lower rate of abuse and diversion than oxycodone and a rate comparable to tramadol.

Methadone

Methadone hydrochloride is a powerful analgesic. It causes less sedation and has a more prolonged action than morphine (half-life 40–90 h, increasing with subsequent doses). It exhibits high oral bioavailability. Absorption from fatty sites (e.g. subcutaneous and epidural) is very slow.

Methadone has been used to wean addicts from morphine and for chronic pain. It is used for the maintenance treatment of patients with an opioid addiction because of the high oral bioavailability (60%–95%), high opioid potency and sustained effect. The use of methadone for acute pain management is limited by the long unpredictable duration of action. Careful dosage titration is required to avoid accumulation and adverse effects.

Methadone is metabolized primarily by the cytochrome P450 group of enzymes and over 50 drug–drug interactions with methadone are described. Concurrent administration of other medicines that are CYP450 inducers may increase methadone metabolism (e.g. carbamazepine, rifampicin, some antiretroviral agents) leading to reduced efficacy or even withdrawal. Conversely, medicines that inhibit CYP450 (e.g. other antiretrovirals, some SSRIs, grapefruit juice) may lead to raised methadone levels and an increase in adverse effects or overdose.[1]

Dextropropoxyphene

Dextropropoxyphene is the only one of the four isomers of propoxyphene to have analgesic activity. It undergoes extensive first-pass metabolism. It has poor analgesic properties on its own and is commonly combined with paracetamol. The use of this compound has been withdrawn in many countries because of not only its low efficacy but also a number of risks associated with it, including QT-interval prolongation and possibility of Torsade des Pointes and cardiogenic death.

Mixed Agonist/Antagonists and Partial Antagonists of Opium

Buprenorphine

Buprenorphine is a powerful, long-acting synthetic thebaine derivative with partial agonist properties. Its duration of action is up to 10 h.

Buprenorphine is used as an analgesic agent and also as an alternative to methadone in opioid replacement therapy in opioid addiction.

There is a ceiling effect for respiratory depression but not for analgesia; however, even buprenorphine alone can cause fatal respiratory depression. If buprenorphine-induced respiratory depression occurs, complete reversal with naloxone is possible, although higher than usual doses and a longer duration of naloxone infusion are required.[1]

Buprenorphine can be used in patients with renal impairment and has less immunosuppressive effects than pure μ-opioid agonists.

The commonly used routes are transdermal and sublingual.

Opioid Antagonists

Specific antagonism to opioids was first described in 1915. Antagonists are usually the n-allyl derivatives of opioid analgesics. The more potent the narcotic, the smaller the dose of its allyl derivative necessary to antagonize opioid-induced respiratory depression. They have high receptor affinity and low receptor activity. They do not lead to addiction. They may cause signs of withdrawal in narcotic addicts. The probable mode of action is competition at receptor sites on cell surfaces. Antagonists counteract the analgesia produced by morphine, pethidine and oxymorphone.

Naloxone

Naloxone, n-allyl noroxymorphone, is derived from oxymorphone. It was first synthesized in 1972. It also antagonizes the respiratory depression caused by pentazocine and dextropropoxyphene.

The short duration of effect of naloxone (1 h) may be less than that of the opioid it is designed to antagonize, so repeat dosage or an infusion may be necessary. It relaxes spasm of the sphincter of Oddi induced by opioid analgesics. With careful titration of dosage, analgesia is not reversed.

Naloxone can be used in the treatment of opioid-induced respiratory depression and in midwifery to reverse fetal respiratory depression due to opioids.

Naloxone reverses the respiratory depression but not the analgesia of intrathecally administered opioids.

Naloxone may raise blood pressure in septic shock, suggesting that endorphins may contribute to this hypotension and can cause acute pulmonary oedema in previously fit patients. It has caused arrhythmia and even sudden death and can be given intramuscularly for a more prolonged effect.

Pharmacokinetics

The half-life of naloxone is 20 min. It is metabolized in the liver.

The dose of naloxone is 0.1–0.4 mg intravenously, repeated as required (0.01 mg/kg in neonates).

Methylnaltrexone

Methylnaltrexone is epoxymorphinan. It has a very long half-life, and its main use is as an aid in maintaining abstinence in opioid withdrawal. It has been suggested that with careful titration of dosage, analgesia is not reversed.

Opioid Overdose

Opioid overdose causes coma, respiratory depression, hypoxia, acidosis and muscle compression (from deep sedation), all leading to rhabdomyolysis and acute renal failure. Pulmonary oedema (noncardiogenic), cerebral oedema, convulsions and aspiration pneumonia also occur. Treatment is by immediate reversal with naloxone and by organ support.

Inhalational Analgesia

Entonox

Entonox is a 50:50 mix of nitrous oxide and oxygen. It can be used for procedures such as bone marrow aspiration, dressing changes, labour contraction pain and in pre-hospital trauma care.

When using this technique the potential haematological and neurological adverse effects of repeated nitrous oxide exposure, disrupting vitamin B_{12} metabolism and methionine synthesis, should be considered.

Methoxyflurane

Methoxyflurane, in low doses, is an effective analgesic agent with a rapid onset. It is used in the pre-hospital setting and a range of procedures in the hospital setting with good safety data (see Chapter 2.3).

NMDA Receptor Antagonists

The NMDA-receptor antagonists ketamine and magnesium have useful analgesic properties.

Ketamine

Ketamine is widely used to provide anaesthesia in out-of-hospital settings and in the developing world, but it is also used in the management of pain at lower doses.

Ketamine is commonly available as a racemic mixture of *R*- (−) and *S*- (+) isomers, with the S- (+) isomer a more potent analgesic (twofold) with a shorter duration of action.

Efficacy

Ketamine has the following properties:

- Perioperative administration reduces postoperative opioid consumption.
- Improves pain relief when added to PCA opioids.
- In low dose improves analgesia in patients with opioid-tolerance.
- Reduces the development of opioid-induced hyperalgesia.
- Reduces the development of persistent pain after surgery.
- Epidural ketamine (without preservative) added to opioid-based analgesia improves pain relief.
- Caudal ketamine (without preservative) in children, in combination with local anaesthetic or as the sole medicine, improves and prolongs analgesia.

Adverse Effects

Ketamine is associated with the following adverse effects:

- Dose-dependent neuropsychiatric effects such as hallucinations and dysphoria – can be reduced by the concurrent addition of benzodiazepines
- Nystagmus, blurred vision and diplopia

Toxicity leads to cognitive impairment and abuse to liver and bladder toxicity.

At low doses ketamine does not cause clinically relevant cardiovascular side effects.

Magnesium

Perioperative intravenous magnesium has an opioid sparing effect.

In combination with spinal anaesthesia, magnesium reduces pain scores and opioid consumption. It also reduces the development of opioid-induced hyperalgesia.

Gabapentinoids

Mechanism of Action

Gabapentinoids bind to the $\alpha2\delta$ subunit of the presynaptic voltage-gated calcium channel in spinal nociceptive neurons. Binding leads to the inhibition of calcium influx and a commensurate reduction in the relative excitatory transmitters in the pain pathway.

Pregabalin is the newer of the two substances and has a linear dose-response relationship, longer half-life and higher oral bioavailability and potency compared to gabapentin.

Efficacy

Gabapentinoids are effective in the treatment of neuropathic pain (NNT 4), including pain due to spinal cord injury, traumatic or postsurgical nerve injury.[1]

Perioperative gabapentinoids improve analgesia and reduce postoperative opioid consumption.

Adverse Effects

These include:

- Sedation, visual disturbance, dizziness
- Weight gain and peripheral oedema

α2-Adrenergic Receptor Agonists

Perioperative intravenous $\alpha2$-adrenergic receptor agonists (clonidine and dexmedetomidine) have opioid-sparing effects and reduce nausea. However, their use in acute pain is limited by side effects such as hypotension and sedation.[1]

Intrathecal clonidine improves the duration of analgesia and anaesthesia when used as an adjunct to intrathecal local anaesthetics.[1]

Clonidine improves the duration of analgesia and anaesthesia when used as an adjunct to local anaesthetic peripheral blocks, but it is associated with increased hypotension and bradycardia.[1]

Antidepressant Medications

The analgesic effect is mainly due to the activation of the inhibitory descending pathways by inhibiting the reuptake of norepinephrine and serotonin (5-hydroxytryptamine, 5-HT).

Amitriptyline (a tricyclic antidepressant) is commonly recommended as first-line for the treatment of acute neuropathic pain. It may cause drowsiness and is best given at night. In elderly patients, it should be avoided as the use of medications with anticholinergic activity increases the risk of cognitive impairment and mortality in this patient group.[1]

Duloxetine is a serotonin-norepinephrine reuptake inhibitor (SNRI) and has an opioid sparing effect perioperatively.

Systemic Local Anaesthetics

Mechanism of Action

Local anaesthetics block sodium channels, thereby stabilizing cell membranes and reducing ectopic discharges which are thought to be a major contributor to neuropathic pain states (see Chapter 4.1)

Efficacy

Perioperative intravenous lidocaine infusion is opioid sparing. It reduces significantly the 'at rest' and 'during activity' pain scores, nausea, vomiting and duration of ileus after abdominal surgery and length of hospital stay.[1]

Perioperative intravenous lidocaine has a preventive analgesic effect, with the beneficial effect of lidocaine significantly outlasting the expected duration of action of the drug.[1]

The use of systemic lidocaine in acute neuropathic pain states is extrapolated from its efficacy in the treatment of chronic neuropathic pain states.

Adverse Effects

These include dizziness, perioral numbness and tingling, tachycardia, cardiac arrhythmias and haemodynamic instability.

Corticosteroids

Dexamethasone reduces postoperative pain and opioid requirements to a limited extent but also reduces nausea, vomiting, fatigue and improves quality of recovery compared to placebo.[1] Mild hyperglycaemia may follow the perioperative administration of corticosteroids.

Capsaicin

Topical capsaicin formulations are effective in patients with peripheral neuropathic pain. Topical capsaicin acts in the skin to attenuate cutaneous hypersensitivity and reduce pain by a process of 'defunctionalization' of nociceptive fibres.

The main adverse effect is local, transient application site reactions, predominantly pain and erythema.

NONPHARMACOLOGICAL TECHNIQUES USED IN ACUTE POSTOPERATIVE PAIN MANAGEMENT

A wide variety of nonpharmacological techniques have been shown to have a beneficial effect in the management of acute postoperative pain but the magnitude of benefit tends to be small.

The effect of listening to music is equivalent to paracetamol 325 mg in reducing pain intensity and opioid requirements. The type of music is not important.

Hypnosis relaxation is an effective adjunctive procedure for a wide variety of surgical procedures, irrespective of patient 'susceptibility'.

Perioperative acupuncture reduces pain intensity, opioid requirements and opioid related side effects for up to 72 h.

Transcutaneous electrical nerve stimulation (TENS) can be used as an adjunctive therapy for minor and procedural pain. Effectiveness is dependent on selection of optimal parameters, and a higher frequency (80–130 Hz) is best for acute pain.

Evidence of benefit of other therapies, including massage, aromatherapy, guided imagery and touch therapies, is lacking.

PRINCIPLES OF ACUTE POSTOPERATIVE PAIN MANAGEMENT

It is important to identify and if possible remove the cause of pain (e.g. distended bladder). Thereafter, treatment may be by pharmacological or non-pharmacological techniques.

In general terms, acute pain is best treated by a multimodal approach, using drug combinations to enhance analgesia and minimize side effects. Paracetamol is the fundamental component, to which NSAIDs (or COX-2 inhibitors) are added in the absence of contraindications, with opioid therapy completing the combination. Other analgesic therapies, including regional blockade, adjuvant agents and nonpharmacological techniques, are valuable additions to this approach.

Pharmacological Techniques

Pharmacotherapy includes the use of simple analgesics either as single or combination preparations, and opioid analgesics, often administered using PCA.

Combination preparations include aspirin-paracetamol, codeine-paracetamol, ibuprofen-codeine and tramadol-paracetamol.

Caffeine, which has been shown to have adjuvant analgesic activity when combined with simple oral analgesics, may be added to simple analgesics. A dose of more than 65 mg is needed. In a large meta-analysis of over 10000 patients, analgesia from paracetamol or paracetamol-and-aspirin with caffeine 65 mg added was approximately 1.4 times more potent than without added caffeine.

Patient-Controlled Analgesia

Patient-controlled analgesia (PCA) refers to the on-demand, intermittent self-administration of analgesic drugs by a patient. PCA is predominantly used to deliver opioid analgesics, but other classes of drugs can be administered in this way. The traditional route of drug delivery has been intravenous (IV-PCA), but subcutaneous (SC-PCA) and epidural (PCEA) routes can also be used.

The quality of analgesia is normally good and allows for wide interpatient variation. The basic variables of PCA are as follows:

- Demand (bolus) dose
- Lockout interval (length of the time between patient demands)
- Background infusion rate (if used)
- Hourly or 4-hourly limit

The use of background infusion in adults is controversial, tending to increase sedation and other side effects without improving analgesia, but is more often used in children (in an appropriately monitored clinical environment).

Most PCA infusers incorporate sophisticated pump technology with a lockable syringe compartment to prevent tampering. Compact ambulatory devices are a further refinement. Alternatively, lightweight disposable infusers that combine an elastomeric pressure mechanism (a cylinder containing the analgesic drug within an elastic balloon) with a non electronic nonprogrammable wristwatch control device are available.

A one-way Y-connector enables use with intravenous infusions. Anti-reflux valves should be used to prevent reflux delivery of drug into gravity-fed infusion tubing in the event of an occlusion.

Preoperative counselling in the use of PCA is helpful.

Opioids administered by PCA are associated with less severe decreases in oxygen saturation than when given as intermittent intramuscular boluses.

Pain control, respiration and sedation should be monitored.

Patients express high satisfaction with PCA. The advantages include not having to bother nurses, rapid pain relief, self-control of their own pain, exact titration of dose and lack of intramuscular injections.

Some patients worry about overdose, addiction, lack of personal contact with nurses and machine dysfunction.

PCA is also useful in children over 5 years of age, in obstetrics and in acute medical diseases (e.g. sickle cell crisis and malignant pain). Parent-controlled analgesia, nurse-controlled and spouse-controlled analgesia have all been described.

Drawbacks of PCA include:

- Problems with patient selection/education
- Opioid side effects, especially respiratory depression (rare 0.019%) and excessive sedation; also nausea, vomiting, itching, ileus and hallucinations
- Complex equipment leading to programming errors – equipment malfunction occurs in 5% of cases
- Underutilization, overutilization and syphoning

Regional Techniques

Regional techniques, either as a single shot or with a continuous infusion catheter, form an important part of the multimodal management of postoperative pain.

They fall into three main categories: central neuraxial block (see Chapter 4.3), peripheral neuraxial block and local infiltration (see Chapter 4.2).

The advantages of these techniques include:

- Better postoperative analgesia
- Reduction in opioid consumption as well as opioid-related side effects
- Better dynamic pain relief compared to opioid analgesia
- Increased patient satisfaction

Nonpharmacological Techniques

A number of nonpharmacological interventions can be used for pain relief, including:

- Transcutaneous electrical nerve stimulation (TENS)
- Acupuncture
- Psychological techniques including information provision, relaxation strategies and cognitive-behavioural interventions
- Complementary and alternative medicine
- Physical therapies including manual and massage therapies

Acute Pain Management for Opioid-Dependent Patients

Opioid dependency can occur in patients on long-term opioid treatment for chronic pain, cancer pain, opioid replacement therapy (e.g. methadone) or those using opioids recreationally. These patients may need review by a specialist acute pain team as their pain may be difficult to control in the postoperative period.[5]

The principles of management are as follows:

- Preoperative counselling and discussion of patient expectation and goals
- Continued perioperative administration of maintenance opioid
- Use of perioperative multimodal analgesic techniques with regional anaesthesia, pharmacological techniques including the use of PCA
- Ketamine to enhance opioid-induced analgesia
- Opioid rotation if pain is poorly controlled postoperatively

ACUTE NEUROPATHIC PAIN

Neuropathic pain can develop after surgery and must be diagnosed promptly and managed correctly to ensure the best outcome for the patient and avoid chronicity. The diagnosis of neuropathic pain can be obtained from the presenting features of burning, stinging or shooting pain, increasing despite apparent tissue healing, with a relative lack of response to doses of opioids used in the postoperative period (this does not imply that neuropathic pain is unresponsive to opioids), and some or all of the features of allodynia, hyperaesthesia and dysaesthesia.

Treatment of acute neuropathic pain should follow guidelines for chronic neuropathic pain with the use of tricyclic antidepressants and gabapentinoids, however, these drugs may take time to have their full effect. Ketamine, intravenous lidocaine and opioids (including tramadol and tapentadol in particular) may offer faster onset of effect than other treatment options.[1]

DELIVERY OF ACUTE PAIN MANAGEMENT

An Acute Pain Service can teach, encourage and oversee the delivery of analgesia. It involves surgeons, physicians, pharmacists, physiotherapists, anaesthetists and nurses working in a concerted manner to reduce pain, facilitate rehabilitation and improve outcome for the patient.

The relief of postoperative pain can be badly managed, simply by neglect. Failure can occur at the point of writing prescriptions and at the point of delivery of analgesia by nurses. Experience with pain teams has heightened awareness of this, but the risk is that the whole of the pain (and fluid and other) management of the hospital may be transferred by default to the team by those surgeons and nurses who previously looked after it. Thus, pain team activity may need to be mainly advisory in continuing effective analgesia and developing even more efficient methods by nurses, surgeons, etc.

Invaluable roles of the pain team include education of patients and staff about pain relief techniques, introduction of treatment protocols based on scientific evidence, regular audit of efficacy and safety of techniques used, and provision of a consultation service for difficult pain management cases.

REFERENCES

1. Schug SA, Palmer GM, Scott DA, Halliwell R, Trinca J. Acute Pain Management: Scientific Evidence. 4th ed. Melbourne: Australian and New Zealand College of Anaesthetists and Faculty of Pain Medicine; 2015. Available at: http://asp-au.secure-zone.net/v2/index.jsp?id=522/2055/8212&lng=en
2. Bromley L, Brandner B, eds. Acute Pain. Oxford Pain Management Library. Oxford: Oxford University Press; 2010.
3. McIntyre P, Schug S, eds. Acute Pain Management. A practical guide. 4th ed. Boca Raton: CRC Press Publishers; 2015.
4. Buvanendran A, Kroin J. Multimodal analgesia for controlling acute postoperative pain. Curr Opin Anaesthesiol 2009;22:588–93.
5. Mehta V, Langford R. Acute pain management for opioid dependent patients. Anaesthesia 2006;61:269–76.

FURTHER READING

Schug SA, Palmer GM, Scott DA, Halliwell R, Trinca J. Acute Pain Management: Scientific Evidence. 4th ed. Australian and New Zealand College of Anaesthetists and Faculty of Pain Medicine: 2015. Available at: http://asp-au.secure-zone.net/v2/index.jsp?id5522/2055/8212&lng5en

Chapter 3.3

Complications of Anaesthesia and the Perioperative Period

Timothy Cook

PERIOPERATIVE COMPLICATIONS IN CONTEXT

A recent review has suggested that anaesthesia is one of the safest clinical specialties with incidences of complications of anaesthesia reported as 1 in 5 for minor complications, 1 in 100 for major complications and 1 in 100,000 for death.[1]

Effective patient-centred care requires a focus on what is important to the patient, rather than the doctor or other health care practitioner. Patients may experience complications in the perioperative period as a consequence of surgery, anaesthesia or the interaction between the two. Increasingly, anaesthetists and surgeons are considering perioperative care in a joint manner.

Up to 300 million patients undergo surgery each year globally. Risk factors for complications and death include patient health (ASA status, comorbidities), age, extent of surgery and emergency surgery.

Mortality within a month of elective in-patient surgery is approximately 0.5%–4%. Mortality after day-care surgery is much lower at < 0.1%.

Postoperative morbidity may be measured by a number of tools including the Postoperative Morbidity Score which captures elements of ongoing medical treatment that prevents patients from being discharged. Complications after elective in-patient surgery affect approximately 20% of patients. Complication rates after surgery are less variable than mortality rates between hospitals, suggesting that it is the failure to identify and successfully manage complications ('failure to rescue') that differentiates poor from well-performing hospitals. Complications and mortality after unscheduled surgery are much higher (≈6% overall). After emergency laparotomy mortality is >10%, increasing to ≈20% in those aged > 80 years and almost all patients experience complications.

Elderly, frail and comorbid patients are likely to experience more complications and are less able to tolerate the physiological stresses they produce, which accounts for increased mortality. Surgical factors increasing complications include duration and extent of surgery. Patients who experience complications are likely to have a more prolonged hospital stay and increased hospital mortality. Further, the lasting impact of complications occurring in hospital is underestimated. Several studies indicate that in-hospital complications are associated with increased mortality for several years, in one study up to 10 years, after surgery.

Over recent years the age and ASA status of surgical patients has increased, whereas perioperative and anaesthetic mortality has decreased. Frailty is an increasingly well-recognized risk factor for complications and death, in the increasingly elderly surgical population, but there is still a challenge in identifying, quantifying and managing it.

Increasing ASA status correlates across numerous studies and a wide range of surgical procedures with increased risk of complications, mortality, hospital length of stay and resource use. ASA ≥ 3 is associated with an up to 10-fold increase in complications, increasing even further in emergency surgery. Despite its limitations, the ASA physical status classification remains a useful risk-stratification tool.

The stress response to surgery is not a 'complication' of either surgery or anaesthesia but it is a physiological consequence of both. Many of the physiological consequences of the stress response create the precursive setting for complications. Surgery and trauma induce a neuro-humoral 'stress response' with increased levels of catecholamines, antidiuretic hormone, gluco- and mineralocorticoids and other catabolic hormones. This response can be blocked or attenuated by the use of regional anaesthesia, high-dose opioids and to an extent by anaesthesia itself, but the benefits of doing so remain unproven. The stress response leads to water and, to a lesser extent, sodium retention, a tendency to hyperglycaemia and catabolism. This needs to be taken into account when considering fluid balance. There is also a relatively prothrombotic state after surgery due to disturbance of all elements of Virchow triad (blood stasis, endothelial wall injury and hypercoagulability) which impacts on both venous thromboembolism and cardiovascular thrombotic events.

Among perioperative complications, respiratory complications are very frequent and can range from minor to life-threatening. Cardiac, renal, infectious and neurological complications have a lower frequency but high impact.

When considering 'complications related to anaesthesia', it is worth noting that many may be missed, judged to be or contribute to 'surgical complications'. Efforts to improve patient experience and outcome require a collaborative approach to reduce the burden of complications, of whatever aetiology, in all patients. Awareness of the risks of anaesthesia and surgery plays a major part in deciding the proposed anaesthetic technique for an individual patient.

This chapter is laid out by system and by diagnosis. In clinical practice the initial presentation of problems is often more complex and the diagnosis is not always obvious. The immediate management of all acute complications must follow a structured approach and for serious complications the airway, breathing and circulation (ABC) approach remains a good start.

COMPLICATIONS AND THE PATIENT PERSPECTIVE

When asked which perioperative complications they associated with anaesthesia and wished to avoid, the top ranked items by patients were (in order): vomiting, gagging on the tracheal tube, incisional pain, nausea, recall without pain, residual weakness, shivering, sore throat and somnolence. More recently in a study of patient reported outcome measures (PROMS) related to anaesthesia in >15,000 patients, the commonest identified 'worst features' of the perioperative period were anxiety (34%) and pain (17%). Factors associated with low rates of satisfaction included dissatisfaction with the process of waking up, management of pain or postoperative nausea and vomiting (PONV), or 'general dissatisfaction with anaesthesia care'.

When expert anaesthetists were asked which complications they wished to avoid and which were most common, the five items with the highest combined score were incisional pain, nausea, vomiting, preoperative anxiety and discomfort from i.v. insertion. The complications anaesthetists considered most important to prevent irrespective of frequency were death, recall with pain, peripheral nerve injury, recall without pain and corneal injury.

The pattern of litigation in anaesthesia is perhaps indicative of complications that are important to patients and cause unexpected harm (but the pattern is quite different from the pattern of patient safety incidents). One study found that anaesthetists are involved in around two-thirds of hospital admissions but litigation against anaesthetists accounts for approximately 2.5% of claims and 2.5% of costs related to litigation, making anaesthesia a low-risk specialty in medicolegal terms.[2] The (nonexclusive) categories associated with the highest number of claims against anaesthetists are regional anaesthesia ($\approx$45%), obstetrics ($\approx$30%), inadequate anaesthesia ($\approx$20%), drug administration including anaphylaxis ($\approx$10%) and airway management ($\approx$10%). Claims relating to positioning, venous cannulation, wrong side procedures and consent each account for <5% of claims but should not be ignored. Claims related to airway management and central venous cannulation are more often associated with severe patient outcomes and high claim-related costs, whereas the converse was true with claims related to regional and obstetric anaesthesia. Clinical themes in claims include the following:

- Regional anaesthesia – central neuraxial blockade (80%), epidurals more than spinals and both more than peripheral nerve blocks. Peripheral blocks; ocular blocks prominent, nerve injury and inadequate anaesthesia with >50% of claims obstetric. Many claims of low harm and low cost.
- Obstetrics – regional anaesthesia (80%), inadequate anaesthesia and issues around consent. Many claims of low harm and low cost.
- Inadequate anaesthesia – approximately 40% awareness, 40% inadequate regional anaesthesia and 20% inadvertent brief paralysis without anaesthesia (i.e. muscle relaxant given in error). The latter group associated with 100% payout and highest costs.

- Airway – hypoxic brain injury and death, airway trauma. Clinical area with highest costs and highest mortality per case.
- Drug administration – drug errors leading to awareness, opioid overdose, administration of known allergen, severe anaphylaxis.
- Venous access – serious morbidly and mortality from CVC insertion. Clinical area with second highest costs per claim.

Conversely, patient safety incidents are more likely to feature problems with breathing system (disconnections, misconnections and leaks), drug errors (overdosage, underdosage, wrong drug), airway management problems (failed intubation, oesophageal and bronchial intubation, premature or accidental extubation, aspiration) and equipment failures (laryngoscopes, intravenous infusion devices and breathing system valves). Some of this data is old and complications related to misplaced and displaced tubes and ventilation failures should now be much reduced by improved technology and widespread use of capnography.

A recent prospective study of 15,000 patients used a validated tool to measure anaesthesia-related patient reported outcome measures (ROMS). The predominant causes of anaesthesia-related discomfort were thirst, drowsiness and operative pain. PONV was less common that hoarseness, sore throat or cold (Table 3.3.1).

TABLE 3.3.1 Anaesthesia-Related Patient Reported Outcome Measures of Discomfort

Anaesthesia-Related Discomfort	None (%)	Moderate (%)	Severe (%)	Overall Incidence (%)
Postoperative thirst	30	51	19	70
Drowsiness	35	54	10	64
Pain at surgical site	51	37	11	48
Hoarseness	65	29	4	33
Sore Throat	69	26	3	30
Cold	75	19	4	23
Nausea and vomiting	82	13	3	17
Confusion	83	15	1	16
Shivering	85	11	3	14
Pain at injection site	86	12	1	13

Source: With permission from Walker EMK, Bell M, Cook TM, Grocott MPW, Moonesingh SR. Patient reported outcome of adult perioperative anaesthesia in the United Kingdom: a cross-sectional observational study. Br. J. Anaesth. 2016;117:758–66. doi: 10.1093/bja/aew381.

HUMAN FACTORS AND QUALITY IMPROVEMENT IN PREVENTION OF COMPLICATIONS

Although the underlying health of a patient and the surgery undertaken are major determinants of risk of complications, it is widely accepted that patients also experience complications due to variations in quality of care and due to human error (omission, commission). Up to 10% of in-patients are reported to experience iatrogenic harm, with 50% of this is considered preventable and 1 in 10 such complications contributing to death.

In a large study, the commonest human factors associated in anaesthetic critical incidents were inattention/carelessness, inexperience, haste, failure to check equipment, unfamiliarity with equipment, poor communication, restricted access, failure of planning, distraction, lack of skilled assistance, lack of supervision, fatigue and decreased vigilance. All these factors were also seen in the UK National Audit Projects (NAPs) reporting major anaesthetic complications (see Sources of Audit Data on Complications below).

Clinical human factors science describes the impact on health care delivery of the manner in which humans interact with their environment. This includes environmental, organizational and job factors and individual characteristics which influence behaviour. There is increasing recognition that a focus on human factors can improve reliability of health care delivery (which is rarely >60% reliable, compared to industrial processes >99.99% reliable). Quality improvement programmes often focus on implementing evidence-based, locally evaluated care bundles and efforts to improve reliability of care delivery. Enhanced recovery programmes are one example and have been shown to improve efficiency of care and patient outcomes.

There is no doubt that improved communication within theatre teams, shared understanding, shared goals, appropriate use of checklists and protocolized care can improve reliability, reduce clinician-centred variation and improve patient care. The use of the World Health Organisation (WHO) surgical checklist is a good example of this.

Sources of Audit Data on Complications

Large-scale audit projects can provide robust data particularly on rarely occurring events. The National Audit Projects (NAPs) are a series of UK studies examining rare, clinically important complications of anaesthesia. These studies combine a year-long national registry of events with a national activity survey to provide both quantitative data (prevalence, incidence) and qualitative data on these complications. The following complications have been studied:

- Major complications of central neuraxial blockade – NAP3[3]
- Major complications of airway management – NAP4[4,5]
- Accidental awareness during general anaesthesia (AAGA) – NAP5[6]
- Life-threatening perioperative anaphylaxis – NAP6[7]

With high rates of case ascertainment and almost 100% national involvement they provide a rich source of data. The NAPs are referred to as appropriate in specific sections.

SPECIFIC COMPLICATIONS

Death and Cardiac Arrest

Death caused by anaesthesia alone is uncommon and decreasing in incidence (3.6 per 10,000 pre-1970, 0.5 per 10,000 1970–1980s and 0.3 per 10,000 after 1990). Anaesthetic mortality in developed countries was reported to be 25 per million (compared to surgical mortality for ASA 1 and 2 patients being 600 and 1400 per million operations). In reality, anaesthesia-related actions, omissions and complications probably contribute to many more deaths than are captured by such estimates. Due to this, and its rarity, death is a relatively blunt measure of anaesthetic quality. An ASA score ≥3 raises mortality approximately five-fold compared to ASA 1–2.

Case mix with impact on mortality risk and the baseline ASA of patients presenting for surgery has increased over the decades. Age impacts on the risk of events, and patients younger than 1 and older than 65 years are more likely to suffer critical incidents, cardiac arrest and death. ASA impacts on harm, with patients ASA 4–5 considerably more likely to experience harm or death when such incidents occur.

A study of >1 million ASA 1–2 patients undergoing elective and emergency anaesthesia reported rates of critical incidents, cardiac arrest and death of approximately 600, 100 and 30, respectively, per million cases. Rates of cardiac arrest and death solely caused by anaesthetic management were 18.7 and 1.4 per million cases. In a recent study of >1 million ASA 1–2 patients, the risk of death or other serious complication from anaesthesia was also about 10 per million anaesthetics; main event types were airway problems (40%) and hypovolaemia (30%), with other causes including bronchospasm, myocardial infarction and primary cardiac arrest.

A 2003 study of >2 million anaesthetics reported the risk of cardiac arrest to be 100 per million anaesthetics. Causes were as follows:

- Drug overdose or selection error – 15%
- Serious arrhythmia – 14%
- Myocardial infarction or ischaemia – 9%
- Airway management problems – 8%
- High spinal – 7%
- Inadequate vigilance – 7%
- Massive haemorrhage managed badly – 5%
- Overdose of inhaled anaesthetic – 3%
- Suffocation, aspiration –3%
- Dis/or misconnection – 2%

Most studies of mortality come from the developed world. There is evidence that anaesthesia-related mortality is many-fold higher in less developed and less resourced centres with airway management and haemorrhage management being prominent causes in these settings.

Airway and Respiratory Complications

These include the following:

- Procedural complications
- Pulmonary aspiration of gastric contents
- Failure of routine airway techniques
- Upper airway obstruction
- Lower airway obstruction
- Postoperative pulmonary complications
- Obstructive sleep apnoea
- Airway trauma
- Pulmonary barotrauma and pneumothorax
- Airway fire and oxygen cylinder fire

Procedural Complications

Currently the best evidence of the frequency and nature of harmful airway complications (death, brain damage, emergency surgical airway, unanticipated intensive care unit admission) occurring during anaesthesia and in ICU and emergency departments is provided by NAP4,[4,5] which reported 46 events per million general anaesthetics or 1 in 22,000. Among ≈3 million anaesthetics, airway events led to 16 deaths and 3 episodes of persistent brain damage; a mortality rate of 5.6 per million general anaesthetics or 1 in 180,000. Rates for different airway devices are given in Table 3.3.2.

TABLE 3.3.2 Complication Rates for Different Airway Devices

Type of Event	Events	Death and Brain Damage
All	1 in 22,000	1 in 150,000
TT events	1 in 12,000	1 in 110,000
SAD events	1 in 46,000	1 in 200,000
FM events	1 in 22,000	1 in 150,000

TT, tracheal tube; SAD, supraglottic airway device; FM, facemask.

Source: Cook TM, Woodall N, Harper J, Benger J; Fourth National Audit Project. Major complications of airway management in the UK: results of the Fourth National Audit Project of the Royal College of Anaesthetists and the Difficult Airway Society. Part 2: intensive care and emergency departments. Br J Anaesth 2011;106:632–42.

In three-quarters of fatal cases, care was judged to be poor, indicating a high rate of human factors. A follow-up study identified human factors impacting on every case with an average of four factors per case. Important themes in NAP4 (many of which are not new) were as follows:

● Poor airway assessment – assessment of potential airway difficulty and aspiration risk were equally important.
● Poor planning – a coordinated, logical sequence of plans that aim to achieve good gas exchange and prevention of aspiration is recommended.
● Failure to plan for failure – outcome was generally poor.
● Awake fibreoptic intubation (AFOI) indicated but not used – suggests lack of skill or confidence, poor judgement and lack of suitable equipment.
● Difficult intubation managed by multiple attempts at intubation – deteriorates to a 'cannot intubate cannot oxygenate' situation (CICO).
● Supraglottic airway devices (SADs) used inappropriately – resulting in both nonaspiration events and aspiration.
● SADs used to avoid tracheal intubation in patients with a recognized difficult intubation, with subsequent problems and patient harm.
● Anaesthesia for head and neck surgery featured prominently.
● Poor management of the obstructed airway.
● Obese and morbidly obese patients were over-represented.
● High failure rate of emergency cannula cricothyroidotomy during CICO ≈60% – in contrast a surgical technique for emergency surgical airway was almost universally successful.
● Aspiration was the single commonest cause of death.
● Unrecognized oesophageal intubations due to failure to correctly interpret a capnograph trace.
● One-quarter of events occur during emergence or recovery – airway obstruction is the commonest cause.
● Poor judgement, education and training were the commonest causes.
● Airway management was poor in more than a third of events.
● One in four major airway events occur in ICU or the emergency department – outcome was more likely to lead to permanent harm or death.
● Failure to use capnography in ventilated patients contributed to more than 70% of ICU-related deaths.
● Displaced tracheostomy, and to a lesser extent displaced tracheal tubes were the greatest cause of major morbidity and mortality in ICU.
● Most events in the emergency department were complications of rapid sequence intubation.

The NAP4 report recommends that anaesthetists should be skilled and practised in surgical (now referred to as 'scalpel') cricothyroidotomy.

Pulmonary Aspiration of Gastric Contents

Aspiration occurs in approximately 1 in 1000 emergency patients and 1 in 5000–10,000 elective patients. There is little strong evidence to suggest choice of airway device impacts on this rate in routine clinical practice, but this is clearly biased by clinical decision-making intended to reduce such events. Despite its rarity, aspiration remains the commonest cause of airway-related deaths and brain damage.

If aspiration occurs or is suspected, the patient should be given 100% oxygen, tilted head-down, turned on to one side and pharyngeal and tracheal suction done. Where a SAD is in place, this need not be removed unless the clinical situation dictates, as this may lead to further aspiration. The stomach should be emptied. Bronchoscopy may be needed, along with supportive treatment such as bronchodilators and physiotherapy.

Consequences

Food particles can physically block airways and lead to rapid mortality. Acid with a volume of greater than 25 mL and a pH below 2.5 is traditionally quoted as sufficient to cause lung damage. Acute chemical trauma to bronchial and alveolar epithelia results in acute exudative pneumonitis or Mendelson syndrome. Controlled ventilation may worsen the effects of aspiration. Steroids do not provide benefit.

In the majority of cases aspiration does not cause harm. Patients who have not developed clinical signs (cough, wheeze/bronchospasm, hypoxia, respiratory distress, chest signs, abnormal chest X-ray) 2 h after an aspiration event are unlikely to develop major complications. Conversely those who develop an aspiration pneumonitis can develop all these symptoms and signs and require ICU admission. Approximately half to two-thirds of these patients recover rapidly, whereas the others may go on to develop ARDS and multi-organ failures (MOFS). Death can occur from acute airway obstruction, pulmonary oedema, ARDS or MOFS.

Infection may develop and can be primary (although gastric contents are normally sterile) or secondary to lung injury. Antibiotics should be restricted to cases with evidence of infection. Foreign material gravitates into the dependent apex of the lower lobe (usually the right) with the patient lying supine and into the dependent upper lobe with the patient on their side, and these are the commonest sites of local infection.

Prevention

There is no fool-proof method of prevention, but the following are well-established practices:

- Assess all patients for risk of aspiration and manage appropriately.
- Gastric ultrasound may be used to assess the state of the stomach and stratify risk.
- Use a regional anaesthesia and allow the patient to remain awake with full protective reflexes; if general anaesthesia is needed:
  - Adequate preoperative starvation – 6 h for solids and 2 h for clear fluids.
  - If a nasogastric tube is in place, use it to remove liquid from the stomach, but this will not remove solids.

- Metoclopramide 10 mg is prokinetic and may hasten gastric emptying.
- Inhibit secretion of gastric acid by giving H2 antagonists, such as ranitidine 150 mg orally, or a proton pump inhibitor such as omeprazole 20–40 mg orally, the night before and on the morning of operation. Neutralize residual acidity with antacids, sodium citrate (15–30 mL of 0.33 M solution) immediately preoperatively.
- Avoid heavy preoperative sedation, which may result in aspiration in the ward before or after operation.
- Perform an awake fibreoptic intubation under topical anaesthesia.
- Rapid sequence induction of anaesthesia. If there is a modestly increased risk of aspiration and an SAD is to be used a second generation device (i.e. one with design features to reduce the risk of aspiration) is appropriate.
- Extubate when fully awake. If this is not possible, extubate with the patient in the lateral position, perhaps head-down, and leave in that position until airway reflexes have fully returned.

Rapid Sequence Induction

This technique is aimed at providing prompt intravenous anaesthesia and a short period of unconsciousness between induction and establishing a secure airway with a cuffed tracheal tube (TT) (see Chapter 2.6). There is controversy about the technique in general and particularly about cricoid force. It is a misconception that RSI enables rapid wake-up in the event of airway difficulty; if this occurs, active management of the airway is required to prevent hypoxaemia and further complications.

The technique involves adequate pre-oxygenation, a predetermined dose of intravenous induction agent followed by a rapidly acting muscle relaxant. Cricoid force is applied to prevent aspiration of regurgitant matter. A force of 10 N (1 kg) is appropriate as the patient loses consciousness, increasing to 30 N (3 kg) with loss of consciousness. Higher forces provide no benefit and distort the airway. The risk of difficult laryngoscopy is increased several-fold during RSI and videolaryngoscopy may be helpful to improve laryngeal view and observe application of cricoid force.

Failure of Routine Airway Techniques

Most major airway complications arise from failed, difficult or delayed tracheal intubation. Most cases of CICO are originally 'cannot intubate, CAN oxygenate' before deteriorating after multiple attempts at airway instrumentation. The following failure rates are reported for routine airway management in the elective anaesthetic setting:

- Face-mask ventilation < 1 in 700
- Insertion and ventilation via SAD < 1 in 50
- Tracheal intubation < 1 in 1500
- Cannot intubate, cannot oxygenate < 1 in 5000
- Requirement for front of neck access (FONA) ~ 1 in 50,000

Secondary complications such as airway trauma and aspiration also increase during airway difficulty and failure. Multiple repeated attempts at the same procedure without changing something significantly have a <20% chance of success and increase the risk of failure of other techniques.

Importantly when one airway technique fails, the likelihood of failure of other techniques is markedly higher. This is termed 'composite airway failure'. Several airway techniques have predictors of failure in common, e.g. obesity, reduced mouth opening, Mallampati class 3-4 and neck rigidity, and this explains some of the failure.

- When intubation fails, mask ventilation may fail in up to 10% of cases.
- When mask ventilation is difficult (DMV), the risk of failed intubation increases more than 10-fold.
- When SAD insertion fails, the risk of DMV is increased three-fold.
- After multiple attempts at intubation, the risk of airway obstruction, failed rescue with a SAD or facemask and the risk of CICO all increase.

As a consequence, any patient who presents risk factors for difficulty with one mode of airway management must be assessed carefully for predictors of ease or difficulty with the techniques planned to be used if the first choice fails. This data also emphasizes the importance of 'first attempt success' in minimizing complications and failure. Use of modern airway equipment such as second-generation SADs and videolaryngoscopes has an important role in this respect.

Management of Failed Intubation

Failed intubation precedes many airway disasters. It is essential to distinguish 'cannot intubate, can oxygenate' from 'cannot intubate, cannot oxygenate' (CICO). The priority is to maintain oxygenation and avoid airway trauma that may lead to progression to an unrecoverable condition.

Cannot intubate, can oxygenate occurs in around 1 in 1500 anaesthetics. It should be managed in a protocolized manner with emphasis on (a) patient safety, (b) application of a preplanned airway strategy and (c) good communication to the team around. Multiple attempts at laryngoscopy should be avoided. Guidelines have been produced that provide extensive practical guidance.[8]

Failure rates of repeated attempts are ≈80%.

Videolaryngoscopy improves the view at laryngoscopy and reduces the incidence of difficult or failed intubation.

When tracheal intubation fails task fixation must be avoided and it is essential to recognize when techniques are failing: algorithms and cognitive aids may help. The vortex approach advocates up to three attempts (or one 'best attempt') at each of the facemask ventilations, SAD placement and laryngoscopy. If these have all failed to rescue the situation, it is time to transition to FONA even if oxygenation remains adequate, as it will inevitably deteriorate over time.

Cannot intubate, cannot oxygenate (CICO): This was previously described as 'cannot intubate, cannot ventilate' (CICV), but 'cannot intubate, cannot oxygenate' (CICO) better describes the problem and the priority.

CICO is rare during routine anaesthesia (<1:5000 with FONA required in 10%). It occurs more often in emergencies, ENT cancers, trauma, obesity, obstetrics, outside the operating room, but the elective setting probably occurs most commonly after multiple attempts at intubation in patients in whom ventilation was previously possible.

Death after CICO is more often due to failure to act than complications of rescue techniques, which are infrequent.

Front of neck access (FONA): Surgical/scalpel FONA techniques have a higher success rate than cannula cricothyroidotomy and it is recommended that all anaesthetists are educated and practised in 'scalpel cricothyroidotomy'.[7]

Use of cannula-based techniques retain a role for those who are expert in them, but it is notable that high pressure source ventilation ('jet ventilation') is associated with high rates of failure and complications.

Upper Airway Obstruction

Upper airway obstruction is a medical emergency that may present before, during or after anaesthesia. It is diagnosed by:

- Increased work of spontaneous breathing and use of accessory muscles of inspiration.
- Excessive abdominal movement and paradoxical movement of the chest wall (see-saw movement) in the spontaneously breathing patient.
- Noisy breathing, especially inspiration (stridor), unless obstruction is complete when no sound is heard.
- Progressive hypoxaemia and hypercapnia.
- During anaesthesia, reduced or absent movement of the reservoir bag, high airway pressure during intermittent positive-pressure ventilation (IPPV) and an absent or diminished capnograph trace.

Awake patients with upper airway obstruction often adopt a 'best-breathing position' which they find most comfortable. It is useful to establish the positions in which the patient feels most comfortable and which they avoid, as this is relevant during anaesthesia.

Patients who have chronic upper airway obstruction may have adapted to the obstruction and may present with considerably less distress and abnormal physiology than those with acute upper airway obstruction. These airways may be especially challenging to manage.

Subatmospheric intrathoracic pressures generated by upper airway obstruction may cause acute pulmonary oedema (especially after the obstruction is relieved; post-obstructive pulmonary oedema), which can be mistaken for aspiration and can cause prolonged hypoxia requiring ICU admission.

Causes and Management

Blocked circuits and other equipment faults: Causes include equipment faults such as misplacement, kinking or obstruction of an anaesthetic circuit/filter/ connector, TT or SAD. Fatalities have occurred as a result of foreign bodies (e.g. caps for intravenous tubing, clear plastic packaging) obstructing connectors and filters, or circuits obstructed by the wheel of an anaesthetic machine.

Less common faults are absence of fresh gas flow due to empty cylinders (e.g. in remote locations without piped gases) and blockage within the machine itself. Modern anaesthetic machines are increasingly complex; they may have multiple fresh gas outlets and it is essential to ensure that gas is flowing from the outlet in use. Modern machines also have electrical rather than mechanical switches and malfunction can lead to loss of or misdirection of gas flow.

Checking the complete anaesthetic circuit for patency and gas flow and all airway devices that are to be inserted, for patency, before every case reduces these risks considerably and should be routine practice. If obstruction is suspected immediate disconnection and ventilation via a separate device (e.g. a bag-mask-valve and fresh filter/catheter mount) should rapidly determine whether the problem is proximal to the TT/SAD or distal. The next step is to change the airway device to determine whether it is a TT/SAD or a patient problem. Capnography is central to assessing ventilation during this process.

Obstruction above the glottis: In the supine position in the unconscious patient, gravity leads to the lips, cheeks, soft palate, tongue and epiglottis all falling backwards. There is a general loss of airway tone, as a result of loss of consciousness, and reduced respiratory drive or apnoea. This leads to a fall in calibre of the pharynx and potential airway obstruction by the soft palate (nasopharynx), tongue base (oropharynx), epiglottis (trachea/laryngopharynx) or all three.

Airway obstruction can be managed by:

- Keeping the patient's dentures *in situ*
- Positioning the airway in the sniffing position (lower cervical spine flexed – often omitted – and upper cervical spine extended)
- Chin lift, progressing to jaw thrust if not effective
- Oropharyngeal airway
- Nasopharyngeal airway
- Face mask ventilation with positive pressure and a good seal
- Insertion of a SAD (as a temporizing or definitive airway)
- Tracheal intubation

Anaesthetizing the patient in the sitting position will reduce gravitational airway obstruction but risks haemodynamic instability.

Foreign bodies such as swabs, dislodged teeth, saliva, vomitus or blood must be removed, usually by suction or Magill's forceps. Very rarely, dislocation of the epiglottis or cysts or tumours of the epiglottis are encountered.

In patients with known masses or abnormalities above the glottis that increase the risk of airway obstruction, or decrease the likelihood of successful management of obstruction it is prudent to secure the airway awake before inducing anaesthesia. AFOI or awake videolaryngoscopy are appropriate techniques.

Obstruction at the glottis: Causes of glottis obstruction include:

● Laryngospasm
● Misplaced or displaced SAD
● Foreign body
● Swelling/trauma/tumour
● Nerve injury

The commonest complication leading to glottic obstruction is laryngospasm. This describes closure of the vocal cords with partial or complete airway obstruction. It causes inspiratory stridor, increased work of breathing, tracheal tug and paradoxical chest movement. If not treated it will cause desaturation and, particularly in children, bradycardia. It occurs commonly in light planes of anaesthesia or during intense surgical stimulus (e.g. dilatation of sphincters) or at extubation. Reported rates are 1% in adults but as high as 25% in children undergoing ENT surgery. Risk factors include children, recent upper respiratory tract infection, smokers, asthmatics, ENT/airway surgery. Blood, debris or secretions in the airway increase the likelihood of laryngospasm. Total intravenous anaesthesia (TIVA) may reduce the risk.

Treatment is administration of 100% oxygen, application of continuous positive airway pressure, increasing depth of anaesthesia, suction of the oropharynx and Larson's manoeuver (firm pressure applied behind both mandibular condyles). Small doses of propofol (0.5 mg/kg) or brief paralysis may be needed: 0.1–025 mg/kg succinyl choline may be sufficient. Airway management once laryngospasm is resolved is a clinical judgement, but if it has been severe there is a risk of post-obstructive pulmonary oedema.

A poorly placed or misplaced SAD may lead to glottic obstruction either by down-folding of the epiglottis, placement of the tip of the SAD in the glottis or partial closure of the glottis due to the presence of the SAD in the hypopharynx (compression and rotation of the arytenoids). Displacement is a particular risk in smaller children (< 15 kg). Good insertion technique, careful securing of the device and avoidance of traction on the proximal end of the SAD should prevent the problem. Controlled ventilation will overcome minor degrees of dysfunction but replacement is a better choice.

Lower Airway Obstruction

This is caused by:

● Bronchospasm
    ● Surgical stimulation, or airway stimulation (e.g. intubation or carinal stimulation during light anaesthesia) especially in smokers and children

- Asthma and COPD
- Anaphylaxis
- Aspiration (gastric contents, blood)
- Foreign body
- Pulmonary oedema
- Tension pneumothorax
- Respiratory infection
- Tracheal tube cuff herniation
- Endobronchial intubation (unilateral obstruction)

The underlying cause must be treated. Airway suction and deepening anaesthesia (especially with a volatile) may resolve minor bronchospasm. Severe bronchospasms can be treated according to standard protocols. Administration of aerosol and nebulized β adrenergic agents may be logistically difficult and early recourse to intravenous salbutamol, magnesium, aminophylline and epinephrine may be necessary.

Postoperative Pulmonary Complications

Atelectasis is collapse of dependent areas of the lung. It is caused by alveolar and small airway collapse and may be contributed to or worsened by inadequate coughing due to pain, residual neuromuscular block or sedatives. Anaesthesia also impairs mucociliary transport in the lungs due to inhalation of cold, dry and irritant gases.

Postoperative pulmonary infection may arise because of atelectasis or separate from it, but the clinical signs are difficult to distinguish (hypoxia, increased respiratory rate, increased work of breathing, collapse and crackles on chest examination, chest X-ray changes and organ dysfunction if severe). Respiratory failure after major surgery may occur in 5%–20% of cases and is a common cause for unplanned ICU admission.

Risk factors that at least double the risk of postoperative pulmonary complications include:

- Increasing age (age >70 years is a four- to six-fold higher risk than <50 years)
- ASA ≥2 (two- to four-fold increase)
- Lack of preoperative independence
- Congestive heart failure
- Abdominal, thoracic, vascular, and head and neck surgery
- Prolonged surgery
- Emergency surgery
- General anaesthesia
- Serum albumin <30 g/L

Obesity, COPD, obstructive sleep apnoea (OSA) and smoking also have an impact though this is less fully established.

Efforts to reduce the risk of postoperative pulmonary complications include:

- Minimally invasive surgery and incision planning (e.g. subcostal rather than midline)
- Avoidance of general anaesthesia
- Avoidance of opioid medication
- Optimal multimodal analgesia
- Epidural analgesia (proven to reduce respiratory failure)
- Early mobilization
- Early rehabilitation and nutrition (enhanced recovery)
- Physiotherapy (including incentive spirometry)
- Secretion management pre- and postoperatively

More recently lung-protective ventilation has been shown to have benefit in reducing postoperative pulmonary complications, ICU admission and length of stay. Lung protective ventilation comprises (a) pressure controlled ventilation limiting peak pressure to < 30 cmH_2O, (b) low tidal volumes 6–8 mL/kg ideal body weight, (c) PEEP and (d) recruitment manoeuvres every 30–60 min.

Obstructive Sleep Apnoea

Sleep apnoea may be caused by airway obstruction (obstructive sleep apnoea – OSA) or central respiratory depression (Ondine's curse). OSA is common (reports of 9%–24% of population), whereas the latter is rare. OSA is defined as a condition affecting the airway during sleep such that there is cessation or reduction of airflow in the presence of continued breathing effort. OSA is primarily a problem of obesity but is also increased in those with airway abnormalities and especially in children undergoing adenotonsillectomy.

Patients with OSA have an increase in cardiac comorbidities (hypertension, arrhythmias, myocardial ischemia and infarction, pulmonary hypertension, heart failure) and are at increased risk of perioperative problems (difficult/failed mask ventilation, SAD insertion and tracheal intubation, difficult airway rescue, short safe apnoea time, hypoxia) and postoperative problems (immediate: delayed or failed extubation, obstructive hypoxia, need for re-intubation, post-obstructive pulmonary oedema; delayed: exacerbation of cardiac comorbidities, stroke, prolonged recovery, prolonged length of stay, unplanned admission and re-admission, hypoxic brain injury and death).

Detection, patient selection and perioperative management are keys to reducing the risk of complications. The vast majority ($>75\%$) of patients with OSA are not diagnosed at the point they attend for surgery. Surgeons ($>90\%$ missed) and anaesthetists (60% missed) are poor at detecting OSA or its severity. The STOP-BANG questionnaire is an effective screening tool (Box 3.3.1). Increasing scores suggest higher risk and degree of OSA. Polysomnography (sleep study) is required to formally diagnose and quantify its severity.

Minimally invasive surgery is optimal. General anaesthesia should be avoided where possible. If general anaesthesia is required, avoidance of opioids (pre- and

---

BOX 3.3.1 STOP-BANG

Score 1 for each positive answer, high risk variously reported as ≥3 or ≥5

Snoring: Heavy, audible in next room
Tired: Daytime somnolence
Observed: Apnoea during sleep
Blood Pressure: Hypertension
BMI: >35 kg/m^2
Age: >50 years
Neck collar: >40 cm/16 inch
Gender: Male

Source: Adapted from Chung F, Yegneswaran B, Liao P, et al. STOP questionnaire: A tool to screen patients for obstructive sleep apnea. Anesthesiology 2008;108:812–21.

postoperatively) and use of drugs with rapid offset is ideal. Patient's home CPAP/ BiPAP should be used postoperatively and need for enhanced monitoring (oximetry, capnography) may necessitate HDU admission. Ambulatory surgery may be possible in patients with optimized OSA and stable comorbidities.

OSA is common in children undergoing adeno/tonsillectomy. It should be screened for, based on history and sleep study if indicated. Severe OSA leads to pulmonary hypertension, right heart hypertrophy and increased risk. In-patient stay may be required.

Airway Trauma

Minor oral soft tissue and dental trauma is common and is frequently caused by poor intubation technique.

Major trauma is a significant cause of medicolegal claims accounting for 1 in 20 claims against anaesthetists, mostly associated with TT insertion and adjuncts (bougies or rigid stylets). Airway trauma causes both direct injury (e.g. perforation, bleeding) and increases the risk of problems during emergence.

Major airway trauma leading to litigation has the following distribution:

- Larynx: 33%–35%
- Pharynx: 15%–20%
- Oesophagus: 14%–18%
- Trachea: 15%
- Temporomandibular joint (TMJ): 10%

The majority of pharyngeal, oesophageal and tracheal injuries are perforations, with tracheal and oesophageal perforations having a mortality of up to 20%.

Curved videolaryngoscopes have introduced a new risk of pharyngeal injury, as they require the use of a stylet to guide the tube to the larynx and during insertion the tube tip may pass out of view into a 'blind spot' before re-emerging into the view of the camera. Selection of a device with the smallest blind spot and careful technique should reduce the risk of injury to close to zero.

Avoidance of unnecessary tracheal intubation and use of SADs is likely to decrease airway trauma. Use of appropriate volumes and manometry for monitoring SAD cuff pressure should prevent airway trauma and neuropraxia. Airway trauma with a TT is reduced by use of small tracheal tubes, avoidance of blind intubation techniques, not advancing any device beyond the carina (≈23 cm from teeth) and avoiding high pressures during ventilation. Use of high-volume, low-pressure tracheal tube cuffs reduces the risk of ischaemic injury. Importantly, although tracheal and oesophageal trauma occurs more frequently during difficult tracheal intubation, most laryngeal and TMJ injuries occur during easy airway management.

Pulmonary Barotrauma and Pneumothorax

Alveolar trauma can occur if the alveoli are overinflated or exposed to excessive pressure (volutrauma and barotrauma). Barotrauma leading to macroscopic injury (pneumothorax, pneumomediastinum or surgical emphysema) is usually due to grossly elevated intrathoracic pressure. Patients at increased risk are those with emphysematous lung disease and especially if there are large bullae.

Positive pressure ventilation may reveal or worsen an existing pneumothorax caused by trauma, laparoscopic surgery, peripheral nerve block (e.g. supraclavicular, interscalene, intercostal and paravertebral blocks) or central venous access (subclavian or internal jugular). Rarely this may convert a simple pneumothorax into a tension pneumothorax. Management of a closed pneumothorax is by insertion of a chest drain.

Open pneumothorax may be caused by upper abdominal, thoracic or neck surgery when the parietal pleura is opened. The lungs should be inflated to expel pleural air and the pleural defect closed.

Airway Fire and Oxygen Cylinder Fire

This is a rare but serious complication and occurs when diathermy or laser causes ignition of flammable material (e.g. airway device, swab or tissue). Lasers pose a particular risk and this should be considered whenever they are used near the airway. Fire requires ignition, a fuel and a gas that supports combustion (e.g. oxygen, nitrous oxide).

Risk of airway fire is reduced by:

- Briefing and awareness of risk before using lasers
- Safe use of lasers
- Wet flame-retardant swabs around operative areas
- Use of nonflammable tracheal tubes ('laser-safe' TTs, though these are bulky and may not be practical for all circumstances)
- TT cuff inflation with saline
- A good tracheal cuff seal
- A minimal FiO_2
- Avoidance of nitrous oxide

Airway fire is usually easy to recognize. It causes harm by (a) heat trauma locally and distal spread into the lower airway, (b) release of toxic chemicals from burning plastic causing a lung injury and (c) airway obstruction may occur.

Management includes stopping the laser or diathermy, extinguishing the fire and cooling the upper airway with saline, removing damaged airway devices, briefly stopping ventilation and reducing FiO_2 as tolerated. Anaesthesia should be maintained (intravenously) and the upper and lower airway inspected and debris removed as necessary. Intubation and ICU care will be required in most cases, as airway swelling and lung injury will follow. Steroids (e.g. dexamethasone 0.5 mg i.v., up to 8 mg, 6-hourly for six doses) may reduce oedema.

Oxygen cylinders themselves pose a small risk of fire. If it occurs it can lead to massive and sudden fire. Fire can occur if there is flammable material in the valve mechanism of the cylinder and is made more likely if lubricants or alcohol gels are used near oxygen cylinders. If the flow controller is opened before the cylinder (on/off) valve is opened, this will lead to a sudden increase in flow and adiabatic changes lead to rapid heating of the exiting oxygen. Risk is reduced by maintenance of cylinders, not placing cylinders on beds, avoiding alcohol hand-rubs and lubricants when handling cylinders and opening the on/off valve with the flow controller closed before slowly increasing flow.

Other rare sources of fire or explosion in theatre include alcohol-based skin preparation solutions, paper surgical drapes, intestinal gases such as hydrogen and methane, and hydrogen produced by diathermy to the bladder. Ignition may be by diathermy, laser, misadventure or poor maintenance of electrical equipment.

Cardiovascular Complications

These include:

- Myocardial ischaemia and infarction
- Myocardial injury in noncardiac surgery
- Hypotension
- Hypertension
- Cardiac arrhythmias
- Stroke
- Complications of vascular access
- Venous thromboembolism
- Air or gas embolism

Myocardial Ischaemia and Infarction

See Chapter 1.2 for factors that predispose to cardiac risk during and after surgery.

Myocardial ischaemia is caused by an imbalance of myocardial oxygen supply and demand.

Factors affecting oxygen supply are as follows:

- Coronary perfusion pressure – the difference between pressure in the aorta and in the ventricles during diastole
- Oxygen content of arterial blood
- Coronary vascular resistance, especially the presence of atheroma
- Tachycardia

Factors affecting oxygen demand are as follows:

- Heart rate
- Ventricular pressure during systole (afterload, can be taken as mean arterial pressure) and diastole (preload, taken as central venous or pulmonary artery wedge pressure)
- Contractility
- Muscle mass (e.g. left ventricular hypertrophy)

Episodes of ischaemia can occur in the absence of major haemodynamic change due to coronary artery spasm, microthrombosis or coronary steal syndrome.

Increasing use of nonsurgical techniques (e.g. stents and longer term antiplatelet therapy) to manage coronary heart disease has, to an extent, added to the anaesthetic complexity of management of these patients and recommendations are regularly updated.

Avoidance of myocardial infarction (MI) and acute coronary syndromes (ACS) during anaesthesia requires the following principles:

- Delay elective surgery for investigation and treatment in patients with unstable coronary syndromes or MI.
- For urgent and emergency surgery the risk of delaying surgery must be balanced against the risk of major adverse cardiovascular events (MACE, MI, ACS, cerebrovascular event (CVE) and cardiovascular death).
- Avoid surgery in those at high risk of coronary stent occlusion (14 days after angioplasty, 30 days after bare metal stent and ideally 6 months after drug eluting stent insertion, though can be considered after 3 months).
- Avoid stopping dual antiplatelet therapy in patients who must undergo surgery. Where this is unavoidable continue aspirin and restart the P2Y12 antagonist (e.g. clopidogrel/ticagrelor/prasugrel) as soon as feasible.
- Bridging with intravenous antiplatelet or anticoagulant agents may be considered, but is not currently recommended routinely.
- Noncardiac surgery is not an indication for preoperative angiography or coronary revascularization in patients who would not have this done without surgery.
- Maintain statins in those taking them.
- Maintain β-blockade in those taking β-blockers.
- Do not start β-blockers on the day of surgery.
- Avoid tachycardia as this decreases oxygen supply and increases demand.
- Avoid and manage hypotension in patients who have had coronary artery grafting or recent angioplasty because of the risk of graft or stent thrombosis.

● Avoid hypertension as this can cause an increase in demand that exceeds reserve. The major sign of intraoperative ischaemia is a fall in the ST segment on the ECG. Newer monitors may display ST segment trends. Arrhythmias may also occur.

Myocardial Injury in Noncardiac Surgery (MINS)

This subject has been of recent interest and follows the finding that the degree of elevation of serum troponin postoperatively was closely correlated with adverse patient outcomes. This has been studied primarily in elective patients. Troponinaemia may be caused by a Type 2 MI (nonocclusive MI due to an imbalance of oxygen demand and supply). An elevated troponinaemia is a more sensitive indicator of myocardial injury than 12-lead ECG or patient symptoms. Raised Troponin, irrespective of the presence of an ischemic feature, independently predicts 30-day mortality.

An elevated troponin is a predictor of both cardiac and noncardiac events, for reasons that are not clear. At present the role of screening for elevated troponin postoperatively is uncertain and the actions to be taken when an elevated troponin is identified are also unclear. Patients with an elevated troponin postoperatively should be considered at increased risk of cardiac and noncardiac complications. There is logic in screening to exclude acute coronary syndrome (e.g. new regional wall motion abnormality). There may be benefit in introducing cardiac medications (β-blockers, statin, ACEI and anti-platelets) to these patients but this is yet to be confirmed.

Hypotension

Hypotension may be due to a low cardiac output, a low peripheral vascular resistance or both, and is common during anaesthesia (depending on definition, up to 80% of cases). The lower limit of cerebral autoregulation is at a mean pressure of 60 mm Hg, but many patients have intercurrent disease, which may make this blood pressure dangerous. ST depression on the ECG and arrhythmias suggests poor myocardial perfusion. Sustained hypotension may lead to organ dysfunction and cardiac arrest. Conversely, there are numerous series of induced hypotension reporting very low rates of complications.

The longer-term impact of intraoperative hypotension is an area of intense current research. Observational data suggests that a MAP <60 mm Hg and especially <55 mm Hg may lead to longer term adverse outcomes including acute kidney injury and myocardial injury. Even short periods of hypotension (as little as 5 min) are implicated in kidney injury, whereas slightly longer periods of hypotension (e.g. >20 min) are associated with myocardial injury.

The impact of prompt reversal of hypotension on these adverse outcomes is currently unknown. A pragmatic approach is to aim to keep the blood pressure within 20% of the patient's normal value and MAP >60 mm Hg, but this may change with emerging evidence.

Common causes of hypotension are as follows:

- Hypovolaemia due to haemorrhage. Blood pressure may not fall in a fit young person until more than 30% of the circulating volume has been lost. Blood loss may be concealed or difficult to measure.
- Other causes of hypovolaemia, such as trauma, burns, dehydration and metabolic causes.
- Drops in cardiac output and peripheral resistance are common effects of anaesthetic drugs, notably induction agents and inhalation agents. In the elderly and those with cardiovascular morbidity, blood pressure can drop precipitously unless care is taken with dose and speed of administration.
- Intradural or extradural administration of local anaesthetics causes vasodilatation by sympathetic blockade, reduced venous return and cardiac output. High blocks, above T4, can also block the sympathetic nervous supply to the heart, reducing contractility and preventing reflex tachycardia.
- In obstetric patients, the combination of aortocaval compression by the uterus coupled with neuraxial blockade can cause profound hypotension.
- In patients with cardiac disease, hypotension from any cause can reduce myocardial perfusion, leading to a drop in cardiac output and a further fall in blood pressure.

Hypertension

Hypertension is common in the perioperative period. It is most commonly caused by pre-existing hypertension and by pain or anxiety. Possible causes of hypertension in the immediate postoperative period include:

- Pain or full bladder – common
- Previously undiagnosed or inadequately treat hypertension – common
- Hypercapnia
- Confusion after anaesthesia, especially in the elderly
- Vasoconstriction after cardiopulmonary bypass and other vascular surgery
- Thyroid crisis – rare
- Unsuspected phaeochromocytoma – very rare
- Malignant hyperpyrexia – very rare

The risks are mainly of increased myocardial oxygen demand. There is often an associated tachycardia, which will also impair coronary perfusion. These two factors may lead to myocardial ischaemia and even infarction. However, in low-risk patients isolated hypertension is often transient. Unless extreme, or associated with evidence of organ dysfunction, there is often greater risk associated with treating it (and precipitating hypotension) than with treating the cause and observing.

If an obvious cause cannot be treated, suitable management includes incremental doses of β-blocker, calcium antagonist or a vasodilator drug such as hydralazine 10 mg. The patient should be monitored and hypotension avoided or treated.

Cardiac Arrhythmias

Cardiac disease is the commonest cause of arrhythmia during anaesthesia and surgery. Common arrhythmias are bradycardia (especially in children and during vagally stimulating surgery), sinus tachycardia (numerous causes) and atrial fibrillation (AF) (most often caused by pre-existing undiagnosed AF or a sign of cardiac disease). Atrial ectopics and occasional ventricular ectopics are usually benign and require no specific treatment other than correction of any reversible cause. Other arrhythmias are increasingly infrequent, in noncardiac surgery, with the fall in use of halothane which was notably arrhythmogenic. Arrhythmias are considerably more common during emergency surgery, because of increased physiological disturbance caused by the underlying emergency condition. Treatable causes include the '4Hs and 4Ts' used in cardiac arrest situations (see Chapter 2.10).

Other causes to remember include hypomagnesaemia, hypercapnia, inadequate anaesthesia, increased surgical stimulus, poorly positioned CVC catheter, arrhythmogenic drugs, local anaesthetic overdose, malignant or other causes of hyperpyrexia.

In anaesthetic practice hypoxia, hypovolaemia and electrolyte disturbances are the commonest causes, often in a patient with existing cardiac disease. The first treatment is correction of the precipitating factor. Several arrhythmias require specific treatment as follows, in line with ACLS guidelines (detailed in Chapter 2.10):

- Ventricular fibrillation and pulseless ventricular tachycardia – there is often a precipitating cause that requires attention.
- Ventricular tachycardia impairs – it is important to check for a precipitating cause.
- Narrow complex tachycardias – usually occur in patients who have a history of paroxysmal tachycardia.
- Sinus or nodal bradycardia.

Stroke

Stroke (cerebrovascular event; CVE) has an incidence of approximately 0.2% after general surgery and anaesthesia in patients without known cerebrovascular disease. It occurs typically from 2 to 10 days postoperatively. The choice of anaesthetic agent is probably of little importance. The causes are sometimes uncertain, but include:

- Emboli when in atrial fibrillation
- Thrombosis due to hypotension
- The hypercoagulable state that occurs after surgery
- Obstruction to a vertebral artery when the neck is rotated
- As a complication of cardiopulmonary bypass
- Air embolus via a patent foramen ovale (rare)

A common query is how long should surgery be delayed after a CVE. Current evidence suggests a previous CVE is a significant risk for major cardiovascular events (MACE: further CVE, MI, cardiovascular death). Risk of these events is 14-fold higher than in those without prior stroke in the first 3 months after a CVE, falling to five-fold higher at 6 months and 2.5-fold at 12 months. Mortality risk is three-fold higher within 3 months, 1.5-fold higher at 12 months. Risk flattens off at 9 months. The extent of surgery does not impact on these risks.

Complications of Vascular Access

Vascular access may lead to numerous complications. Infection is the most commonly cited and often occurs sometime after device insertion. Infection can occur after central or peripheral vascular access and can cause sepsis.

For peripheral access it has become routine to remove and replace after three days use but this lacks an evidence base and is not superior to protocolized care comprising surveillance and replacement when there are clinical signs of inflammation. Short-term central venous access can be managed similarly, but with careful observation the period of time before removal and replacement is usually 7 days. The most important factors for avoiding infection are (a) scrupulous aseptic technique during insertion, (b) use of a clear breathable dressing centred over the skin entry point, (c) scrupulous aseptic technique when accessing the ports of the device and (d) careful patient and device monitoring for signs of inflammation of infection.

Mechanical complications of CVC insertion are significant causes of patient morbidity and occasional mortality. They are an important cause of medicolegal claims, with such claims associated with a high rate of serious harm or death and a high rate of successful claims.

Complications include:

- Vascular injury (highest in subclavian and internal jugular sites):
  - Haemorrhage (e.g. subclavian artery, femoral artery)
  - Compression injury (e.g. carotid artery causing CVE)
  - Embolus (from atrial puncture)
  - Cannulation of the wrong vessel (e.g. carotid artery or vertebral artery during internal jugular approach)
- Loss of guidewire
- Air embolus (during insertion, use or removal)
- Pneumothorax
- Damage to thoracic duct
- Nerve injury (e.g. brachial plexus, cervical nerves, femoral nerve)
- Infection
- Haematoma

Almost all complications are reduced by good technique and training. The use of ultrasound to guide insertion is likely to have reduced complication rates, but this is not proven. Ultrasound also provides an opportunity for safer approaches to vessels than previous landmark techniques (e.g. lateral approach to the axillary vein).

Venous Thromboembolism

Deep venous thrombosis (DVT) can occur before, during or very soon after operation. Thrombosis in the veins of the calf is common, but only likely to result in pulmonary embolism (PE) when it extends into the iliofemoral veins or if it originates in the pelvic veins.

A PE most commonly occurs postoperatively, but can occur during an operation by the detachment of a venous clot in the leg following the application of a tourniquet or a change in the patient's position. Postoperatively there is reduced fibrinolytic activity and increased platelet adhesiveness.

Regional techniques such as central neuraxial blockade (CNB) improve blood flow and reduce the incidence of DVT, although it is a modest effect and it is not certain whether this results in a reduction in mortality due to PE.

Nonthrombotic emboli can occur from fat embolus, renal tumour or amniotic fluid in obstetric patients.

Risk factors for venous thromboembolism include:

- Age over 40 years
- A previous history of DVT
- Immobilization
- Raised BMI
- Oral contraceptives or hormone replacement therapy (HRT) containing oestrogen
- Cancer
- Varicose veins
- Prolonged surgery and anaesthesia
- Pelvic, hip and varicose vein surgery
- Factor V Leiden mutation and similar conditions

Presentation

The classic presentation of PE is the sudden onset of chest pain during the second postoperative week. In practice, symptoms of PE are very varied and include unexplained fever, faintness, dyspnoea, substernal discomfort, pleural pain, haemoptysis and collapse. The onset may coincide with getting up or straining at stool. The diagnosis is often missed or not considered.

Signs of DVT in the calf are those of inflammation; pain, especially on dorsiflexion of the foot (Homan sign), tenderness, redness and swelling. Signs of PE include tachycardia, hypotension, cyanosis, raised CVP, gallop rhythm, pleural rub and signs of consolidation. ECG changes in PE are common, but are nonspecific (e.g. sinus tachycardia, ST segment changes). The ECG is important to exclude other conditions such as ACS. Signs of right heart strain (S wave in lead I, Q-wave and T-wave inversion in lead III; S1, Q3, T3) occur only with a massive PE and are unreliable. Chest X-ray is usually normal but may show linear shadows, effusion or pulmonary oligaemia if the embolus is large. Arterial blood gases show hypoxaemia with a normal or low PCO_2 due to hyperventilation. Plasma D-dimer enzyme-linked immunosorbent assay (ELISA) detects fibrinolysis, but in the perioperative setting it is too nonspecific to be of any value.

Intraoperative PE is rare. Classic signs are hypoxia and decreased or absent capnography despite normal ventilation (increased dead space). Hypoxia, tachycardia, hypotension and ECG changes are a more common, but less specific, presentation.

Clinical symptoms, signs and basic investigations are generally nondiagnostic. A ventilation–perfusion scan was the commonest method of imaging, but a CT pulmonary angiogram is now the definitive diagnostic tool but requires skilled interpretation. Focussed echocardiography has an increasing role, showing right heart dilatation, reduced systolic function and pulmonary hypertension and TOE can potentially image central embolus. Pulmonary angiography is seldom used because it is expensive, invasive and carries a small mortality risk.

Treatment

This follows an ABC approach. ICU admission, ventilation and management of right heart failure may be required.

Anticoagulation is the specific treatment, to prevent recurrence and in an effort to dissipate existing clot, and may be achieved with a number of anticoagulants.

Heparin can be loaded promptly (e.g. 5000 units) and acts rapidly but requires an infusion to maintain an APTT ratio of 2–2.5 times normal. Its main action is to bind to antithrombin III and enhance its anticoagulant effect. Low molecular weight heparin (LMWH) may be given in a full treatment dose. Warfarin and new oral anticoagulants (NOACs) take several days to achieve full effect, so heparin or LMWH is required until they are effective. Acute fibrinolysis with recombinant tissue plasminogen activator (alteplase 100 mg i.v. over 2 h), which converts plasminogen to plasmin and initiates fibrinolysis, remains controversial. Its use is currently reserved for immediately life-threatening PE. There is a significant risk of haemorrhage, including life threatening, especially after recent surgery. Pulmonary embolectomy can only be used with cardiopulmonary bypass and its application is very limited.

Prevention

Hospitals should have local guidelines to prevent DVT and PE. In general, preventive measures include:

- Maintaining ambulation pre- and postoperatively
- Prevention of hypovolaemia by adequate fluid therapy
- Intermittent pneumatic calf or foot compression, replacing the normal muscle pump
- Graded elastic support stockings
- A heel cushion on the operating table, preventing pressure on calf veins

- Stopping oestrogen-containing oral contraceptives and HRT 4–6 weeks before major surgery or surgery to the legs
- Pharmacological prophylaxis for patients at increased risk

The use of drugs altering coagulations can impact on the risk/benefit of regional anaesthesia. Timing of major regional anaesthetic techniques (and removal of RA catheters) needs to be planned carefully to avoid increased bleeding risk. Consideration should be taken of time since last anticoagulant, time between block and next anticoagulant, and use of anticoagulants while a regional anaesthesia catheter is in place.

Air or Gas Embolism

If gas enters the venous circulation, it accumulates in the right side of the heart and pulmonary artery. Since gas is compressible, if the volume of gas is sufficient, the contracting heart simply compresses the gas but does not eject blood from the heart and cardiovascular collapse occurs. The volume of gas required is of the order of 0.5–1 mL/kg. If the gas enters the arterial side of the circulation through a potential right-to-left shunt such as a patent foramen ovale (present in 20% of the population), paradoxical embolism occurs, which usually obstructs coronary or cerebral arteries.

Surgical Causes

Air can enter the circulation if the site of operation is above the heart and atmospheric pressure exceeds the pressure in an open blood vessel (e.g. in operations involving veins in the neck, thorax, breast and pelvis, especially if the patient is tilted; operations on the shoulder, brain and spinal cord in the sitting position, or operations on the heart). Carbon dioxide may enter the circulation during laparoscopy.

Anaesthetic Causes

Air entering the circulation during intravenous techniques from syringes or via central venous catheters left open to atmosphere.

Diagnosis

Features include:

- An abrupt fall of the end-tidal carbon dioxide – an early sign
- A sucking sound in the wound if air enters in large volume
- A loud continuous precordial murmur, the so-called 'mill-wheel' murmur

Clinical signs occur only after a significant amount of gas has entered the circulation. There may be sudden cyanosis, hypotension, tachycardia, engorged neck veins and cardiac arrest. In situations where there is a significant risk (e.g. neurosurgical operations in the sitting position), a Doppler probe on the precordium has been used as a sensitive early detector, although diathermy interferes with this monitor.

Treatment

Treatment includes:

- Prevent further air entering the circulation by compressing veins to raise venous pressure, flood the wound with saline, tilt the patient so that the entry site is below the heart.
- Start CPR if the patient is in cardiac arrest.
- Give 100% oxygen and stop administration of nitrous oxide – diffuses into the gas bubbles and increases their size.
- Place the patient on their left side to reduce risk of bubbles entering the pulmonary artery.
- If a CVP catheter is in place, aspirate directly from the right heart. If no CVP catheter is in place, it is theoretically beneficial to insert one but this should not interrupt resuscitation.

Neurological Complications

These include:

- Inadequate anaesthesia
- Awareness during general anaesthesia
- Delayed recovery from anaesthesia
- Complications of central neuraxial blockade
- Complications of peripheral neuraxial blockade
- Delirium and postoperative cognitive dysfunction
- Convulsions and abnormal muscle movements
- Acute dystonic reactions

Inadequate Anaesthesia

Inadequate anaesthesia includes three separate entities:

- Accidental awareness during general anaesthesia (AAGA)
- Inadequate regional anaesthesia
- Brief awake paralysis – due to inadvertent administration of a muscle relaxant without anaesthesia

All are clinically important patients and all are important contributors to medicolegal claims against anaesthetists. Brief awake paralysis causes the greatest psychological trauma and is associated with almost universal settlement of medicolegal claims.

Awareness during General Anaesthesia (AAGA)

Awareness during general anaesthesia has been reported since the 1950s. It is known to cause distress and psychological sequelae to many patients who experience it. It is important for patients to avoid AAGA.

> **BOX 3.3.2 Brice Questionnaire**
>
> What is the last thing you remember before going to sleep?
> What is the first thing you remember on waking?
> Do you recall anything in between?
> What was the worst thing about your anaesthetic?
> What was the next worst thing about your anaesthetic? (Previously – Did you dream?)

The standard tool for detecting it is the Brice questionnaire (Box 3.3.2), or various modifications.

Using the Brice questionnaire, an incidence of AAGA is fairly consistently detected at 1 in 600–1000 general anaesthetics.

The 'isolated forearm technique' (IFT) involves preventing muscle relaxant from reaching one arm by means of an arterial tourniquet which is inflated before administration and deflated after the neuromuscular blockade (NMB) has worked. This enables an otherwise paralysed patient to respond to simple commands if they are awake. The IFT is used in research but rarely in clinical practice. In the research setting, it may identify 'responsiveness' in up to 1 in 3 general anaesthetics. However, the true value of the IFT is partly obscured by some poor studies and responders in IFT studies do not appear likely to recall awareness or suffer psychological sequelae. This is an area of controversy.

With both the Brice questionnaire and the IFT, there is an apparent disconnect between the incidence detected (very high) and the degree of harm from AAGA observed in the population at large (much lower). It is therefore possible that both the IFT and Brice questionnaire detect something other than 'awareness'.

The causes of awareness include:

- Unintentional administration of too little or no anaesthetic agent:
  - Faulty technique or judgement – common cause
  - Faulty equipment (empty vaporizer, failure of nitrous oxide supply, failure of TIVA delivery)
- Pharmacodynamic variability between patients
- Intentional administration of too little anaesthetic agent (e.g. in a very sick patient)

This last reason should be largely redundant as an acceptable cause given modern methods to support the cardiorespiratory system of very sick patients.

Incidence of Awareness during General Anaesthesia

The incidence of AAGA after ≈3 million general anaesthetics was studied in NAP5.[6] The incidence of certain/probable and possible AAGA was 1 in 19,600 anaesthetics but with considerable variation across techniques and subspecialties. The incidence of AAGA during Caesarean section was 1 in 670. The incidence of 'accidental awareness' during sedation (1 in 15,000) was similar to that during general anaesthesia.

The cases were overwhelmingly reports of unintended awareness during neuromuscular blockade (NMB); the incidence with NMB was 1 in 8200 and without 1 in 135,900.

Two-thirds of AAGA events arose in the dynamic phases of anaesthesia (induction 48%, and emergence 18%). During induction, contributory factors included use of thiopental, RSI, obesity, difficult airway management, NMB, interruptions of anaesthetic delivery during movement from anaesthetic room to theatre. During emergence, residual neuromuscular blockade was perceived by patients as AAGA and commonly due to failures in ensuring full return of motor capacity.

One-third of AAGA events arose during maintenance, most due to problems at induction or towards the end of anaesthesia.

Factors increasing the risk of AAGA included female gender, age (younger adults, but not children), obesity, anaesthetist seniority (junior trainees), previous AAGA, out-of-hours operating, emergencies, type of surgery (obstetric, cardiac and thoracic) and use of NMB. ASA physical status, race and use or omission of nitrous oxide were not risk factors for AAGA.

The report suggested that an anaesthetic checklist as an integral part of the WHO Safer Surgery checklist may help in preventing AAGA, as may the use of BIS monitoring during anaesthesia with TIVA and NMB.

Patients' experiences ranged from isolated auditory through tactile sensations to full awareness. Most (75%) experiences were for <5 min, but 51% of affected patients experienced distress and 41% suffered longer term sequelae. Distress and longer term harm were more common when the patient experienced paralysis (with or without pain). The patient's interpretation of events during AAGA influenced later impact. Explanation and reassurance either during the event or later seemed beneficial to patient recovery.

Not surprisingly AAGA was associated with poor quality care (39% of cases) and was judged preventable in three-quarters of cases. However, in 12% of cases care was judged good and the episode not preventable. AAGA was followed by a complaint in 11% and legal action in 6% of the cases.

The incidence of post-traumatic stress disorder after AAGA reported in the literature is between 0% and 70% with an aggregate incidence of 15%.

If a patient complains of operative awareness some time later, listen, establish the facts, do not disbelieve what the patient says and arrange suitable psychological counselling. It may be helpful to have a witness to your conversation. Make full notes.

Detection of Awareness

Clinical detection: Movement is the commonest sign of inadequate anaesthesia. However, movement occurs much more often than AAGA. In the paralysed patient movement is not possible. Classic signs of AAGA are reported to be sweating, reactive pupils, hypertension, tachycardia and lachrymation. However, in series of cases of AAGA these signs are present in <20% of reported cases, making their absence of little value in excluding AAGA.

Processed electroencephalogram monitors (pEEG): See Chapter 2.2 for more detail. There are several pEEG monitors available designed to monitor 'depth of anaesthesia'. The BIS (bispectrum) monitor is the most widely used and studied. It measures the EEG from the frontal area. Most hypnotic agents (but not ketamine, nitrous oxide or opioids) cause a slowing of the EEG and a left shift of the power-spectrum. There is also an increase in the orderliness of the EEG. The BIS monitor uses several measures of slowing of the EEG (bispectrum, fast-slow synch and burst suppression ratio) in a proprietary algorithm to produce a dimensionless number between 0 (deep unconsciousness) and 100 (wide awake). A BIS value of 40–60 is the target range during anaesthesia. Use of BIS has been shown to reduce the incidence of AAGA in several studies but has not been shown to be more effective than using monitoring and alarms to ensure volatile anaesthetic delivery maintains an end tidal MAC of ≥0.7. BIS is best considered as a monitor of 'cortical suppression' rather than as a direct 'depth of anaesthesia monitor'.

Alternative pEEG monitors include the Narcotrend® and entropy monitors, which have been less widely evaluated. All these monitors are recommended for monitoring patients in whom anaesthetic technique or patient condition leads to an increase in risk from over-dose or underdosing of anaesthetic agents.

Evoked potentials: Evoked potentials may be auditory, visual or somatosensory and their amplitudes and especially the latencies are affected by anaesthetic agents: particularly volatile agents, less so by intravenous agents and opiates. Auditory evoked potentials have most utility in monitoring depth of anaesthesia. Variation between the effects of different anaesthetics can make interpretation difficult.

Other techniques: These are of historical interest and include measures of (a) respiratory sinus arrhythmia which diminishes with increasing depth of anaesthesia, (b) frontalis electromyography which shows a reduction of tonic activity with deepening anaesthesia and (c) lower oesophageal contractions which decrease in rate and pressure with increasing depth of anaesthesia. All are either impractical, unreliable or both.

Delayed Recovery from Anaesthesia

Delayed recovery from anaesthesia may be caused by:

- Sedative drugs taken preoperatively.
- Genetic causes of prolonged neuromuscular blockade – prolonged action of suxamethonium or mivacurium due to pseudocholinesterase deficiency. Incidence ≈1 in 4000 but higher in some ethnic groups, e.g. Arya Vysya in India and Persian Jews. Note the patient will be paralysed but awake.
- Nongenetic causes of prolonged neuromuscular blockade – failure to monitor and reverse appropriately. More common. Note the patient will be paralysed but awake.
- Slow off-set of sedative anaesthetic drugs, e.g. opioids, thiopental, volatile anaesthetic agents.

- Surgical causes (e.g. sepsis, haemorrhage, fat embolism, air embolism, operative trauma in neurosurgery).
- Other anaesthetic causes – hypercapnia, hypoxic episode, electrolyte and acid–base disturbances, fainting (especially in the dental chair), induced hypotension, hypothermia.
- Diseases (e.g. CVE, myxoedema, hypopituitarism, hypoglycaemia, hyperglycaemia, adrenal deficiency, uraemia, liver failure, undiagnosed brain tumour – all very rare).

Complications of Central Neuraxial Blockade (CNB)

Complications of CNB are important to patients and clinicians. They occur infrequently but can be potentially devastating. Medicolegal claims related to CNB are a significant proportion of claims against anaesthetists: 44% of all claims relate to regional anaesthesia, of which 80% relate to CNB and 80% of those to epidural analgesia. Obstetrics is disproportionately represented. Knowledge of complications of CNB is therefore important in determining risk versus benefit and in communicating with/consenting patients. Any consideration of the complications associated with CNB should be balanced by three further considerations: (a) the proven and potential benefits of the technique, (b) the known and potential complications (and benefits) of the analgesic alternatives such as parenteral opioids and non-steroidal anti inflammatory drugs (NSAIDs) and (c) the consequences of less good analgesia. At present the debate often neglects these considerations.

Reported incidences of major complications of CNB range between 1 and 100 per 100,000 procedures. In 2007, two UK studies reported, almost simultaneously, an incidence of epidural abscess following perioperative epidural of 1 in 675 in adults and 1 in 10,000 in children. Previously the two best studies on the topic were Scandinavian. A Finnish study reported an incidence of 1 in 22,000 after spinal anaesthesia and 1 in 19,000 following epidurals. A Swedish study reported an incidence of 1 in 20,000–30,000 after spinal, 1 in 3600 after nonobstetric epidural and 1 in 25,000 after obstetric epidural. The commonest clinical events were arachnoiditis and meningitis.

A more recent study of major complications of CNB is provided by NAP3,[3] which sought evidence of harm as a result of CNB persisting 6 months after the procedure. The complications sought were:

- Serious infections (e.g. vertebral canal abscess, meningitis)
- Vertebral canal haematoma
- Major nerve damage (e.g. paraplegia, cord damage, cord infarction, major neuropathy)
- Death where the procedure was implicated
- Wrong route errors (e.g. intravenous drugs given epidurally/intrathecally or vice versa)

CNB techniques were spinals (46%), epidurals (41%), continuous spinal-epidural (CSE) (6%) and caudals (7%) with all but 1% performed by anaesthetists.

Indications were obstetrics (45%), adult perioperative (44%), chronic pain (6%) and paediatric perioperative (3%).

To allow for clinical uncertainty NAP3 presented incidences as a range from a pessimistic estimate to an optimistic estimate (i.e. from higher to lower incidence).

Among 707,000 CNBs, the overall incidence of harm ranged from 1 in 23,500 to 1 in 50,500 (Table 3.3.3).

Estimates of incidence harm due to indication for CNB are given in Table 3.3.3.

Estimates of incidence permanent harm due to perioperative technique of CNB are given in Table 3.3.4.

The incidence of complications is lower than many would have anticipated and is reassuring for patients and clinicians.

Most initially severe complications recovered within 6 months, and >60% of patients with a neurological deficit made a full recovery. The poorest outcomes followed spinal cord ischaemia, vertebral canal haematoma or abscess. After meningitis and traumatic nerve or spinal cord injury the outcome was better.

Complications occurred most frequently after perioperative CNB. Major harm after CNB for obstetric, chronic pain and paediatric indications were notably low.

In terms of the type of CNB; epidurals and CSEs were higher risk and spinals and caudals low risk. Perioperative epidurals accounted for 1 in 7 CNB and 1 in 2 complications. Because of differences in patient characteristics, the potential benefits of a technique and the benefits or risks associated with omitting the

TABLE 3.3.3 Point Estimates of Incidence of Permanent Harm due to CNB

Indications	Incidence Range[a]
All CNB	
Harm	1 in 23,500 to 1 in 50,500
Paraplegia or death	1 in 54,500 to 1 in 141,500
Death	<1 in 100,000 to <1 in 200,000
Harm by indication	
Perioperative CNB	1 in 12,500 to 1 in 24,000
Obstetric	1 in 80,000 to 1 in 320,000
Chronic Pain	1 in 40,000 to no permanent harm
Paediatrics	No permanent harm

[a]Range from a pessimistic estimate to an optimistic estimate.

Source: Cook TM, Counsell D, Wildsmith JAW on behalf of The Royal College of Anaesthetists Third National Audit Project. Major complications of central neuraxial block: report on the Third National Audit Project of the Royal College of Anaesthetists. Br J Anaesth 2009;102:179–90.

TABLE 3.3.4 Point Estimates of Incidence of Permanent Harm after Perioperative CNB

Technique	Incidence Range[a]
Perioperative epidural	
Overall	1 in 5800 to 1 in 12,000
Paraplegia or death	1 in 16,000 to 1 in 98,000
Perioperative spinal	
Overall	1 in 38,000 to 1 in 63,000
Paraplegia or death	1 in 47,000 to 1 in 95,000
Perioperative CSE:	
Overall	1 in 5500 to 1 in 8300
Paraplegia or death	1 in 8300

[a]Range from a pessimistic estimate to an optimistic estimate.

Source: Cook TM, Counsell D, Wildsmith JAW on behalf of The Royal College of Anaesthetists Third National Audit Project. Major complications of central neuraxial block: report on the Third National Audit Project of the Royal College of Anaesthetists. Br J Anaesth 2009;102:179–90.

technique or use of alternatives, great caution should be taken before comparting between groups.

Litigation and complaints were uncommon. Remediable care was much less common than good practice. Where care was remediable, this included failure to monitor patients, failure to understand or respond to abnormalities promptly (especially postoperatively) and failure to follow existing recommendations.

An important but rare complication is adhesive arachnoiditis after CNB. This has been caused by inadvertent neuraxial administration of high concentrations or volumes of chlorhexidine (experimentally or accidentally). It has also been identified as 'a cause in the absence of other explanations' in some legal cases. Every effort should be made to ensure chlorhexidine, used to prepare the skin, is dry before a central (or peripheral) nerve block is undertaken, and to prevent any chlorhexidine coming into contact with the operator's gloves or equipment. Chlorhexidine 0.5% is currently recommended, 2% solutions should be avoided.

Complications of Peripheral Neuraxial Blockade (PNB)

Neurological Injury

The data on neurological complications after PNB is less robust. Reports of permanent harm range from 1 in 10 to 1.5 in 10,000. As an aide memoire a reasonable approximation is 1 in 30 after 1 week, 1 in 300 require neurological referral and <1 in 3000 permanent injuries. In the largest study of 23,271 blocks success rate was 97%, with immediate complications 2.2% and the all-cause 60-day rate of neurological sequelae was 8.3 in 10,000.

Other complications of CNB include:

- Wrong site block
- Haematoma
- Local anaesthetic systemic toxicity (LAST)
- Mechanical needle-related trauma (e.g. pneumothorax, vascular injury, abdominal organ injury)

The use of ultrasound for PNB has probably been associated with improvements in success and safety, though he latter is difficult to prove. Paradoxically, the use of ultrasound has revealed that intraneural injection is common and relatively benign. Avoidance of subperineural (intrafascicular) injection and avoidance of injection at high pressures (limit to <1 atmosphere injection pressure) is probably key to preventing needle-related nerve injury.

Local Anaesthetic Systemic Toxicity

Local anaesthetic systemic toxicity (LAST) occurs when local anaesthetic is administered either as an absolute overdose (drug dose in excess of known safe levels) or relative overdose (dose inadvertently administered intravenously, or too high a dose for the specific block). Symptoms include (progressively) tinnitus, perioral tingling, hypo- or hypertension, arrhythmia, seizure, loss of consciousness and respiratory or cardiac arrest. Bupivacaine is particularly toxic because of its long duration of action and binding to myocytes where it inhibits mitochondrial oxidative phosphorylation.

Treatment involves stopping administration of the local anaesthetic and resuscitation using standard protocols. Oxygen, fluid, seizure control and CPR where necessary are basic tenets. There is also interest in the use of lipid emulsions in treatment of LAST. The mechanism of action is not clear but it appears to improve successful resuscitation after LAST in animal models and in clinical reports. Proposed mechanisms include drawing local anaesthetic from tissues into the lipid layer of plasma ('lipid sink') or providing a substrate to the myocardial mitochondria and unblocking oxidative phosphorylation. Dose is initially 1.5 mL/kg of 20% lipid followed by an infusion of up to 10 mL/kg over 30 min. However, administration of lipid emulsion should not be allowed to delay standard resuscitative efforts.

Delirium and Postoperative Cognitive Dysfunction

Delirium describes a temporary reduction in cognitive ability and this is common postoperatively affecting up to 15% of in-patients but is much more common in the elderly. Hyperactive delirium is easier to identify than hypoactive delirium. Both can feature hallucinations, delusions, impaired sleep and impaired memory and cognition.

Prolonged deterioration in cognitive ability is termed postoperative cognitive dysfunction or decline (POCD). It can affect up to 10%–40% of patients after discharge and 5%–12% at 3 months. It is not restricted to surgery and anaesthesia and may occur after other major health events. There is no consensus definition, diagnostic criteria or tool for detection. As a consequence, it is under-reported and frequently misdiagnosed.

Risk factors include:

- Old age
- Pre-existing cognitive decline
- Acute illness
- Extent and duration of surgery

The aetiology is unclear. Proposed mechanisms include direct toxic effects of anaesthetic agents or inflammatory cytokines on the brain and micro-emboli, but none of these is supported by strong evidence.

The intensity or type of surgery is variably and inconsistently associated with POCD. Avoidance of general anaesthesia is not clearly protective against POCD, though regional anaesthesia (without general anaesthesia or heavy sedation) may reduce delirium. Reducing the depth of anaesthesia using a pEEG monitor to guide anaesthesia may reduce delirium and POCD but this is unconfirmed. There is conflicting evidence regarding the impact of volatiles or TIVA on POCD. Several drugs have been postulated for prevention or treatment (aspirin, minocycline, magnesium, statins, dexmedetomidine, ketamine, dexamethasone and melatonin) without clear evidence of benefit. Of these, dexamethasone has perhaps shown the greatest benefit. There is a consensus that benzodiazepines should be avoided.

There is currently no known preventative or therapeutic treatment. Exclusion of other causes of delirium or altered cognitive state (e.g. sepsis, anaemia, dehydration, hypoxia, electrolyte imbalance, hyperglycaemia, hypothyroidism, drugs and drug withdrawal) should be part of management of the condition. Maintenance of physiological equilibrium, normothermia and sleep patterns, avoidance of general anaesthesia/sedation where possible, minimally invasive surgery, minimal doses of rapid-offset anaesthesia where needed, avoidance of hypotension, dehydration and centrally active drugs, early rehabilitation, cognitive support while in hospital and early discharge to home are prudent but unproven. As the surgical population becomes increasingly elderly and infirm and more patients with a degree of cognitive impairment present for surgery POCD is likely to become a major concern.

Convulsions and Abnormal Muscle Movements

Several types of abnormal muscular action may occur during anaesthesia:

- Involuntary muscle movements – occur with some induction agents (e.g. etomidate, and propofol). EEG recordings show these are nonconvulsant.

- True convulsions – can occur due to epilepsy, eclampsia, hypoxia, hypoglycaemia or local anaesthetic toxicity.
- Increased activity on the EEG and epileptiform seizures – reported with the now little-used, agents enflurane and methohexital.
- Clonus – rarely seen during light anaesthesia and disappearing when anaesthesia is deepened.
- Shivering – common after volatile anaesthetics even when temperature is normal. Severe myoclonus may occur after volatile agents and may be mistaken for a convulsion.

Acute Dystonic Reactions

Dopamine is involved in the pathways controlling movement. By mechanisms that remain poorly understood, drugs affecting dopamine, including phenothiazines, butyrophenone derivatives such as haloperidol, droperidol and metoclopramide, can cause a variety of acute dystonic movement disorders. Akathisia is an uncontrolled restlessness; oculogyric crisis is a spectrum of blepharospasm, periorbital twitches and protracted staring episodes with a characteristic upward deviation of the eyes. These are more common in the young, especially girls and young women, and the elderly.

These conditions are uncommon and onset may be delayed. The key is recognizing the reaction and withdrawing the offending drug. For acute dystonic states, antimuscarinic drugs such as benzatropine (benztropine) 1–2 mg i.v. or procyclidine 5–10 mg i.v. are useful. The reaction subsides within 24 h of stopping the responsible drug.

Renal and Hepatic Complications

Renal and liver failures as a direct complication of anaesthesia are very rare indeed: idiosyncratic drug reactions may lead to renal failure (e.g. antibiotics), immune-mediated hepatitis (halothane <1 in 10,000, other volatiles <1 in 100,000), or cholestasis (e.g. antibiotics). However, in patients who have renal or hepatic impairment, deterioration of organ function after anaesthesia and surgery is common. Avoidance of organ-toxic drugs and maintenance of organ blood flow and oxygenation are the keys to preventing acute or chronic injury. Pre-existing renal and hepatic disease may significantly alter the pharmacokinetics of many drugs and hepatic disease has important effects on the pharmacodynamics of sedative drugs.

Hepatic blood flow decreases during general anaesthesia and this is especially so in abdominal surgery. Those with pre-existing liver disease have reduced hepatic portal vein blood flow and oxygen delivery (normally 75% blood flow, 50% oxygen supply), making them more reliant on oxygenation from the hepatic artery (25% blood flow). This may lead to deterioration in hepatic function after anaesthesia in those with chronic liver disease. Mortality in severe liver disease is high. The deterioration in liver function is not definitively reduced by use of regional anaesthesia which may be contraindicated because of associated coagu-lopathy. Avoidance of excessively deep anaesthesia, hypovolaemia, hypotension, hypoxia, raised abdominal pressure and surgical traction on the liver are all pru-dent in managing patients with liver disease.

Acute kidney injury (AKI) leads to increased morbidity and mortality after surgery. AKI occurs in up to 5% of noncardiac surgical patients with a higher inci-dence (up to 25%) in cardiac patients but is rarely a direct consequence of anaes-thesia. Pre-existing chronic kidney disease (CKD), especially grade 3 and above (eGFR < 60 mL/min), may be worsened by surgery and anaesthesia. Renal func-tion may commonly be worsened by nephrotoxic drugs, hypovolaemia, hypoten-sion or hypoxaemia. General anaesthesia is likely to reduce glomerular filtration rate through reduced cardiac output. Hypotension (MAP < 55 mm Hg) for as little as 5 min may worsen renal function. Cardiac and major vascular surgeries are high risk. In patients with impaired renal function principles of minimizing deterioration in the renal function are:

- Avoid nephrotoxic drugs (e.g. gentamicin, furosemide, NSAIDs, starch-based colloids, angiotensin converting enzyme inhibitors, radiocontrast media).
- Avoid all hypotension and treat immediately if it occurs.
- Ensure there is no obstruction to urine flow (blocked catheter, retention).
- Avoid significantly raised intra-abdominal pressure (limit to <12 mm Hg during laparoscopy, manage actively in >20 mm Hg postoperatively).
- Maintain normovolaemia and cardiac output wherever possible.
- Epidural analgesia may have a protective effect in major vascular surgery.
- Extrapolating from critical care medicine, there is no benefit to use of dopa-mine or furosemide in terms of preserving renal function, even though the diuresis may facilitate management of fluid balance.

Ophthalmological Complications

These include:

- Corneal abrasions
- Ischaemic optic neuropathy
- Central retinal artery occlusion

Corneal Abrasions

Corneal abrasions are the most common ophthalmological complication of anaesthesia. Injury may result from the eyes drying (protective reflexes are lost and tear production and tear film stability reduced), chemical injury (by any antiseptic except povidone–iodine 10% in aqueous solution, including detergent damage to the iris, ciliary body, lens and blood vessels) or direct trauma. Direct trauma to the eye can occur at any time during anaesthesia (poorly applied face mask ventilation, during use of facemasks postoperatively, cables, oximeter probes, etc., staff or the patient's own fingers and surgical drapes). Prevention is by taping the eyelids closed and vigilance, particularly when the patient is moved. Where taping interferes with surgical access viscous ointments or gels may be instilled to maintain lubrication. Prone positioning requires particular attention to avoid corneal abrasions.

Ischaemic Optic Neuropathy

Blood flow to the eye is determined by the perfusion pressure and resistance. The retinal circulation autoregulates to maintain flow across a range of pressures; however, flow to the posterior part of the optic nerve is not autoregulated and is therefore more vulnerable to ischaemia. Ischaemia can be caused by reduced perfusion pressure from low arterial pressure, elevated venous or intraocular pressure, or increased resistance to flow as seen in diabetes mellitus, hypertension and atherosclerosis.

High-risk procedures are bilateral radical neck dissection, spinal surgery and cardiopulmonary bypass. The risk in radical neck dissection is due to the disruption of venous plexuses and the rise in venous pressure. The prone position for spinal surgery elevates venous pressure, a degree of hypotension is often used to control bleeding and there may be direct pressure on the eye. Eye pads should be used in the prone position. Ischaemic optic neuropathy presents as painless visual loss and requires urgent referral to an ophthalmologist. The aims of treatment are to reduce optic nerve oedema with corticosteroids and diuretics and to maintain normal oxygenation by management of blood pressure and haemoglobin. The prospects of recovery are poor.

Central Retinal Artery Occlusion

Central retinal artery occlusion is caused by emboli and can occur together with ischaemic optic neuropathy. It presents with a painless visual defect, which may improve if treated promptly by an ophthalmologist.

Adverse Drug Reactions during Anaesthesia

Unsurprisingly, adverse drug reactions are an important cause of patient incidents in anaesthesia. Claims related to drug administration accounts for ≈11% of litigation against anaesthetists. Claims relate to drug error (two-thirds) and anaphylaxis (one-third). It is estimated that anaesthetists make an average of 1 drug error for every 600 drug administrations. Analysis of drug error events identifies external contributory factors (human factors) in the vast majority. Although some are clinician related (inattention, distraction, fatigue, rules violation), many are external/systems based (e.g. work overload, poor storage of drugs, poor drug labelling by manufacturers, inadequate drug supply governance, etc.).

Although all drugs must be checked (and labelled) before administration, there is little if any evidence that 'double-checking' significantly reduces the rate of administration errors on the ward or during anaesthesia. Double checking may also introduce errors due to 'involuntary automaticity' when multiple participants in the checking process fail to identify errors, due to the routine nature of the process and the lack of individual responsibility when a task is shared. Avoidance of drug errors requires constant vigilance, a robust process and lack of interruption.

Nonallergic drug-related adverse events with drug errors include:

- Wrong dose
  - Absolute overdose (e.g. administering a drug twice, or more than its known upper safe dose). Duplication is more common when multiple anaesthetists attend one patient, and when drugs which are administered in theatre are inadvertently also administered in the postoperative period (e.g. paracetamol, gentamicin and other antibiotics). These events should be reduced by clear communication and documentation of drug administration.
  - Relative overdose (e.g. administering a dose of drug that is inappropriately high for the clinical circumstance, through administration error or error of judgement).
  - Inadequate dose (e.g. as a cause of awareness), causes include intentional underdosing, failing to include a drug or sufficient drug, in an infusion. Remifentanil (omission) and vasopressors (wrong dilution) are typical examples.
  - Dosing errors are more likely in children as a result of calculation errors.
  - Wrong programme – this is an error that is common with infusions and especially during TIVA. Errors include selecting the wrong patient variables or drug concentration, choosing the wrong pharmacokinetic model or swapping syringes so that remifentanil and propofol are administered using the other drug's programme.
- No dose – omission of necessary drugs' administration (e.g. perioperative antibiotics, failing to connect or start an infusion or turn on a vaporizer).
- Wrong drug.
- Substitution – e.g. syringe swaps. Syringe swaps are potentially harmful as the order in which drugs are used during anaesthesia may be critical to patient safety. The typical harmful syringe swap involves administering a muscle relaxant prior to anaesthesia (most commonly suxamethonium). This leads to unexpected paralysis without anaesthesia. It leads to distress, psychological sequelae and may prompt litigation which is generally indefensible. Improved medicines management and solutions such as coloured syringes or prefilled syringes may provide a solution; wrong route; there are numerous wrong routes that can occur and some are considered 'never events'. Wrong route events with the greatest potential for harm are as follows:
  - Intended epidural medicine administered intravenously – potentially fatal, if the drug is bupivacaine, and a cause of direct anaesthesia death.
  - Intended intravenous drugs administered epidurally – has the potential to cause serious neurological injury, though this route is considerably lower risk than intrathecal administration. Several such cases were reported in

NAP3, mostly in obstetrics including errors by anaesthetists and midwives especially during emergencies.

● Intended intravenous drugs administered intrathecally – a known cause of neurological harm and death when chemotherapy intended only for i.v. use (vincristine) is administered intrathecally. This route of error is very uncommon in anaesthetic practice and no cases were reported in NAP3.

The elimination of wrong route errors has been a focus of considerable interest. Governmental pressure in the UK and legislation in California has led to the development of new 'non-Luer' small bore connectors (ISO 80369-6) for use in regional anaesthetic procedures. Formal testing of this connector has shown it to perform acceptably in clinical practice but to prevent cross connections with Luer connectors. It is likely this connector will soon become routinely used in equipment for regional anaesthesia and neuraxial access and will largely 'engineer-out' the risk of the above wrong-route errors.

● Wrong time – e.g. drugs retained in venous access devices that are inadvertently administered when the line is flushed or used for infusion.
  ● Lines with large dead space (central venous lines, peripherally inserted central catheters [PICCs], peripheral lines with extensions) and in small children are particularly high risk. Remifentanil and suxamethonium may cause problems in adults, whereas any anaesthetic drug may cause problems in small children. Routine flushing of lines and removal of unnecessary lines at the end of anaesthesia eliminates this problem and should be routine practice.

Adverse drug events without drug error include the following:

● Intolerance of known side-effects (e.g. pruritus or nausea with opioids).
● Rare but recognized side-effects (e.g. triggering of porphyria by barbiturates, 'scoline apnoea' with succinylcholine or mivacurium, malignant hyperpyrexia).
● Drug interactions, pharmaceutical, pharmacokinetic or pharmacodynamic – the common interactions are pharmacodynamic, relating to the effects of two drugs on the same body system (e.g. intravenous induction agents and volatile anaesthetics both decrease blood pressure). An important pharmaceutical drug reaction in anaesthesia is the hypertensive crisis precipitated through raised norepinephrine levels in patients taking monoamines inhibitors when administered indirectly acting sympathomimetic drugs (e.g. ephedrine, metaraminol, pethidine). Some modern anti-depressants can have similar effects. Tramadol has a theoretical risk of precipitating a serotonergic crisis (including hypertension and hyperpyrexia) in patients taking selective serotonin reuptake inhibitor (SSRI) antidepressants, but this appears to be extremely rare.

Anaphylactic Reactions

Anaphylaxis is a severe, life-threatening, generalized or systemic hypersensitivity reaction. It is classically mediated by IgE, with antigen-specific antibodies causing degranulation of mast cells to release powerful mediators, including histamine, prostaglandins, leukotrienes and platelet-activating factor. However, such reactions may be allergic (IgE- or IgG-mediated) or nonallergic. The term anaphylactoid is no longer used.

The incidence of anaphylactic reactions related to anaesthesia is considered to be 1 in 10,000 anaesthetics (reported ranges ≈1 in 2000 to 1 in 20,000). Perioperative anaphylaxis accounts for approximately one-third of ICU admissions for anaphylaxis.

The drugs responsible are most commonly neuromuscular blocking agents (especially suxamethonium, rocuronium and atracurium), antibiotics (especially β-lactams and teicoplanin) and less commonly colloids, induction agents and opioids. Other important agents include surgical dyes and chlorhexidine which may be present in a number of preparations used preoperatively (e.g. surgical prep, local anaesthetic gel and coating of central lines). Anaphylaxis from latex is declining, due to increased awareness and avoidance in health care settings. Anaphylactic reactions to local anaesthetics are very rare and to inhalation agents unknown.

Predicting anaphylaxis without a full immunological work-up is difficult and blood tests to detect allergy (antibodies) to specific drugs are relevant only to a few drugs.

A classification of perioperative anaphylactic reactions is given in Table 3.3.5.

TABLE 3.3.5 Classification of Grades of Anaphylaxis[7]

Grade	Denomination	Features
1	Not life-threatening	Rash, erythema and/or swelling
2	Not life-threatening	Unexpected hypotension – not severe, i.e. not requiring treatment and/or Bronchospasm – not severe, i.e. not requiring treatment +/– Grade 1 features
3	Life-threatening	Unexpected severe hypotension requiring treatment and/or Severe bronchospasm requiring treatment and/or Swelling with actual or potential airway compromise +/– Grade 1 features
4	Life-threatening	Fulfilling indications for CPR
5	Fatal	Causing death

Source: Royal College of Anaesthetists. Sixth National Audit Project. Perioperative Anaphylaxis London: Royal College of Anaesthetists; 2016. Available at: http://www.nationalauditprojects.org.uk/NAP6home.

Presentation

Reactions to intravenous drugs normally occur within minutes of exposure, even with small doses. Latex allergy usually occurs 30–40 min after exposure. The commonest presentation of any life-threatening reaction is cardiovascular collapse with some combination of bronchospasm and skin changes. However, cardiovascular collapse is the only feature in 10% of patients, and hypotension which is resistant to treatment should arouse the suspicion of anaphylaxis. The severity of the reaction may be worse in patients with a reduced endogenous catecholamine response; those with asthma, those taking β-blockers and those with CNB.

Immediate Management

Immediate management of anaphylaxis follows an ABC approach and includes the following:

- Withdraw all likely responsible drugs and stop anaesthesia and surgery if possible.
- Summon help and note the time.
- Administer 100% oxygen, ensure airway patency. Intubate early if there is airway swelling and ventilate the lungs if necessary.
- If there is hypotension elevate the legs.
- If there is cardiac arrest start CPR and follow ALS guidelines (Chapter 2.10).
- Give intravenous adrenaline (epinephrine) as a bolus, 50 μg in adults (in children 1 μg/kg), titrated to effect. Do not give undiluted i.v. adrenaline (epinephrine) (1:1000). If repeated doses of adrenaline (epinephrine) are needed, consider an infusion. If intravenous access is not available, it may also be given i.m.: 500 μg in adults/small children, 300 μg in child age 6–12, 150 μg in child aged <6.
- Rapidly infuse intravenous crystalloid, up to 1 L (20 mL/kg in children).
- Consider the need for further drug therapy: antihistamines (chlorpheniramine [chlorpheniramine] 10–20 mg), corticosteroids (hydrocortisone 100–200 mg) and bronchodilators (aminophylline 5 mg/kg slowly or salbutamol 250–500 μg slowly).

Further Management

- Patients with grade 3–4 anaphylaxis should be admitted to ICU for further treatment and assessment.
- Mast cell tryptase levels should be assessed within 1 h and 6–24 h. A rise during the event confirms mast cell degranulation.
- Refer the patient to an allergist at a regional allergy centre for full assessment: history and challenge testing (skin prick tests and intradermal dilutional testing) will be required to identify the causative agent. The presence of specific IgE antibodies can be measured for a few drugs (e.g. suxamethonium, rocuronium, latex, chlorhexidine and penicillins).
- Write full clinical notes and complete adverse drug reaction notification.

- Explain the situation to the patient and encourage the patient to carry a warning card and Medic-Alert bracelet.
- Communicate the plan and any conclusions to the patient and their GP and suggest safe drug combinations for future anaesthesia.

Prevention

A careful drug history is the main preventative factor. There is no evidence to support use of a 'test dose' before the main dose of an antibiotic, because this requires serial incremental challenges spread over a prolonged period to have and sensitivity. For a number of reasons, it is sensible to administer antibiotics several minutes before induction of anaesthesia. There is also no evidence to support the prophylactic use of antihistamines or corticosteroids.

A patient known to be latex-sensitive should be first on the operating list (latex particles persist in the air) and all equipment in contact with the patient must be latex-free. Most modern equipment and modern theatre environments are latex-free.

Outcome

Mortality of up to 5% has been reported historically. A recent Australian database reported no deaths caused by 264 cases of perioperative anaphylaxis (0%, upper 95% confidence limit 1.4%).

Nausea, Vomiting and Regurgitation

Nausea is a sensation of unease and discomfort vaguely referred to the epigastrium and stomach that is characterized by an urge to vomit. Vomiting is an active process that occurs during consciousness. Regurgitation is passive. Aspiration is the movement of (gastric) contents from the pharynx into the lungs. The three are often confused.

Vomiting

Vomiting is an active reflex:

- Sensors are mechano- and chemoreceptors in the gut, including mechanoreceptors in the pharynx, and receptors in the chemoreceptor trigger zone (CTZ) in the area postrema in the posterior part of the fourth ventricle. The CTZ is outside the blood–brain barrier and has numerous receptors including muscarinic, histaminic, serotonergic (5-HT), dopaminergic and opioid. There are sensors in the vestibular system whose protective function is unclear.
- The CTZ communicates with a functionally (but not anatomically) defined area in the medulla, termed the vomiting centre. Within this the 'central pattern generator' coordinates the sequence of physical and autonomic components of vomiting.

● Efferents produce an early wave of nausea, sympathetic and parasympathetic activity, including salivation. The proximal stomach then relaxes, and retrograde giant contraction waves move small bowel contents back into the stomach. Ejection is the movement of gastric contents into the pharynx and out of the mouth. During this phase there is apnoea and closure of the cords to protect the airway.

Vomiting occurs primarily in the awake state but can occur in very light anaesthesia. Base of the tongue or pharynx stimulation (e.g. airway manipulation) may cause it. The larynx relaxes soon after the ejection phase and there is then a significant risk of aspiration.

Regurgitation

Regurgitation is passive movement of gastric contents into the pharynx under the force of gravity. In the upright position a pressure of 40 cm H_2O is required to move gastric contents into the pharynx (hence, prior to RSI, induction of emergency anaesthesia was often performed in the sitting position). When lying flat, regurgitation is normally prevented by the barrier pressure between the stomach and lower oesophagus produced by the cardiac sphincter. This is a functional area, rather than discrete anatomical sphincter, at the gastro-oesophageal junction.

Regurgitation is made more likely by:

● Anaesthesia, which itself reduces the barrier pressure
● Atropine, hyoscine or glycopyrronium
● Head-down position
● Increased gastric pressure (e.g. pregnancy, full stomach, bowel obstruction, gas from facemask ventilation, high intra-abdominal pressure during laparoscopy)
● Incompetence of the cardiac sphincter (e.g. hiatus hernia, achalasia)

Postoperative Nausea and Vomiting

The overall incidence of PONV is usually quoted to be of the order of 25%–30%, but this is an underestimate for some patient groups, such as those undergoing major gynaecological surgery. Early PONV is much less common (severe <5%, moderate/severe <20%) with most PONV being delayed until later in recovery. As well as being profoundly disliked by patients, vomiting raises intraocular and intracranial pressure and may harm areas operated on (abdominal wall, neck surgery and skin flaps).

Causes: PONV may be central (causes acting on the brainstem and higher centres), peripheral (causes acting on the gut), or vestibular.

● Patient factors include those who suffer from travel sickness or previous PONV, nonsmokers, women more than men and the young (especially children) more than the old. Other factors include suggestion and the example of surrounding patients.

- Anaesthetic factors –opioids, volatile agents, nitrous oxide, anticholinergic reversal agents, barbiturates, hypoxia and hypotension are all potential contributors. Poor airway management and filling the stomach with gas can contribute.
- Surgical factors – vomiting is more frequent after major or prolonged operations and after gynaecological, abdominal, eye, ear, throat and neurosurgery. Surgical drugs such as antimicrobials may contribute.

Treatment and prevention: Treatment and prevention include preventing the above factors, using regional techniques when possible and using TIVA rather than volatile agents. The Apfel score allocates one point to female gender, non-smoker, previous PONV or motion sickness and an operation requiring postoperative opioids. Patients with a score of 0, 1, 2, 3 had a probability of PONV of 10%, 21%, 39% and 61%. Patients with a score ≥ 2 should receive anti-emetics routinely and as the score rises multiple interventions are indicated.

Use of a prophylactic anti-emetic reduces the incidence of PONV by $\approx 25\%$. TIVA reduces the incidence by $\approx 20\%$ and avoidance of nitrous oxide by 12%, however if TIVA is used, nitrous oxide does not increase the incidence of PONV. Acupuncture or acupressure may also be useful and are inexpensive, but not widely used. The P6 (pericardium 6) acupuncture point is in the forearm, three fingerbreadths proximal to the proximal wrist crease, between the tendons of palmaris longus and flexor carpi radialis.

Prevention of PONV should be planned for as part of every anaesthetic intervention. If drugs are not given prophylactically they should be made available for the management of PONV if it occurs. As anti-emetics are rather poorly effective (number needed to treat, NNT ≈ 4) multiple drugs may be needed and choosing drugs from different pharmacological groups is logical. Options include:

- Serotonin (5-HT$_3$) antagonists – (e.g. ondansetron 4–8 mg i.v. towards the end of anaesthesia, 4–8 mg orally/i.v. postoperatively). It is effective and potentiates other anti-emetics. It is relatively free of side-effects (headache; number needed to harm, NNH 10). Several 5-HT$_3$ antagonists are available.
- Corticosteroids– dexamethasone 4–8 mg is widely used (in up to 50% of anaesthetics). It raises serum glucose levels so should be avoided or used with careful monitoring in diabetics. Psychosis has been reported, but only rarely, after single doses. There is soft evidence of an increase in cancer recurrence with its use and it should be used with caution in this setting.
- Phenothiazines – act as dopamine antagonists in the chemoreceptor trigger zone (e.g. prochlorperazine 12.5 mg i.m., 5 mg p.o.). They can cause acute dystonic reactions.
- Antihistamines – (e.g. cyclizine 50 mg orally, i.m. or slowly i.v.) can cause sedation and tachycardia.
- Dopamine antagonists – metoclopramide 10 mg (p.o., i.m., i.v.) acts both centrally and peripherally. It speeds gastric emptying time and increases

the tone of the lower oesophageal sphincter. It is a weak anti-emetic and is a prominent cause of acute dystonic reactions, especially in young females. Domperidone 30 mg PR crosses the blood–brain barrier very slowly and so does not usually cause neurological or psychological side-effects.

- Butyrophenone derivatives – droperidol has been reintroduced in the UK, previously withdrawn due to concerns over prolongation of the QT interval. Lower doses are now recommended, e.g. 0.625–1.25 mg i.v.. Haloperidol is used in palliative care. It has a specific effect on the chemoreceptor trigger zone and may cause acute dystonic reactions.
- Anticholinergic drugs – hyoscine hydrobromide 0.4 mg i.m., i.v. inhibits the muscarinic activity of acetylcholine on the gut and may also have a central action.

Other Complications Associated with Anaesthesia

Accidental Hypothermia

Hypothermia is defined as a core temperature of <36°C. Body temperature should be monitored during all but the most minor surgery. Heat loss may be prevented by increasing the environmental temperature (>21°C), keeping the patient covered, the use of active warming blankets (warmed air at 38°C–42°C), warming intravenous fluids (to ≈40°C), and warming and humidifying inspired gases (heat and moisture exchange [HME] device).

Heat may be lost during anaesthesia by:

- Radiation – (≈50%) increased by uncovering parts of the body, low ambient temperature and the vasodilatation caused by many anaesthetic agents
- Convection – (≈30%) increased by frequent air changes in the operating theatre
- Conduction – (5%–10%) due to cold inspired gases and intravenous fluids
- Evaporation – (10%–15%) due to dry inspired gases and evaporation of sweat or body fluids

In anaesthetized patients body temperature falls rapidly. Heat production falls and shivering and normal behavioural mechanisms to conserve heat are totally lost. Vasodilatation occurs and hypothalamic temperature regulatory centres are depressed. The elderly and young – especially infants/neonates – are at increased risk as they cannot raise their metabolic rate to counteract heat loss. Long operations inevitably increase heat loss. The elderly, those who arrive hypothermic and those at increased risk of cardiovascular events, are at greatest risk of hypothermia and its consequences. Accidental hypothermia can infrequently be secondary to conditions such as hypothyroidism, hypopituitarism, adrenal failure, drug overdose and near drowning.

Severe hypothermia (<34°C) can cause severe physiological disturbance including arrhythmias which may be life-threatening.

Lesser degrees of hypothermia also lead to clinically important consequences:

- Reduced basal metabolic rate (approx. 6% for each fall in temperature by 1°C)
- Left shift of the oxyhaemoglobin curve (less delivery of oxygen to the tissues), tissue hypoxia
- Reduced cardiac output and consequent reduced liver and kidney blood flow
- Prolongation of drug effects through reduced metabolism – NMBs especially
- Increased cardiovascular morbidity – including increased myocardial ischaemia, arrhythmias
- Increased bleeding through coagulopathy and impaired platelet function
- Increased rate of infections – especially wound
- Shivering and increased oxygen demand

Hyperthermia

Malignant hyperthermia (MH) is a genetically determined condition (autosomal dominant) in which trigger agents, typically suxamethonium or volatile agents, cause an abnormal rise in intracellular calcium and a subsequent hypermetabolic state (increase in glucose and oxygen consumption and heat production). If the condition is allowed to progress it causes mitochondrial and sarcolemma damage that becomes irreversible and is potentially fatal. MH is genetically heterogeneous. Many, but not all, MH patients have a genetically determined defect in the ryanodine receptor in the sarcoplasmic reticulum that opens to permit the outpouring of calcium into the cytoplasm. The incidence is about 1 in 15,000 patients.

Suxamethonium is thought to cause a brief, marked rise in intracellular calcium and its effects are predominantly related to muscle damage (i.e. myoglobinuria and renal failure). Inhalation agents cause a more sustained rise and their effects are predominantly metabolic owing to the effect of calcium on enzymes of the glycolytic pathway, with hypercapnia, hypoxia, hyperkalaemia and acidosis.

Many patients will be exposed to both types of trigger in the same anaesthetic. For unknown reasons patients do not necessarily react on every exposure to a trigger agent, so previous uneventful anaesthetics with suxamethonium and inhalation agents do not exclude MH.

Over the past decades, prognosis has improved due to awareness of the condition, early detection by improved monitoring (particularly capnography) and early treatment, with dantrolene and aggressive general supportive measures. The mortality rate in the UK from established MH is ≈4%.

Malignant hyperthermia presents with:

- Masseter muscle spasm
- Tachycardia and arrhythmias
- Rise in end-tidal carbon dioxide (often the first sign)

- Tachypnoea if breathing spontaneously
- Unexpected changes in blood pressure
- Hypoxia
- Rising temperature (relatively late)

Serial blood gases show increasing hypoxaemia, rising PCO_2, increasing acidosis and rising serum potassium. Creatine kinase levels are an indicator of the degree of muscle damage. Disseminated intravascular coagulation and cerebral oedema can occur.

Treatment

Specific treatment is dantrolene 1 mg/kg i.v., repeated as necessary every 5 min until the PCO_2 has started to fall, up to a cumulative maximum of 10 mg/kg. Dantrolene is difficult to dissolve and it is wise to assign one person just to this task.

Supportive: Stop the operation if possible and if not possible discontinue the use of volatile agents and continue with TIVA. Cool the patient with external cooling (ice packs to the axillae and groins) and cooled intravenous saline or an intravenous cooling device, if available. Gastric, rectal and bladder lavage with iced saline have also been used.

Monitor and treat hyperkalaemia, acidaemia, coagulopathy and hypoxaemia. Admit the patient to ICU, monitor renal function and use fluids to promote a diuresis to prevent myoglobin-induced AKI. Dantrolene contains 3 g of mannitol per 20 mg ampoule. Monitor the clotting status.

Further treatment: Refer the patient to a MH unit for further investigation by muscle biopsy (under local anaesthetic) and in vitro testing of susceptibility, in which fresh muscle is tested for degree of contracture on exposure to halothane or caffeine (increased contraction in susceptible individuals). The test is ≈95% sensitive and ≈95% specific. Family members will also need to be investigated.

Management if MH Susceptibility Is Known or Suspected

If MH susceptibility is known or suspected:

- Safe drugs include propofol, ketamine, benzodiazepines, opioids, nitrous oxide, NMBs and local anaesthetics.
- Avoid trigger agents (suxamethonium and all volatile agents).
- Use TIVA or regional anaesthesia.
- Remove the vaporizers from the anaesthetic machine, flush with oxygen for 30 min to remove traces of volatile agent and use new anaesthetic circuit.
- Monitor temperature and capnography.
- Have access to a supply of dantrolene – prophylactic treatment is not indicated.

Masseter Muscle Spasm

If a patient develops severe masseter spasm after suxamethonium, lasting several minutes such that it is very difficult to open the mouth to intubate, there is a significant ($\approx$20%–30%) possibility that they may have a susceptibility to MH. Whether to stop the operation or not is a clinical judgement based on whether other signs of MH occur and the clinical urgency of the operation. It may be wise to avoid volatile agents and instead use TIVA. Patients should be closely observed and their blood gases and creatine kinase checked. If there is sufficient clinical suspicion, they should be referred to an MH unit for muscle biopsy and in vitro testing.

Complications of Posture and Positioning

Remaining in any position without movement for a prolonged period risks pressure injury to skin, nervous tissue and possibly muscles, by compression. This is exacerbated by obesity, hypotension or hypovolaemia. Pre-existing vascular, neurological or dermatological conditions will increase the risk of compression injuries. Diabetes is a major risk factor. Padding dependent and at-risk areas is part of routine care. Passive movement or change of position can be used to reduce periods of compression, if it does not interfere with surgery.

Supine Position

The ulnar nerve at the elbow is particularly prone to injury from pressure on or stretching. The elbow should be padded and the forearm supinated, which provides more protection for the ulnar nerve. Legs should be flat on the table and not crossed. The Achilles tendon must not rest on the unpadded edge of the table. A soft pad, raising heels from the table, avoids pressure on the calf veins and may lessen the incidence of DVT.

To prevent injury to the brachial plexus by the head of the humerus, if the arm must be abducted it should not be to greater than a right angle. Turning the head slightly to the side of the arm may also help. The arm should not drop down below the plane of the body.

Changes of Position of the Head and Neck

A patient with a decreased cardiac output or cerebrovascular disease is at risk of reduced cerebral blood flow if changes in position alter the relationships of the vertebral arteries to surrounding bony structures. This is possible on rotation of the head or hyperextension of the neck at the atlanto-occipital joint. Patients with cervical pathology may have nerve symptoms following immobilization from any cause, including surgery.

Trendelenburg Position

The Trendelenburg is a head-down position and is generally well tolerated in anaesthetized patients breathing spontaneously. In obese patients or those with an abdominal mass, pressure on the diaphragm may reduce lung volumes considerably and IPPV may be preferred. Cyanosis occurs in the face and neck of plethoric patients in this position owing to venous stasis, even with adequate ventilation. There is an increased risk of regurgitation.

Steep Trendelenburg may be used for laparoscopic procedures and pros-tatectomy. There is a risk of airway oedema which requires careful manage-ment at extubation. An increase in CVP will cause a fall in cerebral perfusion, particularly if the patient is hypotensive. This can result in cerebral oedema (commonly seen as postoperative agitation) and retinal detachment. If shoulder braces are needed to support the patient, careful positioning is required to avoid brachial plexus injury.

Prone Position

A specifically designed mattress or frame is usually used to ensure that pressure is completely removed from the abdomen and inferior vena cava. This prevents extradural veins becoming unduly distended, reduces the risk of pressure injury including to intraabdominal organs and minimizes the impact on breathing. A cuffed, armoured tracheal tube may be wise to secure the airway, although some experienced anaesthetists use a SAD successfully. There is increased risk of airway dislodgement and whatever airway is chosen there should be a plan to manage displacement.

Skeletal injury readily occurs when turning the unconscious patient. Particular care should be taken when moving the arms to avoid shoulder dislocation.

Corneal abrasions are a particular risk. The eyes should be carefully pro-tected with pads. Retinal arterial occlusion and blindness from pressure on the eye have been reported. Regular inspection of the face and gentle movement to release pressure may reduce the risk of facial (supraorbital and infraorbital) neuropraxias.

Lithotomy Position

When putting a patient in the lithotomy position, both legs should be moved together to avoid strain on the pelvic ligaments. The anterior superior iliac spines should be at the level of the break in the table. The knee should be outside any metal supports to avoid pressure on the lateral popliteal nerves. If the hips are very flexed, sciatic nerve stretch may occur. Hip arthroplasties are at risk of dislocation and use of a Lloyd-Davis position (legs half elevated) may be neces-sary. Lower limb compartment syndrome has occurred after prolonged surgery, and intermittent compression devices should be avoided in the lithotomy posi-tion (see also Chapters 5.5 and 5.17).

Lateral Position

The lateral position impairs spontaneous respiration, especially if a 'bridge' is also used to add lateral flexion. In an anaesthetized patient breathing spontane-ously, more ventilation goes to the upper lung while more blood flow goes to the lower lung, thus causing ventilation–perfusion mismatch and impaired gas exchange. This is made worse by IPPV.

Care should be taken with the position of the arms to prevent nerve com-pression.

Sitting Position

The head must be very carefully secured. The elevated position of the head leads to a risk of hypotension and inadequate cerebral perfusion. Hypotension must be actively prevented or treated. There is a risk of air embolus.

Moving the Patient

The reflexes that maintain blood pressure are greatly reduced in an anaesthetized patient, and hypotension is common during changes in body posture. This is particularly true if the patient is also hypovolaemic or CNB has been used. Movement also risks displacement of airway, vascular and surgical drain devices. All movements should be communicated, coordinated, smooth and gradual.

Nerve Palsies

Nerve palsies are more common in patients with existing risk factors such as diabetes mellitus or multiple sclerosis and in longer operations (>30 min). Nerves may be stretched or compressed as a result of positions that would be uncomfortable if the patient was conscious. Tourniquets can cause problems if excessive pressure is applied over a nerve trunk (especially if >60 min). The cuff should be adequately wide and padded. The pressure for upper limb ischaemia need only exceed arterial blood pressure by 50 mm Hg and for the lower limb by 100 mm Hg.

Patients with established or suspected nerve damage should be referred to a neurologist for conduction studies to establish the site and degree of damage, though performing this test too early (<6 weeks) may lead to unreliable results.

Nerves that may be damaged include:

- Supraorbital and infraorbital nerves – can be compressed by the tracheal tube connector/anaesthetic circuit or when prone, causing forehead numbness or cheek numbness, respectively.
- Facial nerve – compressed between fingers and ascending ramus of mandible when holding a facemask, causing facial paralysis.
- Brachial plexus – particularly at risk from stretching or compression in the Trendelenburg position, but also whenever an arm is abducted. The deltoid, biceps and brachialis are the muscles most commonly affected.
- Radial nerve – stretched if the arm is allowed to sag over the side of the table or compressed by the use of a vertical screen support, causing wrist drop.
- Ulnar nerve – the most frequently damaged nerve in the upper limb – damaged if the elbow is allowed to fall over the sharp edge of the table, so the nerve is compressed against the medial epicondyle of the humerus. If the elbow is extended, it is best to supinate the forearm to provide more protection to the nerve. Injury causes hypothenar weakness, and later 'claw hand'. It is a relatively common injury (1 in 2700) but can occur even if positioning appears to be perfect. Abnormalities of nerve conduction are often found in the other arm.

- Median nerve – may be damaged as a result of intravenous injections in the antecubital fossa, from direct needle trauma or extravasation, causing an inability to oppose the thumb and little finger.
- Pudendal nerve – can be compressed against a poorly padded perineal post during hip surgery with traction to the legs, so that the nerve is pressed against the ischial tuberosity, causing loss of perineal sensation and faecal incontinence.
- Femoral nerve – use of a self-retaining retractor during lower abdominal surgery can result in loss of flexion of the hip and loss of extension of the knee with loss of sensation over the anterior thigh and anteromedial aspect of the calf.
- Sciatic nerve – may be damaged by intramuscular injections not given in the recommended upper and outer quadrant of the buttock. It may also be damaged in emaciated patients lying on a hard table with the opposite buttock elevated, as for hip surgery. Injury results in paralysis of the hamstrings, all the muscles below the knee and sensory loss below the knee.
- Saphenous nerve – compression between a lithotomy pole and the medial malleolus of the tibia when the leg is suspended lateral to the pole, causes sensory loss along the medial border of the foot.
- Lateral popliteal nerve – the most frequently damaged nerve in the lower limb – it can be compressed between the head of the fibula and a laterally placed lithotomy pole, resulting in foot drop.

ENVIRONMENTAL HAZARDS

Electrical Hazards

Electrocution

Skin has a high resistance unless wet (hence the need for gel pads with defibrillators), whereas the interior of the body is a relatively good conductor, particularly nerve and muscle. A passage of several mA of electricity through the body may cause arrhythmias, skin and tissue damage including burns, and gross muscle contractions. The extent and type of damage depends on the path through the body, the duration and the current frequency. A frequency of the mains supply of 50 Hz is particularly likely to provoke ventricular fibrillation.

The basis of safety is to prevent the patient becoming part of an electrical circuit, achieved by either earthing equipment (class I), double insulating it (class II) or using batteries as the power supply. In addition, isolating transformers in the patient circuit protect against electrocution via earth. Microshock can be produced by electrolyte solutions in catheters near the heart when very small currents (50 μA) can cause arrhythmias. Any equipment used near the heart must be designed to avoid this.

Surgical Diathermy

Surgical diathermy uses a radiofrequency (about 3 MHz) alternating current (used continuously for cutting, and in 20 ms bursts at a lower frequency for coagulation). This high frequency allows the use of the heating effect of electricity without affecting excitable tissue. Diathermy has the potential to cause explosions (e.g. pooled alcoholic skin-prep solutions) or interfere with monitors and cardiac pacemaker/defibrillators. When using monopolar diathermy the patient forms part of the circuit, via the earthing plate. Poor contact of this with skin may cause burns and a broken earth plate lead may cause the patient to earth themselves to part of the operating table causing a burn. Unintended use, when the active electrode is touching the wrong part of the patient, a surgeon or assistant, may also cause a burn.

Bipolar diathermy, where the current just passes from one prong of a forceps to the other, is of lower power and efficacy, but interferes least with monitors and pacemakers.

Pollution

Exposure to high levels of volatile anaesthetic agents causes drowsiness in anaesthetists and surgeons. There has also been concern about the effects of chronic low-level exposure. Nitrous oxide is teratogenic in experimental animals and can affect DNA synthesis through inhibition of methionine synthase. The current consensus view is there is no significant risk to long-term health from chronic low levels of exposure. Even so, regulations in many countries limit allowable pollution by anaesthetic agents in the atmosphere of operating rooms, (e.g. in the UK through COSHH [Control of Substances Hazardous to Health]). Maximal suggested levels in different countries range from 2 to 50 ppm for volatile agents, and from 25 to 100 ppm for nitrous oxide. These values may be difficult to achieve in areas such as delivery suites, recovery or if there are substantial leaks in breathing circuits.

Measures to reduce pollution include:

- Adequate ventilation of operating theatres.
- Active scavenging and disposal of waste gases to outside air – for active scavenging an appropriate device is essential to prevent negative pressure being transmitted to the patient circuit.
- The use of low-flow breathing circuits and techniques.
- Use of total intravenous anaesthesia (TIVA) or regional analgesia.
- Careful filling of vaporizers with anti-spill devices.

Ionizing Radiation and Magnetic Resonance Imaging

Ionizing Radiation

X-rays are electromagnetic radiation produced when a beam of particles is accelerated from a cathode to strike an anode and are used for imaging and in the treatment of cancer. When unstable isotopes decay into more stable elements different sorts of radiation may be produced: α particles consisting of a helium nucleus (two protons and two neutrons), β-particles (electrons) and γ-radiation (high-energy electromagnetic radiation, of shorter wavelength than X-rays). Radioactive isotopes are used in cancer treatment and γ-ray-emitting isotopes such as technetium-99m are used in imaging techniques.

All ionizing radiation can cause tissue damage and chromosomal changes, and it is important to minimize the dose. Most protection comes from having safe procedures for handling of isotopes and arrangements to contain spillage.

For anaesthetists the hazard most commonly encountered is X-rays, particularly from image intensifiers in theatres. The intensity of ionizing radiation declines as the square of distance from the source; at a distance beyond 2 m the ionizing dose is low. Lead coats, impervious to X-rays, must be worn by all staff and thyroid protectors are advised.

Magnetic Resonance Imaging

Magnetic resonance imaging does not produce ionizing radiation but presents hazards associated with the intense magnetic field, noise and difficulties in scavenging anaesthetic gases. In particular, ferromagnetic objects can become dangerous projectiles when inside the scanner room where the magnetic field strength exceeds 0.5 millitesla. Strict controls, restricting access to trained, authorized personnel reduce the risk of dangerous events.

Transmission of Infection

Transmissible diseases abound in hospitals. There is a risk of transmission of infection from patients to health care staff, vice versa or more commonly from one patient to another with a health care worker (or their actions) acting as the agent of transmission. Immunocompromised patients are at particularly high risk of all modes of transmission and normally benign microbiological agents may cause invasive infections. In general, transmission of infection is of greater risk to patients than to attending health care workers.

Multiresistant Bacterial Organisms

There is global concern about the emergence of increasing numbers of bacteria which are resistant to multiple antibiotics. The lack of development of new classes of antibiotics compounds this problem. Particularly troublesome organisms in hospitals include those with the following abbreviations:

- MRSA – methicillin-resistant *Staphylococcus aureus*. MRSA is a multidrug resistant Gram-positive bacteria which is a common skin contaminant that can cause skin (surgical site infections), respiratory (pneumonia) and blood-stream infections. Less commonly it causes osteomyelitis or endocarditis. It can contaminate (colonize) skin, nose, urinary and respiratory tracts. MRSA is of relatively low invasiveness but troublesome due to multidrug resistance, difficulty in its eradication, the risk of cross-infection and of serious bloodstream infections. Up to 1 in 3 people have staphylococcal species in their nose and 1 in 50 carry MRSA in their nose, throat or skin. MRSA carriers (patients and staff) require eradication treatment before surgery (nasal mupirocin, chlorhexidine to the skin).

- ESBL – extended spectrum β-lactamases. This refers to the enzyme that leads to resistance to numerous antibiotics. ESBL producing Gram-negative bacteria include *Klebsiella, Proteus and Pseudomonas* species and *Escherichia coli (E. coli)*. Resistance includes penicillins, and cephalosporins including third generation (i.e. 'extended spectrum' cephalosporins) and monobactams. Carbapenems are generally still effective.
- VRE – vancomycin-resistant enterobacteriae. Gut and genital Gram-negative organisms resistant to vancomycin. These may lead to urinary, intra-abdominal or blood stream infections.
- CRE/CPE – carbapenem resistant enterobacteriaceae/carbapenemase-producing enterobacteriaceae. Gram-negative, gut bacteria that have developed resistance to carbapenem antibiotics (second-/third-line antibiotics, e.g. meropenem, imipenem) through development of a carbapenemase that inactivates the drug. Include *Klebsiella* and *E. coli* and *Pseudomonas* species) leading to respiratory, urinary and bloodstream infections. Tend to occur in large metropolitan hospitals.
- *Clostridium difficile.* This is Gram-positive, spore-forming obligate anaerobic bacterium that is widespread in the environment. A cause of outbreaks in hospitals and with the potential to cause death. Predominant in patients who have taken antibiotics, *C. difficile* overgrowth can lead to infective diarrhoea, colitis and septic shock driven by a toxin. Metronidazole is given orally for mild and i.v. for severe infections. Oral vancomycin is added for severe infections. Colectomy may be required.

Scrupulous infection control when dealing with patients with these and other infective illnesses is essential in maintaining the health of the patient and others.

Blood-borne Viruses

Blood-borne viruses represent a potential hazard to staff. However, immunocompromised patients are at great risk from infections and must be treated in the same way as other patients with immune deficiency.

Hepatitis A and E

Hepatitis A and E are commonly transmitted by the faecal–oral route. After an incubation period of a few weeks there is a prodromal illness, which leads to hepatocellular jaundice and resolves without chronic damage. There is a very small risk of infection with hepatitis A after transfusion, if the donor was in a viraemic phase.

Hepatitis B

Hepatitis B is a much more serious condition. Following infection there is usually an acute illness and 5%–10% of patients will go on to develop a carrier state characterized by the presence of hepatitis B surface antigen in the circulation. The long-term consequences include chronic active hepatitis, cirrhosis and primary liver cancer. The presence of the 'e' antigen in blood is a marker of high levels of virus and increased risk of transmission. The prevalence of the carrier state varies between countries; in the UK it is about 0.1%. The risk of infection after a needlestick injury is 1 in 3 for individuals who have not been immunized, as all health care workers should now be.

Hepatitis C

Hepatitis C virus was responsible for most historical non-A, non-B post-transfusion hepatitis. Blood is now screened for hepatitis C antibodies and the risk from transfusion is very low. Of those infected, 40%–85% will go on to develop chronic liver disease. The carrier state has a worldwide prevalence of about 1%. Treatment with interferon, ribavirin and other newer biological agents now offer a good chance of cure of hepatitis C. The risk of infection after a needlestick injury is 1 in 30.

Human Immunodeficiency Virus

Patients with human immunodeficiency virus (HIV) may be completely well and unaware they carry the virus. Conversely full blown acquired immune deficiency syndrome (AIDS) leads to severe immunocompromise, risk of opportunistic infections and other sequelae including development of cancers. The virus is delicate, easily destroyed and has low infectivity. It can be transmitted by blood (needle-sharing drug users and haemophiliacs have been particularly affected), sexual contact and transplacentally. Amniotic fluid, pericardial fluid and peritoneal fluid are also considered as carrying a risk of transmission, whereas faeces, nasal secretions, sputum, saliva, sweat, urine and vomit are not thought to present a risk for transmission. Increasing success with multimodal treatment has transformed HIV into a chronic stable disease for many in the last decade. The risk of seroconversion following a needlestick injury is 1 in 300.

New Variant Creutzfeldt–Jakob Disease (nvCJD)

This disease is caused by a noncellular transmissible protein, a prion, and is the cause of bovine spongiform encephalitis (BSE) in cattle. The misfolded prion proteins lead to misfolding of native proteins in host nervous tissue with loss of function and cell death. In humans, it causes debilitating and rapidly fatal spongiform encephalitis which clinically presents with movement disorders, changes in personality, dementia and death in 6–24 months. It has an incubation period of up to 12 years and is not readily detected in blood. Prions may not be inactivated by standard sterilization procedures and its emergence, especially in the UK, in the late 1980s led to a revolution in infection control procedures, an increase in use of single use equipment and a requirement to track the use of all reusable equipment coming into contact with patients. Brain, spinal cord and corneal tissue of infected patients carry the highest risk of transmission, though transmission by blood transfusion has been reported. For anaesthetists, a particular concern was that prion material was believed to be concentrated in the tonsils. However, a very large study which examined 63,000 surgically removed tonsils for the presence of prion material found no specimens containing prion protein.[9] The risk of transmission of nvCJD therefore appears very low. Despite this, anaesthetists mostly continue to use single-use equipment for adenotonsillectomy, though most surgeons abandoned this practice several years ago.

Prevention of Transmission

Many hospital patients harbour transmissible disease and those with transmissible blood-borne viral or prion disease are often asymptomatic and may not know they are carrying the infection. Screening all patients presenting for surgery is impractical, and even if carried out only for patients considered high risk would miss large numbers of patients and carry difficult ethical problems. The sensible solution is to regard all contact with patients as carrying a degree of risk and adopt Universal Precautions. In particular, every effort must be made to avoid needlestick injuries to oneself and others and observe the following:

- Wear gloves during induction of anaesthesia and while inserting vascular cannulae, setting up infusions, and inserting and removing airways and tubes.
- European legislation has led to the introduction of self-sheathing intravenous cannulae and hypodermic needles with needle-covering hoods. These 'safer' needles may improve safety by reducing needlestick injuries, though additional dexterity may be needed to use them.
- Where substantial spillage of blood is possible, wear a plastic apron, mask and eye protection.
- Dispose of all needles directly into a sharps box and never re-sheath needles.
- Cover cuts and abrasions that might come into contact with body fluids.
- There should be infection control policies and procedures in place for cleaning and sterilizing equipment and the theatre environment.
- All medical staff should be immunized against hepatitis B.
- If a needlestick injury occurs, the puncture or wound should be encouraged to bleed by squeezing the area, then thoroughly washed with soap and water. Splashes into the eye should be washed immediately with sterile eye wash or clean water.
- All hospitals should have procedures for management of a sharps injury and exposure to infected material so that the affected person can receive prompt consultation with an appropriately trained physician. Management may include the use of antiviral drugs – the side-effects of some of these drugs make compliance difficult.

REFERENCES

1. Staender SE, Mahajan RP. Anesthesia and patient safety: have we reached our limits? Curr Opin Anaesthesiol 2011;24:349–53.
2. Cook TM, Bland L, Mihai R, Scott S. Litigation related to anaesthesia: an analysis of claims against the NHS in England 1995–2007. Anaesthesia 2009;64:706–18.
3. Cook TM, Counsell D. Wildsmith JAW on behalf of The Royal College of Anaesthetists. Third National Audit Project. Major complications of central neuraxial block: report on the Third National Audit Project of the Royal College of Anaesthetists. Br J Anaesth 2009;102:179–90.
4. Cook TM, Woodall N, Frerk C. Fourth National Audit Project. Major complications of airway management in the UK: results of the Fourth National Audit Project of the Royal College of Anaesthetists and the Difficult Airway Society. Part 1: anaesthesia. Br J Anaesth 2011;106: 617–31.
5. Cook TM, Woodall N, Harper J, Benger J. Fourth National Audit Project. Major complications of airway management in the UK: results of the Fourth National Audit Project of the Royal College of Anaesthetists and the Difficult Airway Society. Part 2: intensive care and emergency departments. Br J Anaesth 2011;106:632–42.
6. Pandit JJ, Cook TM. Fifth National Audit Project. Accidental awareness during general anaesthesia in the United Kingdom and Ireland: report and findings. London: Royal College of Anaesthetists; 2014. Available at: http://www.nationalauditprojects.org.uk/NAP5report
7. Royal College of Anaesthetists. Sixth National Audit Project. Perioperative Anaphylaxis. London: Royal College of Anaesthetists; 2016. Available at: http://www.nationalauditprojects.org.uk/NAP6home
8. Frerk C, Mitchell VS, McNary AF. Difficult Airway Society 2015 guidelines for management of unanticipated difficult intubation in adults. Br J Anaesth 2015;115:827–48.
9. Clewley JP, Kelly CM, Andrews N, Vogliqi K, Mallinson G, Kaisar M, et al. Prevalence of disease related prion protein in anonymous tonsil specimens in Britain: cross sectional opportunistic survey. BMJ 2009;338:b1442.

Section 4

Regional Anaesthesia

Chapters

Chapter 4.1

Local Anaesthetic Agents

Tim G. Hales, Graeme McLeod

GENERAL CONSIDERATIONS

Local anaesthetics (LA) exert their analgesic actions by reversibly blocking sodium ion (Na^+) channels in the nerve membrane. Local anaesthetics inhibit the transmission of autonomic, sensory and motor impulses, resulting in sympathetic blockade, analgesia and anaesthesia.

The first local anaesthetic introduced into medical practice was cocaine, a naturally occurring ester of benzoic acid that is present in the leaves of *Eythrwylon coca*, a tree growing in the Andes mountains. In 1884, Carl Koller first administered topical anaesthesia to the eye. William Halsted conducted peripheral nerve block using an open surgical technique, applying cocaine directly onto the brachial plexus.

Awareness of the serious adverse effects of cocaine, such as psychological dependence, led to the synthesis of another ester, procaine, introduced by Alfred Einhorn in 1905. The first amide local anaesthetic, lidocaine, was synthesized by Nils Lofgren in 1943 and remains the standard against which other local anaesthetics are compared.

Common to all local anaesthetics is their propensity for toxicity. With local anaesthetics, the relative difference between therapeutic plasma concentrations and life-threatening plasma concentrations is small compared to many other drugs. If given in sufficiently high dose, local anaesthetics may block additional excitable tissue such as brain and myocardium, leading to convulsions, cardiac arrest and death. Clinical application of local anaesthetics for peripheral infiltration, nerve block or neuraxial block requires an understanding of nerve anatomy and physiology and the molecular site of action of local anaesthetics.

Nerve Anatomy and Physiology

Nerves allow long-distance conduction of electrical signals from the central nervous system (CNS) to the periphery and from the periphery to the CNS without loss of information. Myelinated nerves are ensheathed by myelin, which acts as an insulator. Nerves consist of a cell body and an axon, which ends as a presynaptic terminal. The space between a presynaptic terminal and the membrane of another neuron is termed the synaptic cleft, across which pass neurotransmitters such as acetylcholine, γ-aminobutyric acid, glycine, glutamate and norepinephrine (noradrenaline).

Nerve fibres are classified as A, B and C according to their velocity of conduction,[1] A and B fibres are myelinated, whereas C fibres are unmyelinated.

The largest A fibres are subdivided into α, β, γ and δ. Aα fibres supply skeletal muscle, Aβ fibres transmit tactile sensation, Aγ fibres supply skeletal muscle spindles and Aδ fibres transmit stabbing, acute pain.

Type C fibres transmit dull, aching pain from skin and viscera.

Within the myelinated A and B fibres are interruptions of the myelin sheath called nodes of Ranvier. Action potentials pass from node to node rather than continuously down the nerve, as in unmyelinated C fibres.

Two or three adjacent nodes must be blocked to prevent conduction, corresponding to a 6–10 mm segment of nerve fibre. Conduction between successive nodes allows higher transmission velocity than occurs in unmyelinated nerves and conservation of energy because fewer ions move across the nerve membrane.

At rest, an electrical potential of approximately –70 mV exists on the inside of the nerve membrane. Impulse generation along a nerve alters membrane potential by rapid movement of Na^+ inwards and potassium ions (K^+) outwards through highly selective ion channels. Once the membrane potential rises to a threshold of –55 mV an action potential is generated, due to the opening of voltage-activated Na^+ channels. The action potential peaks at +40 mV. There is rapid Na^+ channel inactivation and efflux of K^+ ions repolarizes the nerve back to its resting state.

Molecular Site of Action

The structure of the nerve membrane is that of a bimolecular framework of phospholipid molecules and transmembrane ion channels and transporters.

X-ray crystallography has revealed the three-dimensional structure of a bacterial ancestor of mammalian voltage-gated Na^+ channels (Fig. 4.1.1). Viewed in cross-section, the Na^+-channel protein is bell shaped with transmembrane domains arrayed symmetrically around a central pore allowing the passage of Na^+ between the intra- and extracellular spaces.[2]

Four homologous domains (I–IV) contain six transmembrane α-helices (S1–S6) and an inactivating particle connecting domains III and IV (Fig. 4.1.2). The S5 and S6 segments and the short loops between them form the channel pore. The fourth helix (S4) in each domain has positively charged arginine or lysine residues at every third position and is the voltage-sensitive region of the Na^+ channel.[3] Parts of the local anaesthetic (LA) binding site are located in the

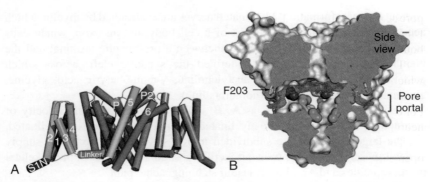

FIGURE 4.1.1   Three-dimensional representation of sodium channel. (A) The arrangement of transmembrane helices in a bacterial homologue of mammalian voltage-activated Na^+ channels. (B) Surface rendering of the bell-shaped structure of a bacterial voltage-activated Na^+ channel solved using X-ray crystallography. This view highlights passageways (red) formed by lateral portals that may enable access of some local anaesthetics into the ion channel's inner vestibule. Several residues implicated in drug binding are also highlighted as is phenylalanine 203 (F203), which may act as a gate keeper for drug access through this route. The alternative entrance is through the inner vestibule (accessible when the channel is in the open state) shown at the bottom of the rendering.[2] *Source:* Reprinted by permission from Macmillan Publishers Ltd: *Nature* 2011;475(7356):353–8. © 2011.

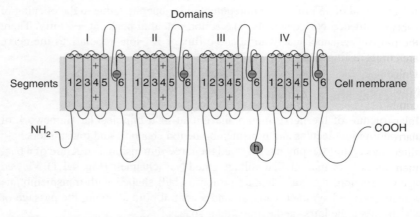

FIGURE 4.1.2   Schematic representation of the topology of the principle membrane spanning α subunit of the voltage-activated Na^+ channel. Domains I–IV, repeating segments 1–6, re-entrant pore loop with selectivity filter (demoted by negative charge) and inactivation gate (represented by 'h') are highlighted. There are nine variants of the α subunit encoded by different genes that exhibit distinctive patterns of tissue expression. Several β subunits have also been identified (not shown), which modify the properties of the ion channel.[3]

pore-lining transmembrane segments 6 of domains I, III and IV (DI-S6, D3-S6, D4-S6). Specific residues within the ion-conducting pore interact directly with bound local anaesthetics.

There are nine genes that encode voltage-gated Na^+ channels in mammals, which all contain the motif for local anaesthetic binding and are therefore vulnerable to block.[4] These genes are differentially expressed in different tissues. For example, $Na_V1.7$ and $Na_V1.8$ Na^+ channels are highly expressed in sensory neurones, whereas $Na_V1.5$ is found in cardiac cells.

Three major conformational states of the Na^+ channel exist (i.e. resting, open and inactivated).

In the resting state, the membrane potential is negative inside because of the presence of larger concentration of potassium ions inside the cell than outside and the permeability of the membrane to K^+. The S4 segments are in the 'down' position, making the channel nonconductive. Outward movement and spiral rotation of the S4 segments moves positive gating charges across the membrane's electric field and opens the ion channel.

Subsequent channel inactivation involves the closure of a hydrophobic inactivation gate or motif (called IFMT; isoleucine, phenylalanine, methionine, threonine) between domains III and IV (Fig. 4.1.2). When all the S4 segments are down, the gate displays little affinity for the mouth of the channel. When the S4 segments are in up position, the affinity of the inactivating particle for the mouth increases and it docks, inducing inactivation.

In contrast to voltage-gated Na^+ channels (which are encoded by nine genes), K^+ channels are a more highly diverse family of membrane proteins with many subtypes. They fulfil a number of roles in peripheral nerves, such as establishing the resting membrane potential and accomplishing repolarization. K^+ channels are configured to allow only potassium ions to pass through the cell membrane. Unlike the principal α subunit of the Na^+ channel, which is a single gene product, voltage-activated K^+ channels require four identical or closely related proteins to combine to produce the four voltage sensors and pore loops that line the extracellular channel pore. The pore presents a wide, nonpolar intracellular opening and narrows on the extracellular side. This region of the pore acts as a 'selectivity filter', which allows only the potassium ions to pass in single file across the cell membrane. As with Na^+ channels, the S4 transmembrane segments form the voltage sensors. K^+ channels exhibit heterogeneous inactivation.

Local Anaesthetic Mode of Action

Local anaesthetics reversibly inhibit peripheral nerve conduction by blocking voltage-gated Na^+ channels. Local anaesthetics cross the membrane gaining access to the inside of the ion channel from the inside of the cell and possibly also through transverse portals enabling access to the channel pore from the membrane (Fig. 4.1.1). As the concentration of local anaesthetic increases, the height of the action potential is reduced, the firing threshold is elevated, the spread of impulse conduction is slowed and the refractory period lengthened. Finally, nerve conduction is completely blocked. Binding is achieved by the ionized moiety of the anaesthetic molecule in a reversible and concentration-dependent manner. The amino acids involved in local anaesthetic binding to Na^+ channels in domain IV, loop S6 have been identified by molecular cloning/mutagenesis studies.

The affinity of Na^+ channels for local anaesthetics is higher in the open or inactivated states than in the resting state. Binding of anaesthetics to open Na^+ channels increases with the frequency of nerve depolarization and is described as use-dependent or phasic block.

Local anaesthetics that bind with higher affinity to open or inactivated channels and therefore dissociate more slowly (such as bupivacaine) will generate a more potent block than lidocaine, which dissociates four times faster. Consequently, bupivacaine accumulation during diastole is likely to delay recovery of cardiac Na^+ channels, prolong conduction and cause re-entry-induced arrhythmias.

Peripheral nerve fibres are differentially sensitive to local anaesthetics. The principle that the smaller the fibre diameter the greater its blockade holds among the myelinated axons. The most susceptible are the Aγ spindle efferents and the Aδ nociceptive fibres. Preganglionic sympathetic nervous system B fibres are easily blocked with low concentrations of local anaesthetics. However, the non-myelinated C fibres are generally less susceptible to block than the myelinated axons and, among themselves, the slowest and smallest conducting C fibres are the least sensitive.

Differential sensitivity to local anaesthetics manifests clinically in two ways.

First, block height is higher according to the modality of testing: sympathetic > temperature (cold) > pain (pinprick) > proprioception (light touch with cotton wool).

Second, during operations under epidural anaesthesia, patients may experience paraesthesia to skin incision (Aδ) and motor block (Aγ), but still experience unpleasant pain (unmyelinated visceral C fibres) and sensation of movement (Aβ).

To minimize unpleasant sensations, adequate anaesthesia for caesarean section should equate to a block height of at least T5 to light touch. Increased sensitivity to local anaesthetics is also found in pregnancy.

Structure of Local Anaesthetics

Local anaesthetic drugs are water-soluble salts of lipid-soluble alkaloids. Each molecule is composed of a lipophilic aromatic ring connected to a hydrophilic amide by an intermediate chain (Fig. 4.1.3).

The lipophilic, aromatic ring aids the molecule's penetration through the perineurium and nerve cell membrane, where dissociation occurs into the ionic and the nonionic forms of the tertiary amine.

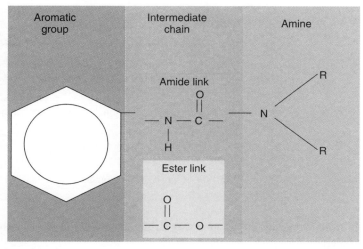

FIGURE 4.1.3 The generic structure of commonly used ester and amide local anaesthetics showing the key features.

Two types of intermediate chain linkers exist – ester and amide (Fig. 4.1.3). Examples of esters are cocaine, procaine, chloroprocaine and tetracaine (amethocaine) and examples of amides are lidocaine, prilocaine, mepivacaine, etidocaine, bupivacaine, ropivacaine and levobupivacaine (*L*-bupivacaine).

Modification of the chemical structure of local anaesthetics alters the pharmacological effect. For example, increasing the length of carbon chains attached to either the aromatic ring, amide linkage or the tertiary amine offers higher lipid solubility, potency and increased duration of action.

Replacement of the tertiary amine by a piperidine ring increases lipid solubility and duration of action; the addition of a butyl group in place of the amine on the benzene ring of procaine results in tetracaine (amethocaine); and the addition of a propyl group or butyl group to the amine end of mepivacaine results in ropivacaine or bupivacaine.

The greater the number of carbons and branching, the greater the potency (and toxicity) up to three to four carbons. After this, the activity drops off, since the analogues are too hydrophobic.

Bupivacaine exists in two forms called enantiomers, which are mirror images of each other. Although structurally identical, enantiomers can exhibit pharmacodynamic and pharmacokinetic differences which manifest clinically as differences in potency or in side effects. The discovery of a stereoselective blockade of cardiac Na^+ channels by the enantiomers of bupivacaine and advances in chiral chemistry led to the creation of two new local anaesthetics – ropivacaine and levobupivacaine. Definitions of chiral terminology are given in Table 4.1.1.

A chiral molecule has no internal plane of symmetry and is nonsuperimposable on its mirror image. Even after rotating one of the molecules it remains

TABLE 4.1.1 Chiral Terminology

Chirality	Spatial arrangement of atoms, nonsuperimposable on each other
Isomer	A molecular entity with the same atomic composition but different stereochemical formulae and hence different physical or chemical properties
Stereoisomers	Isomers that possess identical constitution, but which differ in the arrangement of their atoms in space
Enantiomers	One of a pair of molecular entities which are mirror images of each other and nonsuperimposable
Racemate	An equimolar mixture of a pair of enantiomers

different from its partner in the same way a right hand will not fit properly into a left-handed glove.

Enantiomers can be classified according to their ability to rotate the plane of polarized light through a polarimeter. This is described as optical activity. Right-handed or clockwise rotation is called dextrorotatory, 'D' or '+' and left-handed or counter-clockwise rotation is called laevorotatory, 'L', or '−'. A solution that contains a mixture of the two optical isomers will not change the plane of polarized light, because the effects of the two isomers cancel each other out.

The S and R descriptors are based on the configuration of the four asymmetrical groups around the central carbon atom. An accurate description is determined by the following sequence rules:

- Put the lowest priority towards the back by rotating the molecule
- Look at the direction of highest to lowest – if clockwise, then R (rectus), otherwise is S (sinister)

For the purposes of this chapter S, L and levo (bupivacaine) and R, D and dextro (bupivacaine) are considered the same and are interchangeable.

In vitro studies[5,6] have shown that both ropivacaine and levobupivacaine are less potent blockers of myocardial Na^+ channels, have much lower potency at K^+ channels and are less likely to impair myocardial electrical conduction and contractility than bupivacaine. In vivo animal studies have shown increased convulsive, arrhythmogenic and lethality thresholds and improved resuscitation from cardiac arrest for ropivacaine and levobupivacaine. In a study comparing the effects of intracoronary injection of local anaesthetic in anaesthetized pigs, ropivacaine induced the least QRS and QT widening, but there was no difference in the lethal dose between levobupivacaine and ropivacaine.

Acute tolerance of intravenous infusion of 10 mg/min of bupivacaine, ropivacaine and levobupivacaine has been studied in crossover, randomized, double-blind studies in volunteers previously acquainted with the CNS effects of lidocaine. Bupivacaine impaired myocardial contractility, extended QRS duration and was less likely to be tolerated than ropivacaine. Levobupivacaine had significantly less effect on cardiac stroke index, acceleration index and ejection fraction than bupivacaine.

Pharmacological Properties of Local Anaesthetics

The speed of onset, potency and duration of local anaesthetics is dependent on the pKa, lipid solubility and protein binding, respectively.

pKa

In order to pass through lipid-soluble membranes and then attach to ion channels in their inner vestibule, a drug is required to have the capacity to be both ionized and nonionized (i.e. amphipathic). This property of local anaesthetics is conferred by the tertiary amine.

The dissociation of local anaesthetics is determined by the pH of the solution in which they are dissolved. The pH at which the ionized and nonionized form of a compound is present in equal amounts is defined as the pKa. For bases, such as local anaesthetics, the higher the pKa, the greater the ionized fraction in solution. This relationship is described by the Henderson–Hasselbalch equation.

As diffusion across the nerve sheath and nerve membrane is related to the degree of nonionized drug, local anaesthetics with low pKa have a fast onset of action and local anaesthetics with a high pKa have a slow onset of action. For example, lidocaine (pKa 7.8) has a fast onset in comparison with bupivacaine (pKa 8.1), because at pH 7.4, 35% of lidocaine exists in the nonionized base form compared to only 20% of bupivacaine.

Molecular Weight

Molecular weight has an influence on the rate of nerve membrane and transdural transfer. The smaller the molecular weight the more rapid the transfer.

Lipid Solubility

The lipid solubility of local anaesthetics is expressed as the partition coefficient, which is defined as the ratio of concentrations when local anaesthetic is dissolved in a mixture of a lipid and aqueous solvents. Thus, lipid solubility may also contribute to onset of action because local anaesthetics must diffuse through lipid-soluble membranes to reach their site of action.

Protein Binding

Protein binding influences the duration of action of local anaesthesia, reflecting attachment to protein components of the nerve membrane. Protein binding parallels lipid solubility.

In plasma, amide local anaesthetics bind predominantly to α-acid glycoprotein (AAG), a high-affinity limited-capacity protein, and albumin, a low-affinity large-capacity protein. Thus, the free fraction or bioavailability of local anaesthetics is determined by the availability of plasma proteins: the greater the AAG, the greater the binding of local anaesthetic and the lower the free plasma local concentrations. However, many patients have reduced plasma protein concentrations after surgery, major trauma or malignancy. In these circumstances, the free plasma fraction of local anaesthetic would be expected to rise and increase the likelihood of toxic side-effects. Fortunately, after surgery, trauma or malignancy, AAG levels increase significantly and protect patients receiving local anaesthetic epidural or perineural infusions from anaesthetic toxicity by attenuating rises in the free fraction of local anaesthetics.

In the critically ill, however, hypoxia, hypercarbia and acidaemia all decrease protein binding, increasing free fraction and the risk of toxicity. Neonates and children under 6 months of age have less protein binding of local anaesthetics.

Vasoactivity

Intrinsic vasodilator activity influences *in vivo* potency and duration of action. For example, the enhanced vasodilatatory action of lidocaine compared to that of bupivacaine results in greater vascular absorption and a shorter duration of action.

The newer local anaesthetics have less intrinsic vasoactivity than bupivacaine in the ratio: bupivacaine > levobupivacaine > ropivacaine. All demonstrate a biphasic vasoactive response when measured in the forearm skin of human volunteers, with vasodilatation at anaesthetic concentrations greater than or equal to 0.25% and vasoconstriction at less than 0.25%. Addition of epinephrine (adrenaline) (1:200, 000 to 1:800, 000) increases vasoconstriction prolonging the duration of local anaesthetic action.

Pharmacokinetics

Absorption

The site of injection, dosage, rate of injection, use of epinephrine (adrenaline) and the pharmacological characteristics of the drug influence the absorption of local anaesthetic from its site of injection into the systemic circulation. The order of peak plasma concentration after a single dose is: intrapleural > intercostal > lumbar epidural > brachial plexus > subcutaneous > sciatic > femoral.

All amides show a biphasic absorption pattern, with an initial rapid phase followed by a slow phase.

Following rapid entry of local anaesthetics into the venous circulation, pulmonary extraction limits the concentration of drug that reaches the systemic circulation for distribution to the coronary and cerebral circulations. For bupivacaine, this first-pass pulmonary extraction is dose dependent, suggesting that the uptake process rapidly becomes saturated. For lidocaine, 40% is removed by the lung during a single passage in pigs. The lungs act as a buffer, reducing the arterial plasma concentrations of local anaesthetic after inadvertent intravenous injection.

Distribution

The plasma concentration of local anaesthetic is determined by the relative rate of tissue distribution and clearance of the drug. Tissue distribution is in proportion to the tissue:blood partition coefficient of the local anaesthetic and the mass and perfusion of the tissue. The age, cardiovascular status and hepatic function of patients influence tissue blood flow. Amide local anaesthetics are more widely distributed in tissues than ester local anaesthetics following systemic absorption.

Metabolism

Ester and amide local anaesthetics differ concerning their metabolism and allergic potential.

The amino esters are rapidly hydrolysed in plasma by pseudocholinesterase to the metabolite para-aminobenzoic acid (PABA), which is responsible for allergic reactions in some individuals. Plasma half-life varies from less than 1 min (chloroprocaine) to 8 min (tetracaine [amethocaine]) and is prolonged in the presence of atypical cholinesterase.

In contrast, enzymes in the liver degrade amides more slowly. The initial step is conversion of the amide base to aminocarboxylic acid and a cyclic aniline derivative. Complete metabolism usually involves additional steps, such as hydroxylation of the aniline moiety and N-dealkylation of the aminocarboxylic acid. As they are not metabolized to PABA, allergic reactions with these agents are extremely rare. Metabolism of amides is dependent on hepatic blood flow, decreasing with age, hypovolaemia and congestive heart failure. Drug interactions are few. Metabolism of amides may be reduced by potent inhibitors of cytochrome P450 isoenzymes. Cumulation and systemic toxicity of amides are more likely with prolonged infusions in elderly, sick patients, although the relative increase in AAG offers some protection.

Clearance

Clearance values and elimination half-times for amide local anaesthetics probably represent mainly hepatic metabolism because renal excretion of unchanged drug is minimal. Cumulation of metabolites may occur in renal failure. The rate of metabolism is fastest to slowest in the order prilocaine > lidocaine = mepivacaine > bupivacaine. Poor water solubility of local anaesthetics limits renal excretion of unchanged drug. In heart failure, distribution and clearance of local anaesthetics are reduced.

Placental Transfer

Protein binding determines the rate and degree of diffusion of local anaesthetics across the placenta. Bupivacaine, which is highly protein bound (about 95%), has an umbilical vein/maternal arterial ratio of 0.3 compared to lidocaine, which is less bound to protein (about 70%) and has a ratio of 0.52 to 0.71. Acidosis in the fetus, as occurs during prolonged labour, can result in accumulation of local anaesthetic in the fetus by ion trapping.

Ester local anaesthetics, because of their rapid hydrolysis, do not cross the placenta in significant amounts.

Clinical Preparation of Local Anaesthetics

Local anaesthetics are poorly soluble in water and therefore presented as stable hydrochloride salts with pH from 5 to 6. Alkaline pH destabilizes local anaesthetics.

Improving Clinical Efficacy

Epinephrine (adrenaline), in concentrations of 1:200,000 or 1:400,000, may be added to local anaesthetics to reduce vascular absorption and potential local anaesthetic toxicity. Preparation of 1:200,000 epinephrine (adrenaline) involves dilution of 0.1 mL of 1:1000 (0.1 mg) epinephrine (adrenaline) or 1 mL of 1:10,000 (0.1 mg) epinephrine (adrenaline) to a 20 mL volume of local anaesthetic; 1:400,000 dilutions are made with half the above doses of epinephrine (adrenaline).

Epinephrine (adrenaline)-containing solutions contain a reducing agent, sodium metabisulphite, to prevent oxidation of the epinephrine (adrenaline). In addition, a small amount of preservative and fungicide may be added.

The vasoactive effect of epinephrine (adrenaline) is greater with the more lipid-soluble amides.[7] For example, the recommended dose of plain lidocaine is 3 mg/kg but increases to 7 mg/kg with the addition of epinephrine (adrenaline). However, the addition of epinephrine (adrenaline) to bupivacaine only increases the recommended dose from 2.5 mg/kg to 3 mg/kg.

An acidic tissue environment, such as occurs with infection and inflammation, promotes the quaternary (hydrophilic) configuration causing reduced access of local anaesthetics to their site of action on Na^+ channels, which is accessed from within the cell. Under these circumstances higher doses are required to establish analgesia.

Toxicity

CNS Toxicity

CNS toxicity manifests initially as circumoral numbness, metallic taste, tinnitus, light-headedness and dizziness followed by confusion, slurred speech and then convulsions. Increasing plasma levels lead to respiratory arrest.

Cardiovascular Toxicity

Cardiovascular toxicity manifests as initial excitatory symptoms such as tachycardia and high blood pressure followed by myocardial suppression, peripheral vasodilatation, hypotension, bradycardia, conduction abnormalities, ventricular arrhythmias such as torsades de pointes and finally cardiac arrest.

In order to treat, give oxygen, intubate, ventilate, give intravenous fluids, epinephrine (adrenaline) and cardiac massage if necessary. Resuscitation after the longer acting drugs bupivacaine and etidocaine may be difficult and lengthy.

Inadvertent intravascular injection of local anaesthetics, or frank overdosage and systemic absorption from the site of injection, can block Na^+, K^+ and Ca^{2+} channels within conducting tissue such as in the CNS and cardiovascular system. Cardiovascular collapse, without prodromal CNS symptoms, in six pregnant women following inadvertent intravascular injection of bupivacaine or etidocaine was reported by Albright in 1979.[8]

At a meeting of the USA's Food and Drugs Administration (FDA) in 1983, 53 cases of cardiac toxicity with bupivacaine were reported, 39 after epidural injection and 14 with other regional techniques. Twenty-seven patients received 0.75% bupivacaine. In all, 31 deaths were recorded (24 in pregnancy), 3 patients had a partial recovery and 19 made a full recovery. The medical response to these deaths was twofold. First, bupivacaine was highlighted as a potentially toxic drug (black boxed) and the 0.75% preparation was withdrawn from use in pregnant patients. Second, and most importantly, profound changes in anaesthetic practice occurred, such as slow incremental dosing and the use of test doses.

Incidence of Toxicity

The newer local anaesthetics levobupivacaine and ropivacaine are undoubtedly safer than bupivacaine, but convulsions and cardiac arrest have occurred.[9]

The reasons for continuing toxicity are manifold:

- Ambulatory tumescent liposuction – doses of lidocaine up to 45–50 mg/kg have been administered for pain relief during plastic surgery. A typical regimen consists of 500–1000 mg lidocaine, 0.25–1 mg epinephrine (adrenaline) and 12.5 mmol sodium bicarbonate added to 1 L of crystalloid.
- Plastic surgery – two deaths occurred using 6%–10% lidocaine and tetracaine dermal cream before laser hair removal.
- Accidental intravenous injection – three deaths occurred in the UK when epidural infusions were connected to central venous lines.
- Intravenous lidocaine treatment of acute or chronic pain – typical bolus dose is 1.5 mL/kg and infusion rate is 1.5 mL/kg/h.
- More upper limb regional anaesthesia – the closer the injection to a blood vessel, the greater the risk of toxicity.
- Newer drugs are less sensitive at potential test doses compared to lidocaine.

It must also be remembered that the mode of action of local anaesthetics is also largely the mode of toxicity, blockade of Na^+ channels and that inadvertent intravascular injection can and will occur. In high enough doses, all local anaesthetics can have perilous consequences and clinical vigilance is always necessary. Nevertheless, there continues to be case reports of toxicity after administration of doses of local anaesthetic that are in excess of twice the recommended limit (Table 4.1.2).

TABLE 4.1.2 Maximum Doses of Local Anaesthetics

	Plain	With Adrenaline (Epinephrine)	Over 24 h
Chloroprocaine	800 mg	1000 mg	
Prilocaine	600 mg	600 mg	
Lidocaine	300 mg	500 mg	
Mepivacaine	400 mg	500 mg	
Bupivacaine	175 mg	225 mg	400 mg
Levobupivacaine	150 mg		400 mg
Ropivacaine	225 mg		800 mg

Treatment of Toxicity

Agitation is often a prodromal symptom of local anaesthetic toxicity.

Guidelines for the treatment of systemic toxicity recommend:

- Maintain airway, administer oxygen.
- Control seizures with a benzodiazepine, thiopental or propofol.
- Start cardiopulmonary resuscitation (CPR) if in cardiac arrest.
- If unresponsive give intralipid 20% – 1.5 mL/kg i.v. over 1 min followed by an infusion of 15 mL/kg/h.
- If still unresponsive, a further two boluses (same dose) may be given and the infusion rate doubled.

Double the infusion rate to 30 mL/kg/h if cardiovascular instability persists. The maximum cumulative dose is 12 mL/kg. There are many reports of successful resuscitation using intralipid.[10]

The underlying mechanism of intralipid has not been fully elucidated, although resuscitation may be better when intralipid is administered in the presence of more lipid soluble local anaesthetics such as bupivacaine.[11]

Allergic Reactions

Allergy reactions are rare and may take the form of bronchospasm, urticaria or angioneurotic oedema. They are well documented in association with the use of ester-linked agents. Allergy to amide-linked agents is extremely rare but has been reported. Allergic reactions may be due to methylparaben, which is sometimes used in commercial preparations of local analgesic solutions as a stabilizing agent.

Treatment of allergy reactions is with oxygen, injections of epinephrine (adrenaline) and hydrocortisone.

Reactions to vasoconstrictor drugs include pallor, anxiety, palpitations, tachycardia, hypertension and tachypnoea and may respond to a β-blocker.

Children

In children, the above adult doses do not apply, but the dose can be calculated on a 'dose for weight' basis (e.g. the maximum dose for a 7 kg child would be one-tenth of the adult dose).

DRUGS USED IN LOCAL ANALGESIA

The physicochemical characteristics of commonly used local anaesthetics (in order of discovery) are outlined in Table 4.1.3.

Cocaine

Cocaine is a naturally occurring plant extract. It is an ester of benzoic acid. The alkaloid was isolated in 1855.

Cocaine was first used in surgery (of the cornea) in 1884. It is easily decomposed by heat sterilization. Cocaine is an excellent surface analgesic and vasoconstrictor, 4% being a suitable strength.

Cocaine is a potent drug of abuse which can lead to addiction. Its duration of effect is ≈30 min when administered topically.

Cocaine is a powerful stimulant that causes excitement and restlessness when administered systemically. There is euphoria, agitation, decreased sleep, anxiety, hyperexcitability, psychosis, paranoia, suicidal tendency, violence and confusion.

As cocaine is a powerful vasoconstrictor, epinephrine (adrenaline) added to it is not only unnecessary but also increases the risks of cardiac arrhythmia and ventricular fibrillation. The two drugs should not be used together.

Cocaine inhibits monoamine oxidase and is not destroyed by cholinesterase.

TABLE 4.1.3 Physicochemical Characteristics of Local Anaesthetics

	MW	pKa	Protein Binding (%)	Partition Coefficient	Onset	Duration
Cocaine	303	8.6	98	—	Fast[a]	Short[a]
Chloroprocaine	271	9.1	–	17	Fast	Short
Prilocaine	220	7.7	55	50	Fast	Medium
Lidocaine	234	7.8	64	110	Fast	Medium
Mepivacaine	246	7.7	77	42	Fast	Medium
Bupivacaine	288	8.1	95	560	Moderate	Long
Ropivacaine	274	8.1	94	230	Moderate	Long
Levobupivacaine	288	8.1	95	–	Moderate	Long

[a] Topical analgesia only

Small doses of cocaine increase the pulse rate, raise the blood pressure and potentiate the effects of epinephrine (adrenaline) on capillaries (dilatation or constriction). Arrhythmias may occur but can be reversed by β-blockade. Hypertension and vasospasm may lead to vascular accidents.

Mydriasis occurs with cocaine, perhaps owing to sympathetic stimulation. There is blanching of the conjunctiva from vasoconstriction, clouding of the corneal epithelium and, rarely, ulceration, together with excellent analgesia. Cocaine is used as a 1% solution for analgesia.

Cocaine can be employed usefully as a spray to vasoconstrict nasal mucosa before nasal intubation.

Cocaine is detoxified in the liver, one metabolite being ecgonine, a CNS stimulant. About 10% is excreted by the kidneys unchanged.

Chloroprocaine

Chloroprocaine is an ester that has been in use in the USA since 1952. It has a rapid onset and offset. It undergoes hydrolysis by plasma cholinesterase. Rapid hydrolysis makes it relatively nontoxic and it is not easily transferred across the placenta. Its effect lasts about 45 min.

Chloroprocaine is used as a 2% or 3% solution.

Chloroprocaine is the most acid of local analgesic agents commonly used (3% solution has a pH of 3.3).

Prilocaine

Prilocaine is a secondary amide and was first used clinically in 1959. It is less toxic than lidocaine, and metabolized in lung and kidneys as well as liver, and so has high clearance. Prilocaine is metabolized to ortho-toluidine, which is an oxidizing compound that converts haemoglobin to methaemoglobin. When the dose of prilocaine exceeds 600 mg there may be sufficient methaemoglobin present for the patient to appear cyanotic, and oxygen-carrying capacity is reduced. There is an associated shift of the oxygen dissociation curve of the remaining haemoglobin, which hinders oxygen liberation at tissue level. Methaemoglobin crosses the placenta. Methaemoglobinaemia is readily reversed by the intravenous administration of methylene blue 1–2 mg/kg, injected over 5 min.

Prilocaine is most useful for Bier's intravenous local analgesia in 0.5% solution, for which it is most suitable.

Lidocaine

Lidocaine is the most commonly used local analgesic agent. It is a tertiary amide and was first synthesized in 1943. Solutions are as follows:

- 0.5%–1% for infiltration, with epinephrine (adrenaline) 1:200,000 to 1:400,000
- 4% for topical analgesia, in surgery of throat, larynx, pharynx, etc.

- Nerve block and extradural block 1%–2% with epinephrine (adrenaline)
- Corneal analgesia 4% –causes no mydriasis, vasoconstriction or cycloplegia
- Urethral analgesia 1%–2% in jelly
- Tracheal tubes 5% as an ointment

Lidocaine is less toxic than bupivacaine and is sometimes used for intravenous analgesia, but cardiovascular and CNS symptoms of poisoning may occur. Lidocaine is also used as a class-1b antiarrhythmic agent.

The metabolism of lidocaine is extensive, such that clearance of this local anaesthetic from the plasma parallels hepatic blood flow. The principal pathway of metabolism of lidocaine is oxidative dealkylation in the liver to monoethylglycinexylidide, followed by hydrolysis of this metabolite to xylidide.

The metabolism and volume of distribution of lidocaine are decreased in patients with cardiac failure and cirrhosis of the liver, with increased risk of systemic toxicity.

The clearance of lidocaine is reduced in the presence of propranolol. As in the case of prilocaine, the metabolism of lidocaine can give rise to the formation of methaemoglobin.

Mepivacaine

Mepivacaine, another tertiary amide, was synthesized and first used in 1956. Its structure and pharmacological properties resemble those of lidocaine, but its duration of action is somewhat longer. In contrast to lidocaine, mepivacaine lacks vasodilator activity. Most of the drug is metabolized in the liver and some has been recovered from the urine (increased by acidification).

Mepivacaine is claimed to be a little less toxic than lidocaine and its local analgesic effects last rather longer. When injected into the extradural space of patients in labour it passes rather rapidly into the fetal circulation, where it may cause harm. It would appear to have few advantages over lidocaine.

Bupivacaine

Bupivacaine is an aminoamide local anaesthetic. It is a member of the homologous series of n-alkyl substituted pipecholyl xylidines first synthesized by Ekenstam in 1957 and was used clinically in 1963.

Bupivacaine causes more sensory than motor block. It is not recommended for intravenous regional analgesia. It is metabolized to pipecoloxylidine in the liver.

Levobupivacaine

Levobupivacaine, an enantiomer of bupivacaine (a racemic mixture of both enantiomers), shares the same molecular structure as bupivacaine. The altered spatial arrangement of levobupivacaine compared to dextrobupivacaine (contained in bupivacaine) accounts for differences in their differing pharmacokinetic and pharmacodynamic profiles, manifesting clinically as differences in efficacy and side effects such as motor block. The physicochemical properties of levobupivacaine and ropivacaine are compared in Table 4.1.3 to those of bupivacaine and other commonly used local anaesthetics.

Ropivacaine

Ropivacaine is a single S-enantiomer drug rather than a racemic mixture, which is structurally similar to bupivacaine but with a propyl side chain replacing the butyl group. The smaller side chain contributes less lipid solubility, less toxicity and an increased separation of sensory and motor blockade compared to bupivacaine. It has differential effect on motor and sensory nerves at low concentrations. Most studies have found that onset and duration of sensory block in epidural analgesia are similar to those of bupivacaine, whereas motor block is slower in onset, shorter in duration and less intense with ropivacaine. In animal studies ropivacaine is less cardio-depressant, less arrhythmogenic and less toxic to the CNS than bupivacaine. These findings have been confirmed in human volunteers. The greater lipid solubility of bupivacaine compared to ropivacaine may explain the greater peak plasma concentration and the shorter half-life of ropivacaine. Peak blood levels are unaffected by the addition of epinephrine (adrenaline).

NEW DEVELOPMENTS IN LOCAL ANALGESIA

Slow-Release Formulations of Bupivacaine

Prolonged excellent postoperative analgesia can be achieved by continuous or repeated administration of slow-release formulations of bupivacaine via indwelling catheters for regional, epidural or spinal anaesthesia.[12] However, complications associated with catheterization are not uncommon and include leakage, intravascular injection, catheter migration and infection.

Long-acting anaesthetics placed accurately have the potential to provide long-lasting pain relief and eliminate technical problems and possibly to prevent or reverse hyperalgesia. Strategies in the search for prolonged postoperative analgesia have focused on drug delivery systems for slow release of local anaesthetics held in liposomes.

Liposomes are amphipathic lipid molecules with a polar head and two hydrophobic hydrocarbon tails which form lipid bilayers not unlike a cell membrane when suspended in an aqueous solution. Liposomal function is dictated by size, structure and composition. Possession of both aqueous and lipid environments enables both water- and lipid-soluble drugs to be carried. The likelihood of tissue toxicity being induced by liposome constituents is low because they are biodegradable. A meta-analysis comparing knee infiltration of liposomal bupivacaine for pain relief after knee arthroplasty showed a small improvement in pain relief up to 24 h after surgery but not at 48 or 72 h.[13]

Extending the Duration of Block

Single bolus local anaesthetic limb blocks can provide pain relief between 10 and 18 h. The bigger the dose, the greater the likelihood of motor block. Extending the duration of regional nerve blocks while maintaining limb mobilization is a clinical challenge.[14]

Adjuncts to Local Anaesthesia

Several α2 - adrenergic receptor agonists such as clonidine and dexmedetomidine have analgesic and sedative properties. Trials investigating the addition of dexmedetomidine to spinal anaesthesia or to brachial plexus nerve block demonstrated prolonged spinal block by 2.5 h and sensory block by > 5 h. However, no preferential sensory/motor split was observed.

Comparison of epidural bupivacaine with either dexmedetomidine 1 μg/kg or clonidine 2 μg/kg epidurally showed earlier onset of analgesia, better anaesthesia, cardiovascular stability and improved patient comfort for the former combination.[15] Dexmedetomidine would appear to offer a better clinical profile than clonidine.

Several randomized trials have investigated the addition of dexamethasone to perineural nerve block. Perineural dexamethasone was associated with longer pain relief, and a small reduction in analgesia. There were no reports of persistent nerve injury attributed to perineural injection.[16] Comparison of adjuvant clonidine with dexamethasone for upper limb block is inconclusive. Both drugs prolong sensory block compared to local anaesthetic alone.

It must be remembered that the aforementioned adjuvants are not licensed for perineural administration and the balance of efficacy and potential for serious side effects should be considered, particularly in groups such as diabetics with microvascular disease who are at increased risk of postoperative nerve damage. The mechanism of prolonged analgesia is as yet not known and may be attributable to reduced nerve blood flow. Potential benefit should be judged on clinical significance. Clinical significance should be viewed as extension of pain relief for nerve block by 6 to 12 h. Caution should be given to use of intrathecal adjuvants as drugs act directly on cord tissue.

Effect on Tumour Progression

Laboratory studies suggest a potential benefit of regional anaesthesia on cancer cells, through reduced inflammation and blockade of Na^+ channels on metastatic cancer cells.[17] However, little direct clinical evidence currently exists to support the hypothesis that regional anaesthesia improves patient survival after cancer surgery. Clinical evidence is primarily restricted to retrospective studies.[18,19]

REFERENCES

1. Gokin AP, Philip B, Strichartz GR. Preferential block of small myelinated sensory and motor fibers by lidocaine: in vivo electrophysiology in the rat sciatic nerve. Anesthesiology 2001;95:1441–54.
2. Payandeh J, Scheuer T, Zheng N, Catterall WA. The crystal structure of a voltage-gated sodium channel. Nature 2011;475:353–8.
3. Wang GK, Strichartz GR. State-dependent inhibition of sodium channels by local anesthetics: a 40-year evolution. Biochem (Mosc) Suppl Ser A Membr Cell Biol 2012;6:120–27.
4. Catterall WA, Swanson TM. Structural basis for pharmacology of voltage-gated sodium and calcium channels. Mol Pharmacol 2015 88:141–50.
5. Vladimirov M, Nau C, Mok WM, Strichartz G. Potency of bupivacaine stereoisomers tested in vitro and in vivo: biochemical, electrophysiological, and neurobehavioral studies. *Anesthesiology* 2000;93:744–55.
6. Nau C, Wang SY, Strichartz GR, Wang GK. Block of human heart hH1 sodium channels by the enantiomers of bupivacaine. Anesthesiology 2000;93:1022–33.
7. Newton DJ, McLeod GA, Khan F, Belch JJ. Vasoactive characteristics of bupivacaine and levobupivacaine with and without adjuvant epinephrine in peripheral human skin. Br J Anaesth 2005;94:662–67.
8. Albright GA. Cardiac arrest following regional anesthesia with etidocaine or bupivacaine. Anesthesiology 1979;51:285–87.
9. Mather LE, Copeland SE, Ladd LA. Acute toxicity of local anesthetics: underlying pharmacokinetic and pharmacodynamic concepts. Reg Anesth Pain Med 2005;30:553–66.
10. Weinberg GL, Ripper R, Murphy P, Edelman LB, Hoffman W, Strichartz G, et al. Lipid infusion accelerates removal of bupivacaine and recovery from bupivacaine toxicity in the isolated rat heart. Reg Anesth Pain Med 2006;31:296–303.
11. Zausig YA, Zink W, Keil M, Sinner B, Barwing J, Wiese CH, et al. Lipid emulsion improves recovery from bupivacaine-induced cardiac arrest, but not from ropivacaine- or mepivacaine-induced cardiac arrest. Anesth Analg 2009;109:1323–6.
12. Weiniger CF, Golovanevski L, Domb AJ, Ickowicz D. Extended release formulations for local anaesthetic agents. Anaesthesia 2012;67:906–16.
13. Wu ZQ, Min JK, Wang D, Yuan YJ, Li H. Liposome bupivacaine for pain control after total knee arthroplasty: a meta-analysis. J Orthop Surg Res 2016;11:84
14. Abdallah FW, Brull R. Facilitatory effects of perineural dexmedetomidine on neuraxial and peripheral nerve block: a systematic review and meta-analysis. Br J Anaesth 2013;110:915–25.
15. Shaikh SI, Mahesh SB. The efficacy and safety of epidural dexmedetomidine and clonidine with bupivacaine in patients undergoing lower limb orthopedic surgeries. J Anaesthesiol Clin Pharmacol 2016;32:203–09.
16. Huynh TM, Marret E, Bonnet F. Combination of dexamethasone and local anaesthetic solution in peripheral nerve blocks: A meta-analysis of randomised controlled trials. Eur J Anaesthesiol 2015;32:751–8.
17. Piegeler T, Schlapfer M, Dull RO, Schwartz DE, Borgeat A, Minshall RD, et al. Clinically relevant concentrations of lidocaine and ropivacaine inhibit TNFalpha-induced invasion of lung adenocarcinoma cells in vitro by blocking the activation of Akt and focal adhesion kinase. Br J Anaesth 2015;115:784–91.
18. Baptista-Hon DT, Robertson FM, Robertson GB, Owen SJ, Rogers GW, Lydon EL, et al. Potent inhibition by ropivacaine of metastatic colon cancer SW620 cell invasion and NaV1.5 channel function. Br J Anaesth 2014;113 Suppl 1:i39-i48.
19. Tedore T. Regional anaesthesia and analgesia: relationship to cancer recurrence and survival. Br J Anaesth 2015;115 Suppl 2:ii34–45.

Chapter 4.2

Peripheral Neuraxial Blockade

Pavan Kumar BC Raju, Graeme McLeod

GENERAL CONSIDERATIONS

Peripheral neuraxial blockade (PNB), either alone or in combination with general anaesthesia, has the potential to provide excellent operating conditions and prolong postoperative analgesia, especially when using continuous PNB.

PNB provides more effective analgesia with fewer side effects than opioid and other oral analgesia.

The indications for PNB are dependent on both the patient and the type of surgery.

Identification of Nerves

The first nerve blocks were performed by open surgical exposure. Now, the quality of peripheral nerve blocks is determined by accurate identification of nerves and precise injection of local anaesthetic into an anatomical space.

Eliciting nerve paraesthesia with a needle has been used in the past as a means of finding peripheral nerves, but it is associated with block success rates not compatible with modern clinical expectations and infrequently, with nerve trauma.

Techniques to improve the efficacy and safety of regional anaesthesia include nerve stimulation, percutaneous electrical guidance (PEG), ultrasound, stimulating catheters and computed tomography (CT) scans. Of these, ultrasound is increasingly being preferred for performing PNB as the other techniques have varying success rates. Nevertheless, it is important to remember that new technology merely supplements and does not replace detailed knowledge of regional anatomy.

Principles of Nerve Stimulation

The principle of nerve stimulation is to trigger electrical depolarization of the nerve and stimulate muscular contractions at the proposed site of surgery.

The nerve membrane obeys Coulomb's law and may be considered to behave like a capacitor, whereby the stimulating charge strength is given by:

$$e = k \, (q/r^2)$$

where k is constant, q is the minimum stimulating current and r is the distance of the needle tip from the nerve.

Typical charge strength required to depolarize nerves vary from 120 nano-coulombs (nc) to 1000 nc in elderly diabetics.

The total amount of depolarization or charge transferred across the membrane is a product of the strength and duration of the stimulus, electrode to nerve distance and electrical impedance of the intervening tissues.

An inverse relationship exists between the strength and duration of electrical stimulation but differs according to the type of nerve, as illustrated in Fig. 4.2.1, from which two important parameters may be defined:

- Rheobase – the minimum current that stimulates a nerve, independent of stimulation time
- Chronaxie – the duration necessary to stimulate a nerve when the current is equal to twice the rheobase

The chronaxie can be regarded as a measure of the 'excitability of the nerve'.

Needle-Guided Nerve Stimulation for Peripheral Nerve Block

The rheobase and chronaxie of nerve fibres are dependent on their function.

The Aα motor fibres have the shortest chronaxie (0.05–0.1 ms), whereas the fibres of pain sensation (Aδ and C fibres) require a longer pulse (0.17 ms and 0.4 ms, respectively) at minimum current.

Owing to the differences in chronaxie between motor and sensory fibres, mixed peripheral nerves can be localized with short pulses (0.1 ms) without

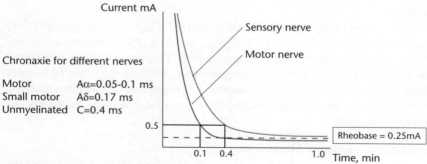

FIGURE 4.2.1 Strength and duration of electrical nerve stimulation. Illustration shows method of calculating chronaxie.

triggering pain sensations. Thus, two different settings of the nerve stimulator are commonly used, depending on clinical circumstance:

- Current 1–2 mA, pulse duration 0.1 ms and pulse frequency 2 Hz – stimulates motor fibres without experiencing pain and positions the needle as accurately as possible
- Current 1–2 mA, pulse duration 0.3 ms and pulse frequency 1 Hz – stimulates paraesthesia, but avoids painful muscle contractions in trauma patients

Needles should be insulated apart from a small area at the tip in order to generate a high current density near the nerve.

When muscle contractions are detected, optimization of needle position should be sought by incrementally reducing the stimulating current.

When a level between 0.2 mA and 0.5 mA has been reached and muscle contractions are still barely visible, the local anaesthetic may be injected after a negative aspiration test. The anaesthetist should always check the current at which contractions cease. Injection of local anaesthetic at a current less than or equal to 0.2 mA may indicate intraneural injection. If the needle position is correct, the muscle response to injection will disappear instantly. When a significant resistance is noted or paraesthesia is felt, the injection must be stopped immediately. Moreover, aspiration checks should be performed repeatedly during the procedure to exclude inadvertent intravenous injection.

Transcutaneous Electrical Stimulation for Peripheral Nerve Block

A variety of transcutaneous electrical stimulation devices have been developed in order to reduce the invasive search for the nerves by optimizing the needle insertion point over the target nerve.

One technique, percutaneous electrode guidance (PEG), uses a cylindrical transcutaneous electrode with a metallic tip less than 1 mm in width. The electrode indents the skin and underlying subcutaneous tissues towards the nerve, thus reducing the distance to the targeted nerve and tissue electrical impedance. After location of the nerve (current < 0.5 mA), a needle is passed through the probe and local anaesthetic is injected. This device is useful for blocking superficial but not deep nerves.

Principles of Ultrasound

Medical ultrasound involves emission of sound waves well above the upper limit of the human audible range ($\approx$ 20,000 Hz), penetration through tissues (traveling at an average speed of 1540 m/s), reflection at tissue interfaces and receipt and interpretation of echoes.

Higher frequencies (10–14 MHz) give a higher spatial resolution with low tissue penetration and are better for blocking superficial plexuses. In contrast, localizing deeper nerves requires a lower frequency (4–7 MHz), but compromising spatial resolution.

The sonographic appearance of peripheral nerves varies according to the plane of ultrasound beam. In the transverse plane, nerves are viewed as round/ovoid shapes consisting of hypoechoic bubbles (fascicles) enveloped by hyperechoic elements (epineurium or connective tissue). This is termed a 'honeycomb pattern' and is seen most often in the trunks and proximal cords.

In the longitudinal plane, hypoechoic parallel bands (fascicles) are bordered by hyperechoic striations (epineurium or connective tissue). This is termed a fascicular pattern.

In the transverse view, small vessels, lymph nodes and muscle fascicles can be mistaken for nerves because they have similar size and echogenicity. Colour Doppler mapping of vascular flow is useful to identify blood vessels.

Direct visualization has revealed that gentle pressure applied to the skin moves nerves considerably within the subcutaneous tissue and that apparent visual needle contact may not necessarily elicit muscle contractions. In this situation, the needle should not be advanced any further but moved gently sideways.

Ultrasound has several potential advantages over the other modalities including:

● Detection of variation in sonoanatomy
● Real-time visualization of needle tip
● Real-time visualization of local anaesthetic solution as it is injected
● Avoidance of intravascular and intraneural injections
● Possible reduction in local anaesthetic dose
● Avoidance of nerve stimulation-induced muscle contraction pain at fracture-sites
● Possible reduction in complications

Ultrasound is associated with faster block performance, fewer needle passes, faster onset of sensory block, greater block success and decreased incidence of vascular puncture.

Ultrasound-Guided Peripheral Nerve Block

Before attempting to perform ultrasound-guided PNB, it is important to understand the basic principles of ultrasound and patient anatomy.

The following are practical tips to achieve not just quick, safe and effective block, but also to decrease the discomfort caused to the patient during the procedure.

Preparation: The following should be undertaken before any PNB.

● Obtain a relevant history and examination
● Identify any contraindications
● Obtain informed consent
● Establish intravenous access and minimum standard of monitoring
● Ensure availability of emergency drugs and trained assistance

PNB should be performed in an awake or lightly sedated patient. The choice of local anaesthetic depends on the desired duration and intended purpose of the block.

Equipment: An appropriate ultrasound machine with a range of transducer selection increases the block success rate. Familiarity with the machine by the operator is important.

Use of sterile aqueous gel as a conducting medium for the ultrasound probe is necessary to prevent air trapping.

Short bevelled needles are used to perform single shot PNBs, whereas Tuohy style needles are preferred for continuous PNB with a catheter; both types of needle can be combined with nerve stimulation. Echogenic needles enhance ultrasound reflection, improving needle shaft and tip visualization and thus improving safety.

Positioning: The operator, patient (anatomical location for the PNB) and the ultrasound machine should be in a straight line in that order. This enables the operator to monitor patient, needle, probe position and sonoanatomy, which improves the success rate.

Confirm block site: 'Stop before you block'. Wrong site block is a 'Never Event'. Before performing any block, it is necessary to confirm correct patient and block site. This step should be repeated immediately prior to needle insertion.

Nerve location: A sterile field should be maintained throughout the procedure. As scanning is a dynamic process, the chances of obtaining optimal image are increased by control of transducer alignment, rotation and tilt (ART) together with adequate pressure.

Nerves are seen as round hypoechoic structures proximally but are hyperechoic distally due to increased connective tissue. Nerve stimulation can aid ultrasound nerve location.

An alternative approach is to identify the fascial plane traversed by peripheral nerve(s) and inject local anaesthetic solution to fill this space.

Needle insertion techniques: There are two approaches to needle insertion:

- Out-of-plane – needle inserted perpendicular to the transducer resulting in visualization of a hyperechoic dot as the needle crosses the ultrasound beam. Patient discomfort is less but identifying the needle tip can be challenging.
- In-plane – needle inserted parallel to the transducer enabling visualization of both needle shaft and tip throughout the procedure. This approach has a better safety profile.

Needle tip identification is aided by hydrolocation whereby small aliquots (0.5–1 mL) of local anaesthetic solution are injected while observing spread on the monitor.

Local anaesthetic injection: Once the correct site is identified, local anaesthetic is injected incrementally. Needle position can be changed depending on the real-time spread of the local anaesthetic in order to obtain circumferential spread.

Ensuring negative aspiration for blood prior to each aliquot of local anaesthetic is necessary to avoid intravascular injection.

Monitoring for high injection pressure is necessary to avoid intraneural injection.

Injecting local anaesthetic solution to fill a fascial plane requires a larger volume than direct nerve block.

Continuous Peripheral Nerve Block

Continuous PNB is associated with superior pain relief, better mobilization, improved patient satisfaction, sleep and cognition, and fewer side effects. Continuous central neuraxial blockade, although providing similar pain relief, limits mobilization and requires urinary catheterization, whereas patient-controlled analgesia (PCA) offers lesser quality pain relief, limited mobilization and increased side effects.

Insertion of a perineural catheter is relatively straightforward. A standard ultrasound-guided PNB is performed and once the desired nerve is located, the perineural sheath is dilated with saline or local anaesthetic. The optimal volume of fluid (if any), to dilate the perineural space or whether all the injectate must be given before or after catheter insertion, is yet to be determined. Administering a large volume, albeit in small aliquots before catheter insertion, has the advantage that if the catheter cannot be threaded then the patient will have received a single shot PNB with pain relief for 6–24 h, depending on the type of nerve block.

Perineural catheters that are echogenic and thus more easily seen with ultrasound than standard catheters have been developed. Recently, e-catheters that are as easy to insert as a single shot technique have been developed but may not be suitable for all types of continuous PNBs.

Local anaesthetic should be administered through the catheter in increments. The practical advantages of incremental injection are as follows:

- Injection at regular intervals ensures catheter patency, preventing small blood clots from blocking the end hole.
- Kinking or blockage is detected by high injection pressures.
- Cardiovascular stability is improved, particularly in frail, elderly, cardiovascularly compromised patients.

If a catheter technique is used for ambulatory surgery, certain criteria must be met:

- Patients should understand instructions.
- Patients should be accompanied by a responsible person.
- Peripheral nerve catheters should be tested for intravascular placement before discharge.
- Dilute concentrations of local anaesthetic should be used.
- Nerves should be protected from pressure damage.

- A nurse should be available 24 h a day to answer questions by telephone.
- Daily follow-up is mandatory.

Infusion pumps should have a reservoir of 200–400 mL, ensure a constant infusion rate, be tamper proof and ideally have the option of a patient-controlled bolus function.

Three modes of infusion have been used:

- Infusion only – simple, inexpensive and can be disposable, but is incapable of dealing with breakthrough pain or motor block.
- Bolus only – ideal for balancing efficacy against side effects but may be associated with nocturnal pain.
- Infusion with patient-controlled bolus – the ideal regimen. Basal infusion combined with patient-controlled boluses provides pain relief equivalent to that of a continuous infusion, but with lower total doses of local anaesthetic.

The optimum concentrations and volumes of local anaesthetics for continuous PNB have yet to be determined. Furthermore, different nerve plexuses may require varying volumes and concentrations, depending on the anatomical characteristics of the nerves and surrounding perineural space. Lidocaine, bupivacaine, levobupivacaine and ropivacaine have all been used as the primary local anaesthetic.

Infusions of 0.2% ropivacaine 5–10 mL/h and 0.125% levobupivacaine 10–15 mL/h are effective in most cases.

Adjuvants

The role of additives to local anaesthetics blocks has still to be defined. The ideal local anaesthetic adjuvant would reduce onset time, increase the density of the block, prolong analgesia and reduce motor blockade.

Additives include opioids, adrenergic agonists (epinephrine [adrenaline] and clonidine), anticholinergics (neostigmine) and N-methyl-D-aspartate (NMDA) antagonists (ketamine).

Addition of buprenorphine has been shown to prolong local anaesthetic axillary block threefold. Addition of epinephrine (adrenaline) both intensifies and prolongs neural blockade by limiting uptake of local anaesthetic into the surrounding vasculature; a concentration of 1:800,000 is as vasoactive as concentrations of 1:400,000 and 1:200,000 epinephrine (adrenaline) for cutaneous infiltration when used either alone or with the local anaesthetics, bupivacaine and levobupivacaine.

Clonidine may prolong motor and sensory block and analgesia but is associated with significant adverse effects, including hypotension, bradycardia and sedation, all of which limit its use, particularly for ambulatory anaesthesia.

In practice, age is actually the main determining factor of duration of complete motor and sensory blockade with PNB, possibly reflecting increased sensitivity to conduction blockade caused by local anaesthetic agents in peripheral nerves in the geriatric population.

REGIONAL TECHNIQUES

Topical Analgesia

The word 'topical' is derived from the Greek word topos, meaning 'a place'. Topical analgesia can be applied:

- On gauze swabs
- As a liquid in a spray
- As a cream, gel or ointment
- As an aerosol
- By direct instillation (e.g. conjunctival sac, nose and trachea)

  Sites for topical analgesia are as follows:

- Conjunctival sac – stinging pain on instillation is eased if the drug is dissolved in methylcellulose
- External ear
- Nasal cavities
- Upper air passages
- Perineum and vagina in obstetrics for spontaneous delivery, or for suture of simple lacerations
- Urethra
- Open wounds before surgical closure

Infiltration Analgesia

A weal of local anaesthetic is raised in the skin and through this a larger needle is used to inject the main bulk of solution. A solution of either 0.5% or 1% lidocaine, each with epinephrine (adrenaline), is ideal for this procedure.

For painless skin incisions, infiltration should be intradermal as well as subcutaneous. A slow, gentle technique is important, and the solution should be injected while the needle is moving to reduce the chances of intravenous injection.

As with all forms of local analgesia, the effect is not instantaneous and several minutes must elapse between injection and incision.

HEAD AND NECK

Scalp and Cranium

The trigeminal nerve (cranial nerve V) supplies the anterior two-thirds and the posterior divisions of cervical nerves supply the posterior one-third of the scalp and cranium. There are five sensory nerves in front of the ear and four behind it. These nerves all converge towards the vertex of the scalp, so a band of infiltration passing just above the ear through the glabella and the occiput will block them all.

Field Block of Scalp and Cranium
Technique Using Anatomical Landmarks

Injections of 0.5% lidocaine with epinephrine (adrenaline) solution must be made in three layers:

● Skin (intradermal)
● Subcutaneous tissues superficial to the epicranial aponeurosis in which the nerves and vessels lie, and also below the aponeurosis
● Periosteum

In addition, solution should be injected into the substance of the temporalis muscle. The dura is insensitive except at the base of the skull.

Eye and Orbit
Nerve Block for Eye Operations

Retrobulbar, peribulbar and sub-Tenon blocks are described in Chapter 5.9.

Ear
Greater Auricular Nerve Block
Technique Using Anatomical Landmarks

The greater auricular nerve is blocked by infiltration of local anaesthetic solution over the mastoid process in the skin fold behind the back of the ear.

Auriculotemporal Nerve Block
Technique Using Anatomical Landmarks

The auriculotemporal nerve is blocked by infiltration of local anaesthetic solution into the skin over the auditory canal in front of the ear. Blockade of the auriculotemporal and greater auricular nerves together is used for pinnaplasty.

Paracentesis of the Eardrum
Technique Using Anatomical Landmarks

Two or three metered doses of lidocaine aerosol spray (10 mg) are applied to the superior wall of the external auditory canal and allowed to trickle down onto the eardrum. This is repeated after 2 min and the incision can be made 3 min later. It is useful in cooperative children.

Nose

The nasal nerve supply is from the first (ophthalmic) division and from the second (maxillary) division of the trigeminal nerve. The skin of the nose is supplied by the supratrochlear branch of the frontal nerve (a branch of the ophthalmic nerve), the anterior ethmoidal branch of the nasociliary nerve (another branch of the ophthalmic) and the infraorbital branch of the maxillary nerve. The maxillary nerve via the sphenopalatine ganglion supplies the lining of the maxillary antrum. The frontal nerve supplies the frontal sinus. The anterior and posterior ethmoidal branches of the nasociliary supply the ethmoid region. The anterior ethmoidal branch of the nasociliary nerve supplies sensation to the anterior one-third of the nasal septum and the lateral wall of the nasal cavity. The long sphenopalatine nerves from the sphenopalatine ganglion supply sensation to posterior two-thirds of the nasal septum and the lateral walls of the nasal cavity.

The sphenopalatine ganglion is situated in the pterygopalatine fossa in the upper part of the pterygomaxillary fissure, lateral to the sphenopalatine foramen. Blocking of the sphenopalatine ganglion causes analgesia of the:

- Lateral nasal nerve
- Inferior palpebral and superior labial nerves
- Posterior, middle and anterior superior alveolar nerves
- Palatal nerves

Together these nerves supply the skin of the upper lip, side of the nose, lower eyelid and malar region, the teeth of the upper jaw and the underlying periosteum, the mucosa of the maxillary antrum and of the hard and soft palate, and the posterior part of the nasal cavity.

Nerve Block for Nasal Operations

Maxillary nerve and sphenopalatine ganglion block are useful for operations on the antrum (e.g. Caldwell–Luc) and on the upper lip, palate and upper teeth as far as the bicuspids.

For radical operation on the antrum a maxillary block together with local infiltration inside the upper lip, over the canine fossa is necessary.

For radical operation on the frontal sinus, anterior ethmoidal and frontal blocks are necessary.

For operations such as dacryocystitis, anterior ethmoidal and infraorbital blocks are required.

Topical Analgesia of the Nasal Cavities

Topical analgesia of the nasal cavities is useful in cooperative patients with reasonably patent nares.

Spray Technique

The nasal cavities are sprayed with a 2.5 mL mixture of 5% lidocaine and 0.5% phenylephrine hydrochloride, aiming dorsally for the mucosa overlying the sphenopalatine ganglion, behind the middle turbinate.

Topical 4% cocaine solution is now rarely used.

Moffett's Method

The traditional Moffett's solution has been modified and now contains a mixture of cocaine hydrochloride, sodium bicarbonate and epinephrine (adrenaline). Application of the solution into the roof of the nasal cavity provides good analgesia without the need for gauze packing.

Anterior Ethmoidal (Median Orbital) Nerve Block

This is a branch of the nasociliary nerve and is blocked in the medial wall of the orbit as it passes through the anterior ethmoidal foramen.

Technique Using Anatomical Landmarks

A weal is raised 1 cm above the caruncle at the inner canthus of the eye. A small needle is introduced along the upper medial angle of the orbit for 3.5 cm keeping near the bone.

Lidocaine, 2 mL of a 2% solution, is usually sufficient.

Frontal Nerve Block

Technique Using Anatomical Landmarks

From the same weal as in anterior ethmoid block, the needle is introduced more laterally towards the central part of the roof of the orbit, where the frontal nerve lies between the periosteum and the levator palpebrae superioris.

Lidocaine, 1 mL of a 2% solution, is injected in close contact with the bone.

Infraorbital Nerve Block

The infraorbital nerve, the terminal portion of the maxillary nerve, divides at the infraorbital foramen into inferior palpebral, external nasal and superior labial branches. These supply the side of the nose, the lower eyelid, the upper lip and its mucosa.

The infraorbital foramen is in line with the supraorbital notch and canine fossa, both of which are palpable, or the second upper premolar tooth; it is 1 cm below the margin of the orbit, below the pupil when the eyes look forward. The mental foramen is in the same straight line, as is also the second bicuspid tooth.

Technique Using Anatomical Landmarks

A needle is inserted through a weal 1 cm below the middle of the lower orbital margin, a fingerbreadth lateral to the ala of the nose. Lidocaine, 2 mL of a 2%

SECTION | 4 Regional Anaesthesia

solution, is deposited near the nerve as it issues from the foramen, not while it is in the foramen. The upper lip and tip of the nose are made insensitive by this injection.

Maxillary Nerve and Sphenopalatine Ganglion Block

Technique Using Anatomical Landmarks

A weal is raised 0.5 cm below the midpoint of the zygoma, which is over the anterior border of the coronoid process. Through it, a needle is introduced at right angles to the median plane of the head until it strikes the lateral plate of the pterygoid process at a depth of about 4 cm. The needle is then moved so that its point glances past the anterior margin of the external pterygoid plate. The needle point should be in the pterygomaxillary fissure. The needle has been known to enter the pharynx or the orbit. If the aspiration test is negative, 3–4 mL of a 1.5% solution of lidocaine is injected and a similar amount as the needle is slowly withdrawn.

The anterior ethmoidal nerve is a branch of the nasociliary nerve and is blocked in the medial wall of the orbit as the nerve passes through the anterior ethmoidal foramen. A weal is raised 1 cm above the caruncle at the inner canthus of the eye. A small needle is introduced along the upper medial angle of the orbit for 3.5 cm, keeping near the bone, and 2 mL of 1.5% lidocaine are injected.

Nerve Block for Throat Operations

Cricothyroid Block

Technique Using Anatomical Landmarks

This block is rarely performed now as topical approaches have become more popular.

The operator stands on the left side of the patient and holds a size 22G intravenous cannula in the right hand. The index and middle fingers of the left hand hold the cricothyroid membrane steady. A single purposeful stab is made in the relatively avascular midline of the membrane and a marked loss of resistance is felt as the trachea is entered. Gentle probing of the membrane is not recommended because the needle will slide off laterally, increase bleeding, and may traumatize structures in the neck.

After aspiration to confirm the presence of air, the patient is asked to inspire deeply and 3 mL of 4% lidocaine is rapidly injected into the trachea.

The needle is swiftly removed after injection because the presence of lidocaine precipitates coughing and spread of local anaesthetic both above and below the vocal cords.

Food and drink must be avoided for 3–4 h after anaesthesia.

Glossopharyngeal Nerve Block

Technique Using Anatomical Landmarks

For glossopharyngeal nerve block, the head is fully rotated to the opposite side with the patient lying supine. At the midpoint of a line joining the tip of the mastoid process to the angle of the jaw, a needle inserted vertical to the skin makes contact with the styloid process 2–4 cm deep. The needle is partially withdrawn and reinserted 0.5 cm deep to and posterior to the styloid process. Injection of 6 mL of solution at this point will produce analgesia of the posterior one-third of the tongue.

An alternative technique is to deposit solution near the jugular foramen. A 5-cm needle is introduced through a weal just below the external auditory meatus, anterior to the mastoid process. It is advanced perpendicularly to the skin until it meets the styloid process 1.5–2 cm deep and passes it posteriorly for a further 2 cm. Successful block results in analgesia of the posterior one-third of the tongue, uvula, soft palate and pharynx. There is no motor block. The gag reflex is suppressed.

Internal Laryngeal Nerve Block

The superior laryngeal nerve divides into the internal and external laryngeal nerves slightly below and anterior to the greater cornu of the hyoid bone.

The internal laryngeal nerve pierces the thyrohyoid membrane and then separates into terminal twigs, which spread superficially below the mucosa of the piriform fossa.

Block of the internal laryngeal nerve causes analgesia of the lower pharynx, the laryngeal aspect of the epiglottis, the vallecula, the vestibule of the larynx, the aryepiglottic fold and the posterior part of the rima glottidis. There is no motor block.

Internal laryngeal nerve block by external injection or internal spray techniques is necessary to provide a tubeless field for laser surgery or bronchoscopy (flexible or rigid) when combined with target-controlled infusions (TCI) of propofol.

When combined with topical anaesthesia of the nose using co-phenylcaine (lidocaine plus phenylephrine) spray, and cricothyroid puncture using 3 mL of 4% lidocaine anaesthesia, excellent conditions are created for awake fibreoptic intubation or tracheal stenting of lung tumours.

Technique Using Anatomical Landmarks

A 25G needle is introduced upwards and medially through the thyrohyoid membrane. After aspiration, to exclude entry into the pharynx, 2 mL of a 2% lidocaine solution is injected.

Alternatively, topical application of 2–3 mL of a 4% lidocaine solution to both piriform fossae with a small disposable spray provides good analgesia of the vocal cords for a variety of airway procedures.

Field Block for Tonsillectomy

The lesser palatine nerve (from the maxillary nerve), the lingual nerve (from the mandibular nerve) and the glossopharyngeal nerve, via the pharyngeal plexus, which gives off filaments that form a plexus called the circulus tonsillaris, supply the tonsil and its immediate surroundings.

Technique Using Anatomical Landmarks

Half an hour before the analgesia is commenced, a tetracaine (amethocaine) lozenge 60 mg is given. Injections of 3–5 mL of 1.5% lidocaine is subsequently administered:

- Into the upper part of the posterior pillar
- Into the upper part of the anterior pillar (both pillars must be made oedematous throughout their whole extent)
- Into the triangular fold, near the lower pole
- Into the supratonsillar fossa, after drawing the tonsil towards the middle line

The patient sits, well supported, in a chair. Adequate time must be given for the anaesthetic to act. Fainting sometimes occurs, and depression of the tongue by the spatula may cause discomfort.

Nerve Block for Maxillofacial Operations

Local Infiltration for Dental Extraction

Local infiltration for dental extraction can be carried out for all teeth with the possible exception of the lower molars. Lidocaine 2% solution with 1: 80,000 epinephrine (adrenaline) solution is commonly used, or alternatively 3% prilocaine with felypressin.

A 26G needle is inserted at the junction of the adherent mucoperiosteum of the gum with the free mucous membrane of the cheek and directed parallel to the long axis of the tooth; 0.5–1 mL of solution is injected superficial to the periosteum on the buccal and either the lingual or the palatal side. Analgesia is tested for after 5 min by pushing the needle down the periodontal membrane on each side of the tooth to be extracted. If required, more solution can be injected.

If there is infection involving teeth in the lower jaw, a 5% solution may give better analgesia than the usual 2%. It has a shorter latency but a similar duration of activity.

Mandibular (Inferior Dental) Block

Mandibular (inferior dental) block may be required for extraction of several teeth of the lower jaw or for removal of the second or third molars. Infiltration cannot always be relied on to make these teeth insensitive.

Technique Using Anatomical Landmarks

A single well-placed injection renders one-half of the lower jaw and tongue anaesthetic, except for the central incisor, which receives some nerve supply from the other side, and the lateral buccal fold and molar buccal alveolar margin and gum supplied from the buccinator nerve. Both these areas can be infiltrated with a small volume of solution to make them painless.

With the mouth open, palpate the anterior border of the ramus of the mandible, the retromolar fossa and the internal oblique ridge. Insert the needle just medial to this ridge, lateral to the pterygomandibular ligament for a distance of 1.5 cm, keeping it parallel to the occlusal plane of the lower teeth with the barrel over the premolar teeth of the opposite side and inject 2 or 3 mL of solution.

In patients whose orbital blood supply is derived from the middle meningeal artery (a rare anomaly), mandibular nerve block may result in transient amaurosis. This may be due to intra-arterial injection of the local anaesthetic/epinephrine (adrenaline) solution.

Lingual Nerve Block

The lingual nerve is the only sensory nerve supplying the floor of the mouth between the alveolar margin and the midline.

Technique Using Anatomical Landmarks

A finger in the retromolar fossa of the mandible will palpate the internal oblique line. The lingual nerve can be injected, just medial to this line, with 2 mL of 2% lidocaine. This is a useful method of analgesia for removing calculi from the submaxillary duct.

Intraoral Nerve Blocks

Infraorbital Nerve

Infraorbital nerve block is achieved by injection in the mucobuccal fold, just medial to the canine tooth; 1–2 mL of local anaesthetic solution is injected, advancing the needle 1 cm. The entire upper lip is anaesthetized. This can be bilateral.

Mental Nerve

Mental nerve block is obtained by injection of 1–2 mL of local anaesthetic solution between the apices of the premolar teeth of the lower jaw. This will anaesthetize the lower lip.

Long Buccal Nerve

The long buccal nerve can be blocked as it crosses the anterior border of the mandible. Injection is immediately in front of the ramus, in the mucobuccal fold opposite the first molar tooth. The needle is inserted just anterior to the margin of the mandible and 2–3 mL of solution is injected while the needle is withdrawn. This is useful for blocking 'crossover' fibres.

Cervical Plexus

The cervical plexus is formed by the anterior primary divisions of the upper four cervical nerves (C1–C4), each one of which, after leaving the intervertebral foramen, passes behind the vertebral artery and comes to lie in the sulcus between the anterior and posterior tubercles of the transverse process of the appropriate cervical vertebra.

Each nerve lies between the scalenus medius (deeper muscle) and the levator anguli scapulae, under cover of the sternomastoid. Each of these four nerves, except the first, divides into upper and lower branches, which form three loops lateral to the transverse processes. The loops are between C1 and C2, C2 and C3, and C3 and C4. The lower branch of C4 joins C5 in the formation of the brachial plexus. The upper loop is directed forwards, the lower two backwards.

Branches of the cervical plexus are superficial (cutaneous), deep (muscular) and communicating. The superficial branches emerging at the posterior border of the sternomastoid, near its midpoint, are as follows:

- Ascending branches – the lesser occipital nerve (C2) and great auricular nerve (C2 and C3), which supply the skin of the occipitomastoid region, auricle and parotid
- Transverse branch – the anterior cutaneous nerve of the neck (C2 and C3), which supplies the skin of the anterior part of neck between the lower jaw and the sternum
- Descending branches – the lateral, intermediate and medial supraclavicular nerves (C3 and C4), which supply the skin of the shoulder and upper pectoral region; C1 has no cutaneous branch

Deep branches of the plexus are as follows:

- The phrenic nerve – C3, C4 and C5
- Anterior (deep) muscular branches
- Posterior muscular branches to sternomastoid, levator scapulae, trapezius and scalenus medius

Communicating branches are as follows:

- Sympathetic – each cervical nerve receives a grey ramus from the cervical sympathetic chain, the upper four nerves from the superior cervical ganglion
- Branch to the vagus
- Branch to the hypoglossal nerve from C1 and C2, the descendens hypoglossi (or superior root of the ansa cervicalis), which joins the descendens cervicalis (or inferior root of the ansa cervicalis) (C2–C3)

The posterior primary divisions of the cervical nerves supply skin and muscles of the back of the neck. Their cutaneous distribution spreads like a cape over the upper thorax and shoulders, and this area is made insensitive in cervical plexus block.

Cervical Plexus Block

Cervical plexus block provides analgesia of the front and back of the neck, the occiput and cape-like area over the shoulders. It is indicated for thyroidectomy and awake carotid surgery.

Superficial Cervical Plexus Block

Technique Using Anatomical Landmarks

A supine patient with the head turned towards the opposite side is common to all approaches of cervical plexus block.

Local anaesthetic 10–20 mL is injected superficial to the investing layer of deep cervical fascia along the posterior border of the sternomastoid near its midpoint.

Technique Using Ultrasound

Alternatively, the plexus can be visualized with ultrasound as hypoechoic (honeycomb appearance) structures lateral to the posterior border of sterno-mastoid muscle. It lies between the prevertebral fascia superiorly and inter-scalene groove. An in-plane technique with a high resolution linear transducer placed at the level of cricoid cartilage is recommended to block these sensory nerves.

Intermediate Cervical Plexus Block

Technique Using Ultrasound

Local anaesthetic, 20 mL, is injected under ultrasound guidance into the fascia between sternomastoid and the levator scapulae muscle.

When combined with perivascular carotid sheath block (3–5 mL of local anaesthetic), overall efficacy is improved.

Deep Cervical Plexus Block

Technique Using Anatomical Landmarks

A line is drawn connecting the mastoid with the transverse process of the sixth cervical vertebra (Chassaignac tubercle). A second line is drawn parallel and 1.5 cm posterior. A needle is inserted to a depth of 1.5–2 cm perpendicular to all planes of the skin so that the transverse processes are contacted.

Inject into the sulcus between the anterior and posterior tubercles of the transverse processes of the second, third and fourth cervical vertebrae (the sixth, seventh and eighth nerves having no sensory branches in the neck, and the first is purely motor). An alternative is a single injection at the level of C3 or C4–C5.

Technique Using Ultrasound

The transverse processes can be easily visualized with ultrasound when the neck is scanned from mastoid to Chassaignac tubercle and local anaesthetic can be injected as described under direct vision, thus avoiding vertebral artery injection.

The deep approach has a relatively higher complication rate and requirement for conversion to general anaesthesia. Complications include:

- Phrenic nerve block – resulting in paresis of the hemidiaphragm
- Intrathecal or intravascular (especially vertebral artery) injection – leading to life-threatening seizures
- Vagus and/or recurrent laryngeal nerve block – resulting in aphonia
- Cervical sympathetic block and Horner syndrome

SHOULDER AND UPPER LIMB

Brachial Plexus

The brachial plexus arises in the neck and travels laterally and inferiorly over the first rib before entering the axilla. It is formed by the anterior rami of C5 to C8 and T1 (roots) with some contribution from C4 and T2 (Table 4.2.1).

Three trunks originate from the roots and are located between the anterior and middle scalene muscles; the C5 and C6 rami unite to form the superior trunk, the C7 ramus continues as middle trunk and the union of C8 and T1 forms the inferior trunk.

At the lateral edge of the first rib, the three trunks separate into anterior and posterior divisions.

The anterior divisions of the superior and middle trunks form the lateral cord, the posterior divisions of all three trunks form the posterior cord and the anterior division of the inferior trunk forms the medial cord.

The lateral cord gives rise to the musculocutaneous nerve and the lateral head of the median nerve; the posterior cord forms the radial and axillary nerves; and the medial cord forms the ulnar nerve, the medial head of the median nerve and the medial cutaneous nerve, which joins with the intercostobrachial nerve to innervate the skin over the ulnar aspect of the arm.

The brachial plexus passes into the axilla, surrounded by a fascial sheath descended from the prevertebral fascia separating the anterior and middle scalene muscles.

Within the axillary sheath, thin septa divide the brachial plexus into separate compartments, thus limiting circumferential spread of injected solutions. Division into compartments accounts for the better results of multiple injection axillary block techniques even with ultrasound, and for the relative failure of single-injection techniques.

A major portion of the brachial plexus is located parallel and lateral to the terminal part of the subclavian and first part of the axillary arteries, just above

TABLE 4.2.1 Motor and Sensory Innervation of the Upper Limb

Nerve Origin	Nerve	Motor Branches	Sensory Branches
Roots	Long thoracic	Serratus anterior	
	Dorsal scapular	Levator scapulae, rhomboids	
	Nerve to subclavius		
Trunks	Suprascapular	Supraspinatus, infraspinatus	
Lateral cord	Lateral pectoral	Pectoralis major and minor	
	Musculocutaneous	Coracobrachialis, biceps, brachialis	Lateral cutaneous nerve of arm
	Lateral head of the median		
Posterior cord	Upper subscapular	Subscapularis	
	Thoracodorsal	Latissimus dorsi	
	Lower subscapular	Subscapularis	
	Axillary	Teres minor, deltoid	Upper lateral cutaneous nerve of arm
	Radial	Triceps, brachioradialis, extensor carpi radialis longus	Posterior cutaneous nerves of arm and forearm, lower lateral cutaneous nerve of arm
	Posterior interosseous branch of radial	Supinator, extensors of fingers and thumb	
	Superficial branch of radial		Skin dorsum of hand
Medial cord	Medial pectoral		Medial cutaneous nerves of arm and forearm
	Median	Pronator teres, flexor carpi radialis flexor digitorum superficialis, palmaris longus, lateral two lumbricals	Palmar cutaneous branch
	Anterior interosseous branch	Flexor pollicis longus, flexor digitorum profundus, pronator quadratus, abductor pollicis brevis, flexor pollicis brevis, opponens pollicis	

Continued

TABLE 4.2.1 Motor and Sensory Innervation of the Upper Limb—cont'd

Nerve Origin	Nerve	Motor Branches	Sensory Branches
	Ulnar	Flexor carpi ulnaris, flexor digitorum profundus, palmaris brevis	Dorsal and palmar cutaneous branches
	Deep terminal branch of ulnar	Flexor and abductor, opponens digiti minimi, four palmar interossei, four dorsal interossei, two lumbricals, adductor pollicis	

and below the clavicle, respectively. At this level the inferior trunk is posterior and the upper two trunks are superior and lateral to the artery.

Brachial Plexus Block

Brachial plexus block is ideally performed with the patient awake or under light sedation. The nerves blocked by the various approaches to the brachial plexus are outlined in Fig. 4.2.2.

Ultrasound has superseded needle-guided electrical stimulation for brachial plexus block.

Interscalene Brachial Plexus Block

Interscalene block provides superior analgesia in comparison with other approaches. As well as the proximal nerve roots and trunks, it also blocks the supraclavicular and suprascapular nerves, both of which emerge before the plexus.

Interscalene block is ideal for surgery involving the shoulder (open and arthroscopic), lateral two-thirds of the clavicle and proximal humerus. Interscalene block is not suitable for distal upper limb procedures due to ulnar sparing (C8, T1).

Although surgery can be performed under interscalene block alone, in the interest of patient comfort and reduced dose of local anaesthetic, it is more commonly combined with general anaesthesia.

Technique Using Ultrasound

The patient lies supine with head turned towards the opposite side. The pillow underneath the head is positioned diagonally to allow adequate space for the transducer and needle manipulation without compromising sterility.

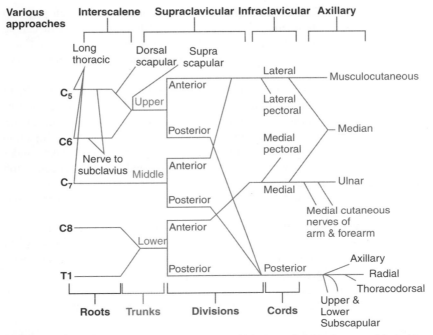

FIGURE 4.2.2 Schematic representation of the brachial plexus showing the nerves blocked by the various approaches.

At the level of the cricoid cartilage, the area between the cricoid cartilage and the supraclavicular fossa is scanned with a high frequency linear transducer (short-axis view) to locate the optimal hypoechoic round images of nerve roots (C5 and C6) and/or upper trunk enclosed in a fascial sheath sandwiched between scalenus medius laterally and scalenus anterior medially (Fig. 4.2.3). A sterile 5 cm nerve block needle is inserted either in-plane (lateral to medial) and parallel to the transducer or out-of-plane (cranial to caudal) and perpendicular to the transducer. For continuous interscalene block the out-of-plane approach is preferred, although the in-plane approach can be performed safely if utilizing an e-catheter. The needle is

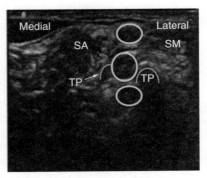

FIGURE 4.2.3 Ultrasound image from a linear probe of the brachial plexus in the interscalene groove, demonstrating the nerve roots (yellow rings) between scalenus anterior (SA) and scalenus medius (SM), in proximity to the transverse processes (TP). *Source:* Pavan Kumar B C Raju, and David M Coventry Contin Educ Anaesth Crit Care Pain 2013;bjaceaccp.mkt059.

advanced until the fascia overlying the plexus is contacted at which point up to 15 mL of local anaesthetic is injected. Alternatively local anaesthetic can be injected after puncturing the fascia. The advantages of not puncturing the fascia include a reduced incidence of direct nerve contact and reduced phrenic nerve blockade.

Injection of local anaesthetic after puncturing the fascia is associated with better spread while permitting the use of a smaller volume and lower concentration. However, it demands careful continuous visualization of the needle tip to minimize direct nerve contact and to prevent intraneural injection. Injection of 0.2% ropivacaine 8–10 mL is sufficient if surgery is to be undertaken under general anaesthesia. A larger volume (up to 20 mL) and a higher concentration is required for awake surgery.

Co-administration of dexamethasone intravenously may prolong the duration of block.

As the likelihood of phrenic nerve block, resulting in paresis of the hemi-diaphragm, increases with increasing volume of local anaesthetic, the lowest possible volume should be injected. A distal approach (lower in the neck where nerve separation is greater) will also minimize the risk.

Care needs to be taken in patients with compromised respiratory function. These patients should be nursed in a semi-recumbent position in the postoperative period.

Horner syndrome due to cervical sympathetic blockade, hoarseness due to recurrent laryngeal blockade or laryngeal hyperaemia have all been reported.

Serious complications such as epidural or intrathecal spread, direct injury to the spinal cord, intervertebral local anaesthetic injection have been reported but are extremely rare.

Supraclavicular Brachial Plexus Block

Supraclavicular block has the widest application of all the brachial plexus approaches, providing analgesia for procedures from the area between mid-humerus proximally to the hand distally. It provides dense, effective, rapid onset block. There has been a resurgence in the popularity of the supraclavicular approach, due to improved safety with ultrasound-guided techniques.

Technique Using Ultrasound

The patient is positioned as for the interscalene approach. A high frequency linear transducer is placed in the supraclavicular fossa slightly obliquely to visualize subclavian artery, first rib, pleura and plexus. The nerve trunks and divisions are tightly packed in the fascia lying superior and posterolateral to the subclavian artery and are visualized as round/oval hypoechoic images, described as 'a bunch of grapes', in the short-axis view. A 5 cm nerve block needle is inserted in-plane (lateral to medial) and placed within the tightly packed fascia paying careful attention to avoid direct contact of needle tip with nerves. Local anaesthetic is injected using the hydrolocation technique and gentle needle manipulation to ensure that the whole plexus is bathed in the solution. The minimum effective volume of local anaesthetic to achieve a rapid and dense block is 25–30 mL.

It can be a challenge to obtain an optimal view in morbidly obese patients.

Complications include pnemothorax due to the proximity of the plexus to pleura, phrenic nerve block (up to 30% of patients) and ulnar sparing due to reluctance of the operator to deposit local anaesthetic close to the first rib.

Infraclavicular Brachial Plexus Block

This is the least preferred approach prior to the widespread use of ultrasound, due to its complexity and variability of landmarks. The infraclavicular fossa is bound anteriorly by pectoral muscles, medially by ribs and intercostal muscles, laterally by humerus and superiorly by clavicle and coracoid process.

Infraclavicular block provides analgesia for procedures on elbow, forearm and hand and is associated with less tourniquet-induced pain than the axillary approach.

Ultrasound enables visualization of axillary artery and cords without the need for arm abduction, useful in patients with shoulder discomfort or upper limb fractured.

Due to the anatomical location, it is the preferred site for continuous nerve blockade.

Technique Using Ultrasound

The patient is positioned as for the interscalene approach. Both linear and curvilinear high frequency ultrasound probes can be used. The area below the clavicle medial to the coracoid process is scanned to visualize the short-axis view of the axillary artery in a parasagittal plane (pericoracoid approach). The three cords are located lateral, posterior and medial to the artery and are seen as bright round structures. The axillary vein is medial to the artery (Fig. 4.2.4). A 5 cm nerve block needle is inserted below the clavicle (superior to the transducer) in an in-plane approach. As the plexus is deep steeper needle insertion is required, thus making the visualization of needle tip challenging. The needle is advanced and local anaesthetic is injected posterolateral to the artery, described as double bubble sign. The needle is advanced further to deposit more local anaesthetic posterior to the artery to ensure all three

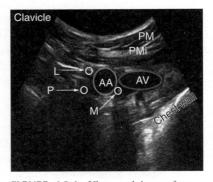

FIGURE 4.2.4 Ultrasound image from a curved-array probe of the brachial plexus in the infraclavicular fossa, demonstrating the cords of the brachial plexus (lateral cord, L; posterior cord, P; medial cord, M), underneath the pectoral muscles (pectoralis major, PM; pectoralis minor, PMi) and around the axillary artery (AA) which lies lateral to the axillary vein (AV). *Source:* Pavan Kumar B C Raju, and David M Coventry Contin Educ Anaesth Crit Care Pain 2013;bjaceaccp.mkt059.

cords are blocked. The total volume of local anaesthetic required is in the range of 25–30 mL for an effective block.

Vascular puncture, especially of the artery, is rare when using ultrasound. Application of pressure to haematoma in this area to reduce bleeding can be difficult.

The incidence of pneumothorax and phrenic nerve blockade is markedly reduced with this approach.

Axillary Brachial Plexus Block

In the axilla, branches of the brachial plexus envelope the axillary artery. The median and musculocutaneous nerves together with their sensory branches are anterior or anterolateral (i.e. above the artery), the ulnar nerve is inferior and the radial nerve is below and behind the vessel.

Axillary block is ideal for surgery performed on the elbow, forearm and hand and certain vascular access procedures such as brachocephalic and brachiobasilic fistulae.

Its safety profile also makes it the approach of choice in high risk patients.

Technique Using Ultrasound

The patient lies supine with the arm to be blocked abducted no more than 90° and externally rotated with the elbow flexed. Excessive abduction in the shoulder joint increases the risk of nerve injury by stretching the brachial plexus. A high frequency linear transducer is placed sagittally on the proximal humerus to obtain a short-axis view of axillary vessels along with the various individual nerves. The axillary artery should be easily located and the individual nerves generally surround the artery and appear as hyperechoic round structures. Wide variability exists with the location of these nerves relative to the artery. The median nerve lies superior and lateral to the artery. The ulnar nerve is located underneath the vein which itself is medial to the artery. The radial nerve is generally located inferomedially, lying close to the artery. At the level of the proximal humerus the musculocutaneous nerve is seen in a fascia separating coracobrachialis (inferomedial) and short head of biceps (Fig. 4.2.5). Identification of these nerves is aided by tracing them from their positions in the distal arm.

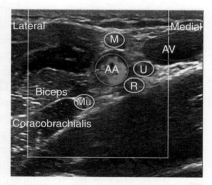

FIGURE 4.2.5 Ultrasound image from a linear probe of the brachial plexus in the distal axilla demonstrating the relationship of terminal nerves of the brachial plexus with respect to axillary artery (AA) and axillary vein (AV). The musculocutaneous (Mu), median (M), ulnar (U) and radial (R) nerves lie around the axillary artery in their typical positions. *Source:* Pavan Kumar B C Raju, and David M Coventry Contin Educ Anaesth Crit Care Pain 2013;bjaceaccp.mkt059.

Both in-plane and out-of-plane approaches can be used. An 8-10 cm nerve block needle is preferred for an in-plane technique, aiming for multiple local anaesthetic injections around the nerves. Musculocutaneous, radial, median and ulnar nerves are blocked in that order with this technique using 25–30 mL of local anaesthetic. A 5 cm nerve block needle is preferred for an out-of-plane technique due to the shorter distances between the insertion site and the nerves.

The brachial approach has the least potential for complications. However, vascular puncture can occur and care should be taken in the form of incremental injections with prior negative aspirations to avoid intravascular injection of local anaesthetic.

Radial nerve may need supplementation more distally in the arm if it is difficult to identify due to its poor visibility.

Distal Nerve Blocks

Distal nerve blocks can be used on their own, to supplement insufficient brachial plexus block or as rescue analgesia. Ultrasound enables the operator to see these nerves along their course anywhere in the arm.

The radial nerve can be blocked at the elbow where it lies between brachialis and brachioradialis muscles, and before it divides into superficial and deep branches.

The musculocutaneous nerve can also be blocked at the elbow where it lies lateral to biceps tendon. This will result in sensory block of the lateral cutaneous nerve of forearm, the continuation of musculocutaneous nerve.

The median nerve can be blocked in the mid-forearm where it lies between flexor digitorum superficialis and flexor digitorum profundus.

The ulnar nerve can also be blocked in the mid-forearm, where it lies medial to the ulnar artery. It is at this level that the ulnar artery becomes deeper to the nerve, making it the best place to block the nerve and minimize the risk arterial puncture.

Each digit is supplied by two palmar and two dorsal nerves. A 25G needle is used to inject 2 mL of plain local anaesthetic solution between bone and skin at the base of the digit on the dorsal and palmar aspect.

Bier's Block

Bier's block can be used for most distal limb procedures of short duration.

Technique

Bier's block two cannulae should be inserted, one in the dorsum of the hand and another in a vein in the other limb in case of toxic signs. Veins in the forearm or antecubital fossa are best avoided.

The limb is drained of blood by elevation for 5 min, with or without compression of the brachial artery. An Esmarch bandage, the Rhys–Davies exsanguinator (an inflatable pneumatic cylinder, which is easier to apply and less uncomfortable) or an orthopaedic pneumatic splint can all be used for this purpose.

A dedicated double cuff is securely placed on the upper arm, and the upper one is inflated to a pressure a little above the systolic blood pressure, before removal of the compression or pneumatic bandage.

Injection of the local anaesthetic solution follows, and after 5–10 min the lower cuff is inflated and the upper one released to minimize discomfort. A tourniquet that does not occlude the brachial artery throughout the operation may result in congestion of the limb, absorption of the drug and imperfect analgesia. Close attention to detail and to the efficiency of the apparatus is most important.

The patient is ready for operation after an interval of 10 min. Analgesia and motor weakness continue while the tourniquet remains inflated but Bier's block does not provide post procedure analgesia.

The tourniquet can be very uncomfortable.

Bier's block has been used successfully in children, and also on the lower limb, in which case the cuff should be placed on the mid-calf.

Local Anaesthetic Solutions

Preservative-free 0.5% lidocaine and prilocaine are effective and relatively safe; the usual volume required is 3–4 mg/kg. In contrast, bupivacaine is efficient but potentially toxic and should never be used.

Cuff Deflation

Cuff deflation should not be attempted for at least 30 min after inflation and is best done in stages, although an interosseous leak may occur. Local anaesthetic drug is released into the circulation in a biphasic manner. There is an initial fast release of 30%, but 50% may still be present in the limb 30 min later.

Toxic signs include drowsiness, twitches, jactitations or convulsions and bradycardia proceeding to asystole, hypotension and ECG abnormalities. The patient should be carefully observed during the 10 min following release of the cuff. Reinflation may be considered if signs of toxicity arise.

Contraindications

Contraindications for Bier's block include Raynaud disease, sickle cell anaemia and scleroderma.

Bier's block is not suitable for major surgery.

HIP AND LOWER LIMB

Although a number of lower limb procedures can be performed under PNB alone, the majority of procedures involving hip and lower limb are performed under a combination of general anaesthesia and one or more PNBs.

Lumbar Plexus

The lumbar plexus is formed from the anterior primary rami of T12 to L4 and is enveloped within a sheath between the psoas major muscle and the quadratus lumborum muscle.

The anterior root of L1 divides into the ilioinguinal nerve and the iliohypogastric nerve and sends a contribution to the genitofemoral nerve.

The L2, L3 and L4 roots divide into anterior and posterior divisions. The anterior division of L2 joins with L1 to form the genitofemoral nerve. The anterior divisions of L2, L3 and L4 descend as the obturator nerve. The posterior divisions of L2, L3 and L4 converge to form the lateral cutaneous nerve of thigh and the femoral nerve.

Iliohypogastric Nerve (L1)

The iliohypogastric nerve leaves the psoas major, crosses the quadratus lumborum, perforates the transversus abdominis and then divides into lateral and anterior cutaneous branches. Its lateral cutaneous branch supplies the skin on the anterior part of the gluteal region after piercing the internal and external oblique muscles 5 cm behind the anterior superior iliac spine and just above the iliac crest, whereas the terminal part of the nerve supplies the skin over the pubic bone after piercing the aponeurosis of the external oblique, 2 cm medial to the anterior superior iliac spine. It does not divide into anterior and posterior branches.

Ilioinguinal Nerve (L1)

The ilioinguinal nerve accompanies the iliohypogastric nerve in its early course, lying just inferior to it in close relationship to the iliac crest. About 2 cm anterior and just below the anterior superior spine, it pierces the internal oblique and runs medially behind the aponeurosis of the external oblique. It then passes with the spermatic cord through the inguinal canal and supplies the skin of the upper and medial part of the thigh and the adjacent skin covering the external genitalia. It has no lateral cutaneous branch, unlike the iliohypogastric nerve, and in the inguinal canal is sensory.

Genitofemoral Nerve (L1, L2)

The genital branch of the genitofemoral nerve supplies the skin of the scrotum or labium majus and is motor to the cremaster muscle. The femoral branch supplies an area of skin on the middle of the anterior surface of the upper part of the thigh.

Lateral Cutaneous Nerve of the Thigh (L2, L3 – Posterior Divisions)

The lateral cutaneous nerve of the thigh, purely sensory, supplies the skin of the anterolateral aspect of the thigh as far as the knee anteriorly but laterally not quite so low after passing behind the inguinal ligament and the sartorius muscle, just medial and slightly inferior to the anterior superior iliac spine.

Femoral Nerve (L2, L3, L4 – Posterior Divisions)

The femoral nerve emerges from the psoas major, passes between it and the iliacus, and enters the thigh behind the inguinal ligament and just lateral to the femoral artery, from which it is separated by a slip of the psoas major. It has anterior and posterior divisions, the former giving rise to the saphenous nerve, which extends to the medial lower leg and the medial and intermediate cutaneous nerves of the thigh. The femoral nerve supplies the hip joint and knee joint, the skin of the anterior part of the thigh and the anteromedial part of the leg. It is motor to the quadriceps femoris, the sartorius and the pectineus (Table 4.2.2).

Obturator Nerve (L2, L3, L4 – Anterior Divisions)

The obturator nerve emerges from the medial border of the psoas muscle where it is a posterior relation of the external iliac vessels. After running forwards on the lateral wall of the pelvis it pierces the obturator canal and divides into anterior and posterior branches; the former supply the adductor longus and brevis and the gracilis, with a branch going to the hip joint; the posterior branch supplies the adductor magnus and the hip joint.

The obturator nerve supplies an area of skin on the medial aspect of the thigh and sends a small branch to the knee joint.

An accessory obturator nerve is present in about 25% of people and runs a variable course across the superior pubic ramus.

TABLE 4.2.2 Lower Leg Muscle Innervation and Function

Nerve	Muscle	Function
Femoral	Quadriceps femoris	Flexes hip, extends knee
Obturator nerve	Adductors of thigh	Adduct thigh
Tibial nerve	Biceps femoris muscle	Flexes knee and rotates leg laterally
	Semimembranosus muscle	Flexes knee
	Semitendinosus muscle	Extends thigh, flexes leg and rotates it medially
	Flexor hallucis longus	Flexes foot
	Flexor digitorum longus	Flexes toes
Common peroneal nerve	Tibialis anterior, extensor digitorum muscles, extensor hallucis muscles, peroneal muscles	Dorsiflexion and inversion of foot, extend, evert and pronate the outer foot

Lumbar Plexus Block

Lumbar plexus block is a deep block that provides effective analgesia for procedures involving hip, anterior thigh and knee. The popularity has diminished due to the development of other superficial ultrasound-guided approaches.

The plexus lies within the psoas major muscle in three-quarters and between psoas and quadratus lumborum in the remaining quarter of patients. Due to the high vascularity of psoas major, analgesia lasts around 6 h. Hence, a continuous block is preferred for prolonged analgesia.

Technique Using Nerve Stimulation

The technique of Capdevila is recommended when using a nerve stimulator to identify the plexus.

With the patient in the lateral decubitus position and operative side up, the needle is inserted 3 cm caudal and 5 cm lateral to the spinous process of the fourth lumbar vertebra, two-thirds of the distance between the midline and the intercostal line, which runs vertically through the posterior superior iliac spines. It is important to contact the transverse process of the fourth lumbar vertebra in order to judge the depth of needle insertion. The needle is then redirected underneath the transverse process.

The lumbar plexus lies 1–2 cm beyond the transverse process of the fourth lumbar vertebra. The median lumbar plexus depth is 8.5 cm in men and 7 cm in women, but the same distance beyond the transverse process. Contraction of the quadriceps muscle indicates close proximity to the lumbar plexus, and 30 mL of local anaesthetic solution is injected when muscle contraction is stimulated using an electrical current between 0.2 and 0.5 mA. A plexus catheter is then advanced 3–5 cm past the needle orifice for a continuous block.

Technique Using Ultrasound

Due to the depth of the plexus, a relatively low frequency (3–6 MHz) curvilinear transducer is required when using ultrasound to identify the plexus.

The patient is positioned as for the nerve stimulator technique. The transverse processes of L2 and L3 or L3 and L4 vertebrae are located either in longitudinal or transverse axes. The needle is introduced either in-plane or out-of-plane and advanced into the posterior part of the psoas major muscle. Local anaesthetic to a total volume of 20–30 mL is injected in increments with intermittent negative aspiration.

Complications

Lumbar plexus block should be avoided in patients with abnormal coagulation due to its depth, high vascularity, possibility of retroperitoneal haematoma and high risk of systemic toxicity.

Total spinal anaesthesia and epidural spread, the latter being more common, have been reported as has visceral injury including renal puncture.

Femoral Nerve Block

Femoral nerve block is a superficial block that is used to provide analgesia for procedures involving anterior thigh and knee. However, as injection of even large volumes of local anaesthetic does not reliably spread to block the other nerves of the lumbar plexus, femoral nerve block is usually performed in combination with lateral cutaneous nerve of thigh and obturator nerve block or with sciatic nerve block.

Technique Using Nerve Stimulation

The patient should be supine with the area below the inguinal crease exposed. The needle is inserted 1.5 cm lateral to the femoral artery, approximately 2 cm below the inguinal ligament and 30° to the skin and advanced in a cranial direction. Contractions of the quadriceps femoris muscle and movement of the patella are necessary to locate the femoral nerve accurately. Injection of 15 mL is sufficient for femoral block alone.

Technique Using Ultrasound

The patient is positioned as for the nerve stimulator technique. A high frequency linear transducer is placed on the inguinal crease and manipulated until the femoral artery is recognized by its pulsations. Immediately lateral to the artery the femoral nerve is identified as a triangular or an oval shaped hyperechoic structure below the fascia iliaca and medial to medial border of iliopsoas muscle. A 5 cm nerve block needle is inserted using an in-plane technique and positioned just underneath the nerve, lifting and enhancing it when local anaesthetic is injected. A single shot technique requires 10–15 mL of local anaesthetic solution.

Fascia Iliaca Block

Fascia iliaca block is used as an analgesic supplement for procedures involving hip, anterior thigh and knee. It is a technically simple procedure that can be performed using anatomical landmark technique or more reliably using ultrasound.

Technique Using Anatomical Landmarks

The patient should be supine with the area below the inguinal crease exposed. The needle is inserted at the meeting point of the lateral and middle third of a line joining the pubic tubercle and the anterior superior iliac spine. The needle is advanced until two pops are felt as the needle pierces fascia lata and iliaca.

Technique Using Ultrasound

The patient is positioned as for the nerve stimulator technique. An in-plane approach with high frequency ultrasound is used. A relatively large volume of local anaesthetic 30–40 mL is placed underneath the fascia iliaca compartment, and it spreads and blocks the lateral cutaneous nerve of the thigh and femoral nerve.

Adductor Canal Block

The adductor canal also called subsartorial or Hunter's canal is a triangular canal bound anterolaterally by vastus medialis, medially by sartorius and posteriorly by adductor magnus. It contains femoral vessels and branches of femoral nerve, namely, saphenous nerve and nerve to vastus medialis.

Adductor canal block is a technically simple block. It is rarely used on its own but when combined with sciatic block it provides analgesia for knee procedures and when combined with popliteal block it provides analgesia for foot and ankle procedures.

Technique Using Ultrasound

The patient lies supine with the knee slightly flexed and the thigh abducted and externally rotated to expose the medial side of thigh.

A high frequency linear transducer is placed transversely in this area to identify the femoral artery lying in the canal under the sartorius muscle. Insert the needle in an in-plane technique aiming to position the tip under the sartorius muscle. Local anaesthetic is injected in small aliquots after confirming negative aspiration until the local anaesthetic spreads around the femoral artery filling the canal; local anaesthetic 5–10 mL is required to provide an effective block. The saphenous nerve may appear brighter with local anaesthetic injection.

Complications

Vessel puncture and systemic toxicity is rare but can occur. Occasionally, proximal spread of local anaesthetic can result in motor blockade.

Sacral Plexus

The sacral plexus is composed of the lumbosacral trunk (L4, L5) and the ventral rami of the upper four sacral nerves (S1–S4). They lie on the posterior wall of the pelvic cavity between the piriformis and the pelvic fascia and have in front the ureter, the internal iliac vessels and the sigmoid colon on the left. The sacral plexus passes out of the pelvis through the greater sciatic foramen.

Posterior Cutaneous Nerve of the Thigh (S1–S3)

The posterior cutaneous nerve of the thigh supplies the skin of the lower part of the gluteal region, the perineum and the back of the thigh and leg.

Sciatic Nerve (L4, L5, S1–S3)

The sciatic nerve is the largest mixed peripheral nerve in the body. The sciatic nerve leaves the pelvis through the greater sciatic foramen and passes in an arc below the gluteal muscles and down the posterior aspect of the thigh midway between the greater trochanter of the femur and the ischial tuberosity. From the lower margin of piriformis, it passes into the buttock on the posterior surface of the ischium.

From midway between the greater trochanter and the ischial tuberosity, deep to gluteus maximus, the sciatic nerve passes vertically downwards into the hamstring compartment. It lies posterior to obturator internus, the gemelli, quadratus femoris and adductor magnus but is crossed posteriorly by the long head of biceps femoris. It supplies all the hamstring muscles.

At the upper angle of the popliteal fossa (or occasionally within the pelvis) the sciatic nerve separates into the tibial nerve and the common peroneal nerve; in approximately 3% of people the two may separate at higher levels in the pelvis.

Tibial Nerve

The tibial nerve passes down the leg deep to soleus, and at the ankle divides into medial and lateral plantar branches which supply the muscles and deep structures of the sole of the foot. The tibial nerve also gives rise to the medial calcaneal nerve, which supplies the heel (Table 4.2.2).

Common Peroneal Nerve

The common peroneal nerve turns round the neck of the fibula and divides into the deep peroneal (or anterior tibial) and superficial peroneal nerves.

The superficial peroneal nerve supplies peroneus longus and brevis and emerges between them to supply the skin of the lower leg and much of the dorsum of the foot (except the skin of the first web space and the lateral side of the fifth toe).

The deep peroneal nerve passes into the anterior compartment of the leg to supply the anterior compartment muscles.

Perforating Cutaneous Nerve (S2 and S3)

The perforating cutaneous nerve supplies the skin over the medial and lower parts of the gluteus maximus.

Pudendal Nerve (S2, S3 and S4)

The pudendal nerve leaves the pelvis through the greater sciatic foramen, crosses the ischial spine medial to the pudendal vessels and goes through the lesser sciatic foramen. With the pudendal vessels it passes upwards and forwards along the lateral wall of the ischiorectal fossa, in Alcock's canal, a sheath of the obturator fascia. It gives off:

- The inferior rectal nerve supplying the external anal sphincter and the skin around the anus
- The perineal nerve supplying the skin of the scrotum or labium majus
- The dorsal nerve of the penis or clitoris
- The medial and lateral posterior scrotal (or labial) nerves
- Visceral branches supplying the rectum and bladder

Sciatic Nerve Block

Sciatic nerve block can be used to provide analgesia to the hip and knee joints and the whole of the foot with the exception of an area of skin over the medial malleolus supplied by the saphenous branch of the femoral nerve.

Several posterior, lateral and anterior approaches to the sciatic nerve have been described. Posterior approaches include the transgluteal (Labat), parasacral and subgluteal. These approaches tend to be performed with the help of electrical stimulation, as proximally the sciatic nerve is deep and obtaining an optimal sonoanatomy can be challenging.

Technique Using Nerve Stimulation

Transgluteal Approach

In the transgluteal approach the patient is placed in the lateral position, with the leg to be blocked uppermost. The other leg is extended and a pillow placed between the legs for comfort. The upper leg is bent approximately 30–40° at the hip joint and approximately 90° at the knee joint. A line is drawn 5 cm perpendicularly from the midpoint of the line connecting the greater trochanter and the posterior superior iliac spine and a needle is inserted perpendicularly. Often gluteal muscle contraction will be observed before dorsiflexion of the foot. In thin patients, the sciatic nerve may be palpable.

Lateral Approach

Lateral approaches (Guardini) to the sciatic nerve block have also been described. As the patient remains in the supine position, the lateral approach is a convenient alternative to the posterior approach. A line is drawn distally from the greater trochanter, on the posterior margin of the femur. Three to five centimetres distal from the greater trochanter, a 12–15 cm needle is inserted through the skin perpendicular to the major axis of the limb, connected to a peripheral nerve stimulator and advanced to contact the bone. The needle is then redirected posteriorly to slide off the bone and advanced under the femur to elicit contraction of the calf or dorsal flexion of the foot, usually at a depth of 8–12 cm. The heads of the biceps femoris may be stimulated while advancing the needle, causing contractions in the thigh and confusing the operator.

Anterior Approach

The anterior approach to the sciatic nerve is helpful in patients who cannot be placed in the lateral recumbent position. The line connecting the anterior superior iliac spine and the symphysis is marked and divided into thirds. The greater trochanter is then identified and a line drawn inferomedially and parallel to the first line. From the first line, a perpendicular line is drawn from the junction of the medial and middle thirds to intersect the second guideline. The puncture is made at this point of intersection and passes between the sartorius laterally and the rectus femoris medially and reaches the sciatic nerve below the lesser trochanter. Internal rotation of the leg may help location of the sciatic nerve and reduce trauma to the femoral nerve and vessels.

Technique Using Ultrasound

Continuous sciatic and popliteal blocks can be utilized for above or below knee amputations.

Although the proximal sciatic nerve can be deep and difficult to visualize (it can also be difficult to locate using electrical stimulation), it is easily visualized in the mid-lower thigh region where it is large and more superficial.

Sciatic Nerve Block

The patient should be positioned either laterally with slight flexion of hip and knee and ensuring the side to be blocked is uppermost, or prone with the side to be blocked clearly marked. Catheters can be inserted using the lateral approach which has the advantage of more secure placement of the catheter away from the mobile knee joint.

A linear or a curvilinear transducer probe is placed transversely over the popliteal fossa. Proximal to the popliteal crease, the popliteal vessels are identified. The tibial and peroneal nerves are found above and behind the artery. The probe is used to trace the two nerves proximally until they merge into a single hyperechoic structure (the sciatic nerve) around the mid-thigh area. As the sciatic nerve is traced higher in the posterior thigh, the shape changes from oval to round to triangular before disappearing deeper. An 8-10 cm nerve block needle is inserted either using in-plane or out-of-plane approach at any point along the course of the sciatic nerve. While ensuring that spread is circumferential, 15–20 mL of local anaesthetic solution should be injected.

Popliteal Block

The patient is positioned as for sciatic nerve block. Popliteal block is performed similarly with the only difference being the position of the needle tip. The needle tip is aimed at the level of bifurcation of the sciatic nerve and local anaesthetic 15–20 mL is deposited around the nerves. Tibial and peroneal components can be blocked separately if required.

Ankle and Foot

Anatomy

The sole of the foot is supplied by the medial (L4 and L5) and lateral (S1 and S2) branches of the tibial nerve, supplying the medial and lateral anterior part of the sole, the sural nerve supplying the posterior and lateral part of the sole and heel, and the tibial nerve (S1 and S2) supplying the medial part of the heel.

The dorsum of the foot is supplied by the medial terminal branch of the deep peroneal nerve (the adjacent sides of the first and second toes); the sural nerve innervates the lateral side of the fifth toe; the superficial peroneal supplies the remainder.

The medial side of the foot is supplied by the saphenous nerve from the femoral nerve. It is also supplied by the medial plantar branch of the tibial nerve.

The lateral side of the foot is supplied by the sural nerve from the tibial and common peroneal nerves, which goes to the fifth toe and lateral side of the foot.

Ankle Block

Ankle block can be performed using traditional landmark technique. However, with the development of ultrasound, these small peripheral sensory nerves can be visualized and blocked in an in-plane approach.

Compared with landmark techniques, a lower volume of local anaesthetic 10–15 mL is required when using an ultrasound technique.

Deep Peroneal Nerve (Anterior Tibial Nerve – S1 and S2)

Technique Using Anatomical Landmarks

The deep peroneal nerve is blocked by inserting a needle midway between the most prominent points of the medial and lateral malleoli, on the circular line of infiltration in front of the ankle joint. It is directed medially towards the anterior border of the medial malleolus and local anaesthetic solution, 10–15 mL is injected between the bone and the skin. Instead of blocking this nerve at the ankle, its parent trunk, the common peroneal nerve, can be blocked at the neck of the fibula, where it can be rolled under the finger.

Technique Using Ultrasound

Under ultrasound (the transducer is placed transversely right over the ankle joint and scanned proximally until the best image is visualized), the nerve is generally seen as a small honeycomb structure rolling over the anterior tibial vessels. One to two millilitres of local anaesthetic can result in an effective block.

Saphenous Nerve (L3 and L4)

Technique Using Anatomical Landmarks

The saphenous nerve is the terminal branch of the femoral nerve and accompanies the long saphenous vein anterior to the medial malleolus, where it can be blocked by the injection of 10 mL of local anaesthetic solution. It supplies an area of skin just below and above the medial malleolus.

Technique Using Ultrasound

The saphenous nerve can be visualized lying very closely to the long saphenous vein under ultrasound and can be blocked along the course of the nerve.

If the nerve cannot be visualized, a perivenous injection can be performed. It is important to pay attention to the pressure applied with transducer ensuring the vein is not compressed. Two millilitres of perivenous local anaesthetic injection is sufficient to provide good analgesia and anaesthesia.

Superficial Peroneal Nerve (S1 and S2)

Technique Using Anatomical Landmarks

The superficial peroneal nerve, a branch of the common peroneal nerve, can be blocked immediately above the ankle joint by a subcutaneous weal extending from the front of the tibia to the lateral malleolus. It supplies the dorsum of the foot (with the exception of the small area innervated by the tibial nerve).

Technique Using Ultrasound

The transducer is placed transversely above the lateral malleolus and scanned proximally in an anterolateral aspect. The nerve can be seen lying at the junction of extensor digitorum longus (distally) and peroneus brevis in a fascial plane. The limitation is the absence of vascular landmarks to guide the nerve localization. One to two millilitres of local anaesthetic is enough to provide effective analgesia and anaesthesia.

Sural Nerve (L5, S1 and S2)

Technique Using Anatomical Landmarks

To block the sural nerve a subcutaneous injection of 5–7 mL is made between the lateral malleolus and the calcaneal tendon; care is necessary to avoid intravenous injection into the short saphenous vein.

Technique Using Ultrasound

Sural nerve lies in close proximity to short saphenous vein in the distal third of the leg and this property is exploited in blocking this nerve using ultrasound with the transducer being placed in the posterolateral aspect of the leg, proximal to lateral malleolus. One to two millilitres of local anaesthetic is again sufficient to block this small nerve. Care must be taken not to compress the short saphenous vein.

Tibial Nerve (S1 and S2)

Technique Using Anatomical Landmarks

The tibial nerve is blocked by 10 mL of solution introduced through a point on the circular weal just internal to the calcaneal tendon, deep to the flexor retinaculum near the palpable posterior tibial artery. It is easiest with the patient lying prone. The needle is inserted forwards and slightly outwards towards the posterior aspect of the tibia, near which the solution is deposited.

An alternative technique uses bony landmarks. The sustentaculum tali is a semilunar-shaped prominence and can be palpated about halfway between the medial malleolus and the medial border of the heel. Insert the needle at right-angles to the skin down onto its bony surface, withdraw slightly and then inject 5–7 mL of local anaesthetic. The local anaesthetic spreads under the medial retinaculum of the ankle joint and gives a reliable block of all branches of the tibial nerve.

Technique Using Ultrasound

A high frequency linear transducer, ideally with a small footprint such as hockey stick transducer, is placed just above medial malleolus. The tibial nerve is usually seen lying posterior (rarely anterior) to the posterior tibial vessels. It can be difficult to differentiate tibial nerve from flexor hallucis longus tendon at this level. When scanned proximally, the nerve will be lying adjacent to the belly of the muscle. Five millilitres of local anaesthetic is injected around the tibial nerve at the level where the image has the best visibility.

ABDOMEN AND PERINEUM

Abdomen

The xiphoid is on a level with the body of the ninth thoracic vertebra. The subcostal plane is at the third lumbar vertebra. The highest part of the iliac crest is on a level with the interspace between the third and fourth lumbar vertebrae.

The superficial fascia in the upper abdomen is a single fatty layer, but from a point midway between the umbilicus and the pubis two layers are described, the deep layer (Scarpa' fascia) and the superficial layer (Camper's fascia).

Camper's fascia passes over the inguinal ligament and is continuous with the superficial fascia of the thigh. It is continued over the penis, spermatic cord and scrotum, where it helps to form the dartos muscle. In the female it is continued into the labia majora.

Scarpa's fascia is tougher. It blends with the deep fascia of the thigh and, like Camper's fascia, is continued over the penis and helps to form the dartos. From the scrotum it becomes continuous with Colles' fascia over the perineum. There is no deep fascia covering the abdomen.

Muscles of the Abdominal Wall

The external oblique is the largest and most superficial of the muscles of the anterior abdominal wall. The aponeurosis is attached below to the anterior superior spine and to the pubic crest and tubercle, it thus forms the inguinal ligament. In the midline it forms the linea alba, which runs from the symphysis pubis to the xiphisternum. The subcutaneous or external inguinal ring is an opening in the aponeurosis. The fibres of the external oblique pass downwards and inwards, like those of the external intercostal muscles.

The internal oblique is a thinner layer than the external oblique. The fibres of this muscle run upwards and inwards.

The fibres of transversus abdominis run transversely. Between it and the external oblique run the lower intercostal, iliohypogastric and ilioinguinal nerves.

Below the level of the iliac crest the fibres of these three muscles (external oblique, internal oblique and transversus abdominis) are aponeurotic and run downwards and medially.

Each rectus abdominis muscle arises from the crest of the pubis and from the ligaments in front of the symphysis and is inserted into the anterior aspects of the fifth, sixth and seventh costal cartilages and into the xiphisternum. Three tendinous intersections cross the muscle and are firmly attached to the anterior layer of its sheath, but not to the posterior layer. One is at the level of the xiphisternum, one at the umbilicus and the third one midway between.

Pyramidalis is a small muscle on each side, within the rectus sheath. It serves to strengthen the linea alba.

The rectus sheath contains, in addition to the rectus and pyramidalis muscles, the superior and inferior epigastric vessels and the terminations of the lower six intercostal nerves and vessels. The nerves pierce the lateral margin of the sheath and run in relation to its posterior wall before they enter the substance of the muscle.

The abdominal muscles are supplied by the anterior rami of the lower six thoracic nerves and by the iliohypogastric and ilioinguinal nerves. They are accessory muscles of expiration and help to compress the abdominal viscera, such as in defecation, straining and coughing. They are not muscles of normal inspiration.

The transversalis fascia is a thin membrane, continuous with the iliac and pelvic fasciae. In the inguinal region it is stronger and thicker than elsewhere and through it, at the abdominal inguinal (internal inguinal) ring, passes the spermatic cord or the round ligament.

Sensory Nerve Supply of the Abdominal Wall

Sensory nerve supply of the abdominal wall is provided by the anterior primary rami of the lower six thoracic nerves, via the intercostal nerves:

- T5 supplies the skin in the region of the nipple.
- T7 nerve supplies skin in the epigastrium.
- T10 supplies skin in the region of the umbilicus.
- T12 supplies skin midway between the umbilicus and the pubis.
- The skin of the groin is supplied by the iliohypogastric nerve (L1).

Intercostal nerves and the last thoracic nerve pass under the costal margin between the slips of the diaphragm and run forwards between the internal oblique and the transversus abdominis before they pierce the lateral margin of the rectus sheath. After lying behind the rectus muscle, they pierce its substance and supply it, and end as anterior cutaneous nerves.

Vessels of the Abdominal Wall

The only vessels likely to be injured by the anaesthetist are the superior and inferior epigastric arteries and veins. The superior epigastric artery is the termination of the internal mammary artery and enters the rectus sheath posterior to the seventh costal cartilage. The inferior epigastric artery arises from the external iliac artery and enters the rectus sheath behind the arcuate line of Douglas.

Rectus Sheath Block

Rectus sheath block is an excellent method for providing analgesia when the incision is to be midline or paramedian and it is usual to do both sides. Although it was initially described to provide muscle relaxation, it is more commonly used as an analgesic technique for umbilical or incisional hernia repairs and for procedures involving midline incisions. It results in blocking the ninth to eleventh intercostal nerves after they penetrate the posterior wall of the rectus muscle. Perforation of the peritoneum should be avoided, but in the absence of peritonitis or adhesions no serious harm is likely to result.

Bilateral continuous rectus sheath blocks can be used to prolong postoperative analgesia.

Technique Using Anatomical Landmarks

The anterior layer of the rectus sheath is detected by the needle throughout its whole extent, but the posterior layer only for about 7.5 cm above and below the umbilicus.

Local anaesthetic solution is placed posterior to the muscle so that the intercostal nerves supplying it, together with the zone of skin medial to its outer border, are blocked.

Technique Using Ultrasound

A high frequency transducer is placed transversely 2–3 cm from the midline and the layers of rectus sheath and muscle identified. The needle is inserted and the tip position confirmed between the posterior wall of rectus muscle and posterior rectus sheath. Care should be taken to avoid puncturing the inferior epigastric vessels, which lie in this space. Local anaesthetic 15–20 mL is injected on each side.

Ilioinguinal and Iliohypogastric Nerve Blocks

The nerve supply of the inguinal region is from the last two thoracic and the first two lumbar nerves via the iliohypogastric, the ilioinguinal and the genitofemoral.

The last two thoracic nerves run downwards and inwards, just above the anterior superior iliac spine, between the internal oblique and transversus muscles. They end by piercing the rectus sheath.

The iliohypogastric and ilioinguinal nerves come from the first lumbar root. They are inferior to the last two thoracic nerves and curve round the body just above the iliac crest, gradually piercing the muscles and ending superficially. The ilioinguinal nerve traverses the inguinal canal, lying anterior to the spermatic cord, and becomes superficial through the external ring and supplies the skin of the scrotum. The iliohypogastric nerve, after running between the internal oblique and the transversus abdominis, pierces the internal oblique just above the anterior superior iliac spine and supplies the skin over the pubis.

The genitofemoral nerve comes from the first and second lumbar nerves and divides into a genital and a femoral branch. The genital branch enters the inguinal canal from behind through the internal ring.

Technique Using Anatomical Landmarks

The anterior superior iliac spine is identified and a point is marked 2 cm cephalad and 2 cm medial to it. A nerve block needle is inserted perpendicular to the skin and advanced carefully until a first loss of resistance (pop) is encountered as the needle pierces the external oblique aponeurosis. Local anaesthetic 5–10 mL is injected after negative aspiration. The needle is advanced deeper until another loss of resistance is encountered as it pierces the internal oblique and a further 5–10 mL of local anaesthetic is injected into the space between internal oblique and the transverse abdominis muscle.

Technique Using Ultrasound

A high frequency transducer is placed along the line joining the anterior superior iliac spine and umbilicus. The plane between internal oblique and transverse abdominis muscle is identified and a needle is inserted using an in-plane technique. Local anaesthetic 15–20 mL is injected after confirming intermittent negative aspiration.

Transverse Abdominis Plane Block

The transversus abdominis plane (TAP) is a myofascial plane between transverse abdominis (deeper) and internal oblique. It encloses nerves from T7 to L1.

TAP block can be used to provide analgesia for procedures involving the lower abdomen including gynaecological and urological procedures.

It has a variable success rate and carries the risk of bowel and visceral injury.

Technique Using Anatomical Landmarks

The landmark technique is based on the 'triangle of petit', the boundaries of which are formed by external oblique anteriorly, lattismus dorsi posteriorly and iliac crest inferiorly.

A nerve block needle is inserted immediately above the iliac crest and in front of lattismus dorsi. Two losses of resistance need to be appreciated as the needle is advanced: the first as the external oblique is pierced and the second after piercing the fascia covering internal oblique. Local anaesthetic solution

20–30 mL is injected slowly after the second loss of resistance incrementally once negative aspiration is confirmed.

Technique Using Ultrasound

A high frequency transducer is placed transversely along the mid-axillary line between the subcostal line and the iliac crest. The fascial plane between internal oblique and transverse abdomnis is identified. An in-plane approach is recommended so that the needle shaft and the tip is constantly visualized throughout the procedure. Local anaesthetic injection is performed in a similar manner to landmark technique.

Quadratus Lumborum Block

Quadratus lumborum (QL) block can be used to provide analgesia for abdominal surgery above and below the umbilicus. However, bilateral block is necessary for a midline incision.

Technique Using Ultrasound

A high frequency transducer is placed near the posterior axillary line, below the coastal margin and above the iliac crest. The potential space medial to the abdominal wall muscles and lateral to the QL muscle is identified. The block needle can be inserted in plane either from anteromedial to posterolateral or from posteromedial.

There are three approaches to injecting local anaesthetic.

QL1 block (also called posterior TAP block) involves depositing local anaesthetic at the anterolateral margin of the QL muscle at the junction with the transversalis fascia.

QL2 block involves depositing local anaesthetic at the posterior margin of the QL muscle.

QL 3 (transmuscular) block involves the needle passing through lattismus dorsi and QL before depositing local anaesthetic anterior to the QL muscle, where it meets psoas major.

Erector Spinae Block

Erector spinae block involves depositing local anaesthetic in the plane between rhomboid major and erector spinae muscles. As the erector spinae muscle extends along the length of the thoracolumbar spine, extensive spread of local anaesthetic solution in this plane can result in analgesia over multiple dermatomes from thorax to upper abdomen.

Perineum

The penile sensory nerves are derived from the terminal branches of the internal pudendal nerves. The dorsal penile nerves run beneath the pubic bone, one on each side of the midline, lying against the dorsal surface of the corpus caverno-sum. The skin at the base is supplied by the ilioinguinal and the genitofemoral nerves. In addition, the posterior scrotal branches of the perineal nerves run paraurethrally to the ventral surface and fraenum. So, there are four nerves to be blocked.

Penile Block

Technique Using Anatomical Landmarks

For penile block an intradermal and subcutaneous ring weal is raised around the base of the penis; the subcutaneous infiltration should precede the intradermal. The dorsal nerve is blocked on each side by injecting 5 mL of solution into the dorsum of the organ just below, but not deep to, the symphysis so that the needle point lies against the corpus cavernosum. If the needle pierces the corpus caver-nosum, pain is experienced.

For the ventral injection of the paraurethral branches, the penis should be pulled upwards and 2 mL of solution injected near the base into the groove formed by the corpora cavernosa and the corpus spongiosum.

Infiltration of 5 mL of 1% lidocaine or 0.5% bupivacaine into each dor-sal nerve provides good postoperative analgesia. In infants, smaller volumes are used. Postoperative pain can be relieved by repeated penile block in awake patients, even in children, without undue discomfort. Epinephrine (adrenaline) must not be used because it may cause penile necrosis.

Care must be taken not to cause haematoma formation because this may contribute to gangrene of skin; subpubic injection must be avoided.

Pain following circumcision under general anaesthesia can be relieved by sacral extradural analgesia or by infiltrating each dorsal nerve at the root of the penis with 1–3 mL of local anaesthetic solution (e.g. 0.5% bupivacaine, without epinephrine [adrenaline]). This is a satisfactory alternative to extradural sacral block, with fewer complications. Lidocaine spray or gel applied topically gives useful relief.

THORAX

The Thoracic Wall

The thorax constitutes the upper part of the trunk and consists of an external musculoskeletal cage, the chest (or thoracic) wall and an internal cavity contain-ing the viscera.

Cutaneous Nerves of the Trunk

Anteriorly the cutaneous nerves of the trunk are the lateral, intermediate and medial supraclavicular branches of the superficial division of the cervical plexus (C3–C4), the anterior rami of the thoracic nerves, excluding T1 and the iliohypogastric and ilioinguinal nerves (L1).

Posteriorly the cutaneous nerves of the trunk are the posterior rami of C2–C5, T1–T12 and L1–L3 and the five sacral and the coccygeal nerves.

Spinal Nerves

Typical intercostal nerves are the third to sixth thoracic nerves. Each nerve is formed by the union of the anterior (motor) and the posterior (sensory) root – the posterior root has a ganglion on it.

The mixed spinal nerve soon divides into anterior and posterior primary divisions (rami). The thoracic or dorsal nerves are then distributed as follows.

The posterior rami are smaller than the anterior. They turn backwards and divide into medial and lateral branches (except C1, S4 and S5, coccygeal), which supply the muscles and skin of the back.

The anterior rami in the thoracic region of the second to sixth nerves are each connected to the lateral sympathetic chain by a grey and a white ramus communicans. Each crosses the paravertebral space between the necks of contiguous ribs and then enters the subcostal groove where it lies below the vein and artery in a triangular space, bounded above by the rib, the posterior intercostal membrane and the internal intercostal muscle until it reaches the anterior axillary line, at which point the nerves come into direct relationship with the pleura, as the innermost intercostal muscle terminates. There is a communication between each space and those contiguous to it. Each intercostal nerve supplies muscular branches to the intercostal muscles and lateral and anterior cutaneous branches to supply the skin of the chest and abdomen. The seventh to eleventh nerves pass below and behind the costal cartilages, between the slips of the diaphragm running between the internal oblique and transversus muscles (again between the second and third layers) to enter the posterior layer of the rectus sheath. They run deep into the rectus, pierce and supply it, and end as anterior cutaneous nerves (Figs 4.2.6 and 4.2.7).

The lateral cutaneous branch emerges in the mid-axillary line and divides into anterior and posterior branches, which supply the skin on the lateral wall of the chest as far forward as the nipple line.

The anterior cutaneous branch is the termination of the intercostal nerve; it supplies the skin on the front of the chest, internal to the nipple line.

Exceptions

The first intercostal nerve supplies most of its fibres to the brachial plexus and gives neither lateral nor anterior cutaneous branches, the skin over the first intercostal space being supplied by the descending branches of the cervical plexus (C3–C4).

The lateral cutaneous branch of the second intercostal nerve crosses the axilla and becomes the intercostobrachial nerve, supplying the skin on the medial aspect of the arm.

The lateral cutaneous branch of T12, which does not divide into anterior and posterior branches, crosses the iliac crest to supply the skin of the upper part of the buttock as far as the greater trochanter.

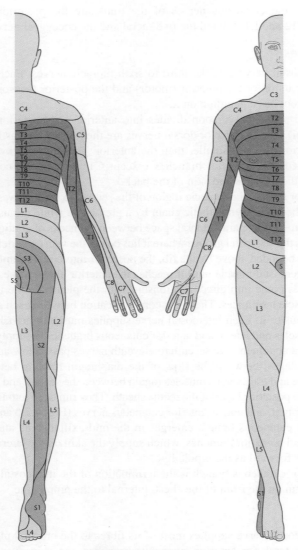

FIGURE 4.2.6 Sensory dermatomes.

T12 and L1 nerves supply sensory branches to the anterior chest and anterior abdominal wall, the parietal pleura and the parietal peritoneum. T10, lateral and anterior cutaneous branches, supplies the area of the umbilicus. T9, T8 and T7 supply the skin between the umbilicus and the xiphisternum. T11, T12 and L1 supply the skin between the umbilicus and the pubis.

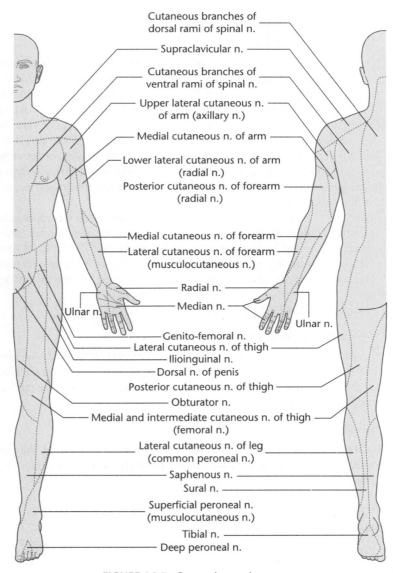

Cutaneous branches of
dorsal rami of spinal n.

Supraclavicular n.

Cutaneous branches of
ventral rami of spinal n.

Upper lateral cutaneous n.
of arm (axillary n.)

Medial cutaneous n. of arm

Lower lateral cutaneous n. of arm
(radial n.)

Posterior cutaneous n. of forearm
(radial n.)

Medial cutaneous n. of forearm

Lateral cutaneous n. of forearm
(musculocutaneous n.)

Radial n.

Median n.

Ulnar n.

Ulnar n.

Genito-femoral n.

Lateral cutaneous n. of thigh

Ilioinguinal n.

Dorsal n. of penis

Posterior cutaneous n. of thigh

Obturator n.

Medial and intermediate cutaneous n. of thigh
(femoral n.)

Lateral cutaneous n. of leg
(common peroneal n.)

Saphenous n.

Sural n.

Superficial peroneal n.
(musculocutaneous n.)

Tibial n.

Deep peroneal n.

FIGURE 4.2.7   Sensory innervation.

Intercostal Nerve Block

Intercostal block is useful in enabling deep breathing and coughing in patients
with postoperative abdominal pain especially if the incision is subcostal. It can
also been used for rib resection, pain relief for fractured ribs and insertion of an
intercostal chest drain.

Technique Using Anatomical Landmarks

At the Angle of the Ribs

At the angle of the ribs the intercostal nerve becomes relatively superficial, lateral to the erector spinae muscle. The patient is placed in the lateral position and two lines are drawn, four fingerbreadths from the vertebral spinous processes, extending from the spines of the scapulae to the iliac crests. At a point where the lower border of the eleventh rib on the patient's upper side crosses the line, a needle is introduced until it makes contact with the rib. It is then partially withdrawn and advanced until it slips past the lower border of the rib for 3 mm; 2–3 mL of local anaesthetic solution with epinephrine (adrenaline) is then injected. A zone of solution thus surrounds the intercostal nerve as it lies in the subcostal groove.

The T6 to T10 nerves are blocked in the same manner on the upper side, followed, after turning, by the lower seven nerves on the patient's other side. T12 nerves are deeper and require special care. Before T6 and T7 can be blocked the patient's scapulae must be drawn laterally by crossing his or her arms over his chest.

The needle pierces the trapezius, the latissimus dorsi and the two intercostal muscles.

Analgesia can last for up to 12 h.

In the Posterior Axillary Line

Intercostal nerve block in the posterior axillary line is carried out with the patient supine and arms abducted to a right-angle. In this position the ribs, and hence the intercostal nerves, are not so deeply placed. A block in the midaxillary line misses the lateral cutaneous nerve.

In the Midaxillary Line

It has been shown that the intercostal nerves can be blocked at the level of the midaxillary line in supine patients as effectively as at the posterior angle of the ribs.

Complications

Complications of intercostal block include

- Pneumothorax
- Damage to intercostal vessels
- Toxicity due to excessive absorption of local anaesthetic and associated epinephrine (adrenaline)

Intercostal block is the technique associated with the highest systemic absorption of local anaesthetic and requires patient monitoring for at least 20 min after injection.

It has been proposed that more complications follow intercostal nerve block performed from inside the thorax than percutaneously.

Other Chest Wall Blocks

These rely on placing local anaesthetic between the muscles of the thoracic wall.

Pectoralis Plane Block

Pectoralis plane (PEC) blocks consist of injecting local anaesthetic into the interfascial plane between pectoralis major and minor muscles, can be used to provide analgesia for breast and axillary surgery, tumour resection and chest trauma.

Technique Using Ultrasound

PECS 1 block: A linear high frequency transducer is placed in the infraclavicular area similar to the position used while performing infraclavicular block. The interfascial plane between pectoralis major and minor is identified at the level of the third rib. The lateral pectoral nerve lies next to thoracoacromial artery (colour Doppler can be used to identify this vessel). Local anaesthetic 20–30 mL is injected into this plane.

PECS 2 block: Indicated for more extensive chest wall surgery. In addition to a PECS 1 block the space between the pectoralis minor and serratus anterior muscles at the level of the third and fourth ribs is identified and a further 20 mL of local anaesthetic is injected.

Serratus Plane Block

Provides analgesia for latissimus dorsi flap reconstruction and multiple rib fractures.

Technique Using Ultrasound

The transducer is orientated in the mid axillary line at the level of the 5th rib. Two planes are identified in relation to serratus anterior and local anaesthetic is deposited above (deep) and below the muscle.

Thoracic Paravertebral Space

The paravertebral space is a wedge-shaped compartment, bounded:

- Superiorly and inferiorly by the heads and necks of adjoining ribs.
- Posteriorly by the costotransverse ligament.
- Medially it communicates with the extradural space through the intervertebral foramen.
- Laterally it is bounded by the parietal pleura and its apex leads into the intercostal space.

The posterolateral aspect of the body of the vertebra and the intervertebral foramen and its contents forms the base. The upper aspect of the spinous process coincides with the transverse process of the lower vertebra.

There is no direct communication between one paravertebral space and another, but an indirect communication exists medially through the intervertebral foramen with the extradural space.

Spread from one paravertebral space to another, across the extradural space, is frequent and may involve nerves on the same or opposite sides of the body.

When the first thoracic to second lumbar nerve roots are blocked, their rami communicantes are blocked too.

Thoracic Paravertebral Block

Thoracic paravertebral block is used to provide pain relief after unilateral thoracic, breast or abdominal surgery and for fractured ribs, chronic pain, refractory angina and cancer pain. Pain relief is comparable with epidural anaesthesia performed at the same spinal level but with reduced complications. Paravertebral infusions have been used to provide postoperative pain relief for ambulatory surgery. Thoracic paravertebral block involves injecting a local anaesthetic close to the vertebral column where the nerve trunks emerge from the intervertebral foramina.

Technique Using Anatomical Landmarks

For thoracic paravertebral block skin weals are raised 4 cm from the midline. In the thoracic region, the injection point is 2–3 cm lateral to the superior aspect of the spinous process. Through each weal, an 18G block needle is inserted perpendicularly 3–5 cm to strike bone near the lateral extremity of the transverse process. It is then redirected to pass below the transverse process and at this point local anaesthetic solution is injected. Insertion of the block needle in a caudal direction reduces the risk of pneumothorax compared to insertion in a cranial direction because the block needle is much more likely to hit the corresponding rib. The block needle is more likely to penetrate pleura when inserted in a cranial direction.

Never disconnect the syringe to the extension tubing because there is a risk of pneumothorax.

Aspiration tests are essential. If there is resistance to injection, progress 3 mm through the costotransverse ligament.

If several levels are to be blocked, a large 15 mL volume can be injected. The placement of a catheter in turn allows the continuous administration of 3–4 mL/h. The anaesthetic solution spreads in the intercostal, interpleural and epidural directions.

Technique Using Ultrasound

A low frequency (3–6 MHz) linear transducer is placed 4–5 cm from the midline in a sagittal plane. Once pleura, ribs and the posterior intercostal membrane have been identified, the transducer is moved medially. This dynamic scanning should reveal the transition of rib to transverse process (always more superficial than rib) and pleura. At this point, the needle is inserted in out-of-plane approach and advanced until the tip is in the potential space between the costotransverse ligament and pleura. Local anaesthetic is injected into this space after confirming negative aspiration.

Complications

Complications of thoracic paravertebral block include

- Local anaesthetic toxicity
- Pneumothorax ($<1\%$)
- Epidural diffusion (1%)
- Hypotension ($<5\%$)
- Intravascular injection

Horner syndrome indicates achievement of C6–T1 sympathetic block – in such situations the patient should be closely monitored for possible phrenic and/or recurrent laryngeal nerve block.

FURTHER READING

Brown DL, editor. Atlas of regional anesthesia. 4th ed. Philadelphia: Saunders Elsevier; 2010.

Siegfried P, Gruber H, editors. Atlas of peripheral nerve ultrasound. Berlin: Springer-Verlag; 2013.

Raju PKBC, Coventry DM. Ultrasound-guided brachial plexus blocks. Contin Educ Anaesth Crit Care Pain 2014;14:185–91.

Stoneham MD, Stamou D, Mason J, Hardman JG. Regional anaesthesia for carotid endarterectomy. Br J Anaesth 2014;114:372–83.

Munirama S, McLeod G. Ultrasound-guided femoral and sciatic nerve blocks. Contin Educ Anaesth Crit Care Pain 2013;13:136–40.

Purushothaman L, Allan AGL, Bedforth N. Ultrasound-guided ankle block. Contin Educ Anaesth Crit Care Pain 2013;13:174–78.

Tighe SQM, Greene MD, Rajadurai N. Paravetebral block. Contin Educ Anaesth Crit Care Pain 2010;10:133–37.

Chapter 4.3

Central Neuraxial Blockade

Ayman Mustafa, Graeme McLeod

Intrathecal anaesthesia has been practised for over 100 years. The intrathecal use of cocaine was first described by August Bier in 1898 and the use of intrathecal opioids was first described in 1901 by a Romanian surgeon, Nicolae Racoviceanu-Pitesti. In 1979, Mourad Behar and colleagues published the first report on the extradural use of morphine. Intradural and extradural anaesthesia is widely practised for both surgery and obstetrics.

This chapter outlines the anatomy of the spinal column and the pharmacodynamics of local anaesthetics and opioids, and describes the different modes of spinal and extradural anaesthesia, indications for intervention, clinical efficacy, side effects and outcomes associated with neuraxial block.

ANATOMY

Vertebral Column

The vertebral column consists of 7 cervical, 12 thoracic, 5 lumbar, 5 sacral and 4–5 coccygeal vertebrae. The vertebral column has four curves – the anterior convexity of the sacrum, the lumbar lordosis, the thoracic kyphosis and the cervical lordosis.

In the supine position the fourth lumbar vertebra marks the highest point of the lumbar curve and the fourth or fifth thoracic vertebra is the lowest point of the dorsal curve.

At least one-quarter of the length of the vertebral column is made up of intervertebral discs, each consisting of an outer cover, the annulus fibrosis, enclosing a core of gelatinous material, the nucleus pulposus. The discs give flexibility to the column and act as shock absorbers.

The vertebral bodies and intervertebral discs are held together throughout the length of the spine by the anterior and posterior longitudinal ligaments. Posterior to the vertebral bodies and posterior longitudinal ligament are the vertebral canal and the spinous processes.

466

The spinous processes of the cervical, upper thoracic and lumbar vertebrae are almost horizontal and lie posterior to the bodies of their respective vertebra. The other spinous processes are inclined downwards, their tips being opposite the bodies of the vertebrae immediately below. Maximal inclination is present in the midthoracic region (between the fifth and eighth thoracic vertebrae).

The spinous processes are held vertically together by the interspinous ligament, except in the cervical spine, where it is absent. Anteriorly, it fuses with the ligamenta flava and the laminae. Posteriorly, the interspinous ligament blends with the strong supraspinous ligament that runs along the tips of the spinous processes and blends with the ligamentum nuchae at its superior end. In the elderly the ligament can become ossified, making a midline approach to the extradural space difficult.

The vertebral canal is bordered posteriorly by the spinous processes and interspinous ligaments, laterally by the pedicles and posterolaterally by the laminae and ligamenta flava, a thick, yellow elastic structure that passes from lamina to lamina and connects in the midline. The lateral halves of the ligamenta flava meet variably in the midline at an angle less than 90° and form a steeply arched roof over the lumbar posterior extradural space.

A midsagittal gap between the ligamenta flava in the midline is common (50%) in the thoracic and cervical regions. It may contribute to a variable loss of resistance when the midline approach is used to enter the extradural space.

The vertebral canal ends superiorly in the foramen magnum and inferiorly in the sacral hiatus.

The vertebral canal consists of spinal cord, spinal membranes, adipose tissue, blood vessels, cerebrospinal fluid (CSF) and the roots of spinal nerves.

Degenerative joint disease and ageing can narrow the intervertebral foramina and prevent the spread of local anaesthetic out of the foramina, resulting in greater longitudinal spread in the extradural space.

Spinal Cord

The spinal cord is the extension of the central nervous system (CNS) into the upper two-thirds of the vertebral canal. It is 45-cm long in the average adult, extending from the upper border of the atlas to the upper border of the second lumbar vertebra. At its upper end, the spinal cord is continuous with the medulla oblongata and below with the conus medullaris, from which the filum terminale descends as far as the coccyx. There are two enlargements of the cord, one in the cervical, the other in the lumbar region, corresponding to the origins of the nerves of the arms and legs.

In adult life, the cauda equina consists of vertical lumbar and sacral nerves bathed in CSF that descend to meet their respective foramina.

The spinal cord receives its vascular supply from three arteries, one anterior and two posterior. The anterior spinal artery, a single vessel lying in the substance of the pia mater overlying the anterior median fissure, arises at the level of the foramen magnum from the junction of a small branch from each vertebral artery. It receives communications from the intercostal, lumbar and other small arteries and supplies the lateral and the anterior columns, comprising three-quarters of the substance of the cord. Thrombosis of this artery causes anterior spinal artery syndrome.

The posterior spinal arteries, two on each side, branch from the posterior inferior cerebellar arteries at the level of the foramen magnum. They supply the posterior columns that carry fibres responsible for position, touch and vibration sense. Communicating branches at the level of the first and eleventh thoracic vertebrae are larger than the others (arteries of Adamkiewicz) and help to supply the cervical and lumbar enlargements of the cord. The artery at the level of the eleventh thoracic vertebra supplies the cord both upwards and downwards, and at the level of the first thoracic vertebra only downwards from this level.

Three membranes (dura, arachnoid and pia mater) ensheath the spinal cord. The dura is the outermost membrane. It is a strong fibrous sheath consisting of collagen and elastin fibres. Dural fibres are actually arranged in a complex, overlapping lattice, suggesting that the position of needle bevel has little influence on the size and shape of the dural hole.

Within the cranium, the dura is composed of an outer endosteal component that lies against the bone of the cranium and an inner meningeal layer. Both layers are tightly adherent except where they divide to form the venous sinuses. Within the vertebral column, the dural layers separate. The inner, meningeal layer of the cerebral dura mater forms the spinal dura mater and the cranial endosteal layer continues as periosteum lining the vertebral canal, thus forming the extradural space, closed off from the cranial vault. The extradural space communicates freely with the paravertebral space through the intervertebral foramina and caudally ends at the sacral hiatus.

Epidural Space and Meninges

The extradural space contains loose areolar connective tissue, fat, lymphatics, arteries, an extensive plexus of veins and the spinal nerve roots as they exit the dural sac and pass through the intervertebral foramina.

The anteroposterior dimension of the posterior extradural space varies markedly throughout the length of the extradural space. In the cervical region the posterior extradural space averages 1–2 mm, whereas in the lumbar region it averages 5–6 mm.

The lumbar extradural space has been anatomically described as segmented and discontinuous due to the predominance of lumbar extradural fat, wedged between dura and the side walls of the vertebral canal, dividing the extradural space into anterior, lateral and posterior segments.

Segmentation may impede the passage of an extradural catheter and promote coiling and misplacement. In addition, direct injection of local anaesthetic into extradural fat may account for a prolonged latency of clinical effect. In contrast, the thoracic extradural space is more continuous; it has less fat than the lumbar region and dura is less likely to contact bone. Thus, extradural catheters placed in the midthoracic interspaces may pass with greater ease.

Segmentation of the extradural space not only impedes extradural catheter placement but also causes maldistribution of local anaesthetics and unilateral or patchy anaesthesia. The greater the volume of injectate, the more homogenous the spread as channels open up. Injected solution travels preferentially towards the nerve roots and through the intervertebral foramina, although with some restriction exerted by the fascia of the posterior longitudinal ligament.

A network of valveless veins connecting the head and the pelvis fills the anterior thoracic extradural space. Venous return from the pelvis passes through the extradural venous plexus to the azygos vein, bypassing the inferior vena cava (IVC). Thus, any obstruction to IVC flow from an increase in intra-abdominal pressure (coughing or straining) or an intra-abdominal mass (pregnancy or tumour) redirects venous return through the vertebral venous plexus.

Dilated extradural veins pose many problems for the anaesthetist. In particular, the risk of entering veins during extradural catheter insertion and inadvertent intravenous injection is increased. Dilatation of veins decreases extradural space volume, distributing local anaesthetics more widely and increasing the extent of anaesthetic block.

The arachnoid membrane is a membrane of flat, overlapping cells with tight junctions closely applied to the dura. Although only eight cells thick, the arachnoid membrane presents the greatest barrier to drug transport from the extradural space to the cerebrospinal fluid (CSF).

The space between the dura and arachnoid is termed the subdural space. Although a potential space, malposition of an extradural needle and injection of local anaesthetic between the dura and arachnoid creates a hydrospace, extending widely into thoracic and lumbar regions and providing rapid clinical pain relief. If suspected, the extradural catheter should be immediately removed as migration through the thin arachnoid mater into CSF can easily occur and precipitate total spinal anaesthesia.

The pia is a fenestrated, single layer of flat epithelial cells that is tightly adherent to the spinal cord and sends delicate septa into its substance. From each lateral surface of the pia mater a fibrous band, the denticulate ligament, projects into the subarachnoid space and is attached by a series of pointed processes to the dura as far down as the first lumbar nerve. The pia mater is separated from the arachnoid by CSF within the subarachnoid space, a continuation of the ventricular system CSF at the base of the brain.

Cerebrospinal fluid lies between the arachnoid and the pia within the spinal canal. The total volume of CSF, including CSF within the ventricles and around the cisterns of the brain, is between 100 and 150 mL.

Cerebrospinal fluid is formed from the choroid plexuses of the four cerebral ventricles at a rate of 800 mL/day, five times the total volume of CSF. The choroid plexus is a protrusion of blood vessels covered by a thin epithelial layer. Compared to plasma, sodium and chloride ion concentrations are greater, and glucose and potassium concentrations are lower in CSF. The pH of CSF is 7.32 but is very responsive to change in CO_2. CSF is reabsorbed by arachnoid villi, which project into the venous sinuses of the brain and veins of the spinal cord.

Lumbosacral CSF volume varies considerably between 40 mL and 80 mL and is the principal determinant of intrathecal spread of drugs.

Spinal Nerves

There are 31 pairs of spinal nerves: 8 cervical, 12 thoracic, 5 lumbar, 5 sacral and 1 coccygeal. Each main spinal nerve is formed in the intervertebral space from the convergence of anterior and posterior roots. The perineurium of the spinal nerves is formed from pia and arachnoid membranes and the epineurium is formed from the dura. The spinal nerve trunks subsequently divide into anterior and posterior primary divisions.

Nerve roots differ in size between the thoracic and lumbar regions. The diameter of thoracic roots is half that of lumbar roots, although much variability in root sizes occurs between individuals.

Arachnoid granulations up to 3 mm in diameter cluster around the nerve roots in the dural cuff region. They emerge through the dura and press into surrounding veins and extradural fat. Arachnoid granulations clear the CSF of foreign particulate material by emptying directly into the extradural venous plexus or by lymphatic drainage. Transport of drugs back into the CSF by this route does not occur.

Sympathetic Chain

Efferent fibres arising from cell bodies in the lateral columns of the spinal cord between the first thoracic and the second lumbar segmental levels travel in the anterior primary rami of spinal nerves then pass in white rami communicantes to the sympathetic chain.

The sympathetic chain consists of two long nerve strands, one on each side of the vertebral column, that extend from the base of the skull to the coccyx. Each trunk consists of a series of ganglia, interconnected by bundles of nerve fibres (interganglionic rami) to form a chain. The sympathetic ganglia contains the cell bodies of postganglionic sympathetic effector neurons. The nonmyelinated axons of the postganglionic neurons are distributed to the periphery by a variety of routes: grey rami communicantes back to the spinal nerves, prevertebral plexuses in front of the vertebral column and periarterial plexuses.

The cervical part of the sympathetic trunk consists of three interconnecting ganglia, the superior, middle and inferior. The latter is fused with the first thoracic ganglion to form the stellate ganglion, positioned between C7 and T1 in front of the seventh cervical transverse process and neck of the first rib.

Interruption of preganglionic input or postganglionic outflow from the stellate ganglion produces Horner's syndrome, which includes dropping of the upper eyelid (ptosis), a small pupil, and absence of sweating on the affected side of the head and neck.

The sympathetic trunks enter the thorax from the neck, descend in front of the heads of the ribs and enter the abdomen by piercing the crura of the diaphragm. In the thorax, each trunk has 11 or 12 separate ganglia of varying sizes, including the stellate described above.

The thoracic sympathetic trunks give rise to delicate cardiac and pulmonary mediastinal branches and to larger branches called splanchnic nerves. In the abdomen and pelvis, the two sympathetic trunks descend on the vertebral column, adjacent to the psoas major muscles. The right trunk lies behind the IVC, the left one beside the aorta. The trunks continue into the pelvis, where they lie on the pelvic surface of the sacrum.

Postganglionic fibres within the abdomen form plexuses such as the coeliac plexus, intermesenteric plexus and the superior hypogastric plexus. The coeliac plexus spreads down the abdominal aorta and all its branches, giving rise to subsidiary perivascular plexuses, named according to the blood vessels along which they pass.

Peripheral nerves are comprised of thousands of nerve fibres. They contain either sensory or motor fibres of the somatic and autonomic nervous systems, but sometimes both in combination.

CENTRAL NEURAXIAL BLOCKADE

Central neuraxial blockade is obtained by:

- Intradural anaesthesia
- Extradural anaesthesia
- Combined intradural and extradural anaesthesia
- Continuous intradural anaesthesia

Intradural Anaesthesia

Single-injection intradural (spinal) anaesthesia is simple to administer, with rapid onset and offset of sensory and motor block. It is used as a single technique for ambulatory surgery and for major surgery when combined with long-acting intrathecal opioids, extradural anaesthesia or regional lower limb block. Spinal anaesthesia has a faster onset of action and fewer complications than epidurals, and a more predictable onset, duration and offset than regional limb blocks. The rapid onset of spinal anaesthesia reduces the need for general anaesthesia for urgent caesarean section, thus minimizing the risk of failed intubation and acid aspiration. General anaesthesia in pregnancy is associated with a tenfold increase in failure to intubate the trachea and has been shown, since the first audit of maternal morbidity and mortality in 1950, to have contributed to maternal and fetal death.

Extradural Anaesthesia

Extradural (epidural) analgesia is the central neuraxial method of choice for relieving pain in labour, particularly when combined with opioids such as fentanyl or sufentanil.

The advantage of lumbar extradural analgesia is that extension and increased depth of the extradural block for operative delivery is readily obtained by injection of local anaesthetic. Potential side effects include visceral pain from traction of the peritoneum during caesarean section and local anaesthetic toxicity (convulsions, torsades de pointes) after inadvertent intravascular injection.

In contrast, placement of an extradural catheter into a thoracic interspace provides anaesthesia for abdominal when combined with general anaesthesia. Postoperative titration of analgesia provides optimal pain relief on awakening from surgery and for several days without recourse to intravenous opioids. Sufficient freedom from pain to allow deep breathing and coughing without restriction goes some way towards attenuating the incidence of hypoxaemic episodes and pulmonary complications experienced after surgery.

Combined Intradural and Extradural Anaesthesia

Combined spinal epidural (CSE) anaesthesia is a combination of intradural and extradural techniques. It has a faster onset of action than extradural analgesia for the provision of pain relief in labour.

For CSE, the overall balance of benefit versus risk improves when analgesia is requested in late labour or for long arduous labours (dystocia). Combined spinal extradural would not seem to offer significant advantage in terms of mode of delivery compared to low dose extradural analgesia.[1,2]

Continuous Intradural Anaesthesia

Continuous spinal anaesthesia (CSA) combines the advantages of a single-dose spinal with that of a continuous technique. Advantages include direct application of local anaesthetic and opioid to the CSF, attenuation of the neurohormonal stress response, titration of profound anaesthetic block, relative cardiovascular stability when used in small doses and little risk of toxicity.

CSA allows the use of regional anaesthesia when extradural anaesthesia is relatively contraindicated (severe cardiac disease) or might be difficult (severe obesity). However, catheters may unknowingly travel caudad or cephalad. Lidocaine administration via a caudal micro-catheter has led to cauda equina syndrome. A retrospective review has shown no serious complications associated with intrathecal catheters. The failure rates were

3% for intentional placements and 6% following accidental dural puncture. However, postdural puncture headache (PDPH) occurred in two out of five patients.[3]

PREPARATION FOR CENTRAL NEURAXIAL BLOCKADE

Preparation for central neuraxial blockade consists of:

- Assessment, explanation, consent and examination of the patient
- Obtaining venous access
- Commencing intravenous infusion
- Establishing monitoring of the patient (oxygen saturation, ECG, noninvasive blood pressure, etc.)
- Checking the anaesthetic machine
- Ensuring that the operating table tilts
- Making sure that anaesthetic drugs are available (thiopental or propofol, suxamethonium, atropine)
- Ensuring that a defibrillator is available

The patient can be positioned in the sitting or lateral position. If heavily sedated or ill, the patient should be placed in the lateral position with his or her back parallel to the edge of the table and knees and head flexed. For caesarean section, intrathecal injection is frequently performed in the right lateral position to avoid unilateral left-sided spinal anaesthesia when women are turned supine with a left lateral tilt after the injection. Many anaesthetists find the sitting position easier than the lateral position. The patient is placed across the table or bed with their feet resting comfortably on a stool and the spine should be flexed with the chin pressed on to the sternum. A pillow on the knees gives helpful support to the arms.

Site of Insertion for Central Neuraxial Blockade

Spinal anaesthesia, CSE and continuous spinal catheters should be placed between the third and fourth lumbar vertebrae. Tuffier's line joining the posterior superior iliac spines is unreliable because as a guide it does not always pass through the body of the fourth lumbar vertebra. The tip of the conus usually lies between the first and second lumbar vertebrae, but it may extend further.

Thoracic extradural catheters should be inserted at the interspace corresponding to the middle of the surgical wound. Although the decision to perform regional anaesthesia on a patient under general anaesthesia remains contentious, it is preferable to perform thoracic extradural anaesthesia while the patient is lightly sedated. Insertion of a spinal or extradural needle in an awake patient has two principal benefits; lancinating pain warns the anaesthetist of any potential neurological damage, and the extent of sensory analgesia can be measured before inducing general anaesthesia. Classic landmarks are the root of the spine of scapula at the level of the third thoracic vertebra and the inferior angle of scapula at the level of the seventh thoracic vertebra. Always count up interspaces from that between the third and fourth lumbar vertebrae as a check.

An aseptic technique should be used for all neuraxial blocks. The technique should be the same as for any invasive surgical procedure: hat, mask, handwashing, donning of sterile gown and gloves. The insertion site should be carefully prepared and draped and sterility maintained throughout the procedure. Pain can be minimized by the infiltration of local anaesthetic into the subcutaneous and deeper tissues, especially during the paramedian approach, onto the lamina through the Touhy needle.

Preparation of all drugs should be with a filter needle. It is important to physically separate skin preparation fluid such as chlorhexidine from local anaesthetics to prevent contamination and neural toxicity. Injection of intrathecal drug is easier with a Luer lock 3 mL syringe. This prevents dripping and loss of contents on injection.

Approach for Intradural Anaesthesia

Two approaches exist to the intrathecal or extradural space: midline or paramedian. In the elderly, supraspinal and interspinal ligaments are often calcified, and intervertebral spaces are narrowed. The author's preference is to use the paramedian approach for spinal anaesthesia in the elderly. The spinal introducer is inserted 1–1.5 cm lateral to the midline at the inferior aspect of the intervertebral space and directed slightly caudally about 20° to the midline.

Approach for Extradural Anaesthesia

For extradural anaesthesia, the midline approach is no more difficult in the lower thoracic region compared to lumbar epidurals because of the similar angulation of the spinous processes. In the mid and high thoracic regions, however, extreme upward angulation of the Tuohy needle directed through a small space makes insertion more difficult in the midline. The inferior tip of the spinous process corresponding to the vertebra above should be palpated and, 1 cm lateral to this point, local anaesthetic injected into both skin and the lamina of the vertebral body below. The approach of the needle is about 15° to the midline and 60-65° from the coronal plane. It may be preferable to use the paramedian approach because the bony lamina of the vertebra below acts as a depth finder and there is a definite 'rubbery' feel as the Tuohy needle passes from bony lamina to ligamentum flavum. The thoracic extradural space is identified by two methods, loss of resistance to saline/air or hanging drop. Use of saline is associated with a reduced dural puncture rate.

Ultrasound Imaging for Central Neuraxial Blockade

Preprocedural ultrasound imaging has a role in facilitating neuraxial block, particularly in patients with difficult surface anatomic landmarks. Preprocedural ultrasound helps identify the correct anatomical level for needle insertion and estimates the distance between skin and ligamentum flavum both in the midline and via the paramedian acoustic window.[4]

Ultrasound imaging reduced the risk of failed lumbar punctures and extradural catheterization. Ultrasound imaging also reduced the number of insertion attempts.[5,6]

Contraindications to Central Neuraxial Blockade

Absolute

Absolute contraindications to central neuraxial blockade are as follows:

- Raised intracranial pressure (papilloedema, cerebral oedema, tumours in the posterior fossa, suspected subarachnoid haemorrhage)
- Coagulopathy, blood dyscrasias or full anticoagulant therapy
- Skin sepsis or marked spinal deformity
- Patient refusal
- Hypovolaemia

Relative

A relative contraindication to central neuraxial blockade is mildly impaired coagulation. The risk of spinal haematoma should be weighed against the benefits of avoiding general anaesthesia in patients with platelets less than 80,000/mL. If coagulation is impaired, spinal anaesthesia should be preferred over extradural anaesthesia because of the reduced risk of haematoma formation.

Bioavailability of Drugs Used for Central Neuraxial Blockade

The extent to which drugs reach their site of action is termed bioavailability. Bioavailability is determined by the pharmacological properties of drugs and the relative hydrophobic and hydrophilic properties of tissues. Pharmacological properties of a drug include not only its lipid solubility but also the amount of free, nonprotein-bound unionized drug available to diffuse down a concentration gradient. The higher the pKa of a local anaesthetic or opioid, the greater is its ionization at physiological pH and the less nonionized drug available to diffuse through tissues.

Although the dura is a relatively tough, avascular fibrous membrane, the arachnoid, with its tight overlapping cells, represents 90% of resistance to drug permeability and keeps CSF confined to the subarachnoid space. Drugs are removed primarily from the rich capillary network of subdural vessels apposed to and supplying the underlying arachnoid.

Within the CSF, drugs move by diffusion and bulk flow. Diffusion is proportional to the temperature of solution and inversely to the square of mass. As the mass of drugs administered into CSF is similar, diffusion alone does not explain movement in CSF. Why drugs move cephalad in CSF is attributable to the movement of CSF itself. As arterial blood flows into the brain, compression of the cranial CSF pushes spinal CSF caudally down the posterior surface of the spinal cord then cephalad up the anterior surface of the spinal cord.

The differences in rates of respiratory depression between intrathecal opioids are attributable to clearance into the dorsal horn. Clearance into the dorsal horn or systemic vasculature is dependent on lipid solubility. Lipid-soluble drugs, such as fentanyl, penetrate poorly into the dorsal horn and keep to lipid-soluble white matter. Their volume of distribution is high owing to partitioning within white matter, or into plasma. Water-soluble drugs, such as morphine, penetrate deep into grey matter (lacks myelin) where opioid receptors exist. Thus, water-soluble drugs such as morphine have a greater potency when injected into CSF than do lipid-soluble drugs such as fentanyl.

The common doses of fentanyl and sufentanil used with an extradural or intradural technique in labour analgesia are safe for neonates up to 24 h after delivery.[7]

Clinical Efficacy of Central Neuraxial Blockade

Selective Central Neuraxial Blockade

Intradural and extradural anaesthesia with local anaesthetic blocks the following:

- Autonomic (sympathetic) preganglionic b fibres
- Sensory fibres (Aβ, Aδ, C, conveying temperature, pinprick, touch, pressure, vibration and proprioception)
- Motor fibres (Aα, Aγ)

During central neuraxial blockade, the height of the sympathetic, sensory and motor block follows the same order. Thus, sympathetic block is higher than sensory block, the extent of which varies according to testing modality. A block of T5 to light touch is recommended for confirmation of adequate anaesthesia before caesarean section. However, the corresponding block heights to testing modalities such as ice or pinprick in the same patient may be two to three sensory segments higher. The duration of sensory block is greater than that of motor block.

The rank order of sensitivity to neural block is in the order Aγ > Aδ = Aα > Aβ > C, with faster conducting C fibres (conduction velocity >1 m/s) more sensitive than slower ones (conduction velocity <1 m/s).

INTRADURAL ANAESTHESIA

Efficacy of Intradural Anaesthesia

Spread

The best predictor of spread of intrathecal solutions is CSF volume. This parameter cannot be measured in practice. Clinically, spread of intrathecal local anaesthetic is determined principally by the baricity of the solution and the position of the patient. Baricity is the density of solution relative to CSF. The density of a solution is the mass of drug in g, per mL of solution. Other determinants of spread of local anaesthetic include age, height, body mass index, pregnancy, spinal anatomy, site of injection, direction of needle aperture and tissue fixation.

There is a tendency to increased spread of spinal anaesthesia with increased age, probably owing to decreased CSF volume and increased susceptibility to local anaesthetic block in the elderly. There is no significant correlation between height and spread of spinal anaesthesia within the normal range of adult heights. At the extremes of height, there is a tendency to increased spread because the solution has greater distances to cover. Body mass expressed as the relative weight to surface area (kg/m^2) has an effect on the spread of spinal anaesthesia. Increased spread occurs in obese patients owing to engorgement of extradural veins and compression of the subarachnoid space, and reduction in CSF volume.

Pregnancy

Pregnant patients have a more extensive cephalad spread of spinal block than nonpregnant patients. Several factors may account for this. Progesterone is found in greater amounts in CSF and sensitizes nerves to local anaesthetics. IVC obstruction by the pregnant uterus redirects cardiac return via the extradural venous plexus to the azygous vein and, as in obese patients, compresses CSF. Venous return via the IVC is favoured if the patient lies in a lateral position. The density of local anaesthetics only influences spread of block height in the lateral decubitus position because the effect of IVC obstruction is minimized. However, if the patient is placed in the left tilted 15° position, IVC obstruction becomes the predominant influence on spread and overwhelms the effect of density. Solutions of hypobaric, isobaric and hyperbaric bupivacaine spinal agents all spread to similar high sensory dermatomes in the pregnant patient although heavier solutions had a more rapid onset of action.[8]

Technique

Anatomy of the Spine and Site of Injection

During pregnancy there may be kyphosis, with flattening of the lumbar curvature, or alternatively accentuation of the curvature in addition to the wider female pelvis. Injection in the lateral decubitus position at the interspace between the second and third lumbar vertebrae has a tendency to higher block. However, as with all hypobaric plain solutions, the interindividual spread is irrespective of the chosen interspace. For caesarean section no differences exist between right lateral and left lateral positions and spread of spinal block.

Direction of the Needle Aperture

The direction of the orifice of a pencil-point needle influences the spread of anaesthesia. Spread is less when local anaesthetic is injected caudally compared to cranial orientation of the needle opening. Combined spinal extradural is associated with greater spread, and a greater incidence of hypotension and vasoconstrictor administration than are single-injection spinals.

Fixation

Intrathecal local anaesthetic takes 1–2 h to fix to tissues, not 15 min as was previously thought.

Factors Influencing Onset, Spread and Duration of Spinal Anaesthesia

Baricity of Local Anaesthetic

A hypobaric local anaesthetic is defined as a solution with a density more than three standard deviations (SD) below mean human CSF density. Hypobaric solutions manifest as an unpredictable median sensory block height with a large interindividual spread and are occasionally associated with block failure when the spinal block has not spread high enough for surgery. Hyperbaric solutions are technically solutions with a density more than 3 SD above mean human CSF density. Human CSF density is not uniform and varies according to age, sex, pregnancy and illness (Table 4.3.1).

Density of Local Anaesthetic

All plain solutions of bupivacaine and ropivacaine are hypobaric at 37°C (>3 SD from the density of CSF). The density of levobupivacaine 0.5% with and without dextrose is significantly greater than the corresponding densities of bupivacaine 0.5% and ropivacaine 0.5% at both 23°C and 37°C. The mean density of levobupivacaine 0.75% is 1.00056 g/mL, and it can be regarded as an isobaric solution.

Factors Influencing Density of Local Anaesthetics

The density of local anaesthetics is influenced by temperature, electrolyte composition and the addition of dextrose and opioids. Although changes in density

TABLE 4.3.1 Density of CSF

Group	CSF Density (g/mL) (SD)
Men	1.00067 (0.00018)
Postmenopausal women	1.00060 (0.00015)
Premenopausal women	1.00047 (0.00008)
Pregnant women	1.00033 (0.00010)

may seem minimal and clinically unnecessary, a change in density as low as 0.0006 g/mL may influence spread of local anaesthetic.

Temperature: As the temperature of bupivacaine, levobupivacaine or ropivacaine is reduced, density increases. All concentrations of bupivacaine and ropivacaine are hypobaric when measured at 37°C, but hyperbaric when measured at 23°C.

Electrolyte composition: There is a 13% additional contribution to osmolarity by levobupivacaine compared to bupivacaine. Ampoules of 0.75% levobupivacaine contain 7.5 mg/mL free base (26.0 mmol/L), whereas corresponding ampoules of 0.75% bupivacaine contain 6.66 mg/mL free base, and 7.5 mg hydrochloride (23.1 mmol/L), and ampoules of 0.75% ropivacaine 6.63 mg/mL 7.5 mg hydrochloride (24.1 mmol/L).

Dextrose: Addition of a small amount of dextrose to local anaesthetics increases the density of injectate and provides a reliable and sufficient sensory block within a small range of median maximal block height.

Opioids: Opioids such as fentanyl are hypobaric (0.9933 g/mL), and when added to a local anaesthetic will render the subsequent mixture even more hypobaric. The degree to which this occurs is proportional to the respective densities and volumes of individual drugs.

Spread of Spinal Block

The clinical efficacy of a local anaesthetic may be measured as:

● Time of onset (usually time to attain predefined dermatomal level or maximal block height)
● Duration of action (usually time to predefined block height or time to complete resolution of block)
● Upper and lower sensory levels to sensory testing over time (usually pinprick)

Duration of Spinal Block

The duration of spinal anaesthesia is dependent on the mass of drug – the greater the mass of local anaesthetic injected, the longer the duration. For ambulatory surgery, very small doses of bupivacaine (5 mg) have been successfully used, with duration of block of 60 min. On the other hand, the mean duration of spinal anaesthesia after 20 mg of bupivacaine is 3–4 h. For caesarean section, doses of 10–12.5 mg provide adequate anaesthesia, whereas doses below 10 mg are associated with peritoneal pain.

Potency of Intrathecal Local Anaesthetics

There is little difference between bupivacaine, levobupivacaine and ropivacaine with regard to onset, duration and offset.

Intrathecal Local Anaesthetics

Lidocaine

Lidocaine has a rapid onset of action, intermediate duration and low toxicity with minimal side effects, allowing rapid discharge and high levels of patient satisfaction. There is a dose-dependent increase in duration. Reduction of the intrathecal dose of lidocaine 2% to 40 mg decreased the duration of anaesthesia for outpatient surgery without compromising the quality of spinal block. Disadvantages include its neurotoxicity, with transient neurological symptoms (TNS) as frequent as 33%. TNS are less frequent in the pregnant population.

Prilocaine

A new hyperbaric preparation of prilocaine 2% is available clinically. It has a rapid onset of action and duration limited to 60–90 min. Its primary use is within the day surgery setting.[9]

Chloroprocaine

Chloroprocaine is an ester with similar clinical profile to prilocaine when used for intradural anaesthesia. It is licensed in Europe for surgical procedures up to 40 min. It has a significantly shorter duration of action than lidocaine and is significantly less toxic. Chloroprocaine in doses between 30 mg and 50 mg has a rapid onset time of 3–5 min and a time to ambulation of 90 min.

Bupivacaine

Bupivacaine is the amide local anaesthetic most commonly used for spinal anaesthesia for caesarean section. It exhibits a sensory/motor split but is toxic in overdose. Its relative toxicity compared to that of lidocaine is greater than its relative potency. The frequency of TNS after plain or hyperbaric bupivacaine is small. It is also safe in CSA. In low concentrations (0.1%–0.125%) it can also be used alone or in combination with opioids to provide postoperative analgesia.

Levobupivacaine

Very little difference exists in the spread, duration and offset of intrathecal block between bupivacaine and levobupivacaine as the plain or hyperbaric solutions over a range of doses from 4 mg to 12 mg.

Intrathecal Opioids

Addition of opioids such as fentanyl (12.5 μg), sufentanil (2.5–5 μg), morphine (100–200 μg) and diamorphine (300 μg) improves analgesic quality, prolongs sensory block, reduces local anaesthetic requirements, reduces the duration of motor blockade and improves haemodynamic stability. Intraoperative analgesic supplementation in caesarean section is reduced from 24% to 4%. All increase the duration of postoperative analgesia.

Morphine

Morphine improves the quality of spinal anaesthesia and postoperative pain relief lasts over 18 h. The small dose of morphine used in local anaesthetics for spinal has an additive effect.

Diamorphine

Diamorphine is only available in the UK. Diacetylmorphine breaks down quickly to morphine within the spinal cord. The CSF clearance is twice that of morphine.

Fentanyl

Fentanyl has high lipid solubility, a very large volume of distribution in the spinal cord and rapid clearance from the CSF. The dose is 10–25 µg. Pruritus is common with a higher dose. The addition of 10 µg fentanyl to 5 mg bupivacaine for day-case surgical knee arthroscopy increased success from 75%–100% without prolonging discharge time or time to micturition. It may decrease the incidence of TNS with lidocaine. There is little difference in the extradural and intrathecal doses of fentanyl and sufentanil. It does not reduce patient-controlled analgesia (PCA) morphine consumption. Some studies have shown an increase in PCA requirements after intrathecal fentanyl compared to controls.

Sufentanil

Sufentanil has high lipid solubility, a very large volume of distribution in the spinal cord and rapid clearance from CSF. Intrathecal sufentanil in 2.5–7.5 µg doses has been found to relieve labour pain and improves the quality of caesarean section spinal anaesthesia.

EXTRADURAL ANAESTHESIA AND ANALGESIA

Site of Injection

Spread depends on the site of injection and type of operation:

- Lumbar extradural for labour[10]
- Lumbar extradural for caesarean section
- Thoracic extradural for abdominal surgery
- Lumbar extradural for abdominal surgery

Insertion of a lumbar extradural for abdominal surgery may compromise outcome compared to a well-managed thoracic epidural. Lumbar sensory block for abdominal surgery is difficult to maintain, rescue analgesia is required more often and motor block is inevitable. As sympathetic blockade is extended to the lower limbs, baroreceptor-mediated reflex vasoconstriction is limited to areas cephalad to the block, increasing the likelihood of coronary vasoconstriction and myocardial ischaemia. Furthermore, following large blood loss, decreases in mean arterial pressure, systemic vascular resistance and base excess are significantly larger in the presence of extensive thoracolumbar blockade compared to selective thoracic blockade or general anaesthesia alone. The Bezold–Jarisch reflex, characterized by bradycardia, vasodilation and hypotension is also more common with extensive lumbar epidural blocks. Only by restricting spread to the lumbar and low thoracic regions can lumbar epidural block restrict splanchnic sympathetic blockade, maintain venous return and lessen hypotension. Therefore, the evidence suggests that lumbar epidural anaesthesia should be avoided in patients undergoing abdominal or thoracic procedures.

Outcomes

Neuraxial anaesthesia for lower-limb revascularization is associated with reduction in the incidence of postoperative pneumonia.[11] A summary of Cochrane systematic reviews of neuraxial blockade revealed that, compared with general anaesthesia, neuraxial block reduced the 30-day mortality (risk ratio [RR] 0.71) based on 20 studies. Neuraxial blockade also decreased the risk of pneumonia (RR 0.45) based on five studies.[12]

Dose of Extradural Local Anaesthetic

Traditionally, mass (the product of volume and concentration) has been regarded as the primary determinant of extradural spread and efficacy although newer studies have shown that efficacy is also concentration dependent. Clinically, a large concentration and small volume of levobupivacaine given as a continuous thoracic extradural infusion provides an equal quality of postoperative analgesia as a small-concentration and large-volume infusion and induces less motor blockade and fewer haemodynamic repercussions.

Mode of Delivery

Three modes of delivery of local anaesthetic can be used:

- Continuous infusion
- Patient-controlled extradural analgesia (PCEA)
- Intermittent bolus

Continuous infusion, despite being the most popular means of administration, is associated with sensory block regression, particularly with local anaesthetic alone. Addition of opioid increases the time to first analgesic rescue. The continued popularity of infusion stems from the perception that it is has fewer cardiovascular and respiratory side effects than bolus alone.

PCEA, usually with a background infusion, allows patient self-titration and sparing of local anaesthetic consumption by up to one-third. The main advantage of PCEA compared to infusion is comparable efficacy, but with a marked reduction in side effects. However, this technique is dependent on an awake, cooperative patient and is not suitable for patients sedated following general anaesthesia. PCEA using large boluses (15 mL) of bupivacaine 0.1% plus 2 μg/mL, without a background infusion, is recommended for labour pain.

Intermittent bolus administration at fixed time intervals has been shown to minimize block regression compared to the same concentration of local anaesthetic given as an infusion after pelvic surgery and during labour.

Choice of Local Anaesthetic

The choice of local anaesthetic may vary when used for:

- Labour
- Caesarean section
- Surgery

Extradural solutions of bupivacaine, levobupivacaine and ropivacaine provide similar onset, quality and duration for pain relief in labour and after surgery.

Combinations of Extradural Drugs

The combination of local anaesthetic and opioid provides best analgesia during labour and after major abdominal surgery. The optimal combination is a mixture of bupivacaine 1-1.25 mg/mL (0.1-0.125%) plus fentanyl 3 μg/mL at infusion rates between 7 and 9 mL/h.

Alternative adjuvants include clonidine, epinephrine (adrenaline) and ketamine. Clonidine, an α2-adrenergic agonist, administered in a dose of 5 μg/h, provides additional pain relief and spares local anaesthetic dosing, reducing motor block. Epinephrine (adrenaline) 1:400,000 has a similar effect when added to mixtures of local anaesthetic and fentanyl.

Ketamine is an N-methyl-D-aspartate (NMDA) receptor antagonist and has been used as an adjuvant to opioids and local anaesthetics within the extradural space. However, evidence now exists that intravenous intraoperative administration of ketamine reduces secondary hyperalgesia at 6 months following surgery. This does not occur with extradural ketamine.

Potency of Extradural Local Anaesthetics

Sequential allocation studies (Fig. 4.3.1) of the minimum effective local analgesic concentration (MLAC) for extradural analgesia in the first stage of labour have shown the EC50 of levobupivacaine to be 0.083%.

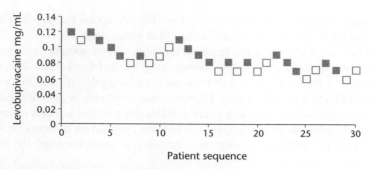

FIGURE 4.3.1   Example of sequential allocation technique. The *y*-axis represents the concentration of local bupivacaine. The *x*-axis shows each successive patient. The blocked squares represent successful block, the empty squares represent unsuccessful block. *Data from Ninewells Hospital.*

Using the same methodology, the EC50 for ropivacaine was between 0.111% and 0.156% whilst bupivacaine was between 0.067% and 0.093%. Recent direct comparisons of levobupivacaine and ropivacaine have shown respectively a 2% and a 19% difference in potency.

Potency of Extradural Adjuvants

The effect of adding epinephrine (adrenaline), fentanyl and sufentanil has also been shown using sequential allocation. The addition of epinephrine (adrenaline) 1:300,000 reduced the EC50 of bupivacaine by a third. Fentanyl at concentrations of 2 μg/mL reduced the EC50 to 0.047%.

Motor Block

Motor block is measured by two subjective scales:

- Modified Bromage scale (0, full power; 1, unable to straighten leg; 2, just able to flex knees; 3, foot movement only)
- Medical Research Council (MRC) straight leg raising score (0, no active contraction; 1, visible palpable contraction without active movement; 2, movement possible with gravity eliminated; 3, movement possible against gravity; 4, movement possible against gravity plus resistance, but weaker than normal; 5, normal power)

Sensory-Motor Split of Extradural Local Anaesthetics

Ropivacaine

An early in vitro study in isolated rabbit vagus nerve was the first to show a preferential blockade of sensory to motor fibres with ropivacaine. The results showed that the depressant effect of bupivacaine was 16% greater than that of ropivacaine on motor fibres, but only 3% greater on sensory fibres. The enhanced differential between sensory and motor blockade was given further standing from an extradural infusion study on volunteers using 0.1%, 0.2%, 0.3% ropivacaine, 0.25% bupivacaine or saline. Over the 21-h study period, sensory block and isometric quadriceps function were measured. The results showed that ropivacaine 0.2% and 0.3% were associated with less motor block than 0.25% bupivacaine.

Levobupivacaine

Widening of the sensory motor split with ropivacaine and levobupivacaine compared to bupivacaine corroborates clinical studies of analgesia in labour using extradural and intrathecal levobupivacaine. Using the same MLAC methodology, and definition of motor block according to the Bromage scale, both ropivacaine and levobupivacaine have been shown to have less propensity for motor block than bupivacaine.

Comparative Potency of Local Anaesthetics for Motor Block

During extradural analgesia for labour, the motor block minimal local analgesic concentration (MLAC) for bupivacaine was 0.33% and for ropivacaine was 0.49%, a potency ratio of 0.66. Whilst the EC50 for levobupivacaine was 0.31% compared to 0.27% for bupivacaine, a potency ratio of 0.87.

The relative importance of motor block depends on the type of surgical procedure, and the depth and duration required of postoperative analgesia. This should be balanced against the clinical properties of each local anaesthetic, such as time of onset, duration of analgesia and motor block and propensity for rescue analgesia. Limb operations, for example, need not only an immobile surgical field, but also postoperative pain relief of such depth that rapid mobilization is possible without motor block to accelerate postoperative function and rehabilitation.

Combination of General Anaesthesia and Extradural Anaesthesia

Induction of general anaesthesia following the establishment of thoracic extradural anaesthesia can precipitate hypotension, particularly with propofol. Hypovolaemia following fasting and/or bowel preparation for surgery will accentuate any drop in blood pressure. Therefore, it is good practice to restore blood volume with intravenous fluids and establish general anaesthesia with intravenous etomidate under direct arterial pressure monitoring. When the patient is anaesthetized, fluids can be titrated according to central venous pressure or oesophageal Doppler monitor. Extradural top-ups of 3–5 mL bupivacaine 0.75% or equivalent are administered judiciously throughout the operation and on wound closure. Alternatively, a constant infusion of extradural solution can be run intraoperatively to minimize fluctuations in blood pressure. Little evidence exists regarding intraoperative management of extradural anaesthesia.

Technical Failure of Extradural Anaesthesia

The benefits of extradural analgesia are limited by technical failure in up to one in seven patients. There are three reasons for failure:[13]

- Primary - epidural never worked 1%–2%
- Secondary - technical problem occurred with the catheter during epidural infusion 7%–10%
- Tertiary - epidural analgesia failed despite a functioning catheter 1%–4%

Leaking at the epidural site after 24 h of infusion is common.

Sacral (Caudal) Extradural Block

Anatomy

The sacrum is a large triangular bone formed by the fusion of the five sacral vertebrae. Its lower extremity is the sacral hiatus, closed by the posterior sacrococcygeal membrane. The hiatus may be many different shapes, ranging from long and narrow to broad. The extradural space below it may range from being deep to excessively shallow – its average length is 10–15 cm.

Technique

An intravenous infusion should be set up, monitoring commenced and the presence of safety resuscitation equipment checked. The patient should be asked to lie in the prone position with hips slightly flexed over two pillows, or in the lateral position with hips flexed. It is important to use a full aseptic technique with cleansing of the skin before insertion of the needle.

The triangular sacral hiatus is palpated at the top of the natal cleft. A 5-cm needle is inserted through the sacrococcygeal membrane at 45°. After aspiration tests for blood and CSF have proved negative, injection is performed. When the needle is correctly placed, injection is easy with no great force being required to depress the plunger of the syringe.

Advantages

Excellent postoperative analgesia is obtained with caudal extradural block. The dose of 0.25% bupivacaine is 0.5–0.75 mL/kg. Caudal extradural block is popular for postoperative analgesia in children (e.g. after circumcision and orchidopexy). It is also useful in adults undergoing haemorrhoidectomy, urological or vaginal procedures, usually combined with light general anaesthesia.

Disadvantages

Disadvantages of caudal extradural block are as follows:

- Length of time taken for development of analgesia.
- Lack of accurate control of height of analgesia.

- Muscular relaxation not maximal in mid and high blocks, although it is excellent in low blocks.
- Technical difficulty if anatomy is abnormal.
- Risk of inadvertent subarachnoid injection if the dura extends downwards.
- Hypotension and possible signs of drug toxicity.
- Complete flaccidity of the anal sphincters (a condition unpopular with some surgeons) has been reported.
- Urinary retention may occur, but is difficult to assess.
- May cause temporary inability to ejaculate in males.

COMBINED INTRADURAL AND EXTRADURAL ANAESTHESIA

The CSE technique was introduced in an attempt to combine the reliability of spinal anaesthesia with the flexibility of epidural anaesthesia.

Historically, four methods of CSE have been used:

- Single-needle, single-interspace
- Double-needle, separate interspaces
- Needle-through-needle, single interspace
- Needle-beside-needle, single-interspace

Combined spinal extradural anaesthesia is used regularly in obstetrics for pain relief in labour and anaesthesia for caesarean section. For labour, the standard needle-through-needle approach (long-shafted spinal needle inserted through standard epidural needle) is taken. Intrathecal injection of 1 mL 0.25% bupivacaine with 15–25 μg of fentanyl provides rapid pain relief, which lasts 45–75 min. Use of sufentanil 5 μg instead of fentanyl extends analgesia up to 120 min. Extradural top-ups with 15 mL bupivacaine 0.1% and fentanyl 2 μg/mL provide extended pain relief. CSE offers a faster onset of pain relief. However compared to low dose epidural,[2] there is no difference in ability to mobilize maternal hypotension, rate of caesarean birth or neonatal outcome.[7]

CONTINUOUS INTRADURAL ANAESTHESIA

Continuous spinal anaesthesia with the needle left in place during surgery was first described in 1907. Hurley and Lambert in 1989 described the continuous spinal microcatheter.

The use of micro spinal catheters in the late 1980s and early 1990s led to 12 cases of cauda equina syndrome, culminating in the banning of microcatheters by the US Food and Drug Administration. The characteristic of each case of neurological injury was poor efficacy of block despite an unremitting requirement for local anaesthetic. The reason was that microcatheters had unknowingly turned caudal and 5% lidocaine was repeatedly given. A pool of high-concentration lidocaine surrounded the cauda equina, leading to irreversible damage to sacral nerves and permanent bowel and bladder dysfunction.

Indications for use of continuous spinal catheters are as follows:

- Analgesia for major abdominal, orthopaedic and vascular surgery
- Treatment of PDPH

Dosing requirements are small. Bupivacaine in doses between 2.5 mg and 5.0 mg is sufficient. If dosing becomes overly frequent and relatively ineffective then suspect a caudal catheter position and the catheter removed.

Paraesthesias have been reported in as many 50% of spinal catheter placements. A retrospective study demonstrated that microcatheters were reliable with failure rates between 2% and 6%[3]. However, PDPH occurred in three out of five cases. Serious complications (meningitis, epidural or spinal abscess, haematoma, arachnoiditis or cauda equina syndrome) were rare.

ADVERSE EFFECTS OF CENTRAL NEURAXIAL BLOCKADE

The recognition of the benefits and risks of sympathectomy with regard to cardiac, respiratory gastrointestinal and metabolic function is necessary to manage patients optimally.

Cardiovascular

Sympathetic activation associated with surgery and postoperative pain manifests as tachycardia, hypertension and increased contractility, all of which serve to increase myocardial oxygen consumption. Injured tissues require more oxygen after surgery for repair. However, the response of patients with coronary atherosclerosis to surgical stress differs from that of healthy patients. Sympathetic stimulation may constrict poststenotic coronary arteries and reduce blood supply to the subendocardium.

Hypotension

Bradycardia, vasodilation and hypotension, is associated with extensive lumbar extradural blocks. Hypotension after spinal or extradural anaesthesia can be attributed to reduction in venous return and/or a fall in cardiac output. Bilateral sympathectomy dilates venous capacitance vessels below the level of the spinal block. As two-thirds of the blood volume is contained within the venous capacitance vessels, venous return decreases and consequently reduces cardiac output.

The physiological response to hypotension is compensatory vasoconstriction of veins above the level of the sympathectomy. Thus, the degree to which hypotension occurs is dependent on the height of the block, the extent of venous pooling, particularly within the splanchnic capacitance vessels, and the degree of upper extremity vasoconstriction.

Unlike the venous vasculature, the arterioles retain a significant degree of vasomotor tone during sympathetic blockade. In young healthy subjects with good myocardial function, systemic vascular resistance decreases only moderately (15%–18%), even with significant sympathetic blockade.

Placement of an extradural catheter in an interspace equivalent to the midline of the surgical incision provides a selective sympathectomy and, in patients at risk of perioperative ischaemia, dilates constricted coronary vessels, decreases heart rate and improves cardiac function by reducing preload and afterload and optimizing myocardial oxygen delivery. Only by restricting spread to the lumbar and low thoracic regions can lumbar extradural block restrict splanchnic sympathetic blockade, maintain venous return and lessen hypotension. Therefore, the evidence suggests that lumbar extradural anaesthesia should be avoided in patients undergoing abdominal or thoracic procedures.

The elderly have a more profound drop in blood pressure owing to an exaggerated decrease in systemic vascular resistance to sympathetic blockade compared to younger patients.

Hypotension during Caesarean Section

Sudden hypotension under spinal anaesthesia has been associated with a decline in uteroplacental blood flow and significant fetal acidosis compared to extradural anaesthesia, which may compromise neonatal well-being.

The incidence of hypotension is no greater in severe pre-eclampsia and spinal anaesthesia may be safely performed in this patient group.

Compression of the great vessels within the abdomen by the pregnant uterus, abdominal tumours or abdominal packs may cause severe hypotension in the presence of central neural blockade. Hypovolaemia or sepsis amplify drops in blood pressure after spinal anaesthesia. Systemic absorption of the local anaesthetic drug can depress vascular smooth muscle and myocardial function, with a fall in cardiac output.

Treatment of Hypotension

Treatment of hypotension should be directed towards the underlying mechanisms of decreased cardiac output and systemic vascular resistance. Clinical interventions include 100% oxygen, elevation of the legs, rapid infusion of fluids and intravenous sympathomimetic drugs and in pregnant patients left uterine displacement.

Fluid Management

Crystalloid: Large volumes (12–30 mL/kg) of crystalloid infusion before spinal anaesthesia have shown no difference in the incidence of hypotension probably because large volumes of crystalloid quickly redistribute from the intravascular to the extravascular compartment.

Sympathomimetics: The four most commonly used sympathomimetics are as follows:
- Epinephrine (adrenaline)
- Phenylephrine

- Metaraminol
- Ephedrine

Epinephrine (adrenaline) has the optimal physical structure for producing α- and β-adrenergic effects and represents the prototype drug among the sympathomimetics. Release from the adrenal medulla stimulates:

- Myocardial contractility
- Heart rate
- Vascular and bronchial smooth muscle tone
- Glandular secretions
- Glycogenolysis and lipolysis

Epinephrine (adrenaline) is the most potent activator of α-adrenergic receptors, being 2 to 10 times more active than norepinephrine (noradrenaline). In increasing doses, it stimulates β2, β1 and α1 receptors.

Epinephrine (adrenaline)-induced stimulation of β2 receptors produces peripheral vasodilation and increased flow to skeletal muscle. Stimulation of β1 receptors increases systolic blood pressure, heart rate and cardiac output. There is a modest reduction in diastolic blood pressure, reflecting vasodilation from activation of β2 receptors. The net effect is an increase in pulse pressure and minimal change in mean arterial pressure. Higher doses stimulate α1 receptors in the skin, mucosa and hepatorenal vasculature, producing intense vasoconstriction.

Phenylephrine is a synthetic noncatecholamine. Structurally, it is a 3-hydroxy phenylethylamine differing from epinephrine (adrenaline) only in lacking a 4-hydroxyl group on the benzene ring. Phenylephrine directly and indirectly (by release of norepinephrine [noradrenaline]) stimulates α-adrenergic receptors ($\alpha1 > \alpha2$). It also has a small effect on β-adrenergic receptors. Clinically, it mimics the effects of norepinephrine (noradrenaline) but is less potent and longer lasting. Central nervous system stimulation is minimal. Intravenous phenylephrine produces intense peripheral vasoconstriction, increased systolic and diastolic blood pressure, and reflex bradycardia.

Metaraminol is a synthetic noncatecholamine that, like ephedrine, acts on α- and β-adrenergic receptors by indirect and direct effects. However, it produces more intense peripheral vasoconstriction and a smaller increase in myocardial contractility than ephedrine. Intravenous administration of metaraminol 0.5–2 mg produces a sustained increase in systolic and diastolic blood pressure that is due almost entirely to peripheral vasoconstriction. Vasoconstriction decreases renal and cerebral blood flow and is accompanied by a reflex reduction in heart rate and cardiac output.

Ephedrine is a nonselective direct- and indirect-acting synthetic noncatecholamine acting on α- and β-adrenergic receptors. Its principal mode of action is increased myocardial contractility and rate due to activation of β1 receptors. Higher doses produce α-receptor-mediated peripheral vasoconstriction. Ephedrine has until recently been the choice of vasopressor in obstetric anaesthesia, given in aliquots of 3–6 mg or as a variable infusion of 60 mg ephedrine in 500 mL crystalloid. Subsequent doses of ephedrine are associated with tachyphylaxis. Ephedrine has been administered intramuscularly to prevent maternal hypotension during spinal anaesthesia. However, ephedrine may contribute to fetal acidosis, and phenylephrine has now been recommended as the vasoconstrictor of choice for caesarean section.

Treatment plan: Hypotensive patients with accompanying tachycardia should be given increments of phenylephrine 100 μg or metaraminol 0.5–1 mg. Hypotension with bradycardia may be treated with intravenous ephedrine (3–6 mg). For severe bradycardia, unresponsive to either ephedrine or atropine or in the setting of a precipitous decrease in heart rate, epinephrine (adrenaline) (10–25 μg) should be administered. Higher doses in increments of 100 μg may be required up to 1 mg for cardiac arrest to perfuse coronary arteries.

Respiratory

The muscles responsible for breathing are the diaphragm, the intercostal muscles and the abdominal muscles. After central neuraxial block, changes in inspiratory function are minimal except for slight decreases in vital capacity. In the absence of sedation, minute ventilation, tidal volume, respiratory rate, mean inspiratory flow rates, arterial oxygen tension or carbon dioxide tensions change little, even with high to mid-thoracic blocks.

In contrast, expiratory muscle function is decreased in proportion to the level of spinal anaesthesia, demonstrated by reductions in maximal expiratory pressure and flow rates due to paralysis of abdominal muscles used in forced exhalation. Thus, coughing and clearing of secretions may be impaired after spinal anaesthesia, particularly in patients with pre-existing lung disease. During spinal analgesia breathing becomes quiet and tranquil, due not only to motor blockade but also to deafferentation, with reduction of sensory input to the respiratory centre.

Hypoxaemia during or after spinal anaesthesia is associated with sedative drugs given intravenously or neuraxially. Monitoring of respiratory rate, oxygen saturation, blood pressure and sedation levels during and after spinal anaesthesia is warranted.

Extradural block attenuates reduction in FRC after abdominal surgery better than intravenous opioids, lessens the work of the heart and tends to relieve any pre-existing pulmonary vascular congestion. The effect of block is largely on the cardiovascular system.

High thoracic extradural anaesthesia increases functional residual capacity by a caudal motion of the diaphragm and a concomitant decrease in intrathoracic blood volume. Diaphragmatic function is impaired by stimulation of inhibitory phrenic nerves within the abdomen.

In the elderly, significant reductions in minute ventilation and tidal volume occur, but the ventilatory responses to hypercapnia and hypoxia are maintained when using thoracic extradural anaesthesia.

The American Society of Anesthesiologists task force on neuraxial opioids and the American Society of Regional Anesthesia and Pain Medicine practice have issued guidelines for the prevention, detection and management of respiratory depression associated with neuraxial opioid administration.[14] They recommended that patients with a history of sleep apnoea, diabetes, obesity, need for opioid medication and any adverse effects with the latter constituted a group at higher risk of postoperative respiratory complications. Moreover, they stated that single-injection neuraxial opioids may be safely used in place of parenteral opioids without altering the risk of respiratory depression or hypoxemia. Patients receiving neuraxial opioids should be monitored by measuring respiratory rate, pulse oximetry and level of consciousness. Continuous infusion or patient-controlled epidural analgesia with neuraxial opioids should be monitored at least once per hour until 12 h have passed then once every 2 h until 24 h and every 4 h thereafter.

Apnoea during Spinal and Extradural Anaesthesia

Causes of apnoea during spinal and extradural analgesia include:

- Inadequate medullary blood flow due to inadequate cardiac output – a serious situation demanding immediate cardiorespiratory support
- Total spinal analgesia with denervation of all the respiratory muscles – true phrenic paralysis is uncommon because the motor roots are large
- Accidental subdural injection: a small volume of solution may travel to an unexpectedly high level in this potential space
- Toxic effects of the local analgesic drug
- Injection of an opioid analgesic drug

Treatment

Treatment of apnoea during spinal and extradural anaesthesia is to:

- Control the airway and ventilate the lungs with 100% oxygen
- Diagnose the cause and monitor other vital signs (e.g. arterial pressure, oxygen saturation, level of consciousness, level of block, pupil size, skin rashes)

Gastrointestinal

Preganglionic sympathetic fibres from T5 to L1 are inhibitory to the gut. Innervation of the oesophagus is vagal. Removal of sympathetic activity to the gut reveals unopposed gut vagal activity; sphincters are relaxed, peristalsis is active and the pressure within the bowel lumen is increased. Stimuli arising in the upper abdomen may ascend along the unblocked vagus and phrenics and cause discomfort if the patient is conscious.

The sympathectomy of thoracic extradural anaesthesia has been shown to benefit bowel function by reducing the duration of postoperative ileus and enhancing bowel blood flow.

Splanchnic blockade may also have deleterious haemodynamic consequences because the splanchnic veins contribute substantially to the control of overall venous capacitance. Hence, sympathetic block during intrathecal and extradural anaesthesia vasodilates mesenteric vessels and is associated with hypotension because of reduced venous return. The degree to which blood pressure falls is dependent on the relative extent of splanchnic sympathetic blockade and the degree of baroreceptor-induced vasoconstriction in unblocked regions of the body.

Hypotension can compromise gut mucosal integrity as well as myocardial blood flow. Translocation of endotoxin from the gut lumen and release of inflammatory mediators are the basis of the systemic inflammatory response, leading to increases in capillary permeability and multiorgan failure. Therefore it is important to prevent gut hypoperfusion.

Ephedrine (mixed α and β) or metaraminol (α) in small aliquots is often used to correct hypotension. A low-dose infusion of dopamine or dopexamine (β and δ) at 3–5 μg/kg/min may also be infused to increase mesenteric and hepatic blood flow.

Nausea and Vomiting

Gastric emptying time is quicker when extradural block is employed for postoperative pain relief than when narcotic analgesics are used. Causes of nausea are as follows:

- Hypotension – correction using a pressor drug may relieve nausea
- Increased peristalsis
- Traction on nerve endings and plexuses, especially via the vagus
- Presence of bile in the stomach due to relaxation of the pyloric and bile duct sphincters
- Opioid analgesics (premedication)
- Psychological factors
- Hypoxaemia

Genitourinary

Sympathetic supply to the kidneys is from T11 to L1 via the lowest splanchnic nerves. Any effects on renal function are due to hypotension. Autoregulation of renal blood flow is impaired if mean arterial pressure falls below about 50 mm Hg. Bladder sphincters are not relaxed during sympathetic block and so soiling of the table by urine is not seen, and the tone of ureters is not greatly altered. The second, third and fourth sacral spinal nerves (S2–S4) contain the afferent and efferent pathways responsible for control of the bladder and urethral sphincters.

After the induction of spinal anaesthesia, the urge to void (normal detrusor function) is abolished. The ability to void normally does not return until sensory anaesthesia has regressed to S3. Prolonged inhibition of normal detrusor function with the use of long-acting local anaesthetics, such as bupivacaine, may allow bladder overdistension and urinary retention.

Postoperative urinary retention may result in hypertension, hypotension, bradycardia and damage to the detrusor, leading to incomplete emptying of the bladder and an increased long-term risk of urinary tract infections.

Metabolic

Muscle wasting occurs after surgery because the rate of muscle protein breakdown exceeds the rate of synthesis. Amino acids provide the substrate for gluconeogenesis in the liver, resulting in an elevation in plasma glucose levels and increased insulin resistance. Sympathetic blockade of adrenal catecholamine release restores the balance between muscle synthesis and breakdown, attenuating the rise in plasma glucose. Provision of oral energy substrates before and after surgery, combined with early mobilization, serves to limit muscle and fat breakdown and accelerate rehabilitation.

Hypothermia

Mild perioperative hypothermia can occur with spinal anaesthesia, particularly in the elderly and with extensive blocks. Perioperative hypothermia has been shown to adversely affect the incidence of myocardial ischaemia, cardiac morbidity wound infection, surgical bleeding and patient discomfort. Core hypothermia with spinal anaesthesia develops primarily from a redistribution of heat from core tissues, which are well-perfused tissues such as the head and trunk, to the peripheral tissues, or arms and legs. Therefore, to minimize the risk of intraoperative hypothermia during spinal anaesthesia, the following strategies are recommended:

- First – core temperature should be monitored.
- Second – active warming with forced air warmers should be used if core hypothermia occurs, or its prophylactic use considered in extended operations or high-risk patients.
- Third – intravenous fluids should be warmed to approximately 37°C if large volumes are to be administered.

Neurological

Three national surveys investigating neurological complications of regional anaesthesia have been undertaken. The first, in France, highlighted that neurological injury was greater with intradural anaesthesia compared to extradural anaesthesia.[15] Two-thirds of patients with neurological deficits had either a paresthesia during needle placement or pain on injection. Of those having atraumatic injection, 75% occurred in patients who had received hyperbaric lidocaine, 5%. Seizures due to local anaesthetic were four times more common after regional blockade.

A second French survey identified 56 major complications in 158,083 regional anaesthesia procedures performed (3.5/10,000).[16] Again, spinal anaesthesia was associated with a greater incidence of cardiac arrest, and lidocaine spinal anaesthesia was associated with more neurological complications than was bupivacaine spinal anaesthesia (14.4/10,000 vs 2.2/10,000).

The third survey, the National Audit Project 3 or NAP3[17], was carried out in the UK. It estimated that >700,000 neuraxial blocks were performed annually divided almost equally between obstetric and perioperative patients. The incidence of permanent nerve injury due to neuraxial block was 1 in 24,000 to 1 in 54,000 and the incidence of paraplegia or death was 1 in 50,000 to 1 in 140,000. In contrast to the French audits, three fifths of major complications were associated with extradural block. Of particular concern was the relatively high contribution of CSE to nerve damage (Table 4.3.2).

Postdural Puncture Headache (PDPH)

PDPH was recognized after first spinal anaesthetic in 1898 by Bier and his surgical resident Hildebrandt, who performed spinal anaesthesia on each other. Typical location of the headache is bifrontal and/or occipital. Occasionally, the symptoms involve the neck and upper shoulders. The intensity ranges from mild to excruciating. PDPH rate is worse in the upright position or during coughing or straining. There is associated nausea, photophobia, tinnitus, diplopia and cranial nerve palsy, and rarely cortical vein thrombosis, subarachnoid haemorrhage or subdural haematoma. It is more common in young pregnant patients, greater depth of the epidural space[18] and with accidental dural puncture rate during epidural anaesthesia using Touhy needles (60%–80%). The incidence of PDPH after spinal anaesthesia has been reduced by the introduction of size 25G and 27G Whitacre pencil-point needles, which replaced cutting needles. The autologous epidural blood patch was first described by Gormley in 1960.

Epidural Blood Patch

The epidural blood patch requires two clinicians and an aseptic technique. The epidural is performed at the same space as the previous spinal or epidural if possible. Once the epidural is in place, withdraw 20 mL of blood from the forearm. The blood is carefully and aseptically transferred to the anaesthetist, who injects it slowly through the epidural needle or until pain is felt in the back. Patients should be placed supine for 1–2 h following the procedure to reduce the leakage of CSF from the dural hole. It is successful in 70% of patients but may have to be repeated.

TABLE 4.3.2 Neurological Complications of Central Neuraxial Block

Syndrome	Onset	Duration	Pain	Neurological Symptoms	Treatment
TNS – transient neurological syndrome	6–36 h	1–7 days	Unilateral or bilateral pain in the anterior or posterior thighs extension into legs	Nil	NSAIDs, opioids, warm heat
Chloroprocaine back pain	Immediate onset after extradural regression	1–4 h	Low back pain	Nil	NSAIDs, oral
Extradural haematoma	0–2 days	Requires surgery	Radicular back pain	Muscle weakness, sensory deficit	CT scan, laminectomy
Extradural haematoma	0–2 days	Requires surgery	Backache, fever	Progressive neurologic symptoms	Antibiotics, possible surgical drainage
Spinal nerve	0–2 days	1–12 weeks	Pain during insertion of needle or catheter	Paraesthesia over distribution of nerve root	EMG
Anterior spinal artery syndrome	Immediate		Painless	Paraplegia	Vasodilator drugs
Adhesive arachnoiditis		Chronic	Pain on injection	Variable degree of neurologic	CT or MRI
Cauda equine syndrome		Chronic		Loss of bowel and bladder function, paraplegia, motor weakness, sensory	

Treatment of PDPH

The largest retrospective study was conducted by Verstraete and colleagues.[19] Of the 29,749 epidural blocks performed over 16 years, 0.43% of patients had an accidental dural puncture with an 18G Tuohy needle. Following known ADP, 39 women had an epidural catheter placed at a different level and 89 had an intrathecal catheter (20G) for at least 24 h. Prolonged intrathecal catheter placement reduced the incidence of PDPH after ADP to 42% compared with 62% in those who have the catheter re-sited epidurally.

Cranial Nerve Palsies

Paralysis of every cranial nerve except I, IX and X has been reported after spinal anaesthesia, and transient deafness or tinnitus is not uncommon. Paralysis of the sixth cranial nerve, which innervates the lateral rectus, causes diplopia. The onset is commonly between the fifth and eleventh postoperative days and is associated with headache. It may be delayed for 3 weeks. Paralysis is never complete. About 50% of patients recover within a month.

Intracranial Subdural Haematoma

Intracranial subdural haematoma is a rare but serious complication. A literature review in the obstetrics population revealed 56 cases.[20] The most important symptom was persistent headache (83%) that did not respond to postural changes and associated focal neurological signs were present in 69% of women. One in ten was left with permanent residual neurological deficit and the mortality was 7%.

Cauda Equina Syndrome

Concerns about the use of spinal lidocaine began in the early 1990s with published reports of cauda equina syndrome after CSA and a case report of four patients who experienced aching and pain in the buttocks and lower limbs after spinal anaesthesia.[21] Of the 11 cases of cauda equina syndrome, 10 patients had received doses of lidocaine up to 300 mg, and one patient had received tetracaine (amethocaine). The cause of toxicity was inadvertent caudal placement of microcatheters and pooling of local anaesthetic around the sacral roots. In response to a lower than expected extent of anaesthesia, large doses of drug were given via the intrathecal catheters and exacerbated sacral pooling. In 1992, because of safety concerns, spinal microcatheters were removed from the US market.

Transient Neurological Syndrome

In 1993 Schneider and colleagues published a case report of patients undergoing spinal anaesthesia in the lithotomy position and who, postoperatively, experienced aching and pain in the buttocks and lower limbs. This is now termed transient neurological syndrome (TNS).

Several different laboratory models have proved that all local anaesthetics can be neurotoxic when applied to neural tissues in clinically relevant concentrations, but that lidocaine and tetracaine (amethocaine) are potentially more neurotoxic than bupivacaine. Neurotoxicity of lidocaine is both concentration- and time-dependent but is not related to sodium channel blockade or the addition of glucose.

Surgical position has an important influence on the incidence of TNS. For example, patients undergoing surgery in the lithotomy position have an incidence of TNS of approximately 30%–36%, patients undergoing arthroscopic knee surgery have an incidence of 18%–22% and patients undergoing surgery in the supine position have an incidence of 4%–8%. It is important to emphasize that if a patient presents with an abnormal neurological examination or motor weakness, causes other than TNS must be eliminated.

Extradural Haematoma

Ehrenfeld and colleagues reviewed 43,000 cases during a 9-year period and estimated the incidence of epidural haematoma to be 1 in 430.[22] Anticoagulants such as heparin, low molecular weight heparin (LMWH) or warfarin are given prophylactically to patients in the perioperative period to prevent deep vein thrombosis. However, if neuraxial anaesthesia is administered when a patient is anticoagulated, catastrophic bleeding may occur within the spinal canal during needle or catheter placement or removal. Bleeding inside the spinal canal may lead to spinal cord compression and untoward motor deficit, necessitating immediate CT scan and surgical laminectomy to prevent paraplegia. In 1998, the US Food and Drug Administration reported 43 cases of spinal haematomas in patients who had received spinal or extradural anaesthesia and who had received enoxaparin 30 mg twice daily. Sixteen patients did not recover from paraplegia despite emergency surgery. This was probably due to higher doses administered (enoxaparin 30 mg twice daily) compared to European protocols (enoxaparin 40 mg once daily). Overall, the incidence of bleeding complications due to neuraxial blocks is estimated to be less than 1 in 150,000 for extradural and less than 1 in 220,000 for spinal anaesthesia. Associated risks include use of anticoagulants, thrombocytopenia, chronic alcohol use, chronic renal failure and difficult blocks.

Heparin

Heparin has a half-life of 1–2 h. Unfractionated heparin inhibits factor II (thrombin) as well as factor X. Its bioavailability is weak and unpredictable because endothelial cells and fibrinogen show a high affinity for the unfractionated heparin molecule. Activity is measured by the activated partial thromboplastin time (PTT).

Low Molecular Weight Heparins

LMWHs have a slow onset (90 min) and a half-life of 4 h. Their effects last 12 h.

LMWHs are the gold standard in the prevention of postoperative venous thromboembolism. They have shorter chains than unfractionated heparin and show no interaction with endothelial cells or fibrinogen. Thus, their bioavailability is higher and more reliable than that of standard heparin. Peak anti-X activity occurs 3–4 h after a subcutaneous injection of LMWH. The plasma half-life of LMWH is two to four times that of standard heparin and increases in patients with renal failure. As their activity is more focused on factor X, monitoring of activated PTT is not recommended. Monitoring of anti-Xa activity is advised only in the elderly and in patients with renal failure.

As the plasma half-life of LMWH is 4 h, 12 h is the recommended safe interval following LMWH prophylaxis for placement of a central neuraxial block or removal of an extradural catheter. Nevertheless, a delay of 24 h is recommended in cases of administration of LMWH in higher doses (e.g. enoxaparin 1 mg/kg twice daily) for treatment of deep venous thrombosis and pulmonary embolism.

Warfarin

Warfarin blocks factors II, VII, IX and X as well as proteins C and S. As the plasma half-lives of these proteins are different (7 h for factor VII, 36 h for factor X and 50 h for factor II), we can observe an early increase in prothrombin time (PT) and international normalized ratio (INR) due to a decrease in factor VII, whereas the fully anticoagulant effect is not achieved before 72–96 h (factors II, IX and X decrease). The INR should be less than 1.4 before performing a neuraxial block and before removal of a spinal or extradural catheter. In patients receiving chronic warfarin medication, the PT and INR require 3–5 days to normalize after discontinuation of the drug. It is mandatory to document normal coagulation status before performing any neuraxial block in such a setting.

Antiplatelet Drugs

The effects of new antiplatelet drugs such as clopidogrel seem more pronounced than those of aspirin or nonsteroidal anti-inflammatory drugs (NSAIDs). In addition, the mechanisms of inhibiting platelet functions differ; aspirin and NSAIDs inhibit cyclooxygenase, leading to a decrease in thromboxane A2 synthesis by platelets and a decrease in prostacyclin synthesis by endothelial cells. Clopidogrel inhibits the ADP pathway necessary for platelet aggregation.

Neither aspirin alone nor NSAIDs without additional factors are considered significant factors for the development of spinal haematoma after central neuraxial anaesthesia. However, when these drugs are associated with other drugs affecting coagulation (heparin, antiplatelet drugs, etc.) or with multiple and difficult punctures, they may increase the bleeding risk inside the spinal canal, thus making possible the occurrence of a compressive spinal haematoma. In elective cases, aspirin and clopidogrel should be stopped 7 and 10 days before surgery, respectively. If the underlying medical disease is serious (e.g. carotid stenosis, recent coronary event), they should be replaced with subcutaneous heparin or LMWH until 12 h before surgery.

Central Neuraxial Blockade and Thromboprophylaxis

The decision to perform neuraxial block should be made on an individual basis, balancing benefit versus risk. The patient's coagulation status should be optimized at the time of spinal or extradural needle or catheter placement, and the level of anticoagulation must be carefully monitored during the period of extradural catheterization. Indwelling catheters should not be removed in the presence of therapeutic anticoagulation because this appears to significantly increase the risk of spinal haematoma. Vigilance in monitoring is critical to allow early evaluation of neurological dysfunction and prompt intervention. Table 4.3.3 summarizes current drugs used for thromboprophylaxis and their recommended conditions of use.

TABLE 4.3.3 Summary of Anticoagulants Available and Recommendations for Practice[23]

Drug	Time to Peak Effect	Elimination Half-Life	Acceptable Time after Drug for Block Performance	Administration of Drug while Spinal or Epidural Catheter in Place	Acceptable Time after Block Performance or Catheter Removal for Next Drug Dose
Heparin					
UFH SC prophylaxis	<30 min	1–2 h	4 h or normal APTTR	Caution	1 h
UFH i.v. treatment	<5 min	1–2 h	4 h or normal APTTR	Caution	4 h
LMWH SC prophylaxis	3–4 h	3–7 h	12 h	Caution	4 h
LMWH SC treatment	3–4 h	3–7 h	24 h	Not recommended	4 h
Heparin alternatives					
Danaparoid prophylaxis	4–5 h	24 h	Avoid (consider anti-Xa levels)	Not recommended	6 h
Danaparoid treatment	4–5 h	24 h	Avoid (consider anti-Xa levels)	Not recommended	6 h
Bivalirudin	5 min	25 min	10 h or normal APTTR	Not recommended	6 h
Argatroban	<30 min	30–35 min	4 h or normal APTTR	Not recommended	6 h

TABLE 4.3.3 Summary of Anticoagulants Available and Recommendations for Practice[23]—cont'd

Drug	Time to Peak Effect	Elimination Half-Life	Acceptable Time after Drug for Block Performance	Administration of Drug while Spinal or Epidural Catheter in Place	Acceptable Time after Block Performance or Catheter Removal for Next Drug Dose
Fondaparinux prophylaxis	1–2 h	17–20 min	36–42 h (consider anti-Xa levels)	Not recommended	6–12 h
Fondaparinux treatment	1–2 h	17–20 h	Avoid (consider anti-Xa levels)	Not recommended	12 h
Antiplatelet drugs					
NSAIDs	1–12 h	1–12 h	No additional precaution	No additional precaution	No additional precaution
Aspirin	12–24 h	Not relevant, irreversible	No additional precaution	No additional precaution	No additional precaution
Clopidogrel	12–24 h	Not relevant, irreversible	7 days	Not recommended	6 h
Prasugrel	15–30 min		7 days	Not recommended	6 h
Ticagrelor	2 h	8–12 h	5 days	Not recommended	6 h
Tirofiban	<5 min	4–8 h	8 h	Not recommended	6 h
Eptifibatide	<5 min	4–8 h	8 h	Not recommended	6 h
Abciximab	<5 min	24–48 h	48 h	Not recommended	6 h
Dipyridamole	75 min	10 h	No additional precaution	No additional precaution	6 h

Continued

TABLE 4.3.3 Summary of Anticoagulants Available and Recommendations for Practice[23] — cont'd

Drug	Time to Peak Effect	Elimination Half-Life	Acceptable Time after Drug for Block Performance	Administration of Drug while Spinal or Epidural Catheter in Place	Acceptable Time after Block Performance or Catheter Removal for Next Drug Dose
Oral anticoagulants					
Warfarin	3–5 days	4–5 days	INR ≤ 1.4	Not recommended	After catheter removal
Rivaroxaban prophylaxis (CrCl >30 mL/min)	3 h	7–9 h	18 h	Not recommended	6 h
Rivaroxaban treatment (CrCl >30 mL/min)	3 h	7–11 h	48 h	Not recommended	6 h
Dabigatran prophylaxis or treatment (CrCl >80 mL/min) (CrCl 50–80 mL/min) (CrCl 30–50 mL/min)	0.5–2.0 h 0.5–2.0 h 0.5–2.0 h	12–17 h 15 h 18 h	48 h 72 h 96 h	Not recommended Not recommended Not recommended Not recommended	6 h 6 h 6 h
Apixaban prophylaxis	3–4 h	12 h	24–48 h	Not recommended	6 h
Thrombolytic drugs					
Alteplase, anistreplase, reteplase, streptokinase	<5 min	4–24 min	10 days	Not recommended	10 days

Notes: APTTR, activated partial thromboplastin time ratio; CrCl, creatinine clearance; i.v., intravenous; s.c., subcutaneous; UFH, unfractionated heparin.

REFERENCES

1. Heesen M, Van de Velde M, Klohr S, Lehberger J, Rossaint R, Straube S. Meta-analysis of the success of block following combined spinal-epidural vs epidural analgesia during labour. Anaesthesia 2014;69:64–71.

2. Simmons SW, Taghizadeh N, Dennis AT, Hughes D, Cyna AM. Combined spinal-epidural versus epidural analgesia in labour. Cochrane Database Syst Rev 2012;10:CD003401.

3. Cohn J, Moaveni D, Sznol J, Ranasinghe J. Complications of 761 short-term intrathecal macrocatheters in obstetric patients: a retrospective review of cases over a 12-year period. Int J Obstet Anesth 2016;25:30–36.

4. Chin KJ, Karmakar MK, Peng P. Ultrasonography of the adult thoracic and lumbar spine for central neuraxial blockade. Anesthesiology 2011;114:1459–85.

5. Chin KJ, Perlas A. Ultrasonography of the lumbar spine for neuraxial and lumbar plexus blocks. Curr Opin Anaesthesiol 2011;24:567–72.

6. Shaikh F, Brzezinski J, Alexander S, Arzola C, Carvalho JC, Beyene J, et al. Ultrasound imaging for lumbar punctures and epidural catheterisations: systematic review and meta-analysis. BMJ 2013;346:f1720.

7. Wang K, Cao L, Deng Q, Sun LQ, Gu TY, Song J, et al. The effects of epidural/spinal opioids in labour analgesia on neonatal outcomes: a meta-analysis of randomized controlled trials. Can J Anaesth 2014;61:695–709.

8. Sng BL, Siddiqui FJ, Leong WL, Assam PN, Chan ES, Tan KH, et al. Hyperbaric versus isobaric bupivacaine for spinal anaesthesia for caesarean section. Cochrane Database Syst Rev 2016:CD005143.

9. Boublik J, Gupta R, Bhar S, Atchabahian A. Prilocaine spinal anesthesia for ambulatory surgery: A review of the available studies. Anaesth Crit Care Pain Med 2016;35:417-421.

10. Grant EN, Tao W, Craig M, McIntire D, Leveno K. Neuraxial analgesia effects on labour progression: facts, fallacies, uncertainties and the future. Br J Obstet Gynaecol 2015;122:288–93.

11. Barbosa FT, Juca MJ, Castro AA, Cavalcante JC. Neuraxial anaesthesia for lower-limb revascularization. Cochrane Database Syst Rev 2013:CD007083.

12. Guay J, Choi P, Suresh S, Albert N, Kopp S, Pace NL. Neuraxial blockade for the prevention of postoperative mortality and major morbidity: an overview of Cochrane systematic reviews. Cochrane Database Syst Rev 2014:CD010108.

13. Hermanides J, Hollmann MW, Stevens MF, Lirk P. Failed epidural: causes and management. Br J Anaesth 2012;109:144–54.

14. Practice Guidelines for the Prevention, Detection, and Management of Respiratory Depression Associated with Neuraxial Opioid Administration: An Updated Report by the American Society of Anesthesiologists Task Force on Neuraxial Opioids and the American Society of Regional Anesthesia and Pain Medicine. Anesthesiology 2016;124:535–52.

15. Auroy Y, Narchi P, Messiah A, Litt L, Rouvier B, Samii K. Serious complications related to regional anesthesia: results of a prospective survey in France. Anesthesiology 1997;87:479–86.

16. Auroy Y, Benhamou D, Bargues L, Ecoffey C, Falissard B, Mercier FJ, et al. Major complications of regional anesthesia in France: The SOS Regional Anesthesia Hotline Service. Anesthesiology 2002;97:1274–80.

17. Cook TM, Counsell D, Wildsmith JA, Royal College of Anaesthetists Third National Audit P. Major complications of central neuraxial block: report on the Third National Audit Project of the Royal College of Anaesthetists. Br J Anaesth 2009;102:179–190.

18. Hollister N, Todd C, Ball S, Thorp-Jones D, Coghill J. Minimising the risk of accidental dural puncture with epidural analgesia for labour: a retrospective review of risk factors. Int J Obstet Anesth 2012;21:236–41.
19. Verstraete S, Walters MA, Devroe S, Roofthooft E, Van de Velde M. Lower incidence of post-dural puncture headache with spinal catheterization after accidental dural puncture in obstetric patients. Acta Anaesthesiol Scand 2014;58:1233–39.
20. Cuypers V, Van de Velde M, Devroe S. Intracranial subdural haematoma following neuraxial anaesthesia in the obstetric population: a literature review with analysis of 56 reported cases. Int J Obstet Anesth 2016;25:58–65.
21. Neal JM, Barrington MJ, Brull R, Hadzic A, Hebl JR, Horlocker TT, et al. The Second ASRA Practice Advisory on Neurologic Complications Associated with Regional Anesthesia and Pain Medicine: Executive Summary 2015. Reg Anesth Pain Med 2015;40:401–30.
22. Ehrenfeld JM, Agarwal AK, Henneman JP, Sandberg WS. Estimating the incidence of suspected epidural hematoma and the hidden imaging cost of epidural catheterization: a retrospective review of 43,200 cases. Reg Anesth Pain Med 2013;38:409–14.
23. AAGBI, OAA, RA-UK. Regional anaesthesia and patients with abnormalities of coagulation. Anaesthesia 2013;68:966–72.

Section 5

Anaesthesia for Various Procedures

Chapters

Chapter 5.1

Abdominal Surgery

David Murray

The provision of anaesthesia for abdominal surgery covers the full range of presentations, from the elective day-case patient to the very urgent patient undergoing emergency laparotomy with subsequent admission to critical care. Minor surgery may take 30–45 min, whereas major colorectal resections may take more than 4 h.

The anaesthetic techniques used have to mirror this diversity. The majority of major elective abdominal surgery is now performed by minimally invasive laparoscopic techniques, with patients receiving care as part of an enhanced recovery pathway. Almost all patients undergoing major surgery will require general anaesthesia, often combined with some form of central neuraxial blockade for analgesia (either continuous epidural analgesia or a single-shot intrathecal injection). Other operations, particularly in the pelvis and on the abdominal wall, can be carried out under central neuraxial blockade.

The preoperative assessment of abdominal surgical patients must be comprehensive. The perioperative period must incorporate close observation and monitoring. Analgesia is vital to the quality of postoperative recovery. Enhanced recovery pathways aim to standardize delivery of care for major surgery and have been successful in reducing length of stay.

GENERAL CONSIDERATIONS

Patient Characteristics

Patients of all ages undergo abdominal surgery, and different pathologies tend to be seen in different age groups. Acute appendicitis tends to predominate in younger patients. Laparoscopic cholecystectomy is commonly required in middle-aged patients. Bowel resection is more common in older patients, especially for cancer and diverticular disease. Emergency bowel surgery is common in the elderly. The comorbidities seen are generally commensurate with the age of the patient.

Indications for Surgery

Patients may require both elective and emergency abdominal surgery for a variety of indications.

Bleeding

Although bleeding may arise from anywhere in the gastrointestinal (GI) tract, 75% occurs in the upper GI tract. Bleeding may be acute, presenting with haematemesis, haemodynamic instability and shock, or chronic presenting with anaemia, particularly from bowel cancer. Common causes of acute bleeding are gastric and duodenal ulcers. However, they are less prevalent with increasing use of proton-pump inhibitors and *Helicobacter pylori* eradication therapy. When acute bleeding does occur, it is predominantly treated by endoscopic techniques. Surgery and anaesthesia is only required when this has failed. These patients are often in extremis due to blood loss, and surgical urgency is such that resuscitation needs to continue alongside active treatment. Oesophageal varices are less common but can result in an emergency presentation with dramatic bleeding, characterized by haematemesis, melaena and varying degrees of shock. Chronic bleeding usually presents with anaemia. Lower GI tract bleeding is more common in the elderly, is more insidious in onset and is usually due to cancer.

Perforation

Perforation of a viscus is often associated with sudden onset of abdominal pain and signs of peritonism. A common cause is perforation of a peptic ulcer, appendix or diverticulum. Malignant or inflammatory bowel disease presenting with perforation has a worse outcome.

Obstruction

Obstruction of a viscus may be acute or subacute and can occur anywhere in the GI tract, most commonly secondary to adhesions, often in the small bowel. Vomiting, constipation and abdominal distension are the classic features. Other causes include hernias, inflammatory bowel disease and malignancies. Patients will often undergo a trial of conservative management, as subacute obstruction may resolve without surgical intervention. Surgery may then proceed if conservative management fails.

Infarction

Infarction of a viscus may be secondary to torsion, strangulation, thromboembolic occlusion or vasculitis. Patients present with pain and signs of peritonism.

Cancer

Colorectal cancers are the most common causes, but gastric and oesophageal cancers also occur. Small bowel cancer is rare. It may be diagnosed following screening programmes, but also present with chronic anaemia, bleeding, perforation, altered bowel habit and pain.

Inflammatory Bowel Disease

Inflammation can occur throughout the GI tract, with some disease involving large parts of the bowel, such as Crohn's disease or ulcerative colitis. Surgery, such as subtotal or total colectomy, or panproctocolectomy, may be required due to failed medical treatment or to prevent cancer. If for the former, patients are frequently unwell due to systemic inflammation and effects of both long-term and acute steroid suppression.

Pain

A variety of conditions feature pain as part of their clinical presentation. In many cases surgery is carried out in an elective setting to relieve ongoing pain, and also prevent longer-term sequelae, e.g. hernia repair, laparoscopic cholecystectomy, haemorrhoidectomy, fistula-in-ano.

TECHNICAL CONSIDERATIONS

Preoperative Preparation for Abdominal Surgery

Preparation for abdominal surgery is as important for elective cases as it is for the high-risk emergency case. The requirements will depend on:

- The age of the patient
- The patient's comorbidities
- Whether it is a minor or a major procedure
- Whether it is day-case or inpatient surgery
- Whether it is elective or emergency surgery

Every patient should be assessed before surgery for fitness for anaesthesia. For elective cases, this is usually carried out in preoperative anaesthetic assessment clinic, frequently by nurse specialists. There should be back-up from consultant anaesthetists who have received specific training in preoperative assessment, and are able to review higher risk patients in person. These clinics allow patients to receive appropriate investigations and provide opportunity for any comorbidity to be optimized prior to surgery. Cardiorespiratory disease and diabetes all benefit from optimization due to the postoperative demand of major surgery. Day-case patients will require appropriate screening and careful selection.

Patients undergoing major surgery may benefit from cardiopulmonary exercise testing to stratify their postoperative risk. 'Prehabilitation', whereby patients undergo a period of exercise to improve general fitness, is also showing promising results in improving outcomes after major surgery. There is no clear evidence on the use of preoperative β-blocking drugs to reduce cardiac morbidity.

Most elective patients are admitted on the day of surgery, even for major surgery. In all cases the standard routine of history, examination and investigation will apply from the outset. Although now used less with enhanced recovery programmes, colorectal patients may have 'bowel prep' before surgery, and patients, in particular the elderly, can be significantly dehydrated.

Emergency patients may require significant resuscitation. Pain, sepsis and dehydration may be significant, with resulting organ dysfunction. There is less opportunity for preoperative preparation and senior input into decision-making is essential.

Principles of Anaesthesia

Monitoring

Before the start of anaesthesia the minimal standard of monitoring is commenced; electrocardiogram, noninvasive blood pressure, oximetry, capnography, oxygen and volatile agent analysis, and airway pressure. Temperature monitoring should be used for all but the shortest procedures.

Induction of Anaesthesia

The inspired/end-tidal oxygen difference is the best monitor of the adequacy of preoxygenation and consequent denitrogenation. An agent most suitable to the condition of the patient should be used for intravenous induction of anaesthesia.

Muscle Relaxation

If paralysis is required, the choice of muscle relaxant will depend on patient factors and the specifics of the abdominal operation. If there is a risk of regurgitation and consequent aspiration, a rapid sequence induction incorporating cricoid pressure is normally used. In order to gain rapid control of the airway, a depolarizing agent such as suxamethonium is traditionally used, although a modified approach might use rocuronium.

Airway Management

Supraglottic airway devices (SADs) may be used when muscle paralysis is not required, providing there is no regurgitation risk. If tracheal intubation is indicated, this should be followed by identification of correct placement of the tracheal tube using both clinical signs and capnography traces. The laryngoscopic reflex can be obtunded by prior injection of an opioid, such as fentanyl or alfentanil.

Maintenance of Anaesthesia

Maintenance of anaesthesia is usually with a volatile anaesthetic agent in either an air/oxygen or nitrous oxide/oxygen mix. Nitrous oxide is now used less often for major surgery because of the increase in bowel distension seen. However, it is still useful for hernia and perineal surgery. A total intravenous technique can be used, commonly propofol and a short-acting opioid such as remifentanil. The use of remifentanil intraoperatively may be associated with high postoperative analgesic requirements due to acute opioid tolerance. Aliquots of muscle relaxants can be given according to the response from the nerve stimulator. Analgesic requirements will depend on the magnitude of surgery and postoperative requirements. A multimodal technique is effective, supplemented by local anaesthesia as appropriate.

Ventilation

Spontaneous breathing via a SAD is suitable for minor surgery. Otherwise ventilation should be controlled. The occurrence of postoperative respiratory complications following major abdominal surgery has long been recognized and many ways have been sought to minimize this potentially serious adverse event. There are multifactorial causes; even the presenting emergency patient can already be compromised by aspiration, splinting of the diaphragm and basal lung collapse from increased abdominal pressure. This can be further compromised by the supine position and postoperative pain, which will contribute to further atelectasis. Minimally invasive techniques using pneumoperitoneum can also influence respiratory function by reducing chest compliance and functional residual capacity. Lung protective strategies with tidal volumes of 6 mL/kg and 5 cm H_2O of PEEP may improve postoperative respiratory outcome. One of the outcome benefits of epidural analgesia is the reduction of postoperative chest complications, but its use needs to be balanced against the potential side effects and complications.

Fluid Management

Patients undergoing major abdominal surgery require careful attention to fluid management during the whole perioperative period. Emergency patients may be significantly dehydrated and require correction of abnormal electrolytes. In elective surgery, preoperative fluid depletion due to the use of purgative bowel preparation and prolonged starvation periods is far less common, predominantly due to the adoption of enhanced recovery programmes. Although the splanchnic circulation receives around 30% of cardiac output, it is often reduced early in hypotension to enable blood flow to be diverted to other organs. This has important implications for anastomotic healing and recovery of bowel function in the postoperative period. Postepidural hypotension and therefore reduction of splanchnic blood flow must be rigorously corrected.

Fluid replacement may be guided by a variety of means. Traditional central venous pressure monitoring has generally been replaced by dynamic methods of cardiac output monitoring that allow goal-directed fluid therapy (GDFT) to be administered. This entails administration of a fluid bolus and monitoring response, via changes in parameters such as stroke volume or pulse pressure variation. However, there is controversy over whether liberal or restrictive regimens should be utilized and which fluid is best used.

Urine output should also be monitored throughout the perioperative period.

Blood loss in major surgery may vary from 300 mL to over 3000 mL especially with extensive pelvic surgery or if there has been preexisting radiotherapy or previous surgery. Blood loss may not be immediately apparent especially in laparoscopic surgery or if it has been collected in swabs rather than in suction containers. Weighing of swabs can provide an accurate estimation of blood loss. Cell salvage may be used during open procedures to reduce the need for allogenic blood transfusion, although concern exists regarding its use in the presence of malignancy. Transfusion triggers and point of care (POC) testing of haemoglobin or haematocrit can aid appropriate blood administration.

Patient Positioning

A variety of different positions may be used for abdominal surgery (Table 5.1.1). Many procedures are carried out with patients supine. Laparoscopic surgery usually requires some degree of lateral and head-up or head down tilt. This improves the view by allowing gravity to assist with moving bowel away from the operative site. In addition, positioning also provides improved retraction of tissues, e.g. right lateral positioning aids dissection of the splenic flexure during colonic surgery. Prone jack-knife positioning may also be used for perineal surgery. It is not unusual for a variety of positions to be used within the same operation. Thus, for laparoscopic abdominoperineal (AP) resection, the patient is first placed in right lateral position while the splenic flexure is mobilized, then placed supine for the remaining pelvic dissection, after which all abdominal wounds are closed. Finally, the patient is placed in prone jack-knife positioning to complete the perineal resection and remove the specimen.

Care must be taken in positioning the patient to ensure pressure areas are adequately protected. Positioning may be challenging in elderly patients due to reduced joint mobility and frail skin.

Thermoregulation

Due to the prolonged nature of abdominal surgery, temperature should be continuously monitored, and steps taken to prevent hypothermia. Hypothermia is exacerbated in general anaesthesia by epidural and spinal anaesthetic techniques

TABLE 5.1.1 Common Positions Used during Abdominal Surgery

Position	Operation
Supine	Most open and laparoscopic procedures
Head-down/head-up/lateral tilt	Laparoscopic surgery Open surgery
Prone jack-knife	Rectal surgery, e.g. Delormes procedure, perineal component of AP resection
Left lateral	Perineal surgery, colonoscopy
Right lateral	Laparoscopic surgery, particularly to mobilize splenic flexure during colonic surgery
Lloyd Davies (legs partially flexed at hips, with head down tilt)	Laparoscopic and open colonic surgery

and also in the elderly patient who has impaired thermoregulation. Active warming with warm air blowers is effective. Reflective drapes can be used on limb extremities when placed in Lloyd Davies or Trendelenburg positions.

Deep Venous Thrombosis Prophylaxis

Prophylaxis against deep venous thrombosis should relate to risk; intraabdominal surgery, especially with cancer surgery, and pelvic procedures, conveys an increased risk. This is reduced by the use of anticoagulants and support stockings or pneumatic compression devices. Most centres use low molecular weight heparin. There must be strict guidelines regarding the use of regional techniques when anticoagulants are used.

Analgesia

Opioids, simple analgesics such as paracetamol and nonsteroidal anti-inflammatory drugs (NSAIDs) are used to provide multimodal analgesia. These can be supplemented by a variety of local anaesthetic techniques, including the use of continuous wound catheters (Table 5.1.2).

TABLE 5.1.2 Summary of Regional Anaesthetic Techniques for Major Abdominal Surgery

Type of Surgery		Required Dermatomal Innervation	Regional Anaesthetic Technique
Upper abdominal	Gastric and hepatic surgery Cholecystectomy Upper abdominal incisions	T4 to L1	Thoracic epidural Transversus abdominis Plane Block
Lower abdominal	Colorectal resections Lower abdominal incisions Pelvic surgery	T6 to L1	Transversus abdominis; plane block Lumbar epidural Subarachnoid block Combined spinal-epidural technique
	Inguinal incisions	T10 to L1	Ilioinguinal and iliohypogastric nerve block
	Perineal and rectal surgery	S2 to S5	Caudal epidural analgesia

Local Anaesthetic Techniques

Local anaesthetic techniques for abdominal surgical operations fall under two main headings:

- Central neuraxial blockade
- Peripheral neuraxial (field) blockade

Central neuraxial blockade may be achieved with epidural analgesia or with spinal analgesia, including caudal epidural injections. Field blockade may be achieved with inguinal, transversus abdominis plane block, interpleural or intervertebral techniques. Central neuraxial and field blocks may be used on their own or to supplement general anaesthesia. Local infiltration may also be effective for inguinal hernia repair.

Epidural Analgesia

Epidural analgesia for open abdominal surgery provides good operating conditions and good postoperative analgesia. There is a reduced neuroendocrine stress response, a shortened period of postoperative ileus and enhancement of bowel blood flow. Thoracic epidurals vasodilate splanchnic veins and the associated hypotension can, if not corrected, compromise gut mucosal integrity. Gut hypoperfusion must be prevented, and vasoconstrictors are more likely to correct bowel blood flow than is excessive fluid resuscitation. The optimal mix of local anaesthetic and opioid remains to be determined. The use of opioid will help reduce the concentration of local anaesthetic, which will enable earlier mobilization of the postoperative patient. The addition of an opioid improves the quality of the block but can lead to respiratory depression. Additional adjuvants, such as the selective α2-adrenergic agonist clonidine, have also been used. The establishment of epidural blockade ideally should occur before commencing general anaesthesia to reduce the incidence of neurological complications. There are several side effects, such as hypotension, urinary retention, respiratory depression and pruritus. The most feared, neurological damage, especially paraplegia, is fortunately rare see Chapter 3.3.

The use of epidurals should be part of strict guidelines involving close monitoring by trained nurses to identify potential dangerous side effects. Local guidance should be enforced for the use of epidurals in patients taking anticoagulants, removal of the catheter being as important an issue as insertion. The most common side effect is a failed epidural, where 20% of patients will experience severe pain. This must be eliminated by having sufficiently trained staff and monitoring by a dedicated pain team. There is proven benefit in the quality of postoperative recovery. The elusive outcome benefit remains controversial. Thus a risk:benefit analysis must be applied to each case.

Spinal Anaesthesia

Spinal anaesthesia is restricted to operations performed below the umbilicus. Unlike with epidural blockade the duration of surgery is an important consideration. Risk:benefit analysis should be made in each case. Many of the contraindications apply to other forms of regional block, including coagulopathy, concurrent anticoagulants, patient refusal, sepsis, hypovolaemia and raised intracranial pressure.

The fine-gauge pencil-point needle is now the most widely used and produces minimal trauma and the smallest hole in the dura. This will reduce the incidence of postdural puncture headache. The insertion site is between the third and fourth lumbar vertebrae, and the extent of the block is determined by the baricity of the solution, the position of the patient and the dose rather than the volume of the local anaesthetic.

Lumbar block using hyperbaric solution (2.5–3 mL 0.5% 'heavy' bupivacaine) is suitable for all lower abdominal surgery, including hernia repair. Saddle (perineal) block is indicated for perineal surgery and can be achieved by establishing the block in the sitting position. Adjuvants such as fentanyl can prolong the duration of analgesia. When coupled with general anaesthesia, a 'single-shot spinal' with 75–200 μg morphine or 200–300 μg diamorphine added to local anaesthetic provides good postoperative analgesia for laparoscopic surgery, and avoids the problems associated with failed epidurals. However, care needs to be taken to observe for postoperative respiratory depression.

Inguinal Field Block

Inguinal field blockade is used for inguinal hernia repair and aims to block the ilioinguinal, iliohypogastric, subcostal and genitofemoral nerves. The first three lie close to each other between the abdominal muscle layers at the level of the anterior superior iliac spine, and they may be conveniently blocked here. This block alone will provide good postoperative analgesia. If the patient is to be awake, there should be additional skin infiltration along the incision site with local anaesthetic agent. Once the spermatic cord is exposed, the cord and hernial sac should be infiltrated with local anaesthetic.

Transversus Abdominis Plane Block

This involves injecting local anaesthetic, often under ultrasound guidance, to block the nerves supplying the anterior abdominal wall (T6 to L1). When performed bilaterally, it can provide good analgesia for midline and port-site incisions. It may be used where epidural anaesthesia is contraindicated although does not provide any modulation of stress response.

Paravertebral Block

Paravertebral block can be used for open cholecystectomy and for thoracotomy (oesophagectomy). The paravertebral space is triangular and situated at the head and necks of the ribs, and the solution can pass over several dermatomes. The space can be found by the 'loss-of-resistance' technique, 2–3 cm lateral to the appropriate spinous process. Once identified, a catheter can be inserted. This block is a useful adjuvant in a multimodal approach when epidural blockade is contraindicated. Paravertebral block may also be performed under direct vision by the surgeons during thoracic surgery.

Conclusion of Surgery

At the end of the procedure, with the guidance of a nerve stimulator, the neuro-muscular blockade is reversed using an anticholinesterase preceded by atropine or glycopyrronium to counteract muscarinic-like effects.

Tracheal Extubation

When spontaneous respiration is established, the tracheal tube is removed after pharyngeal suction and toilet. The patient is then transferred to a recovery area breathing oxygen where close observation and monitoring is continued for as long as necessary. Prolonged close observation may take place in a critical care area (see Chapter 3.1).

Postanaesthetic Care

Analgesia will be required in the postoperative period depending on the magnitude of surgery. Patients with significant comorbidities, and those undergoing major surgery, will benefit from admission to a critical care area for enhanced monitoring of cardiorespiratory status and fluid management. Many patients will receive care as part of an enhanced recovery after surgery (ERAS) programme.

Day Case Surgery

Virtually all general surgical procedures with the exception of major resections are now carried out as day-cases or 23-h stay, including laparoscopic cholecystectomy. The anaesthetic technique should allow patients to be discharged within appropriate timeframes. This will require use of short acting anaesthetic drugs, in combination with multimodal analgesia to reduce the dose of long-acting opioid drugs. Muscle relaxation is not normally required for minor surgery such as inguinal hernia repair and perineal surgery and SADs may be used.

Minimally Invasive Abdominal Surgery

The majority of open abdominal surgical procedures have been replaced by minimally invasive laparoscopic approaches. This has resulted in reduced postoperative pain, reduced inflammatory response to surgery, reduced ileus and faster discharge from hospital. A small open incision may still be necessary to extract the specimen or hand-sew the anastomosis. General anaesthesia intubation and ventilation will be required for laparoscopic surgery. Higher minute volumes will be required to prevent hypercarbia from dissolved CO_2 used to create the pneumoperitoneum. In upper abdominal procedures a nasogastric tube improves the surgical view by reducing gastric volume.

Access to the patient is limited as the arms are usually 'wrapped' to secure them at the patient's side. Hence all intravenous access needs to be secure before surgery, and invasive blood pressure monitoring can be more reliable for longer procedures. Postoperative pain relief is aided by local anaesthetic infiltration of the port sites and local anaesthetics applied directly to the operative site. A 'single-shot spinal' with opioid provides effective pain relief, and epidural analgesia is not generally required.

Pneumoperitoneum

Pneumoperitoneum is achieved by insufflating carbon dioxide via a Veress needle or camera port at a rate of 1–6 L/min into the peritoneal cavity to a pressure of 10–18 mm Hg. This is necessary to create the space to visualize the surgical area through the laparoscope. Carbon dioxide use adds to the safety of the techniques because it is highly soluble in blood and does not support combustion. Carbon dioxide is carried in blood and rapidly eliminated, although an increase in minute volume is usually required to maintain normal CO_2. Trauma to major blood vessels may occur when the pneumoperitoneum is established, with potentially catastrophic consequences.

Changes in respiratory pressures and haemodynamic parameters are caused by the increased intra-abdominal pressures. The respiratory changes are caused by the cephalad displacement of the diaphragm, leading to a reduction in tidal volume and functional residual capacity. There is decreased compliance and greater airway pressures may be required to maintain the same tidal volume. Cardiovascular changes are manifested by a decline in venous return and hence a reduction in cardiac output. Bradycardia can be induced by stretching of the peritoneum. Patients with severe cardiorespiratory disease may not be able to tolerate these effects and open surgery will be required.

Enhanced Recovery Programmes

Enhanced recovery after surgery programmes have been successful in reducing length of stay, and there is some evidence of improved outcomes. They were originally developed for colorectal surgery, and the principles have been extended to other forms of surgery. They consist of several elements:

- Good preoperative assessment and preparation prior to admission
- Preoperative patient education to manage expectations for surgery and recovery, including stoma management
- A structured approach to perioperative and immediate postoperative management, including pain relief
- Reducing the stress response to surgery, with minimally invasive surgical techniques

- Minimal bowel preparation, preoperative carbohydrate loading and GDFT which helps minimize fluid shifts and tissue oedema
- Early postoperative oral nutrition and avoidance of nasogastric tubes aid recovery of bowel function, as does avoidance of systemic opioids where possible
- Early mobilization, aided by minimal use of drains, postoperative intravenous fluids and urinary catheters which would otherwise 'tether' the patient to the bed and drip stands

SPECIFIC OPERATIONS

Upper GI Tract

Oesophagogastrectomy and Gastrectomy

Oesophagogastrectomy and gastrectomy both deliver a major physiological challenge to the patient. There are several approaches for oesophageal surgery:

- An upper midline laparotomy followed by right thoracotomy with anastomosis in the chest (Ivor Lewis procedure).
- A three-stage procedure of right thoracotomy followed by upper midline laparotomy and right-sided cervical incision to allow the anastomosis in the neck.
- A trans-hiatal approach with an incision in the neck, and another in the abdomen, allowing anastomosis in the neck without thoracotomy. This approach does not permit lymph node dissection.

Minimally invasive techniques have also been developed, where the abdominal or thoracic components are performed laparoscopically rather than as open procedures.

Preoperative selection and staging are key to the improved outcome of these patients. The investigations required will be the usual preoperative work-up plus spirometry. Arterial blood gas analysis may be of value if there is chest disease due to the need for one-lung ventilation.

General anaesthesia supplemented by thoracic epidural analgesia is commonly used. A multimodal regimen of analgesia based on the continuous epidural is used postoperatively. Perioperative monitoring is the routine monitoring with invasive arterial blood pressure measurement. Placement of a CVP line facilitates use of vasopressors in the perioperative period, which may be required due to epidural induced hypotension. One-lung anaesthesia is generally required with any thoracic approach to allow optimal surgical access.

There can be several position changes and double-lumen tube placement must be rechecked after movement. Temperature loss can be a problem and great efforts should be made to maintain normothermia. The procedure is prolonged and care of pressure areas must be taken. A nasogastric tube is placed intraoperatively and remains in place postoperatively to allow decompression of the stomach and prevent anastomotic dehiscence. This is usually sutured at the nose to ensure it does not become displaced.

Postoperatively, the majority of patients are extubated and all should be managed in a critical care area. Good analgesia is vital, and this can be provided by thoracic epidural with judicious use of systemic opioids and NSAIDs. Alternative methods of pain relief can be provided by paravertebral, intercostal nerve blocks with patient-controlled analgesia (PCA).

Gastrectomy and other types of upper GI surgery such as Nissan Fundoplication for symptomatic hiatus hernias are usually performed laparoscopically.

Bariatric Surgery

Bariatric surgery is a successful way of managing morbid obesity. Surgery such as gastric bands or bypass is performed laparoscopically and involves either reducing the volume of food that can be ingested or bypassing part of the GI tract to reduce absorption.

Preoperative preparation involves specialized diets to reduce fatty liver. Common comorbidities include cardiovascular disease and diabetes. The latter often resolves immediately after surgery and a reduction in diabetic medication is required. Obstructive sleep apnoea is present in around 5% of patients.

Specialized electric operating tables are used to aid positioning. These are wider and have a higher weight rating than standard tables.

Good preoxygenation is vital. Specialized pillows (such as the Oxford HELP pillow) are used to optimize position for intubation. Difficult intubation is uncommon. An orogastric tube is placed at induction and manipulated to its final position during surgery. Due to arm circumference, an arterial line can provide a more reliable measurement of blood pressure compared to noninvasive cuffs. Drug dosing is based on lean body weight, apart from suxamethonium where actual body weight is used. Intravenous analgesia is sufficient and central neuraxial blockade is generally not required.

Biliary Tract Surgery

This predominantly consists of elective laparoscopic cholecystectomy which is now carried out as day-case or 23-h stay. Open procedures are generally performed if a laparoscopic approach fails (including due to intraoperative complications), if the patient is unfit for pneumoperitoneum, or if there has been previous abdominal surgery where adhesions may be an issue. There is a theoretical effect of opioids on the sphincter of Oddi, but clinically this appears unimportant. Laparoscopic cholecystectomy may also be carried out during periods of acute cholecystitis and biliary tract infection. In these cases it is important to measure coagulation and correct abnormalities preoperatively.

Pancreatic Surgery

Pancreatic surgery is sometimes carried out for necrotizing pancreatitis, chronic pancreatitis, trauma and neoplastic lesions. There has been a reduction in surgical intervention in acute pancreatitis, but necrosectomy may be indicated if necrotizing pancreatitis is detected.

Whipple's procedure involves pancreaticoduodenectomy for lesions in the head of the pancreas.

Diabetes mellitus will complicate the perioperative procedure.

The operation is long and suitable precautions are taken for temperature loss and protection of pressure areas. A thoracic epidural provides good analgesia, and postoperatively patients should be managed in a critical care area.

Lower GI Tract

Colorectal Surgery

Colorectal surgery involves a wide range of surgical procedures of varying complexity for cancer, inflammatory bowel disease and diverticular disease; most involve bowel resection with stapled anastomosis of the remaining segments or formation of an end stoma. A defunctioning loop ileostomy is often formed if there is concern over anastomotic integrity, or for ileal pouch surgery. This allows healing and helps prevent anastomotic leak or breakdown. The latter is associated with a high mortality. A minimally invasive approach now predominates, usually laparoscopic with a small incision to extract the specimen, or small transverse incisions.

The anaesthetic technique will usually be intravenous induction, muscle relaxation with ventilation, central neuraxial analgesia and perioperative monitoring. Nitrous oxide is avoided to prevent bowel distension. Due to the predominance of laparoscopic approaches, thoracic epidural has generally being replaced with single-shot spinal techniques with intrathecal opioid. These provide both intra- and postoperative analgesia.

The large fluid requirements previously seen have generally been minimized with enhanced recovery programmes. GDFT appears to allow better optimization of fluids and improve outcomes, although there is still some controversy over the type of fluid regime and which patient groups benefit the most. Major blood loss will require blood transfusion. However, transfusion in cancer surgery has provoked debate, being linked with increased tumour recurrence and increased infection rates.

Postoperative analgesia can also be provided by opioid PCA. This may be supplemented with simple analgesics. NSAIDs have an opioid-sparing effect, although caution needs to be exercised due to potential fluid shifts, especially in elderly patients. Additional adjuncts such as intrathecal clonidine and intravenous lidocaine have also been used, although the benefits are currently being debated.

Emergency Laparotomy

Acute obstruction and perforation of the small or large bowel is a common surgical emergency. It can affect all ages but is more common in the elderly. Emergency bowel surgery accounts for one of the highest risk patient groups undergoing any type of surgery, after emergency aortic aneurysm surgery, and in the UK it is associated with a 30-day mortality of over 11%, higher in the elderly, compared with a mortality rate of around 2% for elective colorectal surgery. Although the majority of elective major surgery is performed laparoscopically, over 85% of emergency procedures are performed via a midline incision.

Obstruction leads to proximal bowel distension by gas and fluid. The bowel wall becomes oedematous, and eventually there is fluid leak into the peritoneum causing contamination and peritonitis. As further distension occurs, the blood supply becomes compromised, leading to ischaemia, necrosis and eventually perforation. Prolonged vomiting, diarrhoea and fluid sequestration cause fluid and electrolyte imbalances that need to be corrected before surgery. Patients often have a metabolic acidosis due to sepsis and shock. Resuscitation may be carried out in a critical care area. However, this should not delay surgery as mortality is improved when delays to surgery are minimized. Prolonged resuscitation in the presence of sepsis is likely to be futile without effective control of the source of sepsis. The increased intra-abdominal pressure occurring in obstruction can cause diaphragmatic splinting, which can lead to basal lung atelectasis.

Data from the UK's National Emergency Laparotomy Audit (NELA) reveal that:

- 30% of patients have intra-abdominal sepsis
- 25% have perforated at time of surgery
- 35% undergo colorectal resection
- 17% undergo small bowel resection
- 17% undergo adhesiolysis
- Malignancy is present in 20%

Perioperative management involves a multidisciplinary approach involving input from radiology, surgery, anaesthesia and intensive care and elderly medicine for elderly patients. Standards of care have been developed that emphasize:

- Good communication between the multidisciplinary team
- Timeliness of care – antibiotics if septic, preoperative CT scanning, access to theatres without delay
- Preoperative assessment of risk of death to identify high-risk patients (those with predicted mortality >5%)
- Seniority of care for high-risk patients
- Admission to critical care for high-risk cases

Anaesthetic Management

Surgery invariably requires general anaesthesia. Invasive monitoring is advised. An arterial line allows closer monitoring of blood pressure and regular sampling to monitor oxygenation, haemoglobin and acid – base balance. High lactate and base excess is not uncommon. Patients may deteriorate during surgery, and a central venous line allows administration of vasopressors to counter the vasodilatory effects of sepsis. Any nasogastric tube already in situ should be aspirated before induction of anaesthesia and then left on free drainage.

The induction of anaesthesia will involve preoxygenation followed by rapid sequence induction with cricoid pressure to prevent potential aspiration. If not already in place, a nasogastric tube should be inserted. The choice of agents is not important, although nitrous oxide is best avoided. The risk-benefit of an epidural or spinal analgesia is assessed on an individual basis, but concurrent sepsis, coagulopathy and fluid disturbance may tip the balance in favour of PCA morphine for postoperative analgesia. A large-bore cannula is advised as large fluid volumes may be necessary. Unlike elective surgery, the evidence base for cardiac output monitoring and goal directed fluid management is currently unclear. Most patients should be admitted to critical care postoperatively, as there is a high risk of deterioration. A period of postoperative ventilation is not uncommon especially in higher risk patients and those with ongoing sepsis.

Robotic Surgery

Robotic surgery was developed to overcome some of the limitations of laparoscopic surgery. It allows the surgeon to control instruments from a distance with a higher degree of precision and control than is normally possible manually. It has predominantly been used in urological surgery, although its use is increasing for abdominal surgery. The anaesthetic challenges inherent in laparoscopic surgery are generally magnified. Patients are in a steep head-down position for a prolonged period of time. There is limited access to the patient and all intravascular lines need to be secure. Regurgitation of gastric contents is common and may cause ocular burns unless care is taken to protect the eyes. A nasogastric tube should be left on free drainage to minimize these risks.

Perineum and Abdominal Wall

Perianal Surgery

This includes both elective procedures such as surgery for haemorrhoids and fistulas, or rectal prolapse, and emergency procedures for perianal sepsis/abscess. Surgical stimulation during perianal surgery can be significant, which may precipitate reflex responses such as laryngospasm (Brewer–Luckhardt reflex) and bradycardias. General anaesthesia with spontaneous breathing can be used, employing potent analgesic agents such as fentanyl or alfentanil to suppress the painful stimuli. Patient positioning will influence the choice of airway control. The lithotomy or Trendelenburg positions may be used, which can predispose to regurgitation. Lateral and prone positions are also used.

Spinal and caudal extradural anaesthesia have both been used, thus avoiding general anaesthesia and providing good postoperative analgesia. A 'saddle' block aiming to anaesthetize S2–S5 using small volumes (0.5–1.5 mL) of 0.5% heavy bupivacaine is used. Local blocks, such as posterior perineal nerve blockade and local infiltration, can supplement general anaesthesia and provide good perioperative analgesia but in reality are rarely required

Hernia Repair

Hernia repair can occur at several sites in the abdominal wall. A hernia is a bowel protrusion from its normal position through an opening in the abdominal wall. It may occur through a defect in tissue planes or through a previous incision (e.g. incisional hernia and parastomal hernia). After excision of the sac, the defect is repaired with either sutures, polypropylene mesh or biological tissue. The hernia sac may contain significant amount of bowel. There can be an emergency presentation with strangulation, which may require bowel resection.

Inguinal hernia is the most common hernia, accounting for 75%–85% of hernias in both sexes and can occur at almost any age. Early repair is advised to reduce the risk of strangulation. There is a 3% recurrence rate and the procedure for redo repair is more complex and prolonged. Other hernias include femoral hernias, which can strangulate more easily. Paraumbilical hernias are acquired and are associated with middle age, obesity and multiparity. Incisional hernias are a late complication of abdominal surgery. Large incisional hernias frequently occur after previous emergency laparotomy. The repair of these can be technically challenging due to the quantity of bowel and a 'hostile' abdomen due to preexisting peritoneal contamination and adhesions. With the exception of large incisional hernias, the majority of repairs are now performed as daycase procedures. Elective repair can be performed laparoscopically, but at present the benefits over the conventional approach have not materialized.

The anaesthetic technique will depend on presentation, type and size of the hernia. All strangulated hernias are likely to require general anaesthesia with rapid sequence induction and application of cricoid pressure due to the risk of regurgitation of bowel contents. Anaesthesia for large incisional hernias may be more akin to that required for a laparotomy. For other types of repair there is a wide choice of ways to proceed: general anaesthesia with multimodal analgesia based on local field block, field block alone and regional anaesthesia.

FURTHER READING

Saunders D, Murray D, Pichel A, Varley S, Peden CJ; UK Emergency Laparotomy Network. Variations in mortality following emergency laparotomy; the first report of the United Kingdom Emergency Laparotomy Network. Br J Anaesth 2012:109:368–75.

NELA Project Team. Second Patient Report of the National Emergency Laparotomy Audit. London: Royal College of Anaesthetists; 2016. Available at: www.nela.org.uk/

Anderson I, Eddlestone J, Lees N, et al. The higher-risk general surgical patient: towards improved care for a forgotten group. London: Royal College of Surgeons of England; 2011. Available at: www.rcseng. ac.uk/library-and-publications/college-publications/docs/the-higher-risk-general-surgical-patient/

Grocott MP, Dushianthan A, Hamilton MA, Mythen MG, Harrison D, Rowan K, et al. Perioperative increase in global blood flow to explicit defined goals and outcomes after surgery: a Cochrane Systematic Review. Br J Anaesth. 2013;111:535–48.

Simpson JC, Moonesinghe SR, Grocott MP, Kuper M, McMeeking A, Oliver CM, et al. Enhanced recovery from surgery in the UK: an audit of the enhanced recovery partnership programmeme 2009–2012. Br J Anaesth 2015;115:560–68.

Chapter 5.2

Cardiac Surgery

Vivek Sharma

Adult cardiac surgery can be subdivided into the following groups:

- Coronary revascularization procedures
- Procedures involving the cardiac valves and their supporting structures
- Procedures to close defects between the right and left sides of the heart
- Surgery for intractable arrhythmias
- Heart and lung transplantation
- Circulatory support procedures as a bridge to myocardial recovery or transplantation
- Heart failure surgery
- Procedures involving the pericardium and great vessels within the thoracic cavity
- Correction, or revision of a partially corrected, grown-up congenital cardiac (GUCC) anomaly

Interventional cardiology procedures include:

- Arrhythmia ablation
- Pacemaker and indwelling cardio-defibrillator (ICD) insertion/removal
- Transcatheter aortic valve implantation
- Percutaneous mitral valve implantation

GENERAL CONSIDERATIONS

Anaesthetic Problems and Cardiac Surgery

Anaesthetic-related problems in cardiac surgery result either as a direct consequence of the precipitating condition or from associated comorbidities, or as a consequence of the process of cardiopulmonary bypass (CPB).

Effects of the Disease Process

- Impaired ventricular function may be further depressed by anaesthetic agents and exacerbated by hypotension, hypoxia and acidosis.
- Valvular stenosis or regurgitation restricts cardiac output with limited ability to compensate for changes in pre- or afterload.

- Surgical manipulations of the heart may cause arrhythmias and hypotension.
- The function of other organs may be impaired resulting in a reduced ability to maintain normal physiological homoeostasis and excretion of drugs.

Effects of Cardiopulmonary Bypass

Isolation of the heart from the circulation is a necessary requisite for most cardiac surgical procedures. This may:

- Promote a cytokine-mediated systemic inflammatory response
- Affect coagulation and clotting mechanisms adversely
- Result in neurological and/or cognitive dysfunction, either as a result of the effects of CPB or secondary to an embolic event
- Result in myocardial damage due to inadequate myocardial protection during CPB
- Result in an ischaemia-reperfusion injury
- Lead to the development of postoperative arrhythmias

Preparation for Cardiac Surgery

Patients present for adult cardiac surgery following an extensive cardiological assessment and workup. Ideally the preoperative anaesthetic consultation should be conducted in the cardiac preadmission clinic but is commonly performed at the bedside.

History

Presenting Condition

Symptoms of angina can be graded using the Canadian Cardiovascular Society Classification:

- Class 1 – ordinary physical activity does not cause angina. Angina occurs with strenuous, rapid or prolonged exertion.
- Class 2 – slight limitation of ordinary activity. Angina occurs with moderate exertion (walking > 2 blocks on the level or climbing > 1 flight of stairs), or under emotional stress, or during the few hours after awakening only.
- Class 3 – marked limitation of ordinary physical activity. Angina occurs with minimal exertion.
- Class 4 – inability to carry on any physical activity without discomfort. Angina may be present at rest.

When referral for surgery is for angina the following should be ascertained:
- Is the condition stable or unstable with a continuing requirement for anti-anginal medication?
- Is there associated dyspnoea secondary to systolic or diastolic dysfunction?
- Is there a history of recent myocardial infarction or episodes of cardiac failure?

Assessment of the severity of heart failure can be made using the New York Heart Association (NYHA) functional classification:

- Class 1 – patients with cardiac disease without limitation of physical activity
- Class 2 – patients with cardiac disease with slight limitation of physical activity
- Class 3 – patients with cardiac disease resulting in marked limitation of physical activity but comfortable at rest
- Class 4 – patients with cardiac disease resulting in an inability to carry out any physical activity without discomfort although comfortable at rest

Coexisting Disease

Coexisting disease increases the morbidity of cardiac surgery, in particular chronic respiratory disease, peripheral and neurovascular disease, renal impairment and diabetes mellitus.

Drugs and Allergies

The patient's current cardiovascular medications for control of angina, cardiac failure, blood pressure and cardiac arrhythmias should be recorded.

Patients with a recent history of acute coronary syndrome who have undergone a percutaneous attempt at coronary revascularization will have been treated with antiplatelet and/or antithrombotic agents.

Recent guidelines do not recommend withholding aspirin prior to cardiac surgery.

Adenosine diphosphate inhibitors such as clopidogrel and ticagrelor should be discontinued for at least 5 days prior to elective surgery and at least 24 h prior to urgent surgery.

Warfarin should be discontinued 5 days before surgery and substituted with low molecular weight heparin.

Newer oral anticoagulants such as rivaroxaban, apixaban or edoxaban should be discontinued 48 h prior to surgery.

Any history of allergy to heparin, protamine, iodine or antibiotics should be recorded.

For patients receiving a heparin infusion up to the time of surgery, ascertain if there is any evidence of heparin-induced thrombocytopenia syndrome (HITS).

In cases of revision cardiac surgery, ascertain if aprotinin was used at the first operation.

Dentition

Has a dental check been performed in patients presenting for valve replacement?

Oesophageal Disease

If intraoperative transoesophageal echocardiography (TOE) is contemplated any past history of oesophageal disease and/or surgery should be sought.

Examination

A problem-focused full examination of the patient is essential, and of particular relevance are the following.

Cardiorespiratory Reserve

Look for evidence of the severity of any cardiorespiratory disease and the degree of cardiorespiratory reserve.

Bruits

Listen for bruits in the carotid arteries, especially if cannulation of the internal jugular vein is contemplated.

Peripheral Arteries

Where radial arteries are to be used as surgical conduits, it is essential to perform an Allen's test to determine vascular sufficiency.

Airway Assessment for Anticipated Difficult Intubation

Up to 25% of patients presenting for cardiac surgery are diabetic, and this group has a higher than normal incidence of difficult intubation.

Investigations

Routine preoperative investigations should include the following.

Haematology

A full blood count, coagulation and crossmatch profile should be undertaken. Ascertain the cause of any anaemic. Similarly, a cause for neutropaenia and/or thrombocytopaenia should be sought.

Patients who received antiplatelet medications should undergo platelet function testing. A coagulation profile should be requested, especially in patients who have received warfarin.

C-reactive protein concentration (CRP) should be tested if infection is suspected.

Biochemistry

Blood chemistry may be abnormal as a consequence of either the primary disease or drugs used to treat it, e.g. diuretic therapy. Cardiac-specific enzymes, including troponin T, may be elevated where there is a recent history of myocardial infarction.

Brain natriuretic peptide (BNP) concentration is frequently monitored in patients with heart failure.

Electrocardiography

An electrocardiograph (ECG) may demonstrate abnormalities of rate, rhythm or conduction and show evidence of ischaemic injury or ventricular hypertrophy.

Dynamic testing such as exercise tolerance test (ETT) using the modified Bruce protocol, the 6-min walk test and cardiopulmonary exercise testing may be indicated in some patients.

Radiology

The chest X-ray may indicate cardiac abnormalities (e.g. atrial enlargement or cardiomegaly), pulmonary pathology (e.g. chronic obstructive airways disease) or a combination of the two (e.g. cardiac failure).

Cardiac-Specific Investigations

These include cardiac catheterization and echocardiography. Some patients may require further investigations to determine myocardial viability or reserve (e.g. positron emission tomography and thallium scans).

Cardiac catheterization is used to delineate the sites, severity and number of stenotic lesions. Left ventricular function can be assessed allowing an estimate of left ventricular ejection fraction. The valve area and gradient across a stenotic valve can also be measured. Right-sided pressure measurements are helpful in assessing the degree of pulmonary hypertension and for subsequent risk-stratification, preoperative optimization and perioperative management.

Echocardiography is most easily performed via the transthoracic (TTE) route. Further information can be obtained by the more invasive TOE. Echocardiographic investigations give an indication of the severity of valvular pathology as well as allowing an assessment of ventricular systolic and diastolic function.

Echocardiography can also provide information about coexisting congenital heart disease. Typical values are outlined in Table 5.2.1.

Pharmacological stress testing can be used in conjunction with echocardiography to check for regional wall motion abnormalities and changes in ventricular function.

Administrating a radionuclide such as thallium prior to induction of stress (exercise or pharmacological) and detection of subsequent perfusion defects with the use of a gamma camera in patients with stenosed vessels provides further information. A repeat scan is performed 3 h later to gauge reversibility and hence distinguish between viable and nonviable myocardium.

TABLE 5.2.1 Valve Area Measurements and Gradients in Normal and Disease States

Valve	Normal Area (cm^2)	Mild Stenosis Area (cm^2)	Severe Stenosis Area (cm^2)	Gradient
Mitral	4–6	<2	<1	>15
Aortic	3–5	<1	<0.75	>50

Advanced imaging techniques involving the use of ionizing radiation such as computed tomography can be performed to assess coronary anatomy in patients with poor quality angiograms.

Cardiac magnetic resonance (CMR) imaging provides information about the anatomy of the heart as well as perfusion and viability of the myocardium. CMR can be performed in conjunction with pharmacological stress to detect ischaemic areas and with contrast medium such as gadolinium to differentiate between viable and nonviable tissue.

Other Investigations

Pulmonary function tests should be performed in patients with underlying lung disease or neuromuscular disorders. Forced expiratory volume in one second (FEV_1) of less than 50% predicted and lung diffusing (transfer) capacity of carbon monoxide (D_{LCO}; T_{LCO}) of less than 70% predicted are associated with a higher risk of postoperative pulmonary complications.

Carotid Doppler scans should be performed in patients over the age of 65 years and those with history of transient ischaemic attacks or stroke.

Risk Stratification

At least 19 risk-stratification models exist for open heart surgery but the most widely used are the EurosSCORE, the Society of Thoracic Surgeons (STS) algorithms and the Parsonnet score.[1,2]

The following factors have been shown to increase the risk of mortality and morbidity associated with cardiac surgery:

- Demography – female gender and age
- Cardiac status – cardiac failure or cardiogenic shock, ejection fraction less than 40%, valve surgery, left ventricular aneurysm
- Comorbid disease – renal dysfunction, diabetes mellitus, hypertension (systemic or pulmonary) and obesity
- Revision or emergency surgery

Individual and institutional outcome data, using cumulative risk-adjusted mortality (CRAM) or variable life-adjusted display (VLAD) plots to monitor surgical performance, allow realistic predications of outcome.

Premedication

Patients presenting for cardiac surgery have high levels of anxiety. This may result in increased levels of stress-related hormones that may contribute to the development of ischaemia preoperatively.

Provision of Anxiolysis

Provision of anxiolysis is best achieved by the administration of a benzodiazepine hypnotic the night before surgery with a further dose given up to an hour and a half before operation. Alternatively, an opioid-based intramuscular premedication may be administered.

Patients with critical coronary artery disease should receive supplemental oxygen via a facemask following premedication.

A short-acting hypnotic such as diazepam or midazolam can be given to facilitate arterial and central vein cannulation.

Management of Current Medications

All anti-anginal, antiarrhythmic and antihypertensive drugs should be continued up to and including the morning of operation.

Warfarin should be discontinued 5 days before surgery and the international normalized ratio (INR) should be closely monitored. In patients at increased risk of embolism, anticoagulant cover can be provided by newer oral anticoagulants such as rivaroxaban, apixaban or low molecular weight heparins.

If warfarin is not discontinued, its effect can be reversed by administration of oral or intravenous vitamin K. Although the intravenous route achieves a more rapid correction of INR (onset of action within 6–8 h), both routes achieve a similar correction of INR by 24 h. Vitamin K should not be administered subcutaneously or intramuscularly.

For immediate reversal of warfarin, prothrombin complex concentrates (PCC) are preferred to fresh frozen plasma. Advantages of PCC include rapid onset of action, small reconstitution volume, no need for blood group compatibility and minimal rate of transmission of infection and lung injury. Fresh frozen plasma can be used in conjunction with vitamin K to achieve rapid reversal of INR.

Aspirin should be continued until the day of surgery but other $P2Y_{12}$ platelet-inhibiting drugs such as clopidogrel and ticagrelor should be discontinued 5 days prior to surgery. Prasugrel should be discontinued 7 days prior to surgery.

Bridging therapy is recommended for patients at a high risk of thrombosis and subsequent ischaemic events. After discontinuation of the $P2Y_{12}$ inhibitor bridging with tirofiban or eptifibatide should be initiated approximately 72 h before surgery and continued up to 4–6 h from surgery.

Patients with acute coronary syndromes requiring heparin or nitrate infusions should have these continued up until the time of surgery.

Tight homoeostatic control of blood glucose levels has been shown to improve outcome in patients undergoing cardiac surgery. It is important to establish and maintain normoglycaemia (blood sugar levels between 4.5 and 6.0 mmol/L) within the perioperative period for both type 1 and type 2 diabetics. This should start the night before surgery. Intravenous 10% glucose 100 mL/h should be coadministered with an appropriate sliding scale insulin regimen to maintain normoglycaemia. This should be changed to 50% in theatre to reduce the fluid load. The tight control regimen should be continued until the patient is able to resume normal basic activity and be re-established on their preoperative medication.

TECHNICAL CONSIDERATIONS

Prior to Anaesthesia

A standard anaesthetic machine check and set-up as for all procedures is essential, after which the following should be established:

● ECG and pulse oximetry monitoring.
● Oxygen administered via a suitable facemask.
● Insertion of a large-bore peripheral cannula. Supplemental sedation may be required.
● Arterial cannulation – ascertain whether the left, right or both radial arteries are to be used as surgical conduits.
● Insertion of central venous catheter (CVC) – 2D imaging ultrasound guidance is recommended for elective insertion of multilumen CVCs.
● Insertion of pulmonary artery catheter in high-risk patients.
● Insertion of vascular access catheter in patients with established chronic renal failure or acute renal dysfunction.
● Body temperature and urine output monitoring.
● Cerebral oximetry for procedures involving the arch of the aorta where deep hypothermic circulatory arrest (DHCA) is required; also in patients with high grade carotid stenosis.
● External defibrillation pads for patients having revision surgery, high-risk cases and patients undergoing minimally invasive cardiac surgery.
● Depth of anaesthesia monitoring such as bispectral index (BIS) monitoring.

Techniques of Anaesthesia

Patients are almost always induced on the operating table with full invasive monitoring and preoxygenation. Never induce anaesthesia without a surgeon who can put the patient onto CPB present in the operating theatre, nor without a perfusionist and a CPB pump available.

No one anaesthetic technique has been demonstrated to be better for patients undergoing cardiac surgical procedures. The choice lies between an opioid- or an inhalation-based technique.

It is essential to prepare a range of agents to control hypo- or hypertensive episodes. These may be administered by intermittent bolus or by continuous infusion.

Anaesthetic Induction Agents

Traditionally, high-dose opioids were the mainstay of induction and maintenance of anaesthesia. However, 'fast-tracking' post cardiac surgery, coupled with concern regarding intraoperative awareness, has led to alternative approaches. The advantages and disadvantages of some of the commonly used intravenous induction agents are outlined in Table 5.2.2.

TABLE 5.2.2 Commonly Used Intravenous Induction Agents in Cardiac Anaesthesia

Drug	Dose	Advantages	Disadvantages
Propofol	1.5–2.5 mg/kg (reduced in the elderly)	Facilitates early extubation	↓ SVR and cardiac output without compensatory increase in heart rate Bradycardia and asystole can occur
Thiopental	3–7 mg/kg	Fast onset of action	Long context-sensitive half time ↑ heart rate which may be undesirable in patients ↑ airway resistance and bronchospasm
Etomidate	0.2–0.4 mg/kg	More cardiostable than other induction agents	Depression of adrenocortical system Myoclonic movements
Ketamine	1–2 mg/kg	May be used in patients with cardiovascular compensation such as tamponade	Increases myocardial oxygen requirements
Midazolam	0.1–0.2 mg/kg	Less cardiovascular depression	Prolonged recovery time High-dose benzodiazepines are implicated in postoperative delirium in the elderly
Opioids	Dose dependent on the agent used	Stable haemodynamics during induction	Prolonged recovery time if high doses are used Reports of intraoperative awareness

Note: SVR, systemic vascular resistance.

Muscle Relaxants

Pancuronium (0.1 mg/kg) for intubation and maintenance of muscle relaxation has the advantage of causing a slight tachycardia that offsets the bradycardia from opioids.

Shorter-acting muscle relaxants are recommended for 'fast-track' surgery with early extubation.

Prophylactic Antibiotics

Three to five doses of prophylactic antibiotics are prescribed in the perioperative period according to local protocols. Patients suspected of having a methicillin-resistant *Staphylococcus aureus* (MRSA) infection or colonization should be given vancomycin or teicoplanin before skin incision and continued until negative screening results are obtained. In patients with infective endocarditis a longer period of postoperative chemoprophylaxis with appropriate antibiotics is required.

Anti- and Procoagulant Drugs

Heparin

Heparin (300–400 units/kg) by intravenous injection is given for anticoagulation before insertion of the aortic cannula, and in coronary cases following internal mammary artery dissection.

If the patient is not heparinized before CPB, the pump and oxygenator will clot.

Heparin should be given as a bolus over 10–15 s. Always use a central line and aspirate the line before and after administration. Confirm to the surgeon that heparin has been given.

Heparin may adversely affect platelet function and following a period of continuous administration can produce thrombocytopenia (HITS). It can also modulate a number of other processes, e.g. inflammatory response, aldosterone production and lipid metabolism.

The degree of anticoagulation is measured using the activated clotting time (ACT). The control level before heparin administration is 90–130 s, and it should exceed 400 s before starting CPB. Additional heparin during CPB is given according to the ACT.

If heparin cannot be used as the primary anticoagulant (e.g. in cases of HITS), alternative direct thrombin inhibitors such as bivalirudin can be used. There are no reversal agents for bivalirudin but it has a short half-life (20–25 min). The degree of anticoagulation is monitored by an activated partial thromboplastin time (aPTT) of 1.5–2.0 times more than the baseline.

Serine Protease Inhibitors

Coagulation-modifying agents and antifibrinolytics such as aprotinin and tranexamic acid are commonly used to modulate CPB-mediated effects on coagulation and thereby reduce the amount of transfused blood given. Serine protease inhibitors (serpins) produce their action by inhibiting the serine protease-dependent reactions within the clotting cascade.

Aprotinin is administered as an initial intravenous test dose of 2500 units (5 mL), followed by a bolus of 195,000 units (195 mL) and an intravenous infusion of 50,000 units/h until 3 h after surgery. The incidence of anaphylactic reactions with aprotinin is high (1 in 200) and it should be used with caution in patients having had previous exposure to the drug. An ACT > 750 s is required before CPB if aprotinin is being used.

As a result of the BART study, the use of aprotinin was suspended in some countries in 2008.[3] Following an extensive review, aprotinin has now been reintroduced for use in cardiac surgery in patients undergoing CPB for coronary artery CPB grafting surgery.

Lysine Analogues

Tranexamic acid is an antifibrinolytic that competitively inhibits the conversion of plasminogen to plasmin. At higher concentrations it is a noncompetitive inhibitor of plasmin. Tranexamic acid is given as an intravenous bolus before heparinization at a dose of 10–50 mg/kg. Higher doses (>75 mg/kg) have been associated with postoperative seizures.

Protamine

Protamine produces its effect by directly antagonizing the actions of heparin via an electrochemical antagonism.

Protamine (3 mg/kg) should be administered over a period of 4–5 min following separation from CPB. If it is given too fast hypotension may occur due to systemic vasodilatation, or intense pulmonary arterial constriction.

Patients who are allergic to salmon, who have received isophane insulin or have had a vasectomy may be allergic to protamine.

To minimize the risk of potentially fatal administration, protamine should not be drawn up until CPB has been discontinued. Suction devices linked to the CPB machine should be turned off before giving protamine.

The reappearance of anticoagulant activity after adequate neutralization with protamine (heparin rebound) may contribute to excessive postoperative bleeding. Heparin rebound and incomplete heparin reversal are very common after CPB.

ACT is not able to detect residual heparin activity, whereas thromboelastograhy (TEG) analysis (with or without heparinase) can detect heparin rebound.

Vasoactive and Antiarrhythmic Drugs

Anaesthesia, surgery and CPB can promote haemodynamic instability in the patient with cardiac disease.

Vasopressor drugs suitable for bolus administration include metaraminol and phenylephrine. Whilst norepinephrine (noradrenaline) and vasopressin are given by continuous infusion.

Vasodilators include glyceryl trinitrate and phentolamine.

Atropine can be administered to increase heart rate.

In patients with impaired systolic function an infusion of milrinone, epinephrine, dobutamine or dopamine can be used for positive inotropic effects.

Acute arrhythmias during CPB are treated by correcting any precipitating factors and DC cardioversion in cases of haemodynamic instability. Persistent arrhythmias may need to be treated with magnesium or amiodarone (300 mg by slow intravenous injection over 10 min).

General Anaesthesia

Prior to CPB, anaesthesia can be maintained by either a conventional inhalational or a total intravenous anaesthetic (TIVA) technique using controlled ventilation.

Nitrous oxide is generally avoided because of potential problems with expansion of gaseous emboli and intraluminal air in open heart procedures.

Inhalational agents, in particular isoflurane, are known to be cardioprotective and can prevent intraoperative myocardial damage, although some can affect the conduction pathways and precipitate arrhythmias.

During CPB when ventilation is stopped, anaesthesia is maintained by TIVA, most commonly propofol infusion (3–5 mg/kg/h).

Volatile agents can be introduced into the CPB circuit to maintain anaesthesia during extracorporeal circulation. This should only be undertaken where scavenging and exhaust gas monitoring systems are available.

Regional Anaesthesia

Thoracic epidural anaesthesia has some benefit in reducing the risk of perioperative myocardial events in patients with cardiac disease presenting for noncardiac surgery. Controversy exists surrounding the risk-benefit in patients undergoing cardiac surgery with full heparinization.

Monitoring

ECG and Pacing

Use of a five-lead ECG with ST segment analysis is normal. When blood flow to the myocardium is insufficient wall motion abnormality develops within 5–10 s and by 60–90 s ST segment and T wave morphology start to change.

In cases of severe bradycardia an endocardial pacemaker wire may be inserted preoperatively. More commonly, epicardial atrial and ventricular pacing wires are used intra- and postoperatively.

Transoesophageal Echocardiography

TOE is useful in delineating valvular and septal pathologies and allowing real-time assessment of surgical repairs. It provides an early detector of abnormalities of ventricular wall motion. Information about volume and contractile status of the ventricles can help in the choice of inotropic medication or need for mechanical support to wean from CPB, and TOE is able to delineate residual intracardiac air or atrial thrombus.

The TOE probe is inserted at the time of intubation (unless there is a contraindication).

Pulse Oximetry

Peripheral measurement is routine, and mixed venous measurements are available if an oximetric pulmonary artery or CVC is being used.

Arterial Pressure

The dominant radial artery is usually cannulated, although femoral, brachial and ulnar arteries can be used. Flow is nonpulsatile during CPB.

Central Venous Pressure

Central venous pressure (CVP) is an indicator of right ventricular filling pressure. During CPB, a rise in CVP suggests obstruction or malposition of the venous lines. At the end of operation high pressure may be caused by overtransfusion or myocardial insufficiency and low pressure by inadequate transfusion.

Left Atrial Pressure

Left atrial pressure can be measured directly via a surgically sited catheter or more commonly assessed using a pulmonary arterial catheter measurement of wedge pressure.

Cardiac Output

Cardiac output can be measured continuously or intermittently using a pulmonary artery catheter.

Capnography

It is important to maintain normocapnia during all phases of the operation. Rapid alterations of PCO_2 can be harmful and compromise cerebral perfusion.

Temperature

Core temperature is the best monitor for body temperature during cardiac surgery. A number of sites have been used to measure temperature during surgery. These include:

- Pulmonary artery – accurately reflects core temperature
- Oesophagus – good correlation with core temperature
- Nasopharynx – easily positioned but risk of bleeding
- Urinary bladder – may be unreliable in patients with low or no urine output
- Rectum – temperature lags behind other monitoring sites especially during CPB. A loaded rectum may impair accuracy
- Tympanic membrane – good estimate of core temperature but may be difficult to place
- Skin – may differ by up to 2°C from the core; can be affected by cutaneous vasoconstriction

Cerebral blood temperature should not exceed normal body temperature during the rewarming phase of CPB because this can exacerbate cerebral injury.

Maintenance of normothermia is important in off-pump cardiac surgery.

Urine Flow

Urine flow is a simple indicator of adequate renal function. Urine output should be recorded every half hour and should exceed 0.5 mL/kg/h. Initially during CPB the output may be reduced but increases as rewarming occurs and the priming solution is excreted.

Biochemistry

Serum potassium should be maintained at over 4.0 mmol/L to minimize arrhythmias.

Glucose levels should be within normal physiological limits.

Lactate concentration is a marker of peripheral perfusion and an indirect reflector of cardiac output. Serial estimations can indicate whether a patient's condition is responding to a given intervention.

Platelet Function Testing

Platelet dysfunction is a common cause of bleeding after cardiac surgery, especially if patients have received antiplatelet agents. Such patients may have normal platelet count with inhibited platelet function. Assessing perioperative platelet function can help tailor transfusion therapy. Some of the more commonly used methods include:

- TEG® – provides information about interaction of coagulation factors, platelet contribution to clot strength and lysis data but long turnaround time (45 min) and unable to detect specific drug-induced platelet dysfunction
- Platelet mapping assay™ – indicates the degree of platelet inhibition achieved by drugs such as aspirin and clopidogrel but also has long turnaround time
- Impedance aggregometry – involves stimulation of platelet aggregation; has rapid turnaround time (<10 min) and ability to perform specific assays for antiplatelet agents
- Rotational thromboelastometry (ROTEM®) – uses thromboelastometry and impedance aggregometry to assess interaction of coagulation factors and platelet function analysis

Cardiopulmonary Bypass

The extracorporeal circuit incorporates a pump(s), a heat exchanger and a membrane oxygenator for gaseous exchange.

On initiating CPB, cardiac output commonly drops before 'full flow' is achieved.

Optimal, or full, flow is calculated based on the patient's surface area (2.2 L/min/m^2).

Flow is usually nonpulsatile, with mean arterial pressures (MAP) maintained at 50–80 mm Hg. There is no consensus on the optimum MAP to be maintained during CPB, which is influenced by several factors. In general, older patients benefit from a higher MAP during CPB. This pressure can be adjusted with small doses of vasoconstrictor or vasodilator drugs.

Historically most operations were performed under moderate hypothermia at 28°C–32°C but hypothermic CPB does not confer any additional benefit in terms of mortality and major morbidity whereas normothermic CPB (temperature > 34°C) is associated with a lower incidence of blood and blood product transfusion.

During extracorporeal circulation a number of parameters should be monitored continuously and intermittently (Box 5.2.1).[4]

During extracorporeal circulation the anaesthetist should monitor the following:

- ACT
- Blood gases
- Red cell concentration (haemoglobin or haematocrit)
- Serum potassium
- Blood sugar
- Filtrate volume

ACT is measured to confirm anticoagulation status.

As CO_2 is more soluble at low temperatures, PCO_2 will decrease and pH rise if measured values are corrected for body temperature. Consequently, CO_2 is added to the oxygenator gas mixture to avoid this apparent respiratory alkalosis. This is the 'pH–stat' approach.

In practice PCO_2 and pH should not be corrected for temperature and the apparent respiratory alkalosis should be accepted despite the possibility of cerebral vasoconstriction. Allowing PCO_2 to decrease (and pH to rise) as body temperature falls maintains the ratio of H^+ to OH^- constant (electrochemical neutrality), keeping the major buffer systems and enzyme function at their most effective. This is the 'alpha-stat' approach.

The CPB pump is primed with crystalloid and/or colloid (or blood if pre-CPB haemoglobin is <100 g/L) and 10,000 units of heparin. During CPB the target haematocrit is 20%–25%. Red blood cell transfusion is necessary if the haemoglobin decreases to less than 70 g/L during CPB.

BOX 5.2.1 Cardiopulmonary Bypass Parameters Requiring Continuous Monitoring

Venous oxygen saturation of the blood in the venous return line of the CPB circuit

Arterial oxygen tension or saturation of the blood in the arterial line of the CPB circuit

Continuity of the fresh gas flow to the oxygenator using an in-line flowmeter or rotameter

Oxygen concentration of the fresh gas flow to the oxygenator using an oxygen analyser with alarms and sited after the oxygen blender and vaporizer if used

Blood flow rate generated by the arterial pump of the CPB circuit

Arterial line pressure of the CPB circuit

Cardioplegia delivery line pressure when cardioplegia is delivered using the heart-lung machine

Temperature of the blood in the CPB circuit and the water in the heater/cooler system

If a haemofilter/concentrator is being used filtrate volume should be measured.

Other measurements that should be available include:
- Clotting studies, including thromboelastography (TEG)
- Serum calcium, lactate and magnesium

Myocardial Protection

The heart is arrested and the myocardium protected against ischaemic damage by the use of cardioplegia. For short periods of reduced cardiac movement ventricular fibrillation may be induced.

All cardioplegia solutions contain potassium.

Cardioplegia can be delivered as warm or cold, blood or crystalloid solutions, via an antegrade route into the aortic root or retrogradely via the coronary sinus.

For operations on the aortic root involving the coronary ostia and in complex repairs, hypothermic circulatory arrest at 18°C–20°C may be necessary. Under deep hypothermia (18°C) cell metabolism is so low that total circulatory and ventilatory arrest is safe. The period of circulatory arrest should be kept as short as possible to minimize cerebral damage.

On rewarming, the heart can be defibrillated above 30°C–32°C.

Blood Loss

It is important to use a cell-saver at all times during cardiac surgery and to salvage any remaining blood from the CPB circuit. This will reduce the requirements for autologous blood transfusion.

Complications of Cardiopulmonary Bypass

Complications of CPB can be divided into those associated with perfusion and the CPB circuit and those resulting from the process of CPB and its effect on the patient. The former include venous airlock, arterial gas embolism, clotting of the CPB circuit and failure of oxygen delivery. The latter include the following.

Awareness

The risk of awareness is inherent in the technique of CPB.

Anaesthesia can be maintained by a TIVA technique or by having a vaporizer in the CPB circuit.

Depth of anaesthesia can be monitored using bispectral index.

Cerebral Damage, Neurocognitive Dysfunction and Delirium

Cerebral damage may be global or focal, and caused by ischaemia, embolism of gas bubbles, blood clot and calcific fragments from a stenosed aortic valve.

- Emboli may be macro- or microemboli but <50% of the perioperative strokes following cardiac surgery are due to macroemboli (usually originating from the proximal ascending aorta).
- Atherosclerosis is an independent risk factor of postoperative stroke. Epiaortic ultrasound can be used to detect atherosclerosis before aortic cannulation.
- Cerebral hypoperfusion (reduction in MAP of >10 mm Hg during CPB) is associated with a higher incidence of watershed strokes.
- Other causes of include hyperthermia, hyperglycaemia, atrial fibrillation, anaemia and a genetic predisposition.

Delirium is an acute syndrome that involves fluctuating changes in cognition and attention. The incidence of delirium can be up to 50%–67% in patients undergoing cardiac surgery. Risk factors for postoperative delirium include old age, previous psychiatric conditions or cognitive impairment, cerebrovascular disease, perioperative blood transfusion, atrial fibrillation, renal insufficiency and prolonged mechanical ventilation.

Delirium following cardiac surgery is associated with higher mortality, readmission and decreased quality of life.

Lung Changes

Activation of the complement and kallikrein cascades causes neutrophils to aggregate in the pulmonary circulation which can affect vascular tone and capillary permeability.

Gas and particulate emboli can contribute to the development of an inflammatory response, which progresses to adult respiratory distress syndrome (ARDS) in 2%–6% of patients.

Postoperative Bleeding

Postoperative bleeding (Box 5.2.2) occurs especially with repeat or prolonged surgery. Bleeding usually responds to meticulous surgical technique, clotting analysis and targeted replacement of clotting factors and platelets. Further

---

BOX 5.2.2 Possible Causes of Postoperative Bleeding in a Patient Following Cardiac Surgery

Preoperative bleeding diathesis, including treatment with anticoagulant, antiplatelet or thrombolytic drugs
Inadequate neutralization of heparin and heparin rebound
Fibrinolysis and fibrinogen depletion (less than 100 mg/dL)
Platelet sequestration and dysfunction
Failure of surgical haemostasis
Hypothermia

protamine is indicated in the presence of a prolonged ACT. Following chest closure, continued bleeding with clot formation may lead to cardiac tamponade, evidenced by hypotension and a rising CVP.

Renal Dysfunction

Acute renal failure occurs in up to 30% of patients following cardiac surgery. Haemodynamic, inflammatory and nephrotoxic factors are implicated in the pathogenesis of kidney injury following cardiac surgery.

Risk factors associated with acute renal failure following cardiac surgery include haemodilution and haemolysis, prolonged duration of cross clamp and CPB, nonpulsatile flow, low ejection fraction, preoperative heart failure, diabetes and peripheral vascular disease.

In the presence of established renal failure haemofiltration should be employed during CPB.

Separation from Cardiopulmonary Bypass

There are a number of conditions which need to be met (Table 5.2.3) before weaning from CPB can be attempted. Most patients (80%–90%) undergoing first time coronary surgery will wean from CPB without the need for inotropic support. Acceptable parameters following separation from CPB are given in Table 5.2.4.

Inotropic or mechanical support may be required in patients with poor pre-operative ventricular function, prolonged cross-clamp time or inadequate myocardial protection. The choice of inotropic therapy or the need for an intra-aortic balloon pump (IABP) will be guided by experience and possible TOE assessment of the ventricle.

TABLE 5.2.3 Conditions that Need to Be Met before Attempting to Separate from CPB

Condition	Acceptable	Action Required if Not Met
Patient temperature	>36.5°C	Further rewarming
Rhythm	Sinus rhythm > 60 bpm	Pacing to establish atrioventricular synchrony
Serum potassium	>4.0 mmol/L	Give potassium
Acid-base status	Normal	Consider possible causes and correct if necessary
Ventilator	Turned on	
Monitors and alarms	Turned on	
Weaning plan	Agreed	

TABLE 5.2.4 **Acceptable Haemodynamic Variables Following Separation from CPB**

Parameter	Acceptable Level
CVP	<15 mm Hg
Systolic blood pressure	90–110 mm Hg
Cardiac index	2.5–3.0 L/min/m^2
Systemic vascular resistance	~1000 dynes/s/cm^5

In many cases a single dose of a phosphodiesterase inhibitor before weaning from CPB can be effective as the first line treatment for the failing ventricle.

SPECIFIC CARDIAC OPERATIONS

Coronary Artery Revascularization

The indications for coronary artery revascularization on prognostic grounds are as follows:

- Significant (>50%) left main stem stenosis
- Severe (>70%) two or three vessel disease (including the proximal left anterior descending)
- Left ventricle systolic dysfunction

Coronary artery revascularization can be performed either on- or off-pump. Suitable conduits include the internal mammary and radial arteries and the saphenous vein.

Off-pump coronary artery bypass (OPCAB) surgery may have advantages in high-risk patients with significant comorbidities. Anaesthetic management of OPCAB poses two major problems:

- Maintenance of haemodynamic stability with the heart in a nonphysiological and abnormal anatomical position
- Intraoperative myocardial ischaemia, which may develop during the process of grafting

Choice of anaesthetic technique is less important than a good understanding of the procedure itself.

In some patients where a single graft to the left anterior descending artery (LAD) is needed this can be performed by a left thoracotomy without CPB (minimally invasive direct coronary artery bypass; MIDCAB). MIDCAB requires a double-lumen endobronchial tube and one-lung ventilation. External defibrillator pads must be attached to the patient because the heart cannot easily be defibrillated internally via this incision. On-table extubation is usually possible. Anaesthetic management is as for a thoracotomy.

Valvular Surgery

Valvular heart disease may be congenital or acquired, most commonly affecting the left side of the heart. Stenotic lesions are associated with pressure-related disorders haemodynamic disturbance. Regurgitant lesions are associated with volume-related haemodynamic disturbance.

Corrective surgery involves recanalization, repair or replacement of the valve. There is a trend towards conservative surgery.

Mitral Valve Surgery

Closed Mitral Valvotomy

Closed mitral valvotomy is performed in some cases of pure mitral stenosis in the presence of an uncalcified valve. Other closed valvotomies are very unusual.

Mitral Valve Repair

Many surgeons favour mitral valve repair over replacement for mitral regurgitation.

Mitral Valve Replacement

Mitral valve replacement is indicated when repair of a regurgitant valve is impossible, for cases of endocarditis involving the mitral valve and for mitral stenosis.

Aortic Valve Surgery

Indications for aortic valve replacement are similar to those for the mitral valve. Where the ascending aorta is widened with associated valvular dysfunction, it can be replaced with a tissue valve and graft conduit, homograft or a composite graft. In some cases re-implantation of the coronary arteries into the graft may be necessary.

Left ventricular outflow obstruction secondary to subvalvular muscle hypertrophy can mimic aortic stenosis and is treated with a surgical myectomy.

Transseptal Defects

Transseptal defects between the right and left sides of the heart may be congenital or acquired and can be atrial or ventricular in origin.

Atrial communications such as atrial septal defects (ASDs) and patent foramen ovale (PFO) may be amenable to transvenously deployed atrial closure devices.

Ischaemic ventricular septal defects (VSDs) can be anterior or inferior and require surgical closure if associated with haemodynamic instability. This operation is associated with high morbidity and mortality rates.

Arrhythmia Surgery

Accessory conducting pathways causing intractable arrhythmias may be treated by radiofrequency ablation in the cardiac catheter laboratory, alternatively by subendocardial resection or by cryosurgery both of which necessitate CPB.

In patients with persistent atrial fibrillation secondary to atrial enlargement associated with mitral valve disease, surgical scarring of the atria is performed in the Maze procedure in an attempt to interrupt atrial pathways.

Cardiac Transplantation

The main indication for cardiac transplantation is cardiomyopathy, which may be ischaemic, hypertrophic or dilated. Recipients are normally aged < 50 years. Phosphodiesterase inhibitors and mechanical assist devices have been useful in 'bridging' patients to transplantation.

Active infection or malignant diseases are contraindications. Elevated pulmonary vascular resistance is a relative contraindication, and if acute can be treated with prostaglandin infusions or nitric oxide.

Cyclosporin may result in postoperative impairment of renal function.

Anaesthetic problems are similar to those for other cardiac operations in a seriously ill patient.

Heart Failure Surgery

Operative procedures are aimed at remodelling the ventricle in an attempt to improve performance and include the Batista and Dor procedures. These are often coupled with the use of mechanical assist devices and biventricular pacing, with the aim of producing a sustained improvement in cardiac output.

Aortic Surgery

Thoracic Aorta

Thoracic aorta surgery is most commonly performed for aneurysmal dilatation or dissection. The former may be a consequence of aortic stenosis or occur as a result of a connective tissue disorder, such as Marfan syndrome, whereas the latter arises as a result of intimal disease and is associated with hypertension and smoking.

For patients with aortic dilatation in whom the coronary ostia and aortic valve are not involved the aneurysmal section of the aorta can be replaced by an interposition woven graft.

Aortic dissection in the ascending aorta (type A) is a surgical emergency and requires an operation to replace the diseased segment and isolate the dissection flap. Dissections in the arch or descending aorta (type B) can be treated conservatively, or in some cases by endovascular stenting.

Ligation of Patent Ductus Arteriosus

Failure of closure of patent ductus results in blood flowing from the aorta to the pulmonary artery. The left side of the heart dilates to cope with the increased flow through it. Less blood flows down the aorta and the diastolic blood pressure is low. Cyanosis only occurs if pulmonary vascular disease develops or if other congenital abnormalities exist. There may also be pulmonary regurgitation. Endocarditis is a hazard. The ductus is easily torn when it is ligated, resulting in major bleeding.

Coarctation of the Aorta

Surgery for coarctation of the aorta is more risky in an adult than a child because of associated hypertension, coronary artery disease and cerebral aneurysms.

Enlarged collaterals in the chest wall prevent a severe increase in pressure when the aorta is clamped. Induced hypotension can be helpful in reducing blood loss from these collaterals. The blood pressure should be increasing again when the clamps are removed.

If the collaterals are poorly developed and the pressure distal to the coarctation is low, the blood supply to the spinal cord may be at risk.

Pericardium

Constrictive Pericarditis

Constrictive pericarditis limits diastolic expansion of the heart. The rise in atrial pressure leads to venous congestion, ascites, peripheral oedema and sometimes atrial fibrillation. The blood pressure may also decrease on inspiration (pulsus paradoxus).

These patients present considerable anaesthetic risks. Cardiac output may not be able to increase if there is a sudden decrease in peripheral resistance, and intravenous induction agents should be administered with caution. The surgical procedure is lengthy and involves considerable manipulation of the heart. Blood loss can be considerable and should be replaced precisely because the circulation is easily overloaded.

Cardiac Tamponade

Cardiac tamponade is caused by accumulation of fluid, including blood and blood clot, around the heart, resulting in haemodynamic compromise as venous return is reduced. The patient depends on a tachycardia and vasoconstriction to maintain the blood pressure.

Treatment of medical cases is by aspiration and insertion of a pericardial drain.

Open drainage with mediastinal exploration is indicated for trauma and for postoperative tamponade. Intermittent positive-pressure ventilation may cause severe hypotension before the pericardium is opened, and vasopressors may be required.

Chronic pericardial infusions can be drained into the pleural space by creating a pericardial window. This is often performed via a thoracoscopic approach.

Grown-up Congenital Cardiac Disease

Children with congenital cardiac lesions, whether corrected or not, surviving into adulthood may need further revision procedures. Such procedures require specialized multidisciplinary management.

SPECIFIC INTERVENTIONAL CARDIOLOGY PROCEDURES

Most procedures in adult patients are carried out under local anaesthesia with sedation as required. General anaesthesia is required for patients who are unable to tolerate the procedure under local anaesthesia, for complex and potentially prolonged electrophysiological procedures and for all procedures in children.

Arrhythmia Ablation

Cardiac arrhythmias such as atrial flutter and fibrillation, ventricular tachycardia and atrioventricular nodal reentry tachycardias (AVNRT) can be treated by an ablation procedure. Procedures such as AVNRT and supraventricular tachycardia ablation are performed under local anaesthesia since general anaesthesia may supress the incidence of these arrhythmias.

Intracardiac electrograms provide information about the type and origin of the arrhythmia. Catheter navigation systems create a geometry which illustrates a three-dimensional anatomy of the relevant cardiac chamber. Ablation of the arrhythmia involves delivery of energy as radiofrequency or cryotherapy.

The following points are of relevance:

- Procedures are often carried out in locations where access to help is restricted.
- Duration of the procedure can vary from 30 min to 5 h or more so patient positioning and padding of pressure areas is important.
- Maintenance of normothermia particularly during long-duration procedures is important.
- Although procedures involve minimal patient stimulation they necessitate absolute immobility to preserve the geometry acquired by the mapping system.
- TOE may be required to exclude thrombus in the left atrial appendage, guide the ablation catheter into the left atrium and exclude complications but necessitate tracheal intubation.
- Patients may have received therapeutic anticoagulation preoperatively. Also, heparin is administered intraoperatively to achieve an ACT > 300 s.
- Intraoperative hypotension should be treated with a vasoconstrictor. Intractable hypotension due to cardiac tamponade may occur rapidly.

- Fluid overload can occur with injudicious fluid administration as the cardiologists may also administer up to 2 L of intravenous fluid.
- Oesophageal injury can occur following radiofrequency ablation so an oesophageal temperature probe should be inserted.
- Pacing the phrenic nerve and observing diaphragmatic contraction can identify impending cryoballoon ablation-associated phrenic nerve damage but necessitates the use of short-acting muscle relaxants or total intravenous anaesthesia.
- Avoid excessive coughing and straining during extubation which can result in femoral bleeding and haematomas.

Pacemaker and Indwelling Cardio-defibrillator Insertion

Insertion of a permanent pacemaker (PPM) system is usually carried out using local anaesthetic infiltration only. However, intravenous sedation may be required for anxious patients. Insertion of indwelling cardio-defibrillator (ICD), replacement of PPM or pacemaker leads, usually require general anaesthesia with muscle relaxation. Invasive arterial pressure monitoring may be necessary for replacement of PPM. External defibrillator leads are applied for ICD insertion in case the ICD system fails to administer a shock when ventricular fibrillation is induced.

Replacement of PPM leads can be a prolonged procedure and may be associated with significant blood loss, so insertion of a large bore cannula is advisable. A magnet should also be available.

Commonly used anaesthetic agents do not affect pacing voltage theshold, but corticosteroids, including dexamethasone may lower pacing theshold and are best avoided.

Transcatheter Aortic Valve Implantation

Transcatheter aortic valve implantation (TAVI) is indicated for patients considered to be too high a risk for surgical aortic valve replacement. TAVI may be performed under local anaesthesia with sedation or general anaesthesia. The transfemoral approach is most commonly employed for TAVI. Alternatives include axillary, apex of the left ventricle, retroperitoneal iliac artery and ascending aorta.

The haemodynamic goals of anaesthesia management are the same as for patients with critical aortic stenosis undergoing valvular heart surgery.

In addition to routine monitoring for aortic valve surgery, external defibrillator pads should be applied.

Cerebral monitoring may be indicated in patients with cerebrovascular disease or those at risk of neurological events.

Local anaesthesia with lidocaine and sedation with remifentanil infusion may be used to facilitate TAVI.

In patients who may not tolerate local anaesthesia, general anaesthesia is administered. TOE, if used to provide additional information, also necessitates general anaesthesia and intubation.

Rapid ventricular pacing is used to stabilize the balloon and the prosthesis during valvuloplasty and deployment, respectively, but is accompanied by systemic hypotension. Vasopressors may be needed.

Postoperative care is provided in an intensive care unit or high-dependency.

Analgesia requirements with the transfemoral approach are minimal. Patients having a transapical TAVI may benefit from intercostal nerve block, patient-controlled opioid analgesia and regular paracetamol.

Complications of TAVI

● Vascular complications.
● Arrhythmias – AV block associated with balloon dilatation is common and necessitates insertion of a temporary pacing wire.
● Prosthesis malfunction, malposition and embolization – paravalvular leaks requiring reposition of the prosthesis can occur. Inability to reposition will necessitate open heart surgery.
● Neurological complications – over 50% of patients undergoing TAVI show evidence of clinically silent embolic events on diffusion-weighted MRI imaging but < 5% of patients have a major manifestation such as stroke.
● Tamponade.

Percutaneous Mitral Valve Implantation

Patients with severe mitral regurgitation deemed unsuitable for surgery may have a percutaneous MitraClip® device implanted under general anaesthesia or local anaesthesia with sedation.

Access is via the femoral vein and the MitraClip® device is implanted under fluoroscopy and TOE guidance. Some patients may need two clips to obtain sufficient reduction of mitral regurgitation.

Anaesthesia management combines the principles of percutaneous catheter-based procedures as discussed above and those relevant for patients with severe mitral regurgitation. Early tracheal extubation is warranted.

EARLY POSTOPERATIVE CARE

Some patients who have had uneventful coronary artery surgery can be extubated immediately following the end of surgery.

In straightforward cases, patients can be nursed in a postoperative anaesthetic care unit (PACU) and transferred to the ward on the day of surgery. Intensive care is still required for the more difficult cases.

Arrhythmias

Arrhythmias are common in the immediate postoperative period.

Atrial fibrillation is the most frequently occurring post-CPB arrhythmia, affecting up to 30% of patients. The incidence is less in patients who continue their cardiac medications up until the time of operation. Treatment involves correcting any precipitating causes (e.g. hypokalaemia, hypomagnesaemia), followed by pharmacotherapy or DC cardioversion if there is haemodynamic compromise.

Bradycardia can be treated by administering atropine, or if recurrent and associated with hypotension, atrial or sequential pacing.

Ventricular arrhythmias (especially fibrillation) following cardiac surgery may indicate ongoing ischaemia requiring further management.

Blood Product Replacement

In general there is no need to transfuse a patient unless the haemoglobin is < 8 g/dL. In the absence of surgical causes, postoperative bleeding warrants a complete haematological investigation including point-of-care tests (such as TEG) and laboratory investigations such as platelet count, INR and fibrinogen levels. Platelet and clotting factors such as Fresh Frozen Plasma (FFP) and cryo-precipitate can be administered accordingly

Cardiovascular Support

Inotropic drugs and vasodilators are sometimes needed after discontinuing CPB and are usually continued into the postoperative period.

If there is an increased requirement for circulatory support, it is necessary to acquire further information about cardiac status from haemodynamic and echocardiographic data.

Hypotensive episodes are managed by volume loading, followed by vaso-pressor infusions, titrated to a targeted endpoint.

Where impaired ventricular contractility is the cause of a low cardiac output, an inotropic agent will be necessary. Phosphodiesterase inhibitors are preferred to catecholamines but a vasopressor infusion may be required to maintain blood pressure if there is associated vascular relaxation.

Hypertension is managed by sedation and analgesia, followed by infusions of glyceryl trinitrate, or in intractable cases by infusion of a short-acting β-blocker.

Postextubation hypertension can be treated with oral calcium channel blockers such as nifedipine.

If drug therapy fails to maintain cardiac output, mechanical circulatory sup-port should be considered. An IABP can increase the output of a failing heart by 10%–20%, is relatively simple and provides useful but limited assistance. Ventricular support can be provided by the use of an implantable ventricular assist device, allowing manipulation of the ventricular preload to optimize cardiac performance.

Postoperative Hypothermia

Patient temperature tends to fall following separation from CPB. As a result, patients are often admitted to the PACU with a core temperature less than 35°C. To prevent further losses, heat to the patient is provided by warming infusion fluids and the use of forced-air heating blankets.

Postoperative Pain

Pain from a median sternotomy is not severe and is treated by continuous infusion of conventional opioid analgesics supplemented by paracetamol.

Renal Dysfunction

Low urine output is common in the immediate post-CPB period and generally responds to a volume challenge. Where urine volumes are less than 0.5 mL/kg/h in the presence of a normal blood pressure, an adequate filling pressure 5–10 mg of furosemide can be given intravenously to promote diuresis. A sustained diuresis may be achieved by continuous infusion of low-dose furosemide 0.1 mg/kg/h.

The role of 'low-dose' dopamine infusions in preventing renal dysfunction is controversial.

Early haemofiltration is necessary when hypervolaemia, acidosis and hyperkalaemia occur.

REFERENCES

1. Parsonnet V, Dean D, Bernstein AD. A method of uniform stratification of risk for evaluating the results of surgery in acquired adult heart disease. Circulation 1989;79:I3–I12.
2. Roques F, Nashef SAM, Michel P, et al Risk factors and outcome in European cardiac surgery: analysis of the EuroSCORE multinational database of 19030 patients. Eur J Cardiothorac Surg 1999;15:816–23.
3. Fergusson DA, Hebert PC, Mazer CD, Fremes S, MacAdams C, Murkin JM, et al. A comparison of aprotinin and lysine analogues in high–risk cardiac surgery. N Engl J Med 2008;358:2319–31.
4. Curle I, Gibson F, Hyde J, et al. Recommendations for standard of monitoring during cardiopulmonary bypass. London: Association of Cardiothoracic Anaesthetists; 2007. Available at http://www.acta.org.uk/store/docs/publications/cpbrecommendations2007-298972-31-08-2011.pdf

FURTHER READING

Hensley Jr FA, Martin DE, Gravlee GP. A practical approach to cardiac anesthesia. 5th ed. Philadelphia: Lippincott Williams & Wilkins; 2013.
Kaplan JA, Reich DL, Konstadt SN. Cardiac anesthesia. 5th ed. Philadelphia: WB Saunders; 2006.
McKay J, Arrowsmith J. Core topics in cardiac anaesthesia. 2nd ed. Cambridge: Cambridge University Press; 2012.

Chapter 5.3

Day Surgery

Ian Smith

GENERAL CONSIDERATIONS

Indications

Once seen as suitable only for a highly select group of patients and for minor surgery, day surgery should now be regarded as the default treatment for a wide range of elective and a selection of emergency surgical procedures. Assuming that the patient is sufficiently fit to undergo any form of elective procedure, day surgery is only contraindicated where there would be a clear benefit from pre- or postoperative hospital admission. Day surgery affords high quality care, with certainty through booking and choice, thorough preoperative assessment and preparation for surgery, rapid recovery with attention paid to minimizing side effects and providing effective analgesia, preparation for discharge with appropriate information and subsequent support and follow-up. The safety of day surgery remains excellent despite increasing surgical and patient complexity.

Economics

Day surgery avoids the expense associated with an overnight stay, whereas effective preoperative assessment and reduced emergency pressures can reduce cancellations and minimize waste. In some cases, day surgery may require more expensive drugs and equipment, but this is usually outweighed by savings elsewhere. In some parts of the world, enhanced tariffs are payable for some day surgery procedures, and insurance-based health systems may not always cover the additional costs of inpatient treatment where day surgery is the norm. Day surgery does not appear to transfer a significant financial burden into primary care.

Facilities

A variety of facilities are appropriate for day surgery (Table 5.3.1), each one has advantages and disadvantages. The once ideal model of a self-contained

TABLE 5.3.1 Facilities for Day Surgery

Integrated Self-Contained Day Surgery Unit

Description	Self-contained, functionally separate unit within a larger hospital
Advantages	• Efficient and focused • Functional separation from emergency pressures • Unanticipated admissions readily accommodated in the main hospital
Disadvantages	• Finite capacity limit • Duplication of surgical resources for procedures also performed on inpatients • May still be misused during emergency pressures

Freestanding Day Surgery Unit

Description	Self-contained unit remote from other hospitals; sometimes single speciality
Advantages	• Efficient and focused • Complete separation from emergency pressures
Disadvantages	• Finite capacity limit • Unanticipated admissions require transfer to neighbouring hospital • Selection criteria may be conservative to limit perioperative problems

Dedicated Day-Surgery Ward

Description	Modified ward area(s) dedicated to day-surgery patients
Advantages	• Efficient and focused pre- and postoperative care • Flexible and readily expandable with minimal investment • Utilizes existing operating theatre resources, facilitating transfer of complex procedures to day surgery
Disadvantages	• Potential for mixed operating lists reducing quality of care • Susceptible to emergency pressures • Efficiency reduced by distance to operating theatres and shared recovery units

Integrated Day and Short-Stay Unit

Description	Day unit with some overnight capacity adhering to day-surgery principles including nurse-led discharge
Advantages	• Allows operating later in the day and on more complex patients • Readily available beds for unanticipated admissions • Useful where successful discharge after planned day surgery is hard to predict • Helpful in developing new day-surgery procedures
Disadvantages	• Can encourage conservatism where day surgery is not well established • Very susceptible to misuse during emergency pressures • Antisocial hours may deter day-case nursing staff

day unit within a larger hospital remains the most efficient but increasingly lacks capacity as day surgery becomes the more usual form of care. The dedicated ward model is more flexible and avoids duplication of resource but is prone to misuse. Patients should be on dedicated day surgery lists. Mixing with inpatients results in substandard care with the possibility of cancellations if day cases are late on the list and less medical supervision available if they are early. Day cases should not be managed through regular inpatient wards, as they are far less likely to be successfully and comfortably discharged on the day of surgery.

Extended day surgery, or the 23-h stay facility, is an attractive model of care but has disadvantages as well as benefits (Table 5.3.1). This should be seen as a useful additional service for improving the quality of recovery and reducing the length of inpatient stay; however, patients who remain in the hospital beyond the day of surgery do not meet the usual definitions of day surgery. As a fully integrated part of an established day surgery unit, patients who have more complex procedures can be planned as day cases but with the ready availability of an overnight bed if recovery is delayed or complicated.

TECHNICAL CONSIDERATIONS

Selection of Patients

Selection criteria have changed dramatically over the past few years[1] and day surgery is increasingly seen as appropriate for about 80% of all elective surgery. It is still useful to consider surgical, social and medical selection criteria (Table 5.3.2). Laparoscopic and minimally invasive surgery have made more procedures possible, whereas changes in patient management, such as avoiding the use of drains or catheters (or allowing patients home with them in situ for subsequent removal in the community) and more sophisticated forms of analgesia can further extend the range. The British Association of Day Surgery produces a directory, which suggests the proportion of each of almost 200 different surgical procedures, which should be manageable as day surgery, given appropriate facilities and expertise (see Further Reading).

Preoperative assessment should take place as soon as possible after the decision to operate is made. This allows time for further investigation, specialist referral and corrective action to be undertaken, if needed, without delaying surgery. Preoperative assessment is usually nurse run, with appropriate advice from consultant anaesthetists. Preoperative assessment is primarily clinical, involving questionnaires and protocols, with investigations only performed where clinically indicated. Selection for day surgery should not be based on arbitrary limits, such as age, ASA classification or body mass index. Functional limitation and whether there would be a positive benefit from hospitalization are more important. Day surgery should not be cancelled or delayed solely on the basis of increased arterial blood pressure. Although conditions such as morbid obesity may make perioperative management more challenging, it is the effect, if any, on subsequent recovery which should determine the

TABLE 5.3.2 Selection Criteria for Day Surgery (See Also Joint Guidelines from the Association of Anaesthetists of Great Britain and Ireland and the British Association of Day Surgery[1])

Surgical

- Duration of surgery relatively unimportant
- No significant risk of serious complications (such as bleeding, cardiovascular instability) requiring immediate medical attention
- Postoperative pain must be controllable by available analgesia, typically a combination of oral medication and local anaesthetic techniques
- Resumption of oral intake is unlikely to be delayed by more than a few hours
- Surgery should permit mobilization to an adequate extent to permit discharge, with assistance and aids, where necessary

Social

- Following most procedures under general anaesthesia, a responsible adult should escort the patient home and provide support for the first 24 h[1]. This may not be necessary where:
  - The patient has had a brief procedure and made a full recovery
  - Surgery is superficial
  - Bleeding will be obvious and readily controllable with pressure
  - The patient is happy to be alone at home
  - Reasonable access to a telephone, primary care and hospital back-up

Medical

- Fitness for a procedure should not be determined by arbitrary limits, such as ASA status, age or BMI
- Patients with stable chronic disease (e.g. diabetes, asthma, epilepsy) are often better managed as day cases because of minimal disruption to their daily routine
- Main contraindications:
  - Marked dyspnoea on mild exertion or at rest
  - Angina markedly limiting activity or at rest
  - Myocardial infarction or revascularization within 6 months

Note: BMI, body mass index.

suitability for day surgery. Obstructive sleep apnoea is not a contraindication to day surgery, although patients undergoing more invasive surgery involving the chest or airway, or those requiring large doses of perioperative opioids may be less suitable. Patient characteristics are actually poor predictors of the quality of postoperative recovery. Where the planned procedure is compatible with same day discharge, it is preferable to book the patient for day surgery by default. This is because a patient who is prepared for day surgery can always be kept in the hospital should postoperative circumstances suggest that to be safest or most appropriate, whereas an inpatient who recovers faster than anticipated will feel dissatisfied and unsupported if he or she is discharged early at short notice. Paradoxically, day surgery may increase safety. As patients are more active, physiological warning signs, such as breathlessness, dizziness and light-headedness appear earlier and cause patients to seek help sooner than when they are in the perceived safety of the hospital ward.

Modern living standards mean that home circumstances should rarely preclude day surgery. Short travelling times are more comfortable, but distance should not be a barrier provided emergency care is available, not necessarily in the same centre as that performing the surgery. The presence of a responsible carer during the journey home and for about 24 h following anaesthesia has traditionally been seen as an important safety feature of day surgery. However, recent guidelines[1] have relaxed the requirement for a carer where their presence is unlikely to contribute to patient safety (Table 5.3.2). Under these circumstances, patients should not drive themselves home.

Preoperative Preparation for Day Surgery

Preoperative assessment encompasses several important functions (Table 5.3.3). In addition to determining whether there is any benefit from a given patient being kept in a hospital after surgery, it is just as important to ask whether anything can be altered to facilitate day surgery where this might not otherwise have been possible. Preparation includes giving patients information specific to their procedure, which forms part of the consent process. This should include early

---

TABLE 5.3.3 Important Functions of Preoperative Assessment with Examples

Identify Absolute Contraindications to Day Surgery

- Unable to identify a carer where one is required (Table 5.3.2)
- Severe uncorrectable cardiovascular disease
- Patient safety will be compromised by same-day discharge

Identify the Need for Optimization

- Further investigation, therapy or intervention required to improve functional status
- Identify a friend, relative or neighbour to act as a carer

Highlight Issues (for Anaesthetist or Staff) that will Require Management to be Modified

- Potentially difficult intubation requiring advanced airway management skills or equipment
- Susceptibility to malignant hyperpyrexia requiring trigger-free anaesthetic
- Latex allergy
- Obesity requiring specialized equipment
- Vulnerable patients requiring carers, quiet rooms or specialist equipment

Provide Patient Information

- Written information about preoperative preparation, medications, fasting, etc.
- Written information about aftercare including warning signs of major complications

warning signs about potential complications and what to do should these occur; information which should be reinforced shortly before discharge. Patients also need to be told where to come, what to bring and what to expect. Information should be given about regular medication (most should be taken) and fasting, the need for an escort, other postoperative limitations and likely time off work. Information should be both verbal and written. Dehydration is a major cause of postoperative morbidity and patients should be encouraged to drink up to 2 h preoperatively.[2]

Anxiolytic premedication is rarely given to adult day surgery patients because of concerns about limited time for effectiveness and delayed recovery. Greater reliance is placed upon sympathetic explanation and reassurance, as well as moving especially anxious patients to the start of the operating list. Administering oral analgesia shortly before surgery is a good way of ensuring adequate blood levels by the end of the procedure and avoids the disadvantages of rectal, intramuscular and intravenous administration of nonsteroidal anti-inflammatory drugs (NSAIDs). Sustained release preparations are especially beneficial as they achieve effective analgesia for up to 24 h and do not need to be given so soon before the start of surgery in order to retain postoperative efficacy.

Techniques of General Anaesthesia Appropriate for Day Surgery

General anaesthesia should use agents, which are rapidly eliminated and titratable. Intravenous propofol is most commonly used for induction of anaesthesia in adults, but inhaled sevoflurane is also suitable and may be especially beneficial in children, patients with needle phobia or difficult venous access and in the frail elderly. Anaesthesia may be maintained with isoflurane, sevoflurane, desflurane or infusions of propofol. Although all of these have their enthusiastic advocates, good results can usually be achieved with each in experienced hands. Experience, attention to detail and careful titration of the level of anaesthesia to match the degree of surgical stimulation are probably more important than the specific drug used. Meta-analysis shows differences in awakening times after surgery lasting up to 3 h to be small and relatively unimportant, although iso-flurane may delay discharge by 15 min or so. Propofol infusions have consistently been shown to reduce the incidence of postoperative nausea and vomiting (PONV). This too may be of limited significance unless the risk of PONV is especially high and overall the beneficial effect of propofol is similar to single-agent antiemetic prophylaxis. Nitrous oxide is often used as an analgesia supplement, especially with volatile anaesthetics and offers several benefits in day surgery.[3] Although it may increase the incidence of PONV, this effect is negligible for procedures lasting up to 2 h, and practical alternatives, such as opioid analgesics or a deeper level of inhaled anaesthesia, may have the same effect.

The laryngeal mask airway or an alternative supraglottic airway device (SAD) remains simple and effective airway management devices for many day surgery procedures and have the additional advantage of being well tolerated at light levels of anaesthesia. Spontaneous ventilation is usually appropriate and the respiratory pattern may aid in anaesthetic titration, whereas the ability to move protects against awareness. SADs are relatively easy to insert with patients in the prone position, making it a simple way of managing procedures such as pilonidal sinus repair or short saphenous vein surgery. Second generation devices increase the range of patients and procedures suitable for management by SAD. Their use for advanced laparoscopic procedures remains controversial, although their efficacy is well reported, their safety is still not universally accepted. Nevertheless, several advantages are reported, including reduced pain, lower analgesic requirements, less PONV, fewer sore throats, a reduced stress response, shortened recovery and earlier discharge.

Tracheal intubation with controlled ventilation is now more widely used in day surgery in light of increased surgical complexity and is acceptable, provided that neuromuscular blocking drugs of appropriate duration are used and adequate reversal is ensured. Succinylcholine is best avoided because of muscle pains. Nondepolarizing agents are usually suitable alternatives, but for short procedures tracheal intubation can be facilitated by deep propofol-opioid or sevoflurane anaesthesia.

Administering 1–2 L of crystalloid has been shown to substantially reduce drowsiness, dizziness and PONV during the recovery period and into the next day. Reducing the preoperative fluid fasting interval may achieve similar benefits. Intraoperative opioids are a major cause of PONV and their indiscriminate use should be avoided where possible, particularly for minor and intermediate surgery. Intraoperative morphine is especially undesirable, as it may cause somnolence in addition to PONV, but even modest doses of fentanyl or alfentanil substantially increase PONV. Most patients' postoperative pain can be managed by means other avoiding the need for prophylactic opioid administration. The response to intraoperative noxious stimuli can be blunted by adjustment of the main anaesthetic agent. Propofol may give a degree of protection against opioid-induced PONV compared to the use of inhaled anaesthetics. Various other adjuvant drugs have been used in day surgery with limited evidence of unequivocal benefit. Selective $\alpha2$-adrenergic agonists have potentially useful sedative and analgesic properties but at the expense of adverse effects. Despite years of study, they still have no clearly defined role in day surgery.

Techniques of Local Anaesthesia Appropriate for Day Surgery

Many minor day case operations can be performed using local anaesthetic infiltration including adult circumcision and inguinal hernia repair, meaning that virtually every case becomes suitable for day surgery.

A variety of regional nerve blocks may be applicable to several orthopaedic procedures, e.g. shoulder surgery. Spinal anaesthesia may be appropriate for many orthopaedic, urological and gynaecological procedures. It is also often used for inguinal hernia repair, but many consider infiltration anaesthesia to be preferable due to a lower risk of postoperative urinary retention. Spinal anaesthesia permits patients with significant obesity or respiratory disease to undergo day surgery. Care must be taken to ensure that prolonged motor and sympathetic blocks do not delay recovery. One option is to use short-acting agents such as prilocaine or 2-chloroprocaine. An alternative is to achieve selective spinal anaesthesia (SSA) by using a low dose (typically 4–7 mg) of bupivacaine with 10 μg fentanyl, often diluted to a volume of about 3 mL. Fine gauge, pencil-pointed needles can reduce the incidence of postdural-puncture headache to about 1%.

Whatever method of anaesthesia is used, local anaesthesia makes a major contribution to postoperative pain relief. For many operations, simple wound infiltration (or topical application following circumcision) is as effective as a nerve block and may reduce complications. For example, femoral nerve block, which can delay or even prevent discharge, complicates ilioinguinal nerve block in about 5% of hernia repairs. Analgesia can be provided using 0.5% bupivacaine or levobupivacaine in a volume appropriate to the size of the wound. Vasoconstrictors may be added if surgically indicated and may prolong the duration of analgesia, but their effect is probably not that significant. Regional nerve blocks may be useful after extensive shoulder or knee surgery. Catheter-based techniques involving continuous or intermittent delivery of local anaesthesia in the patient's home have been described and may permit more extensive day surgery operations to be performed; however, for a variety of logistical reasons, they have yet to become common and their safety has been questioned.[4] A high-volume local infiltration analgesia (LIA) is a useful alternative.

Alternative Techniques (Sedation, Sedoanalgesia)

The use of local or regional anaesthesia may be made more acceptable by the addition of anxiolytic, sedative and analgesic adjuvants. Simple measures, such as verbal reassurance or music (of the patient's choice) should be tried prior to drug administration. A gentle surgeon is also an important component. A small dose (typically 1–2 mg) of midazolam can provide appropriate anxiolysis and a degree of sedation. If necessary, this may be supplemented by small boluses (10 mg) or a low-dose infusion (1–2 mg/kg/h) of propofol, which allows titratable sedation without compromising recovery to the same degree as a higher dose of midazolam. Pain should primarily be treated with additional local anaesthesia, but systemic analgesia may be useful to overcome the initial pain of injection or from pressure or traction on deeper structures. Small doses of short-acting opioids are usually appropriate, but care must be taken to avoid respiratory depression, which is especially likely with combinations of opioids and benzodiazepines.

POSTOPERATIVE CONSIDERATIONS

Recovery from Anaesthesia

Initial recovery of consciousness, haemodynamic stability and protective reflexes should occur in a properly equipped recovery room (postanaesthesia care unit; PACU). Some patients may reach a satisfactory level while still in the operating theatre and safely bypass the recovery room going straight back to the day surgery unit (fast-track recovery). Prior to discharge, patients should have recovered to the level shown in Table 5.3.4. Scoring systems may sometimes be used, but assessment of recovery is a clinical process and is not aided by psychomotor tests.

Following the regional anaesthesia, patients should have minimal sympathetic or motor block. A self-limiting numb limb or extremity may be acceptable, provided that it can be protected against injury.

Patients must be discharged with information about warning signs of potential complications and the necessary actions they should take. A contact telephone number should be provided for the day unit if open all hours, otherwise to an acute surgical assessment area. Assessment of potential surgical complications through primary care, or even accident and emergency units, can result in inappropriate management and significant delays.

TABLE 5.3.4   Clinical Criteria for Recovery from Day-Case Anaesthesia Sufficient to Permit Safe Discharge

- Oriented to time, place and person

- Haemodynamic stability demonstrated

- Minimal bleeding or wound drainage

- Acceptable control of pain, nausea and dizziness

- Ability to dress and walk where appropriate (able to manage, with help, if a single limb is temporarily incapacitated)

- Has passed urine or low residual volume on bladder scan (only following procedures at high risk of urinary retention)

- Provided with appropriate written information and take-home analgesia

- Responsible adult to take the patient home and provide care for next 24 h (where required)

- Community support arranged (if appropriate)

- Knows when to come back for follow-up (if appropriate)

- Emergency arrangements discussed and contact number (for an acute surgical area) supplied

Most patients are accompanied home in a private car, although a taxi may be considered acceptable, provided a carer, where required, will meet the patient at home. Care should be taken with complex or hazardous tasks until complete recovery has occurred. Alcohol enhances the sedative effects of anaesthesia and analgesia but is not prohibited in moderation. Modern anaesthesia impairs driving performance for at least 6 h and driving is not advised until at least the following day; however, patients should refrain from driving until the pain and immobility due to their operation allow them to safely control their vehicle and perform an emergency stop. This may take several days, e.g. following an inguinal hernia repair. Return to work will depend on the level of pain, the procedure performed and the nature of the patient's work but is frequently possible within two weeks.

Pain Management

Prophylactic analgesia should be administered whenever pain is anticipated. NSAIDs are the drug of choice unless there are contraindications (e.g. known worsening of asthma, recent gastrointestinal pathology). COX-2 selective NSAIDs probably offer little advantage in acute use. Paracetamol and/or codeine compounds are useful alternatives or supplements. Long-acting local anaesthesia should be used wherever possible. Severe postoperative pain should be treated with opioid analgesics if required but with the lowest effective dose, and opioids should not be given routinely. Opioids may play a greater role following more advanced day surgery procedures. Take-home analgesia should be supplied for 3–5 days after most operations unless patients already have a suitable pain relief at home.

Postoperative Nausea and Vomiting

Effective nonopioid analgesia, adequate hydration and careful drug titration all reduce PONV. Patients should be assessed for their risk of PONV, with prophylaxis chosen accordingly. Common risk factors for PONV and for postdischarge nausea and vomiting (PDNV)[5] are given in Table 5.3.5. Dexamethasone, cyclizine or a 5-HT$_3$ antagonist are similarly effective for prophylaxis and their effects are additive. Prophylactic antiemetics should not be administered to those at low risk of PONV (to avoid unnecessary adverse effects), but prophylaxis with single, dual and multimodal antiemetics should be used for those at moderate, high and very high risk, respectively. If PONV occurs, it should be treated aggressively unless it is a transient phenomenon. 5-HT$_3$ antagonists and intravenous fluids are useful. Intractable PONV is usually self-limiting. Admission will not offer a cure if maximal therapy has already been given and patients may be offered the choice of going home, provided they have been adequately hydrated.

TABLE 5.3.5 Common Risk Factors for Postoperative Nausea and Vomiting (PONV) and Postdischarge Nausea and Vomiting (PDNV)

PONV	
Risk factors	• Female gender • Nonsmoker • History of PONV or motion sickness • Perioperative opioid use

Calculation of risk	• Risk increased progressively according to number of risk factors
	• Published data suggest risk approximates to:
	  • 10% for 0 risk factor
	  • 20% for 1 risk factor
	  • 40% for 2 risk factors
	  • 60% for 3 risk factors
	  • 80% for 4 risk factors
	• Published estimates probably overestimate risk with modern anaesthetic techniques, but the gradation of risk still applies

PDNV	
Risk factors	• Female gender • Age <50 • History of PONV • Opioids administered in PACU • Nausea in PACU

Calculation of risk	• Risk increased progressively according to number of risk factors
	• Published data suggest risk approximates to:
	  • 10% for 0 risk factor
	  • 20% for 1 risk factor
	  • 30% for 2 risk factors
	  • 50% for 3 risk factors
	  • 60% for 4 risk factors
	  • 80% for 5 risk factors

Based on Apfel et al.[5]

Unanticipated Admission

Approximately 1%–2% of patients cannot be discharged as planned, surgical reasons being the most common cause. Higher unanticipated admission rates are to be expected following more complex procedures. A similar proportion of patients are likely to be readmitted within 1 month but many for unrelated reasons.

Admission rates, pain, PONV and satisfaction rates should be constantly monitored as performance indicators. Day-case anaesthetists should constantly monitor their own results and follow-up their patients, where possible, prior to discharge.

SPECIFIC OPERATIONS

An increasingly wide range of procedures can be safely and successfully performed as day surgery. However, the proportion of cases carried out as day surgery procedures varies considerably between hospitals and even between different surgeons within the same hospital. This variation cannot be explained solely by the clinical status of the patient and probably reflects conservatism on the basis of an exaggerated perception of the risk of serious complications after discharge. Such risks are reduced when experienced surgeons perform a high volume of cases.

When a particular procedure can be performed as a day case, attempts should be made to continually increase the proportion of patients managed in this way. Defaulting the management's intent of specific procedures to day surgery (see Selection of Patients) is an effective way to achieve this. The development of day surgery is a continually evolving process, with procedures moving from inpatient care to day surgery and others moving out into outpatients and primary care. Developments may require a combination of new surgical techniques, alteration in anaesthetic management, revised working practices and questioning of established practices. Continuous evolution of day surgery involves

- Reduced length of stay of inpatient procedures
- Convert inpatient procedure into overnight stay
- Convert overnight stay into day surgery
- Move minor day surgery into outpatient department or primary care

Nonelective Procedures

Although traditionally confined to elective procedures, a small number of urgent nonelective operations can be managed through a semi-elective day surgery pathway. This is sometimes referred to as 'emergency day surgery'. Some examples of suitable procedures are as follows:

- Incision and drainage of abscess
- Evacuation of retained products of conception
- Tendon repair
- Manipulation of fractures
- Repair of fractures, such as clavicle, mandible, zygoma
- Renal tract stones
- Laparoscopic cholecystectomy
- Laparoscopic appendicectomy

A variety of pathways can be developed to suit local needs and circumstances as given in Table 5.3.6. Emergency day surgery avoids the repeated prolonged fasting and cancellation, which often befalls patients with relatively minor ailments on inpatient emergency lists. Patients appreciate a more guaranteed time of surgery, whereas the hospital benefits from the freeing up beds during the wait for surgery and a reduced length of stay afterwards.

TABLE 5.3.6 Principles of Management for Patients Undergoing Nonelective or 'Emergency' Day Surgery

- Initial assessment:
  - Procedure and patient identified as suitable for day-surgery management
  - Patient can safely be managed conservatively for 1–2 days
  - Pain can be managed with oral analgesia until surgery
  - Suitable list for operation identified
  - Any necessary investigations performed

- Patient discharged with:
  - Standard oral analgesia pack
  - Date and time to return for surgery (within 1–2 days)
  - Written information
  - Plan to follow, if the condition worsens

- Re-admitted to day-surgery unit

- Surgery performed with day-surgery intent
  - Using spare capacity on elective list
  - As planned procedure on an emergency list; usually ring-fenced first case(s)

- Patient discharged, if possible, according to usual day-surgery criteria

Laparoscopic Cholecystectomy

There has been a considerable increase in the adoption of this as a day-case procedure with some units achieving 80% or more. This is largely due to the realization that previous concerns about bleeding and bile leaks were unfounded. In practice, complications are either readily apparent within a few hours and consequently detectable before same-day discharge, or delayed for several days, by the time when even inpatient cases would have been at home. Pain is usually manageable with typical analgesic regimens and morbidity is reduced by avoiding the routine use of drains. Where drains are specifically indicated because of surgical concerns, these can be removed on the day unit when drainage is minimal. Patients undergoing day-case cholecystectomy are often better supported and followed-up than those discharged after an overnight stay in an inpatient ward. Complications leading to increased postoperative pain and conversion to an open procedure are difficult to predict, and there are advantages to managing all cholecystectomies through a day unit, which also has the capacity to keep patients overnight (or even longer), if required.

Laparoscopic Nephrectomy and Pyeloplasty

Still relatively uncommon, but a skilled surgeon can achieve safe and comfortable discharge in a small proportion (10%–20%) of adult patients having laparoscopic nephrectomy for cancer or nonfunctioning kidneys. The principles are the same as those used for cholecystectomy. The main factor limiting same-day discharge is achieving effective pain relief. Pyeloplasty can be managed on a day-case basis in a much higher proportion of cases. The basic management principles are the same, but there is no kidney extraction wound and is usually less painful. In both cases, avoidance of wound drains and urinary catheters, which are an unnecessary source of infective and other complications, is an important aspect of management.

Tonsillectomy

This was previously considered controversial but is now commonly performed as a day case. The arguments are similar to those for laparoscopic cholecystectomy, but again bleeding typically occurs early or very late and the pain is usually manageable. Use of a SAD improves recovery and virtually eliminates the risk of postoperative laryngospasm, although tracheal intubation remains more commonly used because of concerns about obstruction of the airway from the use of surgical gags.

Thyroidectomy

A few centres have reported good results with day-case thyroid and parathyroid surgery in selected patients, but these procedures are still controversial. Careful surgery by experienced, regular surgeons with meticulous control of bleeding is vital to success. In practice, postoperative haematomas are uncommon, few require reoperation and most present themselves early enough to be detectable before patients are discharged. Local anaesthetic techniques appear to be beneficial. Mechanisms to prevent, detect and, if necessary, treat postoperative hypocalcaemia need to be in place.

Mastectomy

Wide local excision has typically been a day-case procedure for some time, but until recently the need for mastectomy usually mandated an inpatient stay. The reasons for this, typically providing support within the hospital, the widespread use of wound drains and the need for physiotherapy, have all been challenged. In practice, patients prefer the support of their family within the familiar home environment to that provided by inpatient wards. The use of surgical drains does not appear to prevent seroma formation and units achieving the highest day surgery rates no longer routinely insert wound drains. Where drains are indicated, they can be managed at home and removed in the community. Physiotherapy exercises can be taught preoperatively and managed outside of the hospital. The widespread use of sentinel node biopsy has reduced the need for axillary clearance and, consequently, morbidity. Lymphoedema is not induced or worsened by using the ipsilateral arm for venous cannulation or blood pressure measurement.

Transurethral Prostatectomy

Conventional prostatectomy results in too much postoperative bleeding to be compatible with routine day surgery. Bipolar diathermy techniques improve haemostasis and appear promising. Greenlight laser prostatectomy reduces bleeding considerably, making day surgery possible in most cases. Many patients can be discharged catheter-free, whereas others can go home with a urinary catheter for subsequent removal in the community. Spinal anaesthesia (using a suitable low-dose technique) provides good surgical conditions, excellent analgesia and is ideal for avoiding the hazards of general anaesthesia in a population where cardiorespiratory disease is common.

FUTURE DEVELOPMENTS

Although many of the developments outlined earlier have come through advances in surgical and anaesthetic techniques, much has also been achieved by challenging myths and conventional wisdom. Patients repeatedly report great satisfaction with day surgery and value the care and support which come from excellent information and preparation. Wound drains and catheters are frequently unnecessary, sometimes harmful, and usually manageable in the community, if needed. Most complications are prevented by a short hospital inpatient stay and the excellent safety record of day surgery has been maintained despite a massive increase in the range and complexity of patients and procedures undertaken. Sceptics frequently state that achievements made elsewhere will not translate to their particular environment for reasons of geography, demographics, facilities, etc. However, successes reported from almost all possible settings result from the application of the same basic day-surgery principles.

New technological developments will bring an even greater range of procedures into the day-surgery arena, while allowing others to be performed in outpatient clinics. Procedures potentially facilitating day surgery include minimally invasive hip replacement, single-compartment knee replacement and stereotactic, awake craniotomy. Radiofrequency or laser ablation of varicose veins and hysteroscopic tubal occlusion are examples of techniques, which have allowed treatments to move from day surgery to outpatient. Radiologically assisted catheter techniques also have the potential to facilitate more day and short-stay surgery, whereas many of the fundamental principles of day surgery are now being applied to the management of elective and emergency medical procedures.

REFERENCES

1. Association of Anaesthetists of Great Britain and Ireland, British Association of Day Surgery, Verma R, et al. Day case and short stay surgery: 2. Anaesthesia 2011;66:417–34.
2. Smith I, Kranke P, Murat I, Smith A, O'Sullivan G, Søreide E, et al. Perioperative fasting in adults and children: guidelines from the European Society of Anaesthesiology. Eur J Anaesthesiol 2011;28:556–69.
3. Billingham S, Smith I. Role of nitrous oxide in ambulatory anaesthesia. Curr Anesthesiol Rep 2014;4:275–83.

4. Pawa A, Devlin AP, Kochhar A. Interscalene catheters—should we give them the cold shoulder? (Editorial). Anaesthesia 2016;71:359–62.
5. Apfel CC, Philip BK, Cakmakkaya OS, Shilling A, Shi YY, Leslie JB, et al. Who is at risk for postdischarge nausea and vomiting after ambulatory surgery? Anesthesiology 2012;117: 475–86.

FURTHER READING

Smith I, McWhinnie D, Jackson I, editors. Day case surgery (Oxford specialist handbook series). London: Oxford University Press, 2012.
British Association of Day Surgery. BADS Directory of Procedures. London. (available from www. bads. co. uk). 4th ed. 2012, but updated periodically.

Chapter 5.4

Endocrine Surgery

Nick Pace, Shubhranshu Gupta

THYROID GLAND

The thyroid gland is the largest endocrine gland. Surgery can vary in complexity, from simple removal of a nodule to excision through a sternal split of a long-standing retrosternal goitre to relieve tracheal compression.

Anatomical Considerations

The close proximity of the thyroid gland to vital structures (see Fig. 5.4.1) requires special surgical attention.

Physiological Considerations

The primary function of the thyroid gland is the secretion of three hormones: thyroxine (T_4), triiodothyronine (T_3) and calcitonin. The vast majority of T_4 and T_3 are bound to plasma proteins such as thyroid-binding globulin (TBG) and albumin. Free (unbound) levels should be measured to distinguish thyroid disease from abnormalities of the carrier proteins (e.g. raised in pregnancy).

The effects of thyroid hormones include regulation of metabolic rate, brain development and function and growth. The feedback mechanism for control of the levels is shown in Fig. 5.4.2.

Pathophysiology and Indications for Surgery

Hyperthyroidism

Hyperthyroidism results from excess circulating T_3 and T_4 hormones. The clinical features include

- General – weight loss, malaise, heat intolerance, cachexia, proximal muscle wasting, pretibial myxoedema (Graves disease)
- Cardiovascular – palpitations, angina, hypertension, breathlessness, tachycardia, atrial fibrillation, hyperdynamic circulation and heart failure; mitral valve prolapse due to papillary muscle dysfunction can occur

Thyroid gland - General topography

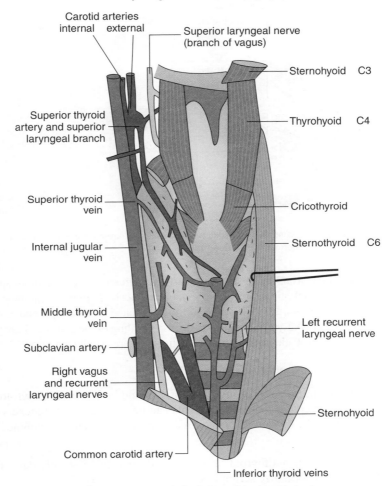

Fig. 5.4.1 Anatomical relations of the thyroid gland.

- Central nervous system – anxiety, irritability and tremor
- Gastrointestinal – hyperphagia, diarrhoea, vomiting
- Ophthalmic – exophthalmos, lid lag, blurred vision

Surgery is usually considered after failed medical treatment in the young and in women who wish to become pregnant. Surgery also has a role in the management of the large toxic goitre or adenoma.

Malignancy

Malignancy of the thyroid gland commonly presents as a thyroid nodule. Papillary and follicular carcinomas are well differentiated and arise from the epithelium. They

Physiology of thyroid hormones

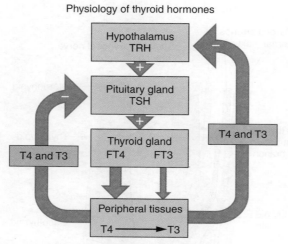

Fig. 5.4.2 Physiological control of thyroid hormones. TRH, thyrotropin releasing hormone; TSH, thyroid-stimulating hormone; FT4, free T4; FT3, free T3.

carry a good prognosis if local and excised early. Undifferentiated carcinomas such as medullary or anaplastic lesions have a poor prognosis. Medullary carcinomas arise from the calcitonin-producing cells and are associated with multiple endocrine neoplasia II (MEN II). Lymphomas cause diffuse swelling of the gland and carry a very poor prognosis. Patients with thyroid malignancy are usually euthyroid.

Implications for Anaesthesia

Patients undergoing surgery for thyrotoxicosis should be rendered euthyroid if possible. In an emergency situation patients can be treated with β-blockers to reduce the risk of a thyrotoxic crisis. Treatment regimes can be combined if required and include

- A titrated dose of antithyroid drug (e.g. carbimazole 15–40 mg daily for 6–8 weeks) to normalize serum levels of T_3, T_4 and TSH
- A block-and-replace regimen of a large dose of antithyroid drug (e.g. carbimazole 40–60 mg) and replacement thyroxine
- Sympathetic overactivity may be blocked with a β-blocker (e.g. propranolol 30–60 mg TDS);
- Oral iodine – for 10 days before surgery in Graves disease has been shown to reduce blood flow in the thyroid and may be considered

Preoperative Assessment

History

The nature of the thyroid pathology should be established. The presence of complications of thyrotoxicosis such as atrial fibrillation, or associated conditions (medullary carcinoma is associated with a phaeochromocytoma) looked for.

Airway Assessment

A significant mass effect is suggested by positional dyspnoea, dysphagia and stridor. Check for tracheal deviation and narrowing on chest X-ray (CXR). Lateral thoracic inlet views may be necessary to exclude retrosternal extension and detect tracheal compression. Tracheal deviation or > 50% narrowing on CXR suggests possible difficulty with intubation. A CT scan is indicated in such cases and can give an accurate assessment of the degree and site of airway distortion; it may also show tracheal invasion by malignancy. Plain X-rays overestimate diameters, owing to magnification effects and are unreliable for predicting the required tracheal tube size. MRI has the advantage of providing images in the sagittal and coronal planes as well as transverse views.

On examination, an enlarged tongue may add to airway difficulty and a lingual thyroid may interfere with laryngoscopy. A large goitre may make emergency tracheostomy difficult and retrosternal spread can cause superior vena caval obstruction.

In malignancy, vocal cord palsies are possible. Distortion and rigidity of the surrounding structures may make it impossible to pass a standard tracheal tube.

Indirect laryngoscopy should be undertaken to assess vocal cord movement and the function of the laryngeal nerves. If this is unsuccessful and a fibreoptic instrumentation is necessary, the anaesthetist should be alerted to the possibility of a difficult intubation.

Investigations

- Routine blood tests – FBC, electrolytes including calcium, thyroid function tests
- CXR, thoracic inlet views, CT scan, MRI
- Nasendoscopy
- Respiratory flow-volume loops – if any evidence of upper airway obstruction

Intraoperative Management

Historically, thyroid surgery was performed under local anaesthesia. Currently, it is almost exclusively performed under general anaesthesia, although uncomplicated unilateral surgery can be performed under superficial and deep cervical plexus block.

The majority of cases are straightforward and, following preoxygenation, can proceed with intravenous induction of anaesthesia, a neuromuscular blocking drug (NMB) and tracheal intubation with a reinforced tracheal tube. The presence of malignancy or patients who have significant respiratory symptoms require careful planning with the consideration of alternative options to secure the airway.

Options to secure the airway include:

- Inhalational induction with sevoflurane or halothane can be used for patients with a potentially difficult airway. However, loss of muscle tone can lead to the loss of the airway and airway obstruction can make it difficult to achieve sufficient depth of anaesthesia.

- Awake fibreoptic intubation (AFOI) is an alternative where a 'difficult airway' is anticipated – this may not be feasible due to a critically narrow airway.
- Tracheostomy below the level of obstruction under local anaesthesia can be performed by the surgeons.
- Ventilation through a rigid bronchoscope can be performed when attempts to pass an endotracheal tube down the trachea fail.
- Useful preoperative oxygenation can be achieved by the use of nasal high flow devices such as Optiflow™.

Maintenance of anaesthesia can be either with volatile or total intravenous anaesthesia (TIVA). Where intraoperative monitoring of nerve function is to be used, long-acting NMBs should be avoided. The neural integrity monitor (NIM)™ electromyography tracheal tube is increasingly used and familiarization with its placement and positioning is useful.

A remifentanil infusion has many advantages: providing a smooth induction and an apnoeic patient (important when a NIM tube is used and NMBs avoided), relative hypotension with a bloodless surgical field during dissection while allowing a quick return to normotension to check for haemostasis on completion of the dissection.

The head and neck are extended by the use of a head ring and a sandbag placed under the shoulders to improve surgical access. If used, the NIM tube position should be rechecked at this stage to ensure that the colour-coded contact band is between the vocal cords. Eye protection with adequate padding is important, particularly if there is exophthalmos. Head up tilt is often used; be aware of the risk of air embolism.

Analgesia is usually achieved by remifentanil and paracetamol intraoperatively but morphine or fentanyl will be required before the end of surgery. Superficial cervical plexus block or local infiltration can provide useful analgesia. Antiemetics are routinely used; dexamethasone also helps to prevents airway oedema.

The surgeon may request a Valsalva manoeuvre at the end of the surgery to check for haemostasis. Occasionally, the need to check the vocal cords may arise. Various techniques can be employed to facilitate smooth extubation, prevent coughing and straining. A laryngeal mask or an alternative supraglottic airway device (SAD) can be exchanged for the tracheal tube at the end of surgery to minimize coughing. Alternatively, 'deep extubation' can be practised; it is prudent to establish the presence of a leak on deflating the tracheal tube cuff to ensure there is no airway oedema.

Postoperative Complications

The potential complications of most concern are those that acutely threaten the airway. Any patient who complains of 'being unable to breathe properly' should be taken seriously. Respiratory difficulty on extubation may require reintubation. Complications include:

- Recurrent laryngeal nerve damage – may be transient or permanent. Unilateral nerve damage may not be clinically apparent due to compensatory over adduction of the opposing cord. However, a voice change and slight stridor can be present and it is possible for glottic incompetence, ineffective cough and aspiration to occur.
- Bilateral recurrent laryngeal nerve damage – uncommon (approximately 1 in 30,000) and may not be immediately apparent on extubation. Stridor and laryngeal obstruction due to unopposed adduction of the vocal cords can result in complete airway obstruction, which requires immediate reintubation and possibly tracheostomy.
- Haematoma – postoperative haemorrhage and haematoma compromise the airway by a direct mass effect. The patient should be reintubated and return to theatre for evacuation of the clot. In extremis, this can be done at the bedside, but it may not be relieved by the removal of skin sutures. Reintubation can be very difficult because of swollen and distorted tissues.
- Tracheomalacia – a long-standing goitre may result in weakening of the tracheal rings, but it is rare for the trachea to collapse. The absence of a leak before extubation should alert the anaesthetist to the possibility of this complication. If present, immediate reintubation is required.
- Laryngeal oedema – usually occurs 24–48 h postoperatively; it may be secondary to a traumatic intubation or extensive surgery. Diagnosis is by indirect laryngoscopy.
- Hypocalcaemia – typically develops 24–48 h postoperatively and is related to damage or resection of the parathyroid glands, most frequently after total thyroidectomy. If the serum calcium is < 2 mmol/L, parenteral calcium replacement is necessary. It is worth remembering that laryngeal stridor progressing to laryngospasm may be one of the first indications of hypocalcaemic tetany.
- Other complications include hypothyroidism, hypoparathyroidism and occasionally hyperthyroidism.

Thyroid Crisis

Thyroid crisis occurs due to uncontrolled release of thyroid hormones. Onset is usually rapid and triggered by surgery, trauma and infection. It is now rare owing to the use of antithyroid drugs but carries a mortality of 20%. It may present 6–24 h postoperatively. Perioperatively it can present with features of malignant hyperthermia (but muscle rigidity is absent).

Clinical Features

- Central nervous system – tremor, agitation, delirium, seizures, coma
- Cardiovascular – hypertension, tachycardia, arrhythmia, congestive cardiac failure

- Respiratory – hyperventilation, hypercapnia, acidosis
- Gastrointestinal – diarrhoea, vomiting, abdominal pain, acute abdomen, fever, hyperthermia

Management

- Oxygen supplementation and active cooling
- β-blockade with propranolol, esmolol or labetolol to decrease heart rate
- Propylthiouracil – inhibits thyroid hormone release and decreases peripheral conversion of T_4 to T_3
- Hydrocortisone – recommended for possible adrenocortical exhaustion
- Judicious use of intravenous fluids
- Magnesium sulphate reduces the incidence and severity of dysrhythmia caused by catecholamines

PARATHYROID GLANDS

Anatomical Considerations

- Four parathyroid glands, two on each side, embedded in the superior and inferior poles of the thyroid.
- Anatomical variations include descent into the thorax along with the thymus.
- Chief cells secrete parathyroid hormone.
- The inferior thyroid artery provides the blood supply; venous and lymphatic drainage is shared with the thyroid gland.

Physiological Considerations

Parathyroid hormone (PTH) is the major hormone responsible for the maintenance of normal calcium metabolism. It has effects on various organs:

- Kidney – increased absorption of calcium and excretion of phosphate; increased bicarbonate and free water clearance
- Bone – increased resorption of bone to mobilize calcium
- Intestine – increased formation of 1,25-dihydrocholecalciferol (vitamin D).

Hyperparathyroidism

Hyperparathyroidism occurs as a result of increased secretion of PTH. It is classified as follows:

- Primary hyperparathyroidism – usually caused by a single parathyroid adenoma.
- Secondary hyperparathyroidism – commonly associated with chronic renal failure as a result of low serum calcium levels.
- Tertiary hyperparathyroidism – development of autonomous hypersecretion of PTH; most commonly in patients with chronic secondary hyperparathyroidism and after renal transplant.

- Ectopic – secretion of a PTH-like peptide by tissues other than parathyroid gland.

Clinical features depend upon the serum calcium but may include:

- Cardiovascular – hypertension, short QT interval, prolonged PR interval
- Neurological – weakness, lethargy, mental status changes
- Musculoskeletal – muscle weakness, osteoporosis, bone pain
- Gastrointestinal – abdominal pain, peptic ulcer, pancreatitis
- Renal – polyuria, polydipsia, severe dehydration, renal stones
- Historically described as a disease of stones, bones, abdominal groans and psychic moans

Indications for Surgery and Surgical Management

The usual indication for surgery is removal of a parathyroid adenoma, the commonest cause of hyperparathyroidism (80% cases). A total parathyroidectomy may be performed for secondary hyperparathyroidism; hyperplasia also often requires removal of all four glands. Carcinoma warrants 'en bloc' dissection.

Surgical management includes minimally invasive parathyroidectomy. This requires preoperative localization and real time intraoperative monitoring of PTH levels. Some centres use frozen section biopsy, alternatively low-dose intravenous Technetium (99mTc) or sestamibi can be used to locate the gland (minimally invasive radio-guided parathyroidectomy). Bilateral neck exploration involves the identification of all four glands and the subsequent removal of the abnormal gland.

Implications for Anaesthesia

Preoperative care includes the correction of hypercalcaemia, a Ca^+ greater than 3 mmol/L should be corrected, wherever time allows. Adequate hydration should be ensured and renal function optimized. When parathyroidectomy is being performed for secondary hyperparathyroidism secondary to renal failure, the patient may need to be dialysed preoperatively.

Intraoperative anaesthetic considerations are similar to that of thyroid surgery. Extra care in positioning for patients with osteoporosis is warranted and a warming device is advisable, as the surgical time can be prolonged especially with difficulties in identification and localization.

Patients may have an unpredictable response to NMBs due to skeletal muscle pathology and raised calcium; the use of a peripheral nerve stimulator is recommended.

Postoperative Complications

A high index of suspicion is warranted for complications such as recurrent laryngeal nerve injury, glottic oedema and metabolic abnormalities – hypocalcaemia and hypomagnesaemia may occur; serum calcium levels should be monitored at 6 h and 24 h postoperatively.

ADRENAL GLANDS

Anatomical Consideration

The adrenal glands are located on the upper poles of the kidneys; the suprarenal glands. The gland is divided into the adrenal cortex and the adrenal medulla. The adrenal cortex is further subdivided into zona glomerularis, fascicularis and reticulosa.

Physiological Considerations

The adrenal cortex secretes glucocorticoids, mineralocorticoids and androgens.

Glucocorticoids are regulated by the pituitary and hypothalamus and mineralocorticoids by the kidney. The adrenal medulla synthesizes and secretes catecholamines (adrenaline:noradrenaline, 70:30). The secretion of catecholamines is triggered by preganglionic sympathetic fibres in response to stress, exercise or emotion.

Pathophysiology of the Adrenal Cortex

Cushing's Syndrome

Cushing's syndrome is a collection of signs and symptoms resulting from excessive levels of corticosteroids. The commonest cause is the prolonged administration of high doses of exogenous corticosteroids.

Cushing's disease occurs due to a pituitary adenoma with increased secretion of adrenocorticotrophic hormone (ACTH), leading to increased levels of cortisol. Other causes of Cushing's syndrome include an adrenal adenoma or carcinoma, or tumours such as oat-cell carcinoma of the bronchus that secrete ACTH. The clinical features include central obesity, hypertension, proximal myopathy, gastro-oesophageal reflux, hypokalaemia and diabetes mellitus (Chapter 1.2). Treatment may involve adrenalectomy for adrenal tumours or hypophysectomy for pituitary adenomas.

Implications for Anaesthesia

Preoperative optimization of complications, such as hypertension and diabetes, are essential. Fluids and electrolyte imbalances should be corrected. Intraoperative emphasis should include careful patient positioning due to obesity and skin fragility. Venous access may be difficult. NMBs should be used with caution due to reduced muscle mass and a peripheral nerve monitor should be used.

Adequate hydrocortisone replacement should be considered intraoperatively where appropriate. Postoperative hydrocortisone replacement, and fludrocortisone, from day 5, will provide adequate glucocorticoid and mineralocorticoid cover for bilateral adrenalectomy.

Conn's Syndrome

Conn's syndrome is caused by the secretion of excessive amounts of aldosterone by an adenoma of the adrenal cortex (75%), or from bilateral adrenal hyperplasia. Secondary hyperaldosteronism occurs due to the activation of the renin–angiotensin–aldosterone axis, secondary to conditions such as renal artery stenosis or cardiac failure. Adenomas are treated surgically, often laparoscopically, whereas hyperplasia is treated medically.

Clinical features include hypertension, hypervolaemia, hypokalaemia and metabolic alkalosis. Muscle weakness and renal tubular damage can occur.

Implications for Anaesthesia

Spironolactone is given preoperatively to correct electrolyte and metabolic imbalance. It is essential that the volume status is corrected before surgery. Intraoperative management may be complicated by cardiovascular instability and refractory hypertension, especially when the adrenal gland is manipulated. A short acting α-blocker should be available to deal with hypertension.

Blood glucose should be monitored – impaired glucose tolerance is common. Postoperative management includes correction of fluid and electrolyte imbalance, hydrocortisone and often fludrocortisone.

Phaeochromocytoma

Phaeochromocytoma are catecholamine-secreting tumours of the chromaffin cells of the adrenal medulla. Phaeochromocytomas are biochemically very active, most commonly producing noradrenaline but also adrenaline and rarely dopamine. Traditionally referred to as the '10% tumour': approximately 10% are familial, 10% bilateral, 10% extra-adrenal and 10% malignant. However, it now appears that a higher proportion of these tumours are malignant (29%), extra-adrenal (24%) or familial (32%). There is an association with multiple endocrine neoplasia syndrome (MEN), von Hippel-Lindau syndrome and neurofibromatosis.

Clinical features often reflect the predominant catecholamine released and include

- Severe hypertension, may be sustained, paroxysmal or both. True paroxysmal hypertension is seen only in 35% of the cases.
- Chronic vasoconstriction causes relative hypovolaemia.
- Paroxysmal crises – with marked hypertension, severe headache, sweating, palpitations, facial pallor, anxiety, tremor, weakness and chest pain.
- Complications include myocardial ischaemia, arrhythmias, neurogenic pulmonary oedema and cerebrovascular events.
- Diagnosis is established by the estimation of urinary and plasma catecholamines.

- Tumours may be identified on CT or MRI scan or using MIBG scintography.
- Early diagnosis is essential – the rare event of a phaeochromocytoma presenting unexpectedly during an unrelated procedure has a mortality rate exceeding 60% compared to less than 2% for elective excision.

Implications for Anaesthesia

Alpha-adrenergic antagonists form the basis of the medical management of phaeochromocytoma, leading to the control of hypertension, progressive restoration of normovolaemia and reversal of catecholamine cardiomyopathy. Commonly used agents include phenoxybenzamine and doxazosin.

Phenoxybenzamine irreversibly alkylates α-receptors and prevents the clinical response to catecholamine release. The dose is titrated to effectively control hypertension. β-blockade is added, following α-blockade, to prevent the resultant tachyarrythmias. However, β-blockade is only started after a complete α-blockade to avoid the unopposed α-mediated vasoconstriction that could occur after antagonism of β_2 mediated vasodilation, which may precipitate a hypertensive crisis. Treatment with phenoxybenzamine is initiated at least 14 days prior to surgery and ideally stopped 24–48 h before surgery. This is to avoid refractory hypotension in the postoperative period.

The selective α_1 antagonist doxazocin may be preferred, as this is not associated with tachyarrythmias and sedation. This regime, however, may offer less cardiovascular stability (see PRESCRIPT trial; http://clinicaltrials.gov/show/NCT01379898).

Phaeochromocytoma surgery should be performed in specialist centres. The majority of procedures are now performed laparoscopically. Laparoscopic surgery allows more precise dissection, diminishes the stress response, minimizes blood loss and leads to a significantly faster recovery and shorter hospital stay. However, creation of a pneumoperitonium can cause a dramatic catecholamine surge possibly as a result of mechanical stimulation of the tumour, increased afterload and chemical stimulation by carbon dioxide absorbed transperitoneally. The most important aspect in the management of a patient with phaeochromocytoma is the close cooperation between the endocrinologist, anaesthetist and the surgeon.

Preoperative Assessment

- Evaluation of cardiovascular and other end-organ effects of hypertension.
- ECG may reveal ventricular hypertrophy, arrhythmias and myocardial ischaemia. Echocardiography is mandatory; up to 50% of patients have cardiomyopathy.
- An elevated haematocrit level indicates significant intravascular volume depletion.
- Roizen criteria for optimal preoperative control are:
  - Consistent blood pressure readings below 160/90 mm Hg
  - Postural hypotension not lower than 80/45 mm Hg
  - Absent ST-T changes on the ECG for 7 days

However, these criteria are now questioned. There is no consensus but tighter blood pressure control is recommended (<130/80 mm Hg) and orthostatic hypotension is not necessary.

Anaesthesia

The primary goal is to prevent haemodynamic compromise and arrhythmias due to catecholamine surges. Invasive monitoring is usually established under local anaesthesia. Central venous access should be considered both for assessing preload and administration of vasopressors if required. If severe cardiomyopathy is present, a pulmonary artery catheter may be considered. Agents that cause catecholamine release, sympathetic stimulation or histamine release should be avoided. Drugs to be avoided include morphine, ketamine, desflurane, atracurium, ephedrine, metoclopramide, droperidol, suxamethonium, naloxone and cocaine.

Catecholamine release is provoked by the following:

● Induction of anaesthesia
● Endotracheal intubation
● Laparoscopic insufflations of pneumoperitoneum
● Tumour manipulation

Benzodiazepine premedication is useful. Epidural analgesia is useful for open laparotomies. Remifentanil infusion is effective for laparoscopic procedures.

Specific aspects of perioperative management include the following.

Management of Catecholamine Surges

● Optimal preoperative medical management
● Attenuate response to laryngyscopy
● Phentolamine (1–5 mg)
● Labetolol (5–10 mg)
● Sodium nitroprusside (0.5–6 μg/kg/min)
● GTN (10–400 μg/min)
● Magnesium (2–4 g/h)

Vasodilators such as phentolamine, sodium nitroprusside or nicardipine infusions should be immediately available. Magnesium sulphate inhibits catecholamine release, exerts a direct vasodilator effect and reduces α-receptor sensitivity.

Management of Tachyarrythmias

● Esmolol (500 μg/kg as loading dose, followed by 50 μg/kg/min maintenance infusion)
● Lidocaine (1 mg/kg)
● Amiodarone (300 mg)

Management of Hypotension after Final Ligation of the Tumour's Venous Drainage

- Fluid boluses – guided by filling pressures, cardiac output monitoring, ECHO
- Vasopressors and inotropes
- Consider angiotensin and steroids

Final ligation of the tumour's venous drainage is often associated with profound and refractory hypotension. The mechanism for this is uncertain but possible mechanisms include the down regulation of α-receptors, suppression of the contralateral adrenal medulla, persistence of preoperative adrenergic-receptor blockage, relative hypovolaemia or catecholamine cardiomyopathy.

Oesophageal Doppler monitoring can be useful to determine systemic vascular resistance and cardiac output. Resistance to vasopressors may be the result of receptor down regulation. Steroid replacement is required if both adrenals are removed and for refractory hypotension.

Postoperative Care

Patients are routinely monitored in a high-dependency unit or intensive care unit depending upon the outcome of surgery. Cardiovascular management, fluid balance, correction of electrolytes are the most important aspects. Patients may develop hypoglycaemia as the α2 mediated suppression of pancreatic β-cell insulin release has been removed.

FURTHER READING

Connor D, Boumphrey S. Perioperative care of phaeochromocytoma. BJA education 2016;16: 153–158.

Farling PA. Thyroid Disease. Br J Anaesth 2000;85:15–28.

Pace N, Buttigieg M. Phaeochromocytoma. BJA CEPD Rev 2003;3:20–23.

Chapter 5.5

Gynaecological Surgery

Mubeen Khan

GENERAL CONSIDERATIONS

Anaesthesia for gynaecological surgery encompasses fit and healthy young women undergoing minor day-case surgery, through to elderly women with significant comorbidity, undergoing radical malignancy surgery.

Remote Location

In vitro fertilization (IVF) procedures often take place in areas not attached to theatre complexes and so the principles of remote location anaesthesia apply (see Chapter 5.15). It is essential to have skilled help, be comfortable with the anaesthetic machine and know the location of emergency drugs and crash trolley prior to anaesthetizing patients.

Positioning

Patient positioning depends upon the individual procedure and the need for surgical access to the operative site.

Lithotomy Position

Lithotomy or Lloyd-Davies positions are commonly used for procedures such as cystoscopy, hysteroscopy, vaginal hysterectomy and IVF. The feet are placed in stirrups, with the legs raised and abducted. If a history of joint disability or osteoporosis is obtained, stretching of hip joints or the pelvic girdle during anaesthesia should be avoided. It is important to have two people, one for each leg, to move the limbs symmetrically and avoid excessive abduction.

The stirrups should allow the calves and legs to hang without pressure, external to the stirrup pole. Padding may be necessary to prevent pressure on nerves and to keep hands and legs away from any metal (to protect from diathermy burns). It is important to avoid undue strain on the lumbar spine due to the exaggerated lumbar pressure associated with this position.

Care must be taken while tilting the table to avoid the risk of patients slipping off the table especially if a sliding sheet, which is used to assist in manual handling, is left in position.

Complications

Complications of anaesthesia in the lithotomy position include:

- Impeded respiratory muscle excursion – respiration needs to be monitored and controlled if necessary.
- Reflux of stomach contents – seen especially during light anaesthesia and surgical stimulation. Adequate depth of anaesthesia and endotracheal intubation where indicated minimizes the chances of aspiration.
- Lower limb compartment syndrome – intermittent compression boots, adequate padding and periodic leg movement help reduce these risks during prolonged surgery.
- Deep vein thrombosis – thromboprophylaxis measures such as graduated elastic compression stockings, intermittent compression boots and pharmacological agents should be used.
- Peripheral nerve injuries – multiple nerves can be damaged, e.g. sciatic, femoral, common peroneal, posterior tibial and saphenous nerves (see Table 5.5.1).

Trendelenburg Position

Laparoscopic procedures require varying degrees of Trendelenburg (head down) positioning to access the pelvic structures. The level of tilt may vary from a gentle 15° tilt to a much steeper incline for robotic access surgery.

TABLE 5.5.1 Potential Nerve Injuries Associated with Lithotomy Position[1]

Peripheral Nerve Involved	Injury Mechanism	Symptoms
Sciatic nerve	Exaggerated knee extension, thigh flexion and hip rotation	Reduced knee flexion and foot drop
Femoral nerve	Adduction and thigh rotation	Weak hip flexion and loss of knee extension
Common peroneal nerve	Compression between fibula and stirrup	Loss of dorsiflexion and foot eversion
Posterior tibial nerve	Pressure from stirrup	Loss of foot inversion; pain and reduced sensation on base of foot
Saphenous nerve	Compression between medial malleolus and stirrup	Loss of sensation on medial side of leg

Complications

Complications of the Trendelenburg position include:

- Airway displacement
- Impeded ventilation due to upward displacement of the diaphragm
- Hypotension due to reduced cardiac return
- Reflux of gastric contents and aspiration in case of an unsecured airway
- Falling from the operating table due to patients not being secured well to the table or slipping on the sliding sheet.

Thromboembolism

Major gynaecological surgery, lasting more than 30 min in women over 40 years of age, is a significant risk for postoperative venous thromboembolism. Deep venous thrombosis (DVT) occurs in the leg or pelvic veins in up to 17% of patients after gynaecological surgery and up to 26% after major gynaecological surgery.[2] Pulmonary embolism is responsible for around 20% of perioperative hysterectomy deaths for malignancy surgery.[3]

Factors increasing risk during gynaecological surgery include effects of positioning and pelvic instrumentation. Pressure on the leg veins (e.g. from stirrups used to elevate the legs or arising from marked flexion at the groin) can cause stasis. Surgical manoeuvres may impede blood flow through the pelvis also leading to stasis. Pre-existing varicose veins, more common in women, add to the risks. The risk of thromboembolism in gynaecological surgery can be graded as low, moderate and high (see Table 5.5.2).

The following are recommendations for thromboprophylaxis:

- Low risk – early mobilization, adequate hydration and graduated elastic compression (GEC) stockings.

TABLE 5.5.2 Thromboembolism Risk in Gynaecological Surgery[4]

Risk Category	Risk Factors
High	• Major gynaecologic surgery, age > 60 • Major gynaecologic surgery, age 40–60 and cancer or history of DVT/PE or other risk factors including thrombophilia
Moderate	• Major gynaecologic surgery, age 40–60 without other risk factors • Minor gynaecologic surgery, age < 40 on oestrogen therapy • Minor surgery, age > 60
Low	• Major gynaecologic surgery, age < 40 without any other risk factors • Minor gynaecologic surgery, age 40–60 without any other risk factors

Source: Reproduced with permission from Cardiovascular Disease Educational and Research Trust. International Consensus Statement (Guidelines according to scientific evidence): Prevention and Treatment of Venous Thromboembolism. International Angiology, Vol 32.2, Page 133.

- Moderate risk – low-molecular-weight heparin (LMWH) along with the aforementioned recommendations.
- High risk – low-molecular-weight heparin should be considered for 4 weeks following surgery, along with aforementioned measures.

If anticoagulation is instituted prior to surgery, this should be stopped in sufficient time to allow a regional block to be performed (e.g. LMWH is stopped 12 h before an extradural nerve block) if appropriate.

SPECIFIC GYNAECOLOGICAL OPERATIONS

Hysteroscopy

Endoscopic equipment enables the gynaecologist to inspect the uterine cavity and explore it with accuracy. Hysteroscopy may be diagnostic to investigate conditions such as infertility and menorrhagia. Therapeutic hysteroscopy can be used to resect fibroids or leiomyomas, treat adhesions and remove lost intrauterine contraceptive devices. Endometrial ablation is a less invasive alternative to hysterectomy for menorrhagia; procedures are shorter, recovery is rapid and there is lower morbidity.

Anaesthetic Concerns

The main indication for diagnostic hysteroscopy is anomalous uterine bleeding – the patient's full blood count should be checked preoperatively in case of anaemia. Hysteroscopy is usually performed as a day-case procedure and under general anaesthesia. It can be done under regional anaesthesia or even a paracervical block, with or without sedation, but the lithotomy position is uncomfortable for a prolonged period and may not be ideal.

For general anaesthesia, a supraglottic airway device (SAD) is common but depends upon various factors such as the length of the procedure, patient's characteristics and aspiration risk.

The technique involves infusion of fluid into the uterine cavity and, as with the transurethral resection of the prostate (TURP), fluid can be absorbed. The amount of fluid used for flushing the hysteroscope during the procedure should be monitored.

Pain after hysteroscopy is rarely severe, a combination of a nonsteroidal anti-inflammatory drug (NSAID), if not contraindicated, with codeine and paracetamol is usually satisfactory.

Complications

Complications include:

- Dilatation of the cervix can lead to autonomic stimulation with laryngeal spasm or bradycardia; additional anaesthetic agents or anticholinergic agents should be available to block these effects.
- Fluid can be absorbed through open venous sinuses leading to hypervolaemia and hyponatraemia as in TURP syndrome (see chapter 5.16). Absorption

depends on the infusion pressure (greater for the uterine cavity than for the prostate), vascularity (the uterus can be atrophic in the midproliferative phase or in response to progesterone analogues), and the duration of surgery.
- Uterine perforation and bleeding; facilities to manage these risks should be available.
- Rarer complications include gas or air embolism.

Assisted Conception

There are two stages at which anaesthetic input may be needed for oocyte retrieval and surgical embryo transfer. For transvaginal oocyte retrieval under ultrasound guidance, a paracervical block and sedation are usually adequate. For invasive surgical embryo transfer (e.g. gamete intrafallopian transfer [GIFT]), a general anaesthetic is required. Spontaneous respiration with a SAD is usual.

Anaesthetic Concerns
- Procedures are carried out in the IVF suite, usually in a remote location.
- There are often numerous cases scheduled in a limited time with resultant time pressures.
- Fasting status should be confirmed as instructions may be misunderstood, especially if the procedure to be performed is under sedation.

Laparoscopy

Laparoscopy has revolutionized modern surgical practice. This minimally invasive technique has transformed gynaecological surgery. What were previously major inpatient procedures have become day-case surgeries, improving patient experience, reducing recovery time and perioperative morbidity. Diagnostic laparoscopy is performed for conditions such as endometriosis and infertility and therapeutic laparoscopy for adhesiolysis, ovarian cystectomy, ectopic surgery and fibroid removal, mostly as day-case procedures. Inpatient laparoscopic procedures include:

- Laparoscopic assisted vaginal and abdominal hysterectomy
- Laparoscopic large fibroid removal.
- Ovarian torsion and cyst removal

Anaesthetic Concerns

Although many laparoscopic procedures are considered relatively minor surgeries, the creation of a pneumoperitoneum is not without risk and should be treated with vigilance to identify potential complications promptly. Insertion of the trocar and insufflation of the abdomen can trigger a vagal reflex, which can result in significant bradycardia. There have been case reports of patients needing cardiopulmonary resuscitation due to profound bradycardia leading to a cardiac arrest. The trocar may be inadvertently inserted into a viscera or a major blood vessel such as the aorta or the vena cava leading to severe haemorrhage, gas embolism or visceral injury.

Pneumoperitoneum

Pneumoperitoneum leads to alteration of physiological parameters:

- Airway – It may result in endobronchial intubation due to upward shift of the diaphragm and lung fields.
- Respiratory – It may lead to increased airway pressures and hypercarbia and hypoxia due to ventilation perfusion mismatch. Upward displacement of the diaphragm may lead to basal atelectasis.
- Cardiovascular – Blood pressure may fall on abdominal insufflation as a result of reduced venous return secondary to aortocaval compression, compounded by increased intrathoracic pressure. Over the course of surgery, increased systemic vascular resistance along with neurohumoral stimulation and activation of renin–angiotensin axis often leads to high systemic pressures.
- Gastrointestinal – Both the patient profile and type of surgery increase the likelihood of postoperative nausea and vomiting; prophylactic antiemetics should be administered.

Airway management for a laparoscopic procedure is usually with a tracheal tube. The use of second-generation SADs is increasing but the potential for regurgitation and aspiration must be assessed carefully. Systemic absorption of CO_2 and raised intra-abdominal pressure necessitates an increased minute volume. Close attention must be paid to airway pressures.

The Trendelenburg tilt may be quite extreme to achieve surgical access to the pelvic organs. The reverse Trendelenburg position may lead to reduced venous return and hypotension.

Postoperative pain after laparoscopy depends upon the procedure. It is more severe after instrumental surgery than diagnostic procedures. It can be reduced by local anaesthetic infiltration of the wound (e.g. 0.25% levobupivacaine 10 mL) or to the surgical site (e.g. fallopian tube). Referred shoulder pain from peritoneal stretching or subdiaphragmatic remnant air is common. Regular NSAIDs and a codeine/paracetamol combination is usually effective. For more extensive procedures, for example, laparoscopic assisted hysterectomy, perioperative analgesia may be provided by a neuraxial block or the use of transversus abdominal plane (TAP) blocks.

Hysterectomy and Myomectomy

Hysterectomies are performed through an abdominal incision or via a vaginal approach dependant on factors such as uterine size, cancerous mass, adhesions, etc. Myomectomy is performed for fibroids that are multiple or too large to be removed laparoscopically.

Anaesthetic Concerns

Patients undergoing vaginal hysterectomy tend to be older and often have comorbidities. A thorough preoperative assessment is essential. In the presence of menorrhagia or postmenopausal bleeding the patient may be anaemic; recent blood results should be checked and group and save performed.

Vaginal hysterectomies can be done using a SAD and spontaneous respiration. A caudal with bupivacaine (20 mL of 0.25%) improves perioperative analgesia. Spinal anaesthesia with or without sedation is an alternative to general anaesthesia. Care must be taken with positioning, as these patients may well have osteoarthritis or have had joint replacement surgery.

Abdominal hysterectomies usually require intubation and controlled ventilation, as muscle relaxation is often needed. A neuraxial block, either a single-shot spinal anaesthetic with diamorphine and bupivacaine or insertion of an epidural catheter to cover postoperative analgesia, should be considered. Alternatively, a TAP block combined with patient-controlled analgesia (PCA) is effective. Postoperative nausea and vomiting is common and prophylactic antiemetics are recommended.

Radical or Wertheim's abdominal hysterectomy is a major procedure, usually performed for uterine or cervical malignancy, associated with greater morbidity and mortality. Surgery can be prolonged and there is the potential for extensive blood loss. Additional efforts should be made to provide protection from the effects of prolonged surgery such as pressure sores or hypothermia. Invasive arterial monitoring is recommended and central venous pressure monitoring or cardiac output monitoring should be considered. Replacement of fluid and blood losses using large-bore, pressurized infusion systems may be required. Neuraxial analgesia is useful for postoperative pain. A postoperative high-dependency unit admission is usual.

ROBOTIC SURGERY

Robotic surgery is a variant of laparoscopic surgery consisting of a telemanipulator, which allows the surgeon to remotely control instruments in a laparoscopic setting, allowing for greater precision. It also enables the surgeon to have a three-dimensional image of the surgical field enhancing visual interpretation. Gynaecological procedures performed robotically include:[5]

- Hysterectomy
- Sacrocolpopexy – where the top of the vaginal vault is suspended from the sacrum by a mesh to treat uterine prolapse
- Myomectomy
- Malignancy staging

High laparoscopic pressures and a steep Trendelenburg incline for prolonged periods can make these procedures unsuitable for patients with significant cardiorespiratory disease. In view of the position, it is important to check the face regularly for evidence of reflux (to avoid facial or conjunctival damage by vomitus) or marked facial oedema. Pressure areas should be wrapped and supported with padding to prevent pressure ulcerations and nerve injury. Perioperative hypothermia can occur due to the prolonged insufflation of gases and active warming is required.

The prolonged pneumoperitoneum can result in cardiovascular instability; arrhythmias or hypotension should be treated promptly. Hypercarbia is common; end tidal CO_2 must be closely monitored and, if a cause for concern or associated with evidence of hypoxia, communicated to the surgeon. Goal-directed fluid therapy minimizes hypervolaemia with subsequent tissue oedema and enhances recovery. In the presence of significant periorbital oedema, care should be taken before extubation, as there is also the possibility of laryngeal oedema and postextubation stridor.

Anaesthetic Concerns

Along with the laparoscopic precautions discussed earlier, other anaesthetic considerations include:

- Additional large-bore i.v. access should be secured in advance; obtaining intravenous access intraoperatively can be extremely challenging.
- Invasive arterial monitoring is recommended to monitor haemodynamics and to allow regular arterial blood gases.
- Maintenance of muscle relaxation is advisable; a still surgical field is very important.
- Agents with a good recovery profile, such as remifentanil and desflurane, should be considered in view of prolonged surgical time.
- Perioperative and postoperative analgesia can be provided using a single-shot spinal with opiates. Alternatively, analgesia can be managed with a combination of paracetamol and a PCA.

GYNAECOLOGICAL ONCOLOGY

Hydatidiform Mole

Hydatidiform mole evacuation can be associated with cardiopulmonary distress, torrential bleeding, embolism, disseminated intravascular coagulation, thyroid storm and, in severe cases, profound hypotension and septic shock. Patients need thorough preoperative assessment and a multidisciplinary approach for surgery.

Ovarian Carcinoma

Preoperative assessment of ovarian carcinoma may reveal multiple medical problems, including ascites, liver metastases, pleural effusion, poor nutrition and renal dysfunction.

REFERENCES

1. Knight DJ, Mahajan RP. Patient positioning in anaesthesia. Continuing Education in Anaesthesia, Critical Care and Pain 2004;4(5):160–63.
2. Nicolaides AN. Prevention of venous thromboembolism. International Consensus Statement. J Vasc Br 2002;1:133–70.
3. Report of the National Confidential Enquiry into peri-operative deaths. 1991-1992. www.ncepod.org.uk/1993report/Full%20Report%201992-1993.pdf
4. Balas P, Nicolaides AN. Prevention and treatment of venous thromboembolism. International Consensus Statement. Int Angiology 2013;32:132–40.
5. Visco AG, Advincula AP. Robotic gynecologic surgery. Obstet Gynecol 2008;112:1369–84.

FURTHER READING

Struthers AD, Cuschieri A. Cardiovascular consequences of laparoscopic surgery. Lancet 1998;352:568–70.

Chapter 5.6

Neonatal and Paediatric Surgery

Peter Brooks

NEONATAL AND INFANT PHYSIOLOGY

Definitions

Definitions relevant to this chapter:

- Preterm – less than 37 weeks' gestation
- Term – 37 to 42 weeks' gestation
- Post-term – over 42 weeks' gestation
- Low birthweight – less than 2500 g
- Infant – 28 days to 1 year
- Child – 1 to 16 years (dependent on local laws of consent)

Respiratory System

Infants have a larger head, shorter neck and larger tongue than older children and adults.

The neonatal glottic inlet is higher, at C3–C4 compared to C5 in the adult, and the infant epiglottis is longer and curved anteriorly. Before puberty, the narrowest part of the larynx is the cricoid ring. At 34 weeks of gestation the true alveoli appear, with further reduction in alveolar membrane thickness. Type 2 alveolar cells produce surfactant, which is necessary to reduce surface tension, stabilize alveoli and prevent the respiratory distress of prematurity.

Ribs in infants are more horizontal than in adults and breathing is diaphragmatic rather than intercostal. The rib cage consists of soft cartilage, resulting in paradoxical chest wall movement in conditions associated with airway obstruction (e.g. laryngo-, tracheo-, broncho-malacia;, croup or bronchiolitis). The neonatal diaphragm has less than 10% fatigue-resistant muscle fibres (25% in adults), increasing the risk of respiratory failure with lung or airway disease.

Functional residual capacity (FRC) lies close to the closing volume (CV) in the infant and the reduction in FRC with anaesthesia or disease can lead to atelectasis and segmental collapse unless positive end-expiratory pressure (PEEP) is applied.

Alveolar ventilation (130 mL/kg/min) and oxygen demand (6.4 mL/kg/min) are much higher than in the adult (60 mL/kg/min and 3.5 mL/kg/min, respectively) but the FRC/V_A (alveolar ventilation) is much lower (half), so the reserves of oxygen in the lung of the infant are lower.[1]

Response to Hypoxia

Unlike in adults, mild hypoxia in the neonate causes hypoventilation leading to apnoea. Many anaesthetic agents exacerbate this. Normal-term neonates up to 52 weeks' postconceptual age have 'periodic breathing' with intermittent apnoeas of up to 5-s duration followed by tachypnoea. This is more pronounced in preterm neonates, with apnoeas of 15-s or more, resulting in desaturation and bradycardia.

Cardiovascular System

Oxygen Transport

At term, red cells contain 70% HbF, which has a higher affinity for oxygen than HbA, with a total Hb of 160–200 g/L, increasing the oxygen-carrying capacity. The HbF proportion declines, such that at 6 months, 90% is HbA.

Fetal and Transitional Circulations

Oxygenated blood from the placenta passes from the umbilical vein through the ductus venosus to the inferior vena cava (IVC). It preferentially streams through the foramen ovale to the left atrium and thence to the ascending aorta. Deoxygenated blood from the superior vena cava (SVC) passes through the right atrium and ventricle and pulmonary artery but is diverted to the descending aorta via the ductus arteriosus.

Three physiological events at birth occur to produce the normal postnatal circulation:

- Loss of the placenta with increased vascular resistance and loss of prostaglandin PGE_2
- Reduction in pulmonary vascular resistance (PVR) that occurs with the first breath, mediated by an increase in PO_2, a decrease in PCO_2 and mechanical factors – the resultant increase in pressure in the left atrium shuts the flap-like foramen ovale
- Closure of the ductus arteriosus caused by increased PO_2, adrenergic stimulation and the loss of PGE_2 from the placenta

Postnatally, life-threatening persistent transitional circulation can occur in conditions causing reopening of the ductus arteriosus, increased pulmonary resistance and right-to-left shunt through the foramen ovale.

The neonatal heart has less organization, less increased connective tissue, fewer myofibrils and immature actin/myosin cross-linking. The Frank–Starling curve is flatter and there is consequently less response to volume loading.

At term, the left and right ventricles are of equal bulk and there is a rightward axis on the ECG. Gradual thinning of the right ventricle (RV) and hypertrophy of the left ventricle (LV) result from the changes in their outflow impedances, resulting in a 'normal' ECG by 6 months.

Cardiac output in the neonate is 200 mL/kg/min, with a heart rate of 100–180 bpm (adult cardiac output is 80 mL/kg/min, with a heart rate of 55–90 bpm).

Nervous System

Neonatal cerebral blood flow (CBF) is proportionately greater than that in adults (infant CBF is equal to one-third cardiac output). Autoregulation exists, but is better adapted to hypertensive surges rather than to hypotension. When MAP decreases below 35 mm Hg, CBF decreases, which may be poorly tolerated by the brain. The high interindividual variability on autoregulatory thresholds, CBF values and cerebral vasoreactivity further complicates clinical decision making.

The blood–brain barrier is immature at birth and central nervous system (CNS) depressant drugs such as morphine can cross more easily, leading to increased drug sensitivity. Crossing of unconjugated bilirubin can produce kernicterus.

At birth, the parasympathetic nervous system is relatively well developed and tends to dominate the sympathetic nervous system. The neonate has limited responses to cold (vasoconstriction rather than shivering) and there is an increased propensity to bradycardia.

Response to noxious stimuli is characterized by a well-developed appearance of pain (grimace, cry and other motor activities) and stress responses. Appreciation of pain is conjectural, but the pathways are present anatomically by 24 weeks of gestation.

Tendencies to intracranial haemorrhages may be exacerbated by unattenuated stress responses to operation or intubation.

Fluid and Electrolytes

Nephrogenesis is complete by 36 weeks of gestation, but the ratio of medullary to cortical nephrons is reduced over the first 6 months after birth, reducing the ability to reabsorb water and solutes. Care must be taken particularly with neonates to ensure adequate sodium and potassium intake, while remembering that electrolyte loads are poorly tolerated. The concentrating ability takes up to a year to become 'mature', although most of the change occurs within the first 6 months.

Extracellular fluid volume forms 40% of body mass at birth, decreasing to 30% within weeks. This contraction is associated with production of relatively dilute urine. Blood volume at birth is 80 mL/kg (depending on the time the cord is clamped), approximately 100 mL/kg in preterm infants.

Water requirements are greater in the neonate than in the older child owing to high urinary and evaporative losses (thin skin, high surface area). This is exaggerated in any preterm neonate. Typical intravenous requirements are:

- 100 mL/kg/day for the term neonate
- Up to 150 mL/kg/day for preterm infants

Additional allowances should be made for the effects of radiant heaters and ultraviolet lights. Additional fluid needs to be added for the effect of pyrexia (10 mL/kg/day for each degree over 37°C).

Daily sodium requirement is 3–4 mmol/kg/day for a neonate up to 10 kg, and the daily potassium requirement is 2 mmol/kg/day for a neonate up to 10 kg.

Metabolism and Thermoneutrality

The basal metabolic rate is higher in infants and children (neonatal oxygen uptake is 8 mL/kg/min, compared to 3–4 mL/kg/min in adults).

Neonatal energy requirements are 500 kJ [120 kcal]/kg/day (for an adult it is 167 kJ [40 kcal]/kg/day). Glycogen stores are relatively low, but brain and myocardium are more glucose dependent (i.e. there is a greater propensity to starvation hypoglycaemia and damage). Calcium homoeostatic mechanisms are less responsive with reduced stores. Transfusion of blood products that contain citrate may require calcium supplementation to prevent hypocalcaemia.

Temperature homoeostasis is aided by the acquisition of subcutaneous fat, which is notably absent in the preterm infant. Babies should be nursed in a thermoneutral environment; a point at which there is minimal metabolic challenge to maintain normal temperature. In the term neonate, naked thermoneutrality is 32°C and clothed, it is 24°C. Shivering does occur in the neonate but is not effective until 3 months. Heat production is reliant on brown fat, but heat loss can rapidly outstrip production.

Drug Responses

Across the paediatric life span, organ size and function change as does body composition and ultimately cellular function and metabolic activity. The neonate is more susceptible than an adult to the effects of CNS drugs. This is due in part to increased drug sensitivity, immaturity of the blood–brain barrier and altered pharmacokinetics (Fig. 5.6.1). In general, however, infants have larger volumes of distribution for most drugs, and even susceptible infants may require larger initial doses of drugs to achieve adequate plasma concentrations.

Anaesthesia-Related Neurotoxicity and the Developing Brain

Animal studies have shown that virtually all general anaesthetics used in clinical practice may lead to neurodegeneration (particularly apoptosis) with functional

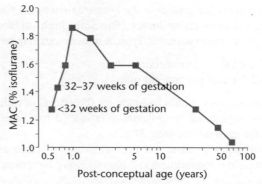

FIGURE 5.6.1   Effect of age on the minimum alveolar concentration (MAC) of isoflurane. MAC decreases with increasing age from 1 year; however, newborn and preterm infants have increased sensitivity to isoflurane with lower MAC. Reproduced from LeDez and Lerman.[2]

deficits in learning and behaviour later in life. Human studies performed so far have been unable to confirm these animal data. A single brief anaesthetic seems safe in infants. Multiple anaesthetic and surgical exposures, however, have consistently been associated with poorer outcomes but these associations are not necessarily causal. There may be other reasons for this than merely the anaesthetics. Currently, there is no need to change anaesthetic clinical practices or to postpone or cancel truly urgent surgeries in young children.[3]

GENERAL ANAESTHETIC CONSIDERATIONS

Preanaesthetic Clinics

Preoperative screening in preadmission clinics is usually questionnaire based with trained paramedics. They are suitable for up to 80% of elective surgery. Haemoglobin and urine analyses are usually not required, except if sickle-cell screening is necessary. The assessor needs to understand the home environment (safety and postoperative care) if same-day surgery is planned. Videos or interactive play can be useful for the psychological preparation, and preoperative family workshops have resulted in a reduction in postoperative maladaptive behaviours.

Preoperative Visit

Key aims of the preoperative visit are confirmation of fitness for surgery, psychological preparation and clear explanations of anaesthesia and postoperative pain relief. Many drugs (such as furosemide [frusemide] and captopril) are better avoided on the day of surgery, but others such as anti-asthmatic medication should be prescribed as normal. Patients with endocrine disorders require careful preoperative management.[4,5]

Psychological preparation is age dependent. Separation anxiety and mistrust of strangers develop at 1 year and can be accompanied later by anger at loss of control. Older children can fear mutilation, pain and death. Individualized plans must be made in conjunction with parents. For example, if a child refuses to be changed into a theatre gown before surgery, normal clothes should be left on until after induction.

Induction of anaesthesia can be intravenous or gaseous, and many children have a strong preference. If intravenous access is planned, clear surface marking of two preferred vein sites is helpful to place local anaesthetic cream effectively. Regional anaesthesia can provide complete analgesia, but the accompanying paraesthesia, numbness and motor weakness can be frightening without explanation. A visit from a pain nurse is helpful if patient-controlled anaesthesia is planned.

Consent is usually established with parents if children are less than 16 years old. However, refusal by the child must be taken into consideration, particularly if he or she is fully aware of the consequences of refusal. Common complications relating to anaesthesia and additional procedures (regional blockade) should be fully discussed. A written documentation of the consent process in the medical notes may be invaluable.

The staff working with paediatric patients may be required to undergo child protection awareness training (CPAT), which in some countries, such as the UK, is mandatory.

Fasting Guidelines

Ingestion of a complex meal can take considerable time to clear the stomach, but clear fluids are normally cleared within 2 h. Neonates and preweaned infants become irritable, dehydrated and hypoglycaemic if starved for extended periods. Prolonged fasting times can result in ketoacidosis with (low) normal glucose concentration in children younger than 36 months of age. For elective surgery, a widely used scheme is:

- Solids – morning case, no solid food overnight; afternoon case, light food at breakfast; no solid food for 6 h before surgery
- Milk – up to 4 h before surgery for bottled milk, up to 3 h before surgery for breast milk
- Clear liquids – up to 2 h before surgery

Children with major organ dysfunction or those acutely ill with infection or trauma should be treated as though they had a full stomach regardless of fasting interval because these conditions are associated with delayed gastric emptying. Small infants should be scheduled first on an operating list to improve planning, but it may still be necessary to commence intravenous fluids. Preliminary data suggest that shorter fasting times for clear fluids might be acceptable. An optimized preoperative fasting management reduces fasting time, decreases ketone body concentration and helps to stabilize mean arterial blood pressure during induction of anaesthesia in children younger than 36 months.[6]

Premedication

Preoperative sedation is rarely given for day-stay surgery, and more emphasis is placed on the calming effects of parental presence in the anaesthetic room together with good psychological preparation. The following patients are likely to benefit from premedication:

● Children with disabilities or special needs, e.g. autism
● Children having major surgery
● Children needing multiple operative procedures
● Children with past history of stormy anaesthetic induction or emergence

The following are some conditions where a careful risk–benefit assessment must be made prior to prescribing sedative premedication:

● Anticipated difficult airway
● Risk of aspiration
● Central or obstructive sleep apnoea
● Raised intracranial pressure
● Acute systemic illness
● Severe renal or hepatic impairment

Benzodiazepines can have an occasional paradoxical effect, with disinhibition and agitation. Intramuscular preparations are no longer used or sanctioned. Rectal sedation with barbiturates is not commonly used. Intranasal dexmedetomidine appears to be a good alternative to intranasal midazolam, particularly if there is a history of dissatisfaction with midazolam but needs more time to work.

Common Premedicant Drugs

Sedation

Benzodiazepines are sedative and anxiolytic and provide anterograde amnesia. Midazolam (0.2–0.5 mg/kg up to a maximum of 20 mg; oral, nasal, sublingual) has a very rapid onset of 20 min and rapid elimination, making it suitable for day-stay anaesthesia. Its bitter lingering taste is hard to disguise. Temazepam (in older children) 10–30 mg, chloral hydrate (30–50 mg/kg up to a maximum of 1 g; oral, rectal) and triclofos (25–30 mg/kg up to 1 g; oral) can provide 'basal narcosis' at high doses and can be useful in highly active children. Other agents include ketamine 2–5 mg/kg orally, clonidine 2–5 μg/kg orally or dexmedetomidine 1–3 μg/kg intranasally.

Analgesia

A loading dose of paracetamol (oral 20 mg/kg up to 1 g) and a nonsteroidal anti-inflammatory drug (NSAID) such as diclofenac or ibuprofen can be given preoperatively to provide effective coanalgesia with opioids or local blocks. The rectal route can also be used effectively for these drugs. In order to be effective, dosing must continue on a regular basis after surgery. Clonidine 0.2–2 μg/kg orally provides both sedation and analgesia but does not induce nausea. Opioids are not usually given before surgery because of vomiting and respiratory side effects.

Topical Local Anaesthesia

EMLA® requires 90 min to be fully effective, whereas tetracaine (amethocaine) cream is more rapid at 60 min. An erythematous rash is quite common with Ametop® (tetracaine (amethocaine) cream) and it can be severe. EMLA® can be used in neonates provided the underlying skin is intact and that excessive doses are avoided. In a busy day-surgery unit, it may be useful to have standing orders to apply the cream immediately on arrival. A promise of pain-free cannulation must be kept if a child's confidence is to be maintained.

EQUIPMENT

Airways

Guedel airways are available in sizes 000, 00, 0, 1, 2, 3 for various sizes of neonate, infant and child. The distance between philtrum and angle of mandible is a guide to size.

Masks

Traditional masks were designed to minimize deadspace (Rendell-Baker–Soucek). Modern masks are light, transparent and disposable, but have a larger deadspace. The rim is made of soft plastic or an inflated ring.

Supraglottic Airway Devices

Supraglottic airway devices such as the laryngeal mask airway (LMA) are useful in short procedures with spontaneous ventilation. They have less resistance than tracheal tubes and are of considerable use in difficult upper airway work and for insertion of fibreoptic bronchoscopes. Approximate sizes are:

- 1 for less than 6.5 kg
- 2 for 6.5–20 kg
- 2.5 for 20–30 kg
- 3 for 30 kg and above

A size 1.5 is also available. Armoured versions have reduced risk of kinking and are longer and narrower. The use of the size 1 has not been widespread because of concerns about secure insertion, increased deadspace and atelectasis. Although it has been used in neonatal resuscitation, it is not yet recommended for controlled ventilation in small children because of the risk of ventilatory impairment from gastric distension.

Breathing Systems

Common breathing systems used in paediatric practice include Ayre's T-piece, Bain and circle. The Ayre's T-piece (Mapleson E) with Jackson–Rees modification remains the mainstay of paediatric anaesthesia. It is compact and light, with low deadspace and airway resistance. It can function in spontaneous or controlled ventilation with or without manual continuous positive airway pressure (CPAP). There is no intrinsic heat/humidity conservation and no pressure-relief valve should the bag become occluded. It requires high fresh gas flows for spontaneous ventilation (2.5–3 times calculated minute ventilation). For controlled ventilation high minute ventilation with limited fresh gas flow and rebreathing provides stable end-tidal carbon dioxide concentrations.

The Bain system behaves like a Mapleson E or F circuit and has been used in all age groups (see Chapter 2.1).

The circle system has become popular for controlled ventilation in paediatrics because of heat and moisture conservation as well as cost efficiencies. Care must be taken to compensate for the compression effect of the system (compliance of tubing, etc.), with controlled ventilation to ensure that tidal volume is adequate.

Ventilators

Accurate capnography and measurement of airway pressure are particularly important during mechanical ventilation because tidal volume and alveolar ventilation cannot always be measured accurately. Most paediatric ventilators used with T-piece circuits are time cycled and are connected on the expiratory limb as a 'bag squeezer' or 'mechanical thumb'. Neonates may require adapted intensive care ventilators to maintain alveolar recruitment. In circle systems, a bag-in-bottle ventilator is used with paediatric bellows.

Laryngoscopes

For infants and small children, straight blades (Robertshaw, Miller) are more useful to control the epiglottis and visualize the higher laryngeal inlet. The age at which the use of curved blades, such as the Macintosh, comes into play depends on individual choice. Videolaryngoscopes are useful for teaching and supervising tracheal intubation in children and as an aid during difficult laryngoscopy.

Tracheal Tubes

Tracheal tubes are made of PVC or polyurethane and marked with both internal diameter (ID) and length graduations in centimetres.

For children older than 1 year:

● The appropriate tube (ID) can be approximately estimated by the formula age/4 + 4.
● The appropriate length for a cut tracheal tube can be approximately estimated by the formula age/2 + 12 oral (+15 for nasal).

In infants:

● Approximate ID sizes for preterms: < 1500 g, 2.5 mm; 1500–3000 g, 3.0 mm; over 3000 g, 3.5 mm.
● Oral length in cm is given by the formula (6 + weight in kg).

The development of a new generation of cuffed tracheal tubes with a thin, polyurethane cuff has caused a transition in the practice with an increased use of cuffed tracheal tubes, even in neonates and infants.

Humidification

Prolonged use of cold dry gases with the Ayres T-piece circuit leads to mucosal damage and mucous plugs. Active heater humidification systems are therefore still used extensively in younger infants undergoing major surgery. Intraluminal heating elements maintain airway temperature distal to the water chamber and prevent condensation ('rainout'). Passive humidification by the use of heat and moisture exchangers (HME) is used in older children combined with microbial filtration. HMEs take up to an hour to develop effective humidification. Commercially available HMEs cover a range of child sizes, and appropriate selection will ensure minimal effect on deadspace.

Vascular Access

Newer plastic technology not only provides peripheral intravenous or intra-arterial catheters as small as 26 stretched wire gauge (swg), but also provides plastic 'memory' and so is less likely to kink and occlude as the child mobilizes. 'Seldinger' kits are available from 24 swg upwards, whereas triple-lumen central venous catheters are available from 4 French Gauge (FG). Intraosseous needles should be available for the shocked child or those with particularly difficult venous access in all acute care areas.

Intravenous Fluid Administration

Controlled, accurate fluid administration is now practical and reliable owing to the widespread availability of volumetric or syringe pumps. However, appropriately rated pumps must be selected for such use. If large-volume replacement is to take place then infusates should be warmed. Recent devices have achieved this effectively by the use of coaxial heat exchangers.

MONITORING

Apnoea Alarms

Apnoea alarms should be used in babies at risk from postanaesthetic apnoea (e.g. all neonates and preterm babies up to 44–60 weeks postconceptual age). The cut-off for this is contentious and may depend on lingering pathology, such as chronic lung disease or previous nervous system insults.

Gas and Vapour Analysis

Gas and vapour analysis is standard practice, but the site of the sampling will affect the result, especially in rebreathing circuits. Tracheal connectors and HMEs are made with side ports and the closer to the patient the better.

Pulse Oximetry

Those paediatric probes should be used that do not compress the circulation in the chosen extremity. Longer term probe application can cause burns. The absorption spectra of HbF and HbA are similar, but meconium on the skin can give a false low reading. In the preterm neonate, it is important to recognize the significance of a difference between pre- and postductal values.

Blood Gases

Mild metabolic acidosis is seen in the first weeks of life owing to immature renal acidification of the urine. Plasma standard bicarbonate may be only 20–22 mmol/L. Normal PO_2 is lower in the newborn (9–10 kPa in air) because of residual atelectasis and extra lung water. Handheld portable gas analysers offer 'real-time' point-of-care testing including a range of other parameters (lactate, Hb).

Transcutaneous Gas Measurement

Transcutaneous gas measurement gives continuous readings of blood gases. There are separate oxygen and carbon dioxide electrodes adherent to skin that operate at 43°C–44°C. This produces the vasodilatation necessary to ensure diffusion of the gases, but thermal injury to the skin will ensue if the electrodes are not moved every 3 h. The oxygen electrode can be affected by volatile agents (false high). Both electrodes become less accurate as the infant's skin thickens with age.

Noninvasive Monitoring of Blood Pressure

Modern automated oscillometric devices have been shown to be reliable, although there is a tendency to underestimate high systolic and overestimate low diastolic pressures. Cuff size is important; for the arm a cuff should be selected that covers two-thirds of the humerus. Recent development of bedside measurement techniques, which enable monitoring of oxygen supply and cerebral circulation, will provide valuable means in the near future to adequately tailor individual patient management.

Invasive Monitoring of Blood Pressure

To measure arterial waveform, the tubing connecting the cannula to the transducer should be rigid and as short as possible. This minimizes damping and reduces harmonics, which can occur at the higher frequency of infant heart rates (≈ 3 Hz).

Cardiac Output

Reliable and practical cardiac output measurement has proved difficult in paediatrics. It can be estimated using oesophageal or transthoracic Doppler techniques. However, its accuracy depends on the assumed aortic cross-sectional area and it may be more useful to track trends rather than absolute values. Other emerging techniques include modified thermodilution, lithium dilution, analysis of the pulse waveform, bioreactance and changes in electrical conductivity.

Electrocardiography

Electrocardiography can accurately track changes and trends in heart rate and can be a guide to the depth of anaesthesia or the depletion of intravascular volume. Although there is less emphasis on ECG morphology in children than in adults, it can be important to identify inadvertent intravascular injection of local anaesthetic, or hyperkalaemia after suxamethonium administration.

Temperature

Central temperature should be monitored for all but the very shortest of procedures. Skin temperatures will be affected by the very measures currently employed to raise it. Nasopharynx, oesophagus, tympanic, rectal and bladder sites are all satisfactory. The nasopharyngeal temperature may be affected by leakage of inspired gases.

Neuromuscular Monitoring

Neuromuscular monitoring in children is similar to that in adult practice. However, it must be noted that in the first month of life the fourth twitch is decreased, even in the absence of neuromuscular blockade.

GENERAL ANAESTHESIA TECHNIQUES

Induction

Gas induction has become increasingly popular since the introduction of sevoflurane. Techniques include:

- Single maximal breath induction
- 'Blowing up a bag or a balloon'
- Using cupped hands or a blanket
- Using a scented mask held by the child or parents

Usually 8% sevoflurane is elected from the outset together with nitrous oxide and oxygen. Parents need to be aware that during induction a phase of excitement and movement may occur.

Opting for intravenous induction depends on the child's preference, suitability of veins, technical expertise and state of the child. Doses should be titrated to effect: neonates and sick infants may require reduced doses, whereas 3–5-year-old children need relatively larger doses than adults. The pain on induction with propofol (2.5–5 mg/kg) can be reduced by adding 20 mg lidocaine to 200 mg propofol. Thiopental (2–7 mg/kg) provides a smooth induction but can delay postoperative recovery.

Maintenance

Most simple short procedures require only spontaneous ventilation under a volatile or intravenous anaesthetic agent and analgesia that will extend into the postoperative period. Neonates are usually intubated and ventilated for surgical procedures to ensure adequate gas exchange, and they are given local anaesthetic blockade where possible to limit CNS depressant drug usage. In complex procedures where postoperative ventilation is planned, high-dose opioid techniques are often used to minimize stress responses.

Volatile Agents

Sevoflurane is expensive and has been associated with delirium and agitation on emergence. Isoflurane remains popular with both circle and T-piece systems. Desflurane, with its irritant properties, is impractical for gas induction. Its low blood gas solubility allows rapid recovery and extubation even after prolonged anaesthesia, making it useful in neonatal anaesthesia. Halothane is arrhythmogenic, particularly in hypercarbia and sympathetic activation, but it is still used extensively worldwide. MAC values are age dependent (see Fig. 5.6.1).

Opioids

Single-dose fentanyl (1–5 μg/kg) has a short clinical effect owing to its rapid redistribution, reducing haemodynamic responses and anaesthetic requirements to surgery and providing some residual analgesia for short procedures. Large doses (25–100 μg/kg) can cause chest wall rigidity and bradycardia.

Morphine given as a loading dose (100–300 μg/kg) followed by a maintenance infusion (10–40 μg/kg/h) provides long-lasting analgesia with sedation. Infusion rates are reduced in neonates (5–20 μg/kg/h).

Remifentanil given by infusion (0.1–1 μg/kg/min) provides intense intraoperative opioid anaesthesia. Hydrolysis by cholinesterases causes ultrarapid time-independent elimination and allows rapid extubation, even in newborns. Consequently, to prevent breakthrough pain, alternative analgesia must be effective before the infusion is stopped.

Muscle Relaxants

Suxamethonium, although used infrequently in routine paediatric practice, should remain immediately available for rapid emergency airway control. Rocuronium (up to 1 mg/kg) is also used for rapid sequence induction because of its fast onset. Vecuronium (0.1–0.2 mg/kg) remains popular owing to its haemodynamic stability and lack of side effects.

Total Intravenous Anaesthesia

Total intravenous anaesthesia (TIVA) is gaining popularity, but it requires individualized adjustment of drug doses based on an understanding of age-related pharmacokinetics. Validated paediatric algorithms are available for propofol target-controlled infusion. Drug combinations include propofol/alfentanil, propofol/remifentanil and propofol/ketamine. They are usually used for longer procedures that require controlled ventilation/muscle relaxation.

Regional Analgesia

Regional blocks reduce intraoperative anaesthesia requirements and provide postoperative analgesia and, unlike systemic analgesia, may provide complete analgesia without systemic side effects, especially in neonates and young infants who have an increased response to opioid side effects. Simple nerve blocks, which can be extended by the use of indwelling catheters, are useful in orthopaedic surgery and thoracic surgery.

Single-dose caudal anaesthesia is well established for lower-body surgery. Less invasive procedures associated with limited postoperative pain (e.g. hernia repair) can be managed effectively for 6–8 h with local anaesthesia alone. This duration is insufficient for more invasive procedures (e.g. orchidopexy). Analgesia can be prolonged by adding clonidine (1–2 μg/kg) or ketamine (0.5 mg/kg for children > 1 years of age) to local analgesia. S-ketamine may be preferable to racemic ketamine in reducing the risk of hallucinations.

Perioperative analgesia for major abdominal and thoracic procedures can be managed successfully in all age groups with indwelling epidural catheters provided tip placement is appropriate.

Local anaesthesia techniques have an excellent safety record in children but carry potential risks from both the instrumentation and the drugs. The stereo-isomers ropivacaine and levobupivacaine have clinical efficacy similar to that of racemic bupivacaine but provide an increased margin of safety from systemic absorption or accidental intravascular injection. Clear guidelines relating to dose and duration of the infusion as well as adequate patient surveillance are mandatory with continuous regional anaesthesia.

Postoperative Pain Management

Acute pain management in children is based on preemptive analgesia, multimodal therapy, close monitoring with early intervention and safety monitoring.

Effective analgesia must be established before the end of anaesthesia. Combinations of drugs or techniques with different modes of action usually improve analgesia and reduce individual side effects.

Maintaining established analgesia requires the identification of early breakthrough pain. Routine monitoring with simple pain tools is useful to alert carers of early analgesia failure. Immediate ward-based treatment must be available, coupled with experienced advice for more difficult issues. Intensive care or high-dependency units need to be considered for patients at increased risk associated with higher risk conditions or with some analgesic techniques.

For major surgery, opioid analgesia remains a cornerstone of postoperative analgesia, with morphine infusions the most popular. Adequate loading with subsequent controlled delivery to optimize analgesia without excessive side effects is essential. Most schemes, whether patient controlled, nurse controlled or parent controlled, usually combine a background infusion with an additional 'demanded' dose. Older children may have less nausea if the background infusion is omitted. Side effects (ventilatory depression, emesis, constipation and pruritus) can be a problem, but the added sedation from morphine analgesia can be beneficial in younger children.

In specialist medical centres, epidural infusions mixtures are used, combining 0.125% bupivacaine with various concentrations of other agents, e.g. fentanyl 0.05–2 μg/kg/h or clonidine 0.1–1 μg/kg/h. Absorption of local anaesthetic agents and toxicity are avoided by limiting the duration of infusion to 48 h and limiting maximum bupivacaine dose to 0.5 mg/kg/h in infants and 0.25 mg/kg/h in neonates.

Paracetamol (acetaminophen) is not potent but can provide useful coanalgesia when given at sufficient dosage to maintain an adequate plasma level. Oral absorption is rapid and less variable than via the rectal route. An intravenous preparation is available. Hepatic dysfunction can occur readily if excess dosage is used.

NSAIDs have a significant opioid-sparing effect and are widely used despite the absence of regulatory data. Early fears about increased bleeding, gastric irritation and renal dysfunction have not been a problem in routine paediatrics.

However, theoretical concerns about impaired bone healing have become a relative contraindication for some orthopaedic procedures.

Fluids

Crystalloids

Intraoperative hypoglycaemia can occur in neonates but is unusual owing to the effects of the stress response on glycolysis and gluconeogenesis. In contrast, excessive perioperative administration of glucose solutions can lead to hyponatraemia, water intoxication and cerebral oedema. Hartmann's solution can be given as a sole agent during surgery, but it is prudent to measure blood glucose hourly during prolonged cases. Alternatively, a fixed maintenance infusion of a glucose-containing solution should be continued throughout, with additional fluid replacement of Hartmann's given independently. A recognized formula for maintenance fluid hourly rates is:

- 10 kg = 4 mL/kg
- 10–20 kg = 40 + 2 mL/kg
- Over 20 kg = 60 + 1 mL/kg

It has been shown that a mixture of glucose 2.5% in Ringer's lactate can maintain normal glucose while avoiding hyponatraemia. Increased replacement fluids may be required if the gut remains exposed.

Colloids and Blood

The threshold for transfusion will vary with the child's overall condition and associated pathologies. For otherwise healthy children, it is acceptable to let Hb drop to 80–90 g/L, but neonates and children with cardiac or pulmonary conditions may benefit from a Hb raised to 100–130 g/L. A volume formula for transfusion is:

(Hb required – Hb actual) × (body weight in kg) × 5
= volume of red cells required (using resuspended SAGM blood)

Fresh frozen plasma and platelets may need replacing earlier than in adults to prevent coagulopathy. These colloids contain citrate and will require additional calcium administration to prevent significant hypocalcaemia if infused quickly.

MANAGEMENT OF COMMON CONDITIONS

Tonsillectomy and Adenoidectomy

Techniques with either tracheal intubation or laryngeal mask are used for tonsillectomy and adenoidectomy. Formal intubation secures the airway, while a laryngeal mask avoids invasion of the subglottis.

Dexamethasone (0.1 mg/kg, up to 10 mg) significantly reduces postoperative nausea and pain and shortens the time to resumption of feeding. Avoiding volatile agents (e.g. TIVA with propofol) can also reduce postoperative vomiting. Regular administration of NSAIDs and paracetamol can eliminate the need for postoperative morphine and its complications. Perioperative analgesia can be effectively provided by intraoperative fentanyl. Delayed administration of NSAIDs until after surgical haemostasis may reduce the risks of postoperative bleeding.

Adenotonsillectomy can be undertaken in children on a day-case basis, but case selection on clinical and social grounds is essential. Children under the age of 3 years often have upper airway obstruction or other chronic conditions that render the day-case approach unsuitable. Children with sleep-disordered breathing have more opioid-related adverse events and need careful titration of postoperative opioids and increased vigilance and monitoring.[7] Post-tonsillectomy pain can also be associated with increased behavioural disturbances, family and social disruption plus increased healthcare use.

Inguinal Herniorrhaphy and Orchidopexy

Inguinal herniorrhaphy and orchidopexy are usually day-stay procedures with general anaesthesia and local blockade. Oral analgesia, paracetamol plus an NSAID is given preoperatively. Alternatively, NSAID suppositories can be given after induction.

A popular regional technique for herniorrhaphy is iliohypogastric/ilioinguinal nerve blockade using a total dose of 0.5 mL/kg of 0.25% bupivacaine. Insert a 22G local anaesthetic (LA) needle one patient's fingerbreadth medial to the anterior superior iliac spine. Pierce the external oblique aponeurosis (palpable click), and deposit one-third to half of the volume. Change the angle inferiorly and laterally to hit the iliac periosteum. Withdraw the needle slowly, depositing another one-third to half of the volume in this track. Any remaining local analgesic can be infiltrated subcutaneously by the surgeon at the end of the procedure.

In orchidopexy, the structures requiring analgesia are more extensive. Afferent nerve supply to testicular structures is as high as T10. Analgesia can be achieved by the use of an adequate volume injected caudally (e.g. 1 mL/kg of either 0.125% or 0.25% bupivacaine), which can be supplemented with clonidine 1 μg/kg or preservative-free ketamine 0.5 mg/kg for children >1 years of age. These adjuvants can double the duration of analgesia. The use of the weaker solutions can minimize postoperative motor blockade. An advantage of caudals is the relative length of postoperative analgesia. Many operators have reported satisfactory results with iliohypogastric and ilioinguinal nerve blockade and local scrotal infiltration for the skin supplied by the pudendal nerve. Some also block the genitofemoral nerve. The total volume used would equate to 0.5 mL/kg of 0.25% bupivacaine, divided in thirds for each nerve. For genitofemoral nerve blockade inject the last one-third volume subcutaneously just lateral to the pubic tubercle. This last volume can also be reserved for pre-operative subcutaneous injection of the posterior scrotum or by the surgeon to infiltrate the scrotal wound. Postoperatively, the parents should be instructed to give the child regular oral analgesia for the next 48 h.

Circumcision

Circumcision is usually performed as a day case with light general anaesthesia and local anaesthetic block. Paracetamol and NSAIDs are given as for herniorrhaphy.

Two types of nerve blockade are commonly employed: A caudal dose of 0.5 mL/kg of 0.25% bupivacaine, with or without clonidine or ketamine or alternatively, a block of the dorsal nerve of the penis is performed. This has been shown to be as effective as caudal analgesia without the side effects of urinary and motor weakness. A ring block of the penis can be performed using 0.25% plain bupivacaine, using sufficient volume to produce a weal and stay within the maximal dose limit (less than 1 mL/kg), but this is less effective and of shorter duration.

For dorsal nerve block the penis is pulled down and a short-bevel 25 or 22 G needle inserted inferiorly to each pubic ramus, the distance between insertion sites equating to the width of the penis. In each case the needle should follow an inferomedial course at 20° to both the transverse and the sagittal planes until both the superficial and Scarpa's fascia are felt to be sequentially punctured. Then, in each of these two sites, 0.1 mL/kg 0.25% plain bupivacaine should be injected after aspiration. Epinephrine (adrenaline) mixtures are contraindicated.

Pyloromyotomy

Hypertrophic pyloric stenosis occurs in 3 in every 1000 births, with a ratio of 4 males to one female. The child will present aged 2–8 weeks with increasing vomiting, which may be projectile and may lead to significant dehydration and a hypochloraemic hypokalaemic alkalosis.

A nasogastric tube should be placed and subsequent gastric losses should be replaced volume for volume by intravenous normal saline (with 20 mmol/L potassium chloride [KCl]). Intravenous maintenance fluids (4 mL/kg/h) should be started, comprising 5% dextrose and 0.45% saline, containing KCl 20 mmol/L, and the estimated fluid deficit is replaced over 24–48 h with 0.9% saline. The operation should be delayed until there is normal skin turgor and perfusion, urine output of 1 mL/kg/h and a serum chloride over 100 mmol/L and bicarbonate of less than 28 mmol/L.

Gastric fluid should be aspirated immediately before anaesthetic induction. Methods of intubation vary; some choose rapid sequence induction with the use of cricoid pressure and suxamethonium, whereas others favour the use of nondepolarizing blockade or even deep inhalational anaesthesia and intubation. The surgical technique (Ramstedt's, paraumbilical or laparoscopic approaches) and the expected anaesthetic time influence the choice of muscle relaxant. Opioids should be avoided if possible, instead using surgical infiltration of the wound with local analgesic and postoperative paracetamol. Early recovery is enhanced if desflurane is used. Surgical practice may require air injection through the nasogastric tube to test mucosal integrity. Patients should receive appropriate monitoring for postoperative apnoea. Feeding is usually commenced soon after surgery, although this is not universal practice.[8]

Strabismus

Key features in relation to strabismus are the oculocardiac reflex in response to surgical movement of the globe, postoperative nausea and vomiting (PONV) and the association of strabismus with occult myopathies and possibly malignant hyperthermia. Surgical conditions are improved by the use of nondepolarizing muscle relaxants that abolish extraneous skeletal muscle activity. Suxamethonium can render the 'forced traction test' invalid and should be avoided.

Antiemesis is improved by the use of propofol on induction and maintenance and by the preemptive use of both 5-hydroxytryptamine inhibitors and dexamethasone, particularly in combination (dexamethasone 150 μg/kg, 50 μg/kg ondansetron). Opioids should be avoided because regular NSAIDs are as effective. Topical NSAIDS (ketorolac 0.5%, diclofenac 1%) have been used with some success.

The incidence of oculocardiac reflex can be reduced by the use of ketamine at induction and by the use of a medial canthal injection of local anaesthetic (2–2.5 mL lidocaine 1%), which also reduces the need for postoperative analgesia.

If bradycardia occurs, the surgeon should release the globe and intravenous atropine 20 μg/kg should be administered. Glycopyrronium 10 μg/kg can be given prophylactically at induction.

Dental

General anaesthesia for dental procedures should be performed in a hospital setting with full facilities.

The vast majority of dental procedures can be performed as day cases. Antibiotic prophylaxis against infective endocarditis is not recommended routinely.

The airway is shared and throat packs are placed by the surgeon to prevent debris and blood entering the airway. In each case, the dental surgeon and the anaesthetist must reach a clear understanding that the pack has been removed before the child is allowed to wake. For short procedures, a specific nasal mask can be used with spontaneous ventilation using volatile agents. For longer procedures, a laryngeal mask can be used, and the reinforced version has a smaller stem and so it helps the surgical view. For longer or more extensive operations, nasal intubation and ventilation may be indicated, but care must be taken in patients with hypertrophied adenoids and bleeding tendencies. Analgesia for single extractions can be provided by paracetamol. More extensive surgery requires infiltration of local anaesthesia by the surgeon, supplemented with NSAIDs for at least 24 h.

The child should be allowed to recover in the left lateral position. Discharge criteria include adequate haemostasis, pain control and toleration of oral fluids. Postoperative nausea and vomiting is not common unless blood has been swallowed.

MANAGEMENT OF SPECIALIZED CONDITIONS

Anaesthesia of the Preterm Infant

Specific preterm pathophysiology must be considered in these high-risk cases. Both brain and lungs are prone to longer-term damage from poorly monitored ventilation. Routine fluid maintenance should continue, but additional replacement fluid should be isotonic (saline or Hartmann's). Hyperoxia must be avoided to prevent retinal damage, and carbon dioxide levels should be kept near awake values. The risks of intraventricular haemorrhage may increase with haemodynamic stress responses to surgery. High-dose fentanyl (25–100 μg/kg) can be used to obtund these.

In the nonventilated infant, general anaesthesia needs to be precise if extubation is planned. Short-term agents are necessary (desflurane, remifentanil, atracurium), and local anaesthetic techniques should be used instead of opioids where possible. Normothermia must be maintained and ventilatory drive preserved by keeping PCO_2 within that individual's normal range (often as high as 8 kPa [60 mm Hg] in infants with lung disease).

Closure of Patent Ductus Arteriosus

The preterm infant with a widely patent ductus arterious develops cardiac failure and fluid overload. These infants are usually ventilated and surgery is usually carried out in the neonatal intensive care unit (NICU). At least one reliable venous access point must be available. Ventilation should be adjusted after administration of pancuronium (0.1 mg/kg) and fentanyl (5–25 μg/kg slowly, observing blood pressure). During surgery, oxygen saturation may drop with lung retraction and surgery may need to be interrupted to restore adequate oxygenation. Blood needs to be available.

Necrotizing Enterocolitis

These neonates may have a major coagulopathy and interstitial fluid losses. Platelets, blood and coagulation factors of adult proportions may be needed intraoperatively. High-dose fentanyl (up to 100 μg/kg) and muscle relaxant combined with low-dose volatile agent are commonly used. Postoperative ventilation is usually necessary.

Diaphragmatic Hernia

Diaphragmatic hernia is not a surgical emergency, the underlying pathology being lung hypoplasia secondary to herniation. The incidence is 1 in 4000, with 75% occurring in the left hemithorax.

Diaphragmatic hernia can be diagnosed antenatally or at birth with respiratory failure and classic radiology. Ventilatory failure may be compounded by severe pulmonary hypertension. Stabilization with conventional or oscillatory ventilation is necessary and low-dose nitric oxide and surfactant may be beneficial. High-dose opioids may prevent a pulmonary hypertensive crisis in response to interventions. Some centres have elected for extra comporeal membrane oxygenation (ECMO) support and early repair, but the results have not been substantially better than with advanced ventilatory support (60%–80% survival). Repair can be carried out in the NICU with high-dose fentanyl/pancuronium anaesthesia.

Tracheoesophageal Abnormalities

The commonest variety of tracheoesophageal abnormality is proximal oesophageal atresia with a distal oesophageal fistula into the trachea, but there are several variants, including the less obvious H-type fistula (4%). The overall incidence is about 1 in 4000. It presents with salivation, choking on feeds and occasionally apnoea and bradycardia and is often associated with other abnormalities (cardiac, skeletal, urogenital), which must be investigated urgently before surgery. A Replogle tube should be left in the proximal pouch on low-flow suction to reduce secretions.

Surgery should be carried out urgently to reduce pneumonitis from gastric contents. Standard neonatal anaesthesia can be used with opioid, volatile agent and muscle relaxant, avoiding nitrous oxide (increasing abdominal gas). Particular care should be taken to avoid insertion of the tracheal tube through the fistula and inflation of the stomach, which can impair ventilation. Minimal inflation pressures should be continued until the fistula is controlled. Some centres carry out bronchoscopy (rigid or flexible) before thoracotomy. Primary repair is usually possible through a left thoracotomy, but with high atresia and/ or a long atretic segment, delayed repair with gastrostomy and cervical oesophagostomy is necessary. After primary repair, the transanastomotic nasogastric tube must remain in situ until the integrity of the repair is confirmed.[9]

Hernia Repair in the Ex-Preterm Infant

Hernial sacs are common in ex-preterm infants and require early repair. Such infants may have significant lung pathology and are prone to apnoea, particularly under 60 weeks postconceptual age. The repair can be carried out awake under spinal anaesthesia. A single injection (0.06 mL/kg + 0.1 mL deadspace (from syringe and needle) of 0.5% bupivacaine) given in a sitting position can produce an adequate block and is well tolerated haemodynamically. However, there is a significant failure rate and the duration of the surgery may outlast the block, particularly for bilateral hernia repair. Adding a caudal block (up to 0.75 mL/kg bupivacaine 0.25%) immediately after the spinal injection augments reliability and duration.

Alternatively, light general anaesthesia with a caudal block may be preferred. After induction (sevoflurane or propofol 2 mg/kg), the infant is intubated (atracurium 0.5 mg/kg) and ventilated, avoiding hypocapnoea. Evanescent volatile agents (sevoflurane, desflurane) are used after induction and opioids are avoided. A standard caudal block (1 mL of 0.25% bupivacaine) is given before surgery.

After surgery, irrespective of technique, apnoea monitoring and close supervision are necessary for 24 h. Caffeine may reduce the risks of postoperative apnoea.

ACUTE ANAESTHETIC PROBLEMS

Vascular Access

Up to 1 week after birth, emergency venous access is easily obtained by cannulation of the umbilical vein using a 5Fr catheter (a sterile feeding tube in an emergency). The stump is trimmed to expose the arteries and vein and a loose ligature is placed around the stump. The catheter is inserted 5 cm and blood is aspirated to confirm its position and flushed with saline. The ligature is tightened. The catheter is further secured with tapes, and an abdominal radiograph will confirm the position of the tip.

Venous access can present serious problems in children. Inhalational induction followed by venous cannulation may help, but airway control may require a second anaesthetist. Access routes to be considered by nonspecialists are femoral veins, external jugular veins and the intraosseous routes.

For intraosseous access, automated and the manual systems are available. The needle should be inserted into the marrow of the anteromedial tibia, 1–3 cm (depending on size of child) below the tibial tuberosity or into the inferolateral femur. The bony cortex can only be breached once in each bone as fluids infused through a second successful attempt will escape through the hole caused by the first.

Respiratory Tract Infections

Runny noses are common in children and not necessarily a contraindication to anaesthesia. However, it is important to establish whether such signs are markers of an active respiratory infection. These include acute changes such as lethargy, insomnia, irritability and anorexia. A pyrexial child (37.5°C) with a new productive cough or with abnormal breath sounds should be postponed. If there is an isolated upper respiratory tract infection then deferment may only be necessary for 2 weeks, but with lower respiratory involvement then an interval of 4 weeks may be indicated to ensure airway oedema and parenchymal infiltrations have resolved. A history of at least two family members having asthma, atopy, or smoking increases the risk for perioperative respiratory adverse events.[10]

Airway Emergencies

Laryngospasm

Laryngospasm can occur on induction of anaesthesia, with surgical stimulation or on emergence, particularly after airway surgery. In all cases, 100% oxygen should be given with positive end-expiratory pressure. During surgery, stimulation should stop and if necessary anaesthesia be increased. If the spasm worsens despite these measures it can be broken with low-dose suxamethonium (0.5–1.0 mg/kg). It may not be necessary to intubate the trachea once the glottis has relaxed if the plane of anaesthesia can be deepened and spontaneous ventilation reestablished. Should another dose of suxamethonium be required, this should be preceded by a dose of atropine 20 μg/kg intravenously. The use of propofol at 0.5 mg/kg to treat laryngospasm has been shown to be safe and free of cardiovascular events; however, some patients may develop transient apnoea which needs airway support and ventilation.[11]

Croup, Tracheitis and Epiglottitis

Croup, tracheitis and epiglottitis have different aetiologies, but present as acute airway obstruction requiring anaesthetic input. Croup (laryngotracheobronchitis) is usually viral and presents in the first to third years of life. Epiglottitis with *Haemophilus* type b has become rare since vaccination programmes began, but still occurs. Tracheitis is either viral or bacterial (*Staphylococcus* and *Streptococcus spp.*).

Medical interference should be kept to a minimum, particularly in epiglottitis. Radiology can be characteristic, but the child should not be moved to obtain these visuals. Disturbance of the child with epiglottis may lead to sudden and disastrous loss of the airway. Anaesthesia may be required to make the diagnosis as well as to secure the airway.

The most experienced anaesthetist available should perform the procedure, and in suspected epiglottitis or extreme tracheitis, it may be valuable to have an ENT surgeon present with a tracheostomy set ready. Inhalational induction is achieved with oxygen and a nonirritant vapour (halothane or sevoflurane). The induction should take place in the child's preferred posture, at least until consciousness is lost.

Laryngoscopy and oral intubation are carried out in the spontaneously breathing child with deep inhalation anaesthesia alone. After successful oral intubation, the tube can be replaced with an optimal nasal tube. This must be strapped securely so that the child cannot easily self-extubate. Further management will be in the paediatric intensive care unit.

Inhaled Foreign Body

Rigid bronchoscopy can be performed under inhalational anaesthesia or titrated propofol/remifentanil TIVA (propofol 200–500 μg/kg/min and remifentanil 0.1–0.2 μg/kg/min) to preserve spontaneous ventilation (positive-pressure ventilation may cause the foreign body to migrate deeper). Premedication with atropine (10–20 μg/kg) prevents bradycardia and excess secretions. The bronchoscope should have a suitable side arm to attach the anaesthetic breathing system. The larynx can be sprayed with lidocaine 3–4 mg/kg. Nitrous oxide is contraindicated because air trapping may be present but undetected. The foreign body can be removed by bronchoscopic forceps and suction. Dexamethasone is commonly given (0.25 mg/kg intravenously) to prevent reactive airway oedema, and a chest radiograph should be performed after the procedure to exclude atelectasis, pneumothorax, etc.

Bleeding Tonsillar Bed

The problems are:

● Potentially significant hypovolaemia
● Swallowed blood in the stomach
● A swollen and bleeding pharynx with a difficult view of the airway

Intravascular volume should be restored before anaesthesia. Classically, the child is anaesthetized in a head-down, left-lateral position with an inhalational agent before securing the airway. However, this may increase venous congestion and bleeding and is not conducive to rapid control of the airway. Alternatively, the child can be anaesthetized after preoxygenation with rapid sequence induction and cricoid pressure. Ketamine (2 mg/kg) may be useful to maintain haemodynamic stability and either suxamethonium 1–2 mg/kg or rocuronium 1 mg/kg used for rapid relaxation.[12]

Malignant Hyperthermia

Malignant hyperthermia (MH) is a rare autosomal dominant condition linked to several chromosomal loci. The crisis is pharmacologically triggered (agents include volatile anaesthetics and suxamethonium), leading to muscle contraction. A hypermetabolic state with respiratory and lactic acidosis ensues, causing hyperthermia, hyperkalaemia and hypercalcaemia. Severe cases have rhabdomyolysis with greatly elevated creatine kinase and myoglobinuria. The condition must be suspected when there is an unexplained rapid rise in expired carbon dioxide and heart rate, possibly associated with supraventricular or ventricular arrhythmias. Hyperthermia is a later sign. Treatment is by immediate cessation of trigger agents, rapid cooling and the administration of dantrolene 1 mg/kg intravenously. Early advice should be sought from a specialized centre for both treatment and later testing.

Latex Allergy

Latex allergy is an immediate hypersensitivity reaction to latex products and is particularly associated with children who undergo operations for spina bifida, possibly owing to repeated latex exposure. Children with a history of food intolerance to vegetables that contain similar proteins (bananas, kiwi fruit, avocado and chestnuts) should also be regarded as at risk. Treatment is initially as for anaphylaxis. Serum should be sent for mast cell tryptase and complement levels (repeated at 6 h and 24 h). To confirm the diagnosis, skin testing and assay for IgE antibodies to latex should be performed 6 weeks after the event. There should be a trolley with latex-free equipment and the children should be looked after in a latex-free environment in hospital.

REFERENCES

1. Trachsel D, Svendsen J, Erb TO, von Ungern-Sternberg BS. Effects of anaesthesia on paediatric lung function. Br J. Anaesth 2016;17:151–63.
2. LeDez KM, Lerman J. The minimum alveolar concentration (MAC) of isoflurane in preterm neonates. Anesthesiology 1987;67:301–7.
3. Hansen TG. Anesthesia-related neurotoxicity and the developing animal brain is not a significant problem in children. Paediatr Anaesth 2015;25:65–72.
4. von Ungern-Sternberg BS, Habre W. Pediatric anesthesia – potential risks and their assessment: part I. Paediatric Anaesth 2007;17:206–15.
5. von Ungern-Sternberg BS, Habre W. Pediatric anesthesia – potential risks and their assessment: part II. Paediatric Anaesth 2007;17:311–20.
6. Dennhardt N, Beck C, Huber D, Sander B, Boehne M, Boethig D, et al. Optimized preoperative fasting times decrease ketone body concentration and stabilize mean arterial blood pressure during induction of anesthesia in children younger than 36 months: a prospective observational cohort study. Paediatr Anaesth 2016;26:838–43.
7. Tait AR, Bickham R, O'Brien LM, Quinlan M, Voepel-Lewis T. The STBUR questionnaire for identifying children at risk for sleep-disordered breathing and postoperative opioid-related adverse events. Paediatr Anaesth 2016;26:759–66.
8. Kamata M, Cartabuke RS, Tobias JD. Perioperative care of infants with pyloric stenosis. Paediatr Anaesth 2015;25:1193–206.
9. Broemling N, Campbell F. Anesthetic management of congenital tracheoesophageal fistula. Pediatric Anaesth 2011;21:1092–99.
10. Rachel Homer J, Elwood T, Peterson D, Rampersad S. Risk factors for adverse events in children with colds emerging from anesthesia: a logistic regression. Pediatr Anaesth 2007;17:154–61.
11. Hampson-Evans D, Morgan P, Farrar M. Pediatric laryngospasm. Pediatr Anaesth 2008;18:303–7.
12. Fields RG, Gencorelli FJ, Litman RS. Anesthetic management of the pediatric bleeding tonsil. Paediatr Anaesth 2010;20:982–6.

FURTHER READING

Special Issue: Neonatal anesthesia: frontier concepts in theory and practice. Paediatr Anaesth 2014;24:1–136.

Good practice in postoperative and procedural pain management, 2nd ed.. Paediatr Anaesth 2012;22:1–79.

Chapter 5.7

Neurosurgery

Hemanshu Prabhakar

Neuroanaesthesia is challenging and an understanding of basic neuroanatomy and physiology essential. Careful titration of anaesthesia and good communication between the surgeon and the anaesthetist are needed for a safe and smooth perioperative course; the vigilance of the anaesthetist cannot be overemphasized. The development of modern surgical techniques has led to advances in anaesthetic techniques and neuromonitoring. 'Awake craniotomy' is gaining popularity, minimally invasive techniques and use of functional neuroimaging are widely practiced. The availability of newer and shorter acting drugs such as dexmedetomidine, remifentanil, propofol, sevoflurane and desflurane have greatly improved anaesthetic practice.

Early emergence and a smooth recovery is one of the goals of neuroanaesthesia practice, to allow prompt assessment of neurosurgical patients.

GENERAL CONSIDERATIONS

Neuroanatomy

The brain is enclosed in the bony cranium surrounded by three meningeal layers: the outer dura mater, middle arachnoid mater and the innermost pia mater.

Cerebral blood flow is derived from two internal carotid arteries (ICA) and two vertebral arteries, which anastomose at the base of the brain forming the circle of Willis (Fig. 5.7.1). Venous drainage is via the dural sinuses ultimately draining into the internal jugular vein.

The blood–brain barrier (BBB) is formed by specialized capillaries in the brain with sealed interendothelial 'tight' junctions limiting the passage even to small ions. Passage across the BBB is determined by lipid solubility; lipid soluble molecules with molecular weight < 500 Da are able to pass. Water-soluble molecules, molecular weight > 180 Da are unable to pass. Amino acids and glucose are transported via carrier-mediated mechanisms. Permeability increases if the BBB is disrupted by disease, e.g. infection, ischaemia or tumour. The circumventricular organs (the neurohypophysis and chemoreceptor zones) lie outside the BBB.

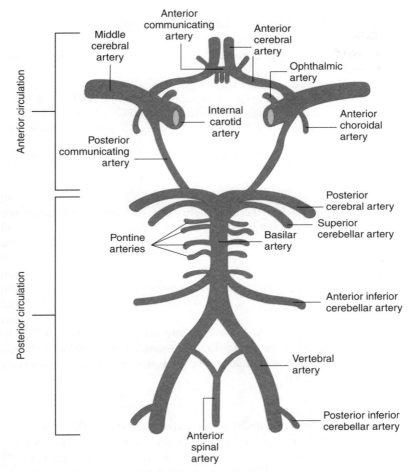

FIGURE 5.7.1   Circle of Willis.

Branches from the trigeminal nerve, vagus nerve, the first three cervical spinal nerves and the branches from the cervical sympathetic trunk supply the dura mater covering the brain and the scalp.[1]

Neurophysiology

Regulation of Cerebral Blood Flow

Although brain comprises only 2% of the body weight, it receives 15%–20% of cardiac output. The normal cerebral blood flow (CBF) is 50–55 mL/100 g/min. It varies with metabolism: grey matter receives approximately 80 mL/100 g/min, whereas white matter receives 20 mL/100 g/min (Box 5.7.1). A CBF below

---

BOX 5.7.1 Normal Values in Relation to the Adult Brain

- Weight: 2% of total body weight
- Metabolic activity: 20% of basal O_2 consumption; 25% of basal glucose consumption
- Blood demand: 15% of cardiac output
- Cerebral metabolic rate of oxygen consumption ($CMRO_2$): 3.5 mL /100 g/min
- Cerebral metabolic rate of glucose consumption (CMRG): 4.5 mg/100 g/min
- Cerebral blood flow: 50 mL/100 g/min (75–80 mL/100 g/min, grey matter and 20–30 mL/100 g/min, white matter)
- Autoregulation limits: 50–150 mmHg

---

20 mL/100 g/min is considered critical; below this, irreversible cellular damage occurs. CBF is influenced by:

- Autoregulation
- Carbon dioxide (PCO_2)
- Oxygen (PO_2)
- Metabolism
- Viscosity

Unlike other body organs, the brain is totally dependent on the glucose for energy. The normal conscious human brain consumes 156 μmol/100 g of tissue oxygen in a minute. Carbon dioxide production is the same, leading to a respiratory quotient (RQ) of 1.0.

Autoregulation

The brain has the ability to maintain a relatively constant CBF over a range of arterial pressures and cerebral perfusion pressures (CPP). This is called cerebral autoregulation (Fig. 5.7.2). CPP is the difference between the mean arterial pressure (MAP) and intracranial pressure (ICP), i.e., CPP = MAP – ICP and is the driving force perfusing the brain. The normal CPP is 80–90 mmHg and becomes critical at 40 mmHg.[2,3] The limits of autoregulation are 50 mmHg, below which CBF decreases and 150 mmHg, above which CBF increases. However, these limits are approximate and are increased by chronic hypertension. Autoregulation is also affected by hypoxaemia, hypercapnia, high-dose volatile anaesthetic agents and pathophysiological states such as severe head injury, subarachnoid haemorrhage and cerebrovascular disease.

The principle mechanisms involved in autoregulation are thought to be:

- Myogenic theory – stretching of smooth muscle cells in the vessel wall results in vasoconstriction.
- Neurogenic theory – mediated by perivascular autonomic innervation.
- Metabolic theory – the ability to maintain local blood blow depends upon on its activity.

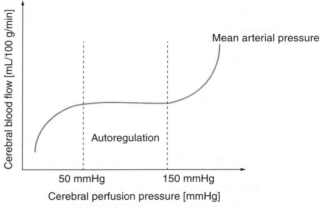

FIGURE 5.7.2   Cerebral autoregulatory curve.

Carbon Dioxide

CBF increases linearly over the range of 3.3–10 kPa PCO_2. This change happens within minutes of the change in PCO_2 and reverts towards normal within a few hours. Reactivity to PCO_2 is attenuated in some patients with carotid stenosis, cardiac failure, severe hypotension and after brain injury. If carbon dioxide reactivity is reduced, a 'steal' may occur in diseased areas as blood is diverted into normally reactive areas when PCO_2 rises.

Oxygen

Hyperoxia has little effect on CBF; hypoxia only begins to increase CBF when arterial PO_2 falls below 8 kPa.

Metabolism

CBF is tightly linked to cerebral metabolism (flow–metabolism coupling). Activation of the cortex results in an immediate focal increase in flow. There is a 10% decrease in CBF during sleep, but rapid eye movement (REM) sleep causes CBF to increase to awake values. Adenosine and nitric oxide may mediate this phenomenon.

Viscosity

Reduced blood viscosity results in increased cerebral microcirculatory flow. Haematocrit is the major determinant of viscosity. A haemoglobin concentration of about 10 g/dL is the best compromise in the cerebral circulation between viscosity and oxygen-carrying capacity.

Intracranial Pressure

Intracranial pressure (ICP) refers to the pressure within the cranial vault, which contains three elements: brain, cerebrospinal fluid (CSF) and the blood within the cerebral vessels. The concept was first proposed by Alexander Munro in

---

BOX 5.7.2 Types of ICP Waves

A waves: Pathological; plateau shaped; last 5–20 min; suggest low compliance of the brain

B waves: Rhythmic oscillations occur every 1–2 min; seen in ventilated patients; suggest poor compliance of the brain

C waves: Rhythmic oscillations occur every 4–8 min; synchronous with spontaneous variations in blood pressure; nonpathological

---

1783, supported by his colleague George Kellie as the Munro–Kellie doctrine. The present doctrine, proposed by Harvey Cushing, states that in an intact skull, the volume of brain, blood and CSF remain constant. An increase in volume of any one compartment must be compensated by the reduction in either one, or both, other compartments.[2,3] However, if compensatory mechanisms are readily exhausted, any further increase in volume of one component will cause a large rise in ICP.

Normal ICP values by age group:

- Adults – 10–15 mmHg
- Children – 3–8 mmHg
- Neonates – 0–6 mmHg

Intracranial waveform analysis provides information regarding ICP and compliance. Waveforms may show one of the three main patterns (Box 5.7.2). Raised ICP can be associated with internal herniation of the brain. The forebrain may herniate into the midbrain, causing third nerve palsy with a large pupil, or the brainstem may herniate through the foramen magnum, causing respiratory arrest.

Brain cavities are filled with CSF, mostly produced by the choroid plexus of the ventricles. CSF drains from the lateral ventricles into the third ventricle via the foramen of Monro and then, through the cerebral aqueduct (aqueduct of Sylvius), to the fourth ventricle. The fourth ventricle is connected to the subarachnoid space by three foramen; the middle foramina of Magendie and, on either side, foramen of Luschka (Fig. 5.7.3). CSF is reabsorbed through the arachnoid villi into superior sagittal sinus by a pressure-dependent process. If the venous pressure is raised, reabsorption decreases. However, normally, production balances reabsorption. The total CSF volume is about 150 mL in adults, divided between the cranial and spinal subarachnoid spaces. In adults, CSF production is about 400–600 mL per day (0.3–0.6 mL/min/g) and is renewed 4–5 times per day. Obstruction to flow may result in hydrocephalus and raised ICP.[2,3]

Neuropharmacology

Anaesthetic Agents

Most anaesthetic agents decrease cerebral metabolic rate of oxygen consumption ($CMRO_2$) and, as CBF is coupled to metabolism, metabolic depression

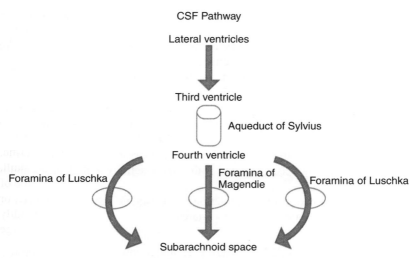

FIGURE 5.7.3 Flow pathway of cerebrospinal fluid in the brain.

results in a secondary reduction of CBF, which may reduce ICP. See Table 5.7.1 for a summary.

Intravenous anaesthetic agents reach the highly perfused and lipophilic tissues in the brain and spinal cord where they produce anaesthesia in single circulation time. All intravenous agents decrease CBF with the exception of ketamine, which produces an increase in CBF but little effect on metabolism.

TABLE 5.7.1 Cerebral Effects of Anaesthetic Agents

Anaesthetic	ICP	CPP	CBF	CMRO$_2$
Thiopental	– –	+ +	– – –	– – –
Propofol	– –	+ +	– –	– –
Etomidate	– –	+ +	– –	– –
Ketamine	+ +	– –	+ +	+
Isoflurane	+/0	–/0	+/0	– –
Sevoflurane	+/0	–/0	+/0/–	– –
Desflurane	+/0	–/0	+/–	– –
Nitrous Oxide	+ +	– –	+ +	+

Notes: +, increase; –, decrease; 0, no effect. See text for further detail.

Ketamine, once regarded as unsuitable for neurosurgery, is increasingly used in trauma patients; recent evidence suggests that its effect on ICP may be limited. In addition, it blocks the excitatory N-methyl-D-aspartate (NMDA) receptor sites and may have neuroprotective effects.[3,4]

Most volatile agents are direct cerebral vasodilators but also depress $CMRO_2$. The overall change in CBF is the balance between these two effects. At low concentrations CBF is reduced along with $CMRO_2$, but above a certain concentration, typically 1 MAC, vasodilator effects predominate. However, at clinically relevant doses, < 1 MAC and with controlled ventilation, the ICP is largely unaffected. Halothane causes the greatest increase in CBF, and sevoflurane the least. Enflurane is associated with seizure activity at high doses and is not used.

There are certain key points in relation to anaesthetic agents which must be remembered during neurosurgical procedures:

- Thiopental decreases CBF, $CMRO_2$, ICP, infarct volume; it has neuroprotective effects, causes burst suppression on electroencephalogram (EEG) and is used for management of status epilepticus.
- Propofol decreases CBF, $CMRO_2$, ICP, intraocular pressure (IOP), has neuroprotective and anticonvulsant effects.
- Etomidate decreases CBF, $CMRO_2$, ICP. It causes minimal cardiovascular depression meaning that CPP is maintained. It enhances somatosensory evoked potentials (SSEPs) and causes minimal depression of motor-evoked potential amplitudes (MEPs).
- Ketamine increases CBF, $CMRO_2$, ICP, IOP and increases the amplitude of SSEPs. As a NMDA blocker, it may have neuroprotective effects. Its role is being re-evaluated.
- Nitrous oxide (N_2O) is a neurostimulant and, administered alone, increases CBF, $CMRO_2$, ICP and IOP. It may have neuroprotective properties due to its NMDA receptor blocking action. It increases the volume of air filled spaces, hence should be avoided in patients with a history of recent craniotomy.
- Isoflurane increases ICP but this can be attenuated by propofol, opioids or hyperventilation. Isoflurane is neuroprotective.
- Sevoflurane appears to have the least effect on CBF and ICP both in animals and humans and in concentrations < 1%–1.2% does not adversely affect autoregulation. The concerns of toxicity during prolonged use have not been substantiated.
- Compared with other halogenated volatile agents, desflurane appears to have greater ICP elevating properties.
- Desflurane causes airway irritability and so unsuitable for induction of anaesthesia.[3,4]

Other Agents

Nondepolarizing muscle relaxants have little effect on cerebral haemodynamics. Suxamethonium causes a small and transient rise in ICP which is clinically unimportant. Opioids have little effect on cerebral haemodynamics at clinically relevant doses. Remifentanil is increasingly popular for neuroanaesthesia, as it provides rapidly titratable analgesia and a prompt smooth recovery.

Dexmedetomidine is a highly selective α2 agonist, which provides sedation without respiratory depression. Other clinical effects include sympatholysis, anxiolysis and analgesia; it does not interfere with electrophysiological mapping. It is increasingly popular in neuroanaesthesia. The use of nonsteroidal anti-inflammatory drugs (NSAIDs) is contentious because of the potential for increased bleeding.

TECHNICAL CONSIDERATIONS

Positioning

Patient positioning is determined primarily by the location of the pathology, but it also has effects on ICP and brain swelling. Four main positions are regularly used for neurosurgical patients; supine, prone, lateral and sitting. The patient's head is stabilized on a horseshoe head rest or a pin-fixation system. Most supratentorial lesions can be operated upon in supine position. Lesions in the brainstem or cerebellopontine angle are usually performed in the prone or lateral positions and those in the posterior fossa in either the prone or sitting position. Each position has its own advantages and disadvantages (Table 5.7.2).

TABLE 5.7.2 Precautions to be Taken during Various Neurosurgical Positions

Position	Specific Precautions
Supine	Adequate padding of pressure points, avoid excessive neck rotation, proper taping of eyelids, additional analgesic and local anaesthetic instillation at pin insertion sites
Prone	Adequate padding of the face and eyes, avoid pressure on the eyeballs, adequate padding of pressure points, avoid pressure on the genitalia, additional analgesic and local anaesthetic instillation at pin insertion sites
Lateral	Adequate padding of pressure points, proper padding of the dependent axilla, avoid excessive neck flexion and rotation, additional analgesic and local anaesthetic instillation at pin insertion sites
Sitting	Adequate padding of pressure points, avoid excessive neck flexion, additional analgesic and local anaesthetic instillation at pin insertion sites

It is important to avoid excessive rotation or flexion of the neck which may impair venous drainage resulting in raised ICP. Excessive neck flexion can also result in injury to the spinal cord. It is a good practice to keep two fingers' breadth between the chin and the sternum at the time of final neck flexion. Complications that may be encountered during various neurosurgical positions include:

- Supine position – venous air embolism (VAE), peripheral nerve injuries
- Prone position – VAE, ischaemic optic neuropathy causing postoperative blindness
- Lateral position – brachial plexus nerve injury
- Sitting position – VAE, peripheral nerve injuries, cervical flexion myopathy, quadriplegia or paraplegia, haemodynamic instability

VAE can occur during any neurosurgical procedure performed in any position, although the incidence is maximum in sitting position.

Fluid Management

Glucose-containing fluids should be avoided in neurosurgical patients; residual-free water, after glucose metabolism, may worsen cerebral oedema and hyperglycaemia exacerbates cerebral ischaemic damage. Hartmann's solution (compound sodium lactate or Ringer's lactate) is effectively hypo-osmolar, compared with serum as the result of aggregation of sodium molecules. 0.9% normal saline has been the crystalloid of choice; it is slightly hyperosmolar but large volumes are associated with a hyperchloraemic acidosis. Alternating bags of 0.9% saline and Hartmann's solution has been suggested.

Blood products are used to replace blood loss to maintain an Hb of >8 g/dL. Hyperosmolar therapy is often required intraoperatively to provide brain relaxation. Mannitol and hypertonic saline are both used, though the superiority of one fluid over the other is not established.

Brain Protection

Both pharmacological and nonpharmacological methods have been tried for brain protection, albeit, with conflicting results. Nonpharmacological methods include the manipulation of physiological variables including: therapeutic hypothermia, glucose control, cerebral perfusion pressure and mean arterial pressures. Pharmacological methods include: intravenous anaesthetics (barbiturates, propofol, ketamine, etomidate), inhalational agents (desflurane, sevoflurane, isoflurane, halothane), calcium-channel antagonists, dexmedetomidine, lidocaine, remifentanil, phenytoin, corticosteroids, magnesium, erythropoietin and hormones.

Neuromonitoring

The choice of monitors in neuroanaesthesia depends upon the procedure and the needs of the surgeon. In addition to standard monitoring, invasive arterial pressure is routine for intracranial procedures. A central venous catheter may be required if vascular instability is likely (e.g. surgery around the brainstem, or severe blood loss). Modern noninvasive blood pressure monitors are satisfactory for many cases. Noninvasive cardiac output monitors may assist in directing therapy in those with cardiovascular instability. Regular estimation of arterial blood gases, glucose and sodium and monitoring of core temperature are also required to optimize treatment strategies.

Besides standard monitors, brain monitoring may be used to detect changes in cerebral haemodynamics, oxygenation and neuronal function. There are various devices to monitor ICP (bolts and catheters) and CBF (radioactive xenon clearance, transcranial Doppler, near-infrared spectroscopy, indocyanine green angiography). Bispectral index (BIS) and spectral entropy can be used to monitor depth of anaesthesia. The use of EEG, evoked potentials (sensory, motor, visual, auditory and somatosensory) and also electromyography (function of cranial nerves: V, VII, IX, X, XI and XII) may be required.

If evoked potential monitoring is needed, propofol infusions give the best conditions, although sensory potentials can be successfully recorded with volatile anaesthesia. Motor evoked monitoring (e.g. transcranial stimulation for spinal cord monitoring or facial nerve monitoring during base of skull surgery) requires muscle relaxants to be avoided, although short-acting agents can be used for intubation.

Preoperative Preparation

Preoperative Evaluation

Preoperative evaluation is extremely important and should include a thorough neurological examination. Involvement of other systems may also be observed in neurosurgical patients, such as endocrine abnormalities and cardiovascular pathologies in patients with pituitary tumours and respiratory system involvement in patients with neuromuscular disorders (myasthenia gravis and Guillain–Barré syndrome), emphasizing the need for complete systematic assessment in these patients. Coexisting medical problems should be optimized and drug history reviewed.

Preoperative investigations should include determination of electrolyte values, blood glucose and a clotting screen where indicated. Review of neuroimaging is mandatory. This is also an opportunity to give an explanation of relevant details of the anaesthetic to the patient and to assess the risks.

Neurological Examination

Assessment of the level of consciousness is the first and most important step, typically using the Glasgow Coma Scale (GCS). A standard measure of global cerebral function, GCS, is based on the best motor, verbal and eye-opening responses to external stimuli. It has a minimum score of three. Patients scoring ≤ 8 are by definition unconscious and need airway protection and ventilation. The GCS has interobserver variability and, because it is calculated from the best response, lateralizing signs such as limb deficits and pupil responses should be documented simultaneously.

Principles of Anaesthesia

Induction

The site and side of surgery should be marked preoperatively and checked with the patient before induction of anaesthesia. Induction should be smooth. Hypnotics, analgesics and muscle relaxants should be titrated to avoid coughing, straining or hypertension. Doses should be chosen to minimize the incidence of hypotension or hypertension, which can cause both brain swelling and increased ICP. This is particularly important when autoregulation might be impaired.

Nonkinking tubes such as the Flexilum™ (Mallinkrodt) are traditionally used and these should be well secured with tape rather than a tie. It should be considered whether there will be a need for nasogastric drainage as it is easier to insert a nasogastric tube at induction than later. A urinary catheter is indicated if surgery is likely to be prolonged, bloody or mannitol may be required.

Brain Relaxation

A relaxed brain during the intraoperative period is essential for a good surgical outcome. If problems arise, use a check list to ensure the following:

- Adequate depth of anaesthesia, good muscle relaxation (in the absence of remifentanil), volatile agents < 1 MAC, consider change to total intravenous anaesthesia
- Care with positioning – reverse Trendelenburg tilt, avoid excessive head rotation, no abdominal compression
- Ventilation to maintain normocapnia and no hypoxia, mild hyperventilation (PCO_2 4.0–4.5 kPa) may be useful for short periods
- Hypertension should be avoided by anticipating episodes of surgical stimuli
- Osmotic agents such as mannitol (0.25–1 g/kg) or hypertonic saline (3–5 mL/kg of 3%) may be considered to achieve good brain relaxation

Emergence

An early, smooth and successful extubation is a prerequisite for a good outcome and should be planned for at the time of the surgical closure with normotension, normocapnia, normothermia and complete surgical haemostasis. Closure of a craniotomy can be painful and stimulating. Anaesthesia should be maintained to prevent hypertension, coughing and premature movement. Analgesics such as paracetamol are useful but opioids may be needed to provide analgesia in patients who have had intraoperative remifentanil and should be administered at least 30 min before the end of the procedure. Local infiltration with 0.5% bupivacaine or a scalp block reduces postcraniotomy pain and opiate requirement.

Patients may be extubated 'awake' or 'deep'. There is no evidence that either is superior. Planning emergence also depends upon other factors such as age, ASA status, preoperative level of consciousness, preoperative neurologic deficits (impaired gag and cough reflex), intraoperative blood loss and massive fluid shifts and duration of the surgery.

Postanaesthetic Care

A rapid recovery allows prompt neurological assessment and detection of complications. Some procedures (e.g. posterior fossa surgery, cranioplasty, complex spinal surgery, ventriculoperitoneal shunt) can be extremely painful. Regular paracetamol is useful and can be combined with regular oral dihydrocodeine and ibuprofen. Morphine can be titrated intravenously in 1–3 mg increments, but oral or intramuscular morphine can also be used and patient-controlled analgesia used, if felt appropriate.

Prophylactic antiemetics are recommended for all patients who have opiates and those who are undergoing posterior fossa surgery, who may need multiple agents.

Postoperative Complications

Minor complications including pain, nausea, vomiting and shivering are relatively common. Postoperative intracranial haematoma can be associated with serious morbidity or mortality. The majority occur within 8 h and virtually all within 24 h. Aspirin is a risk factor, and NSAID use is also a possibility.

After anterior cervical surgery, swelling can occur secondary to haematoma or oedema. Patients complain of not being able to breathe, but rarely have stridor. Oximetry is not a good guide to airway patency. Complete obstruction can occur suddenly. The priority is to open the wound as this may restore the airway.

Electrolyte imbalances are not uncommon in patients with pituitary tumour or aneurysmal subarachnoid haemorrhage. Postoperative visual loss is a rare but well-known complication following surgery in the prone position.[5]

SPECIFIC OPERATIONS

Tumour Surgery

Glioma, meningioma, pituitary tumour or metastatic carcinoma are the usual pathologies. Bleeding is rarely significant except occasionally with a meningioma, but induced hypotension can sometimes facilitate surgery. Remifentanil infusions are useful for this purpose. Dexamethasone decreases ICP by reducing brain swelling associated with tumours, but the hyperglycaemic effect of corticosteroids is unwelcome.

'Awake' craniotomy is indicated for tumours in or adjacent to eloquent areas of brain or for epilepsy surgery. This can be performed under scalp block alone, but more often local infiltration is combined with sedation or general anaesthesia using dexmedetomidine, propofol or remifentanil infusions. Airway control is often with a supraglottic airway device (SAD), which can be removed during the 'awake' phase and re-inserted as necessary.

Posterior fossa lesions present particular challenges including positioning and associated complications (sitting, lateral or prone), potential for brainstem injury (haemodynamic instability), and acute obstructive hydrocephalus. Patients may have impaired gag and cough reflex due to involvement of lower cranial nerves, especially in tumours of cerebellopontine angle. Postoperative nausea and vomiting can be protracted following posterior fossa craniotomy. This should be anticipated and antiemetic strategies implemented.

Pituitary Surgery

Pituitary tumours are often approached through the nose (trans-sphenoidal). Tumour resection is under microscopic vision or with use of endoscopes. Dilatation of the nasal passage is extremely stimulating and profound analgesia is required. A throat pack is recommended. Cushing's disease is associated with significant cardiovascular pathology and acromegaly with glottic stenosis. Severe airway obstruction may occur after extubation in acromegalics and postoperative sleep apnoea may also be a problem in these patients. If throat packs have been inserted, they must be removed before extubation.[3,4]

Vascular Surgery

Interventional neuroradiology is increasingly used to treat aneurysms and arteriovenous malformations (AVMs) using therapeutic devices, such as coils, stents or glue, or to treat vascular complications such as acute ischaemic stroke (AIS) with thrombolytics. Both local and general anaesthesia can be used. For AIS, local anaesthesia is currently preferred where feasible. However, for embolization of aneurysms, the patient must be completely still and general anaesthesia is used.

Interventional neuroradiological procedures can be lengthy and the contrast medium is hyperosmotic, so a urinary catheter is often required. Patients are heparinized for these procedures, which increases the risk of bleeding and may be catastrophic should the aneurysm rupture. Invasive arterial monitoring is required but can be monitored directly using a sidearm of the radiologist's arterial access.

A proportion of aneurysms and AVMs are unsuitable for radiological treatment and proceed to theatre. Normothermia and maintenance of normotension at the patient's preoperative pressure are recommended. Wide fluctuations in blood pressures should be avoided as these increase the risk of rupture. CPP should be maintained and adequate brain relaxation provided to facilitate clipping of the aneurysm. Vasospasm and rebleeding are major concerns in the postoperative period. Any new neurologic deficit should be documented and appropriate measures taken.[3,4]

Neuroendoscopy

Minimally invasive neurosurgery has many advantages, for both surgeons and patients including reduced trauma to normal tissue, preservation of function, quicker recovery, reduced morbidity, shorter hospital stay and reduced cost. Both intracranial and spinal surgeries are now being conducted using this technique. The general principles for management remain the same. During procedures such as third ventriculostomy, excessive use of irrigation fluid may result in electrolyte abnormalities. Robotic assisted neuroendoscopy has shown promising results for management of intracranial and spine lesions.[3,4]

Functional Neurosurgery

Deep brain stimulation is used in the treatment of Parkinson disease, chronic pain, intractable movement disorders, epilepsy and some psychiatric disorders. These procedures are usually performed in 'awake' patients with monitored anaesthesia care.

Spinal Surgery

Surgery is indicated to relieve pressure on the spinal cord or nerve roots typically for disc lesions, spinal stenosis, tumours and occasionally infections or haematomas. Difficult intubation is common with cervical spine pathology. Blood loss from spinal tumours can be marked. Some thoracic spinal lesions have to be approached through the chest and a double-lumen tube is used. Spinal cord monitoring may be required. Postoperative visual loss is a rare complication, most common after prone spinal surgery. Diabetes mellitus, preoperative hypertension, smoking and intraoperative hypotension are risk factors.

Paediatric Neurosurgery

Owing to their developing and maturing physiologic status along with their neurologic disease, paediatric patients pose a special challenge. Common neurosurgical procedures such as CSF diversion techniques for hydrocephalus, repair of neural tube defects, excision of brain tumours (commonly in the posterior fossa) and repair of craniosynostosis are frequently performed.[3,4]

Neuroradiological Procedures

Providing anaesthesia in remote areas is always challenging. Neurosurgical patients are at increased risk due to their altered neurology and rapidly changing physiological status. Diagnostic procedures routinely performed in neurosurgical patients are CT and MRI scans and digital subtraction angiography (see Chapter 5.15).

Interventional procedures are discussed earlier.

Emergency Neurosurgery

Most emergency neurosurgery is performed for evacuation of expanding intracranial extra- or intradural haematoma or for the relief of raised ICP. The aetiology is often trauma, or postoperative acute haematoma or hydrocephalus requiring evacuation or drainage following intracranial surgery. Excision of contused brain and intracerebral haematoma is sometimes indicated. The anaesthetist should maintain CPP without allowing hypertension, which may increase brain swelling and ensure normal arterial blood gases, glucose and temperature.

Chronic subdural haematoma is rarely urgent, although an acute exacerbation can raise ICP. Many patients can be managed with propofol sedation and local anaesthesia for burr hole drainage. If general anaesthesia is required, some suggest returning to spontaneous respiration after opening of the dura, which will allow the PCO_2 to rise and the brain to expand again.

HEAD INJURY

Head injury is the leading cause of death in the first four decades of life and is associated with significant morbidity in survivors.

Pathophysiology

Head injury may involve diffuse axonal injury, focal contusions and space-occupying haematomas. Primary brain injury occurs due to physical disruption of neurons or axons secondary to mechanical trauma at impact. It causes variable degrees of irreversible cell damage that cannot be treated. Secondary brain injury begins from the moment of primary injury and develops over time, causing further neuronal damage and worsening of the ultimate neurological deficit. Secondary brain injury arises from both systemic and intracranial changes. Common causes are hypotension, hypoxaemia and raised ICP.

Resuscitation and Stabilization

Consensus guidelines for the management of patients with severe head injury focus on prevention, recognition and treatment of conditions contributing to secondary brain injury. This includes surgically remedial compressive lesions and the prevention of secondary systemic insults.[6]

Resuscitation is a key point where outcome can be influenced. Initial management is to control the airway, breathing and circulation, followed by a detailed secondary survey to identify other injuries. Unconscious patients should be intubated and ventilated to maintain PO_2 >13.5 kPa and PCO_2 at 4.5–5.0 kPa. Systemic blood pressure must be maintained normal or above, initially by fluid resuscitation. Glucose-containing solutions should be avoided. Blood loss should be replaced by blood products. Hypertonic saline solution may improve outcome in patients with multiple trauma because of its effect on ICP. Extracranial life-threatening injuries should be treated before definitive neurosurgical treatment.

Intensive Care Management

The aim is to prevent and treat secondary physiological insults. Although specialist neurocritical care, with therapy guided by ICP and CPP, appears to benefit patients with severe head injury, there is wide variation in practice.

Monitoring

Invasive cardiovascular monitoring, ECG and pulse oximetry are mandatory. Regular estimation of arterial blood gases, glucose and sodium and monitoring of core temperature are required to optimize treatment strategies.

Cerebral monitors allow measurement of CPP, estimation of CBF and assessment of cerebral oxygenation. Monitoring of several variables simultaneously – multimodality monitoring allows cross-validation between monitors, artefact rejection and greater confidence that treatment is appropriate:

- ICP monitoring using microtransducers placed via an intracranial bolt allows the measurement of ICP, calculation of CPP and detection of abnormal ICP waveforms. ICP may also be measured via an intraventricular catheter (external ventricular drain), which also allows therapeutic drainage of CSF.
- Transcranial Doppler ultrasonography measures blood flow velocity in the middle cerebral artery, an indirect measure of CBF. It can also demonstrate the loss of pressure autoregulation and CO_2 reactivity, indicators of poor prognosis.
- Jugular venous bulb oximetry ($SjvO_2$) is a global measure of cerebral oxygenation and assesses the balance between cerebral oxygen supply and demand. Oxygen saturation can be measured by intermittent sampling or continuously using a fibreoptic catheter. A reduction in $SjvO_2$, or an increase in arteriojugular difference in oxygen content, provides a useful indicator of inadequate CBF. A fall in $SjvO_2$ < 50% is associated with an adverse neurological outcome.

- Near-infrared spectroscopy for bedside noninvasive assessment of cerebral autoregulation/ischaemia.
- Cerebral microdialysis is used to assess evolving brain injury via analysis of brain tissue biochemistry, e.g. glucose, lactate, pyruvate, glycerol and glutamate.

General Care

Maintenance of oxygenation, normocapnia and haemodynamic stability is essential. The hypotensive effect of sedative agents may require additional support with modest doses of vasopressors or inotropes after adequate volume expansion.

Early nutritional support results in better outcome. Enteral administration is preferable. Metabolic monitoring is necessary as hyperglycaemia may lead to secondary ischaemic injury. Blood glucose should be monitored but optimal targets for glycaemic control are yet to be defined. Hypoglycaemia must be avoided.

Patients with traumatic brain injury (TBI) are at significant risk of thrombo-embolic events. Prophylaxis can be provided using mechanical methods such as graduated compression stockings or intermittent pneumatic compression. Pharmacological prophylaxis includes low-dose or low-molecular weight heparin.

Early mobilization is crucial for the best outcome. Skilled neurophysiother-apists must be part of the multidisciplinary team to ensure early rehabilitation.

Maintenance of Cerebral Perfusion Pressure

Raised ICP reduces cerebral perfusion and results in cerebral ischaemia. Consensus guidelines recommend treatment of ICP > 20–25 mmHg. An adequate CPP is required to maintain CBF and tissue oxygenation. Current consensus is a target of > 60 mmHg.[6]

Methods for controlling ICP include:

- Sedation and analgesia – Intravenous anaesthetic agents are routinely used to reduce ICP by a dose-dependent reduction in $CMRO_2$ and CBF while maintaining autoregulation and carbon dioxide reactivity. Propofol is the sedative of choice in most neurointensive care units, but hypotension must be avoided. Adjunct analgesic infusions are often used.
- Posture – A neutral position of the head and neck with moderate head-up tilt (15°–20°) facilitates cerebral venous drainage and reduces ICP.
- Osmotherapy – 0.5 g/kg mannitol reduces ICP in acute settings but chronic use in intensive care is not associated with improved neurological outcome. Hypertonic saline has been used with success. It has fewer side effects and has been shown to control ICP in the patients refractory to mannitol. Various concentrations are available from 1.7% to 29.2% and numerous regimens

described but a dose of 2 mL/kg of a 5% solution is typical. Plasma osmolality should be regularly monitored during therapy.

- Hyperventilation – This can exacerbate cerebral hypoperfusion and consequently is reserved for intractable intracranial hypertension. Aim for PCO_2 4.0–4.5kPa but guided by cerebral monitoring to maintain adequate cerebral perfusion.
- CSF drainage via a ventriculostomy and for failed medical management, decompressive craniectomy can be used to reduce ICP.
- Temperature – Hypothermia has been shown to be neuroprotective in animal studies and has theoretical benefits. However, evidence from studies has failed to demonstrate any consistent or statistically significant reduction in mortality. Moderate hypothermia (32°C–34°C) effectively reduces ICP and is often included in management algorithms.

BRAIN DEATH AND ORGAN DONATION

Advances in medical management, along with better understanding of the pathophysiology, have improved the outcome of neurologically compromised patients in a remarkable way. However, good outcome is not always possible or predictable. Confirmation of death is relatively straightforward in most circumstances; however, developments in resuscitation techniques along with increasing recognition of the medical benefits of cadaveric organ donation have presented new challenges and placed new demands upon the diagnostic criteria for death. Unfortunately there is a lack of consensus in diagnostic criteria between different countries. In the UK and many European countries diagnosis is clinical. In contrast, in some other countries such as the United States, Sweden and the Netherlands, confirmatory testing is recommended or required (Table 5.7.3).

In the UK, a clinical diagnosis of brain death incorporates three sequential but interdependent steps:

- The patient's condition must be due to irreversible brain damage of known aetiology; potentially reversible causes of coma and apnoea, such as drug effects, metabolic, endocrine disturbances or hypothermia are excluded.
- Clinical examination of brainstem reflexes is performed (Box 5.7.3).
- Apnoea testing is performed.

Brainstem death must be diagnosed by two doctors who must be present at each of the two sets of clinical tests that are required to determine death. Although death is not confirmed until the second test has been completed, the legal time of death is when the first test confirms the absence of brainstem reflexes.

Confirmatory tests may also be useful to reduce uncertainty if the preconditions prior to clinical testing are not met, or if it is not possible to perform a comprehensive neurological examination.

BOX 5.7.3 Brainstem Death Tests

- Pupils must be fixed in diameter and not responsive to incident light. **Cranial nerves II, III**
- There must be no corneal reflex (avoid damaging the cornea). **Cranial nerves V, VII**
- Vestibulo-ocular reflexes are absent. No eye movements occur following the slow injection of at least 50 mL of ice cold water over 1 min into each external auditory meatus. Note that the normal reflex is deviation of the eyes away from the side of the stimulus. Access to the tympanic membrane should be confirmed by otoscopy. Injury or pathology may prevent this test being performed on both sides; this does not invalidate the test. **Cranial nerves VIII, III**
- No motor responses in the cranial nerve distribution should occur as a result of stimulation of any somatic area. No limb movement should occur in response to supra-orbital pressure. **Cranial nerves V, VII**
- No gag reflex should occur in response to posterior pharyngeal wall stimulation with a spatula. **Cranial nerve IX**
- No cough or other reflex should occur in response to bronchial stimulation by a suction catheter being passed down the endotracheal tube. **Cranial nerve X**
- No respiratory movements should occur in response to disconnection from the ventilator. Hypoxia should be prevented by pre-oxygenation and insufflation of oxygen through a tracheal catheter. This tests the stimulation of respiration by arterial carbon dioxide tension, which should be allowed to rise to 6.65 kPa – confirmed by arterial blood gases.

TABLE 5.7.3 Ancillary Tests for Diagnosing Brainstem Death

- Electroencephalogram (EEG)
- Evoked potentials
  - Somatosensory (SSEP)
  - Visual (VEP)
  - Brainstem auditory (BAEP)
- Electroretinogram
- Vessel digital subtraction angiography
- CT and MR angiography
- Single photon emission CT
- Tc99 radionucleotide imaging
- Transcranial Doppler

REFERENCES

1. Snell RS. Clinical neuroanatomy. Philadelphia: Lippincott Williams & Wilkins; 2010.
2. Dinsmore J, Hall G. Neuroanaesthesia: anaesthesia in a nutshell. Oxford: Butterworth – Heinemann; 2002.

3. Cottrell JE, Young WL. Neuroanesthesia. Philadelphia: Mosby Elsevier; 2010.
4. Gupta AK, Gelb AW. Essentials of neuroanesthesia and neurointensive care. Philadelphia: Saunders Elsevier; 2008.
5. Prabhakar H. Complications in neuroanesthesia. San Diego: Academic Press Elsevier Inc.; 2016.
6. Brain Trauma Foundation. Management and prognosis of severe traumatic brain injury. J Neurotrauma 2007;24:S1–S106.

Chapter 5.8

Obstetrics

Adrienne Stewart, Roshan Fernando

MATERNAL ANATOMY AND PHYSIOLOGY

The anatomical and physiological changes of pregnancy, with their implications for anaesthesia, are as follows:

- Increased basal metabolic rate – hypoxia occurs faster
- Abdominal mass – decreased oesophageal sphincter tone (regurgitation, aspiration)
- Enlarging uterus - uterine atony, aortocaval occlusion and supine hypotension
- Altered airway anatomy – increased incidence of failure to intubate
- Reduced functional residual capacity (FRC) from 20th week onwards – airway closure and reduced oxygen reserve following pre-oxygenation
- Increased blood flow to uterus and placenta – greater potential for haemorrhage
- Reduced haematocrit (increase in volume of plasma > red blood cell volume) and a hypercoagulable state

In addition, minute ventilation and cardiac output increase throughout pregnancy, reaching 30%–50% above normal by term.

Aortocaval Occlusion (Supine Hypotension) Syndrome

The risk of aortocaval occlusion begins at about 20 weeks' gestation. As the uterus enlarges, it can press on the major vessels in the abdomen resulting in aortocaval occlusion, reduced uterine blood flow and fetal distress. The degree of occlusion depends on both the pressure within the vessel (higher pressure is needed to occlude arteries than veins), and on the position of the vessel in relation to the uterus.

If the IVC is occluded, venous return to the heart may be reduced. This is compensated by vasoconstriction and diverted blood flow through the azygos system via the paravertebral and extradural veins. Regional anaesthesia may impair this compensation (e.g. by sympathetic nerve blockade).

Adding left lateral tilt to avoid IVC occlusion is routine practice during caesarean section (CS). However, it has been demonstrated that aortic volume does not differ significantly between parturients and nonpregnant women in the supine position, and that 15° of left lateral tilt does not effectively reduce IVC compression.

MATERNAL MORTALITY

The most common causes of direct maternal death are thrombosis and thromboembolism, sepsis, haemorrhage and hypertensive disease states. Cardiac disease, sepsis and neurological conditions are common indirect causes.[1] General anaesthetic deaths are few, and historically have been mainly associated with aspiration of stomach contents or hypoxia (failure to intubate, failure to ventilate) and more recently neuraxial anaesthesia (complications of dural puncture and local anaesthetic systemic toxicity). Up to 1% of parturients will require admission to critical care, the most common indications being major obstetric haemorrhage, hypertensive disorders of pregnancy and sepsis.

General Anaesthesia Risks

Aspiration of Stomach Contents

Regurgitation (passive) and vomiting (active) may result in aspiration of liquids or solids. For elective surgery, preparation includes:

- A policy of nil by mouth for at least 6 h for solids and 2 h for clear fluids; may require longer as opioids can delay stomach emptying
- Reduction in gastric acid production (H_2-blockers) and increase in gastric emptying (metoclopramide)

During labour a nonsolids oral regimen will reduce the frequency of complications from aspiration following general anaesthesia. The plan of prophylactic management includes:

- Restriction of food
- Reduction of acid production – ranitidine 150 mg orally or 50 mg intravenously
- Neutralization of any acid produced – clear alkaline solution such as 0.3 mmol/L sodium citrate 30 mL given just before anaesthesia
- Increasing lower oesophageal sphincter tone with prokinetic drugs, e.g. metoclopramide 10 mg intravenously

With these preparations, physically emptying the stomach using a large-bore gastric tube is rarely required for elective surgery, but may be considered for emergency surgery. Protecting the larynx using a cuffed tracheal tube and availability of a functioning wide-bore suction tube and tilting table will reduce likelihood of aspiration.

The clinical features of aspiration may take hours to manifest after the event, and include bronchospasm, dyspnoea, oxygen desaturation, tachycardia, hypotension, hypoxia and metabolic acidosis. Investigations may show radiographic changes, and the differential diagnosis includes pulmonary embolism and asthma. The symptoms and signs may be severe and respiratory support in an ICU may be required.

Failed Intubation

Pregnancy is a contributing factor to failed intubation because it results in an increase in breast size, which impedes laryngoscopy, and an increase in soft tissue mass around the airway making it more difficult to visualize the larynx. An increase in maternal metabolic rate and decrease in the FRC reduces the time to desaturation, increasing the risk of hypoxia if the lungs cannot be ventilated. Guidelines for the management of difficult and failed tracheal intubation in obstetrics have been published.[2]

In CS, if intubation fails the priority is to maintain oxygenation. If adequate oxygenation is maintained with a supraglottic airway device (SAD), it may be appropriate to proceed, as long as surgery is considered safe and essential. If it is not safe or essential, the patient should be woken up and either regional anaesthesia or awake fibreoptic intubation should be considered. If adequate oxygenation is not possible with an SAD then a 'cannot intubate, cannot oxygenate' algorithm should be followed (see Chapter 2.6).

Anaesthetic Outpatient Clinic

Parturients with potential anaesthetic problems such as diabetes, obesity, cardiac, neurological and haematological disease states, should be reviewed before anaesthetic intervention in a specialist multidisciplinary clinic. This will allow optimization of the condition, education about risks involved and delivery planning.

Women who have suffered complications should have time for follow-up and debriefing.

LABOUR AND DELIVERY

Pain Relief

The pain of labour (depending on the stage) is mediated by both visceral and somatic nociceptors. Visceral pain is often accompanied by autonomic symptoms such as nausea and vomiting.

The fetus presenting in the occipito-posterior position, may alter pain patterns because of constant pressure on tissues.

Nonpharmacological

Drugs administered during labour may cross the placenta and enter the fetal circulation, and any method that avoids or restricts their use is potentially attractive.

This is the philosophy of 'natural childbirth' with its focus on the woman's control of breathing and relaxation.

Other nonpharmacological methods include:

- Acupuncture
- Aromatherapy
- Hypnosis
- Massage
- Transcutaneous electrical nerve stimulation (TENS)
- Water immersion (first stage of labour)

Advantages for nonpharmacological techniques include, ease of administration, and minimal side effects; however, there is little evidence to support their efficacy.

Pharmacological

Inhalational Analgesia

Nitrous oxide is safe for the mother and fetus in premixed concentrations of 50:50 with oxygen (Entonox). At higher concentrations pain relief increases, but safety is compromised by an increased risk of sedation and loss of airway reflexes. Other side effects reported include nausea and vomiting. For optimal results with Entonox, inhalation is encouraged to begin at the start of a contraction.

Parenteral Analgesia

Opioids are administered routinely during labour but placental transfer may result in depressant effects in the neonate which necessitate reversed using naloxone after delivery. Therefore, the paediatrician should be warned that the mother has received parenteral opioids during labour.

Pethidine (1 mg/kg intramuscularly) is popular but its efficacy is questionable, providing sedation rather than analgesia. In countries where it is available, diamorphine (5–7.5 mg/kg intramuscularly) is an effective alternative.

Intravenous patient-controlled analgesia (PCA) with fentanyl (20 μg bolus dose, 5 min lockout time) and remifentanil (0.25–0.5 μg/kg bolus dose, 2–3 min lockout time) has been used. Both the parturient and the neonate need careful monitoring. Remifentanil PCA is used as an alternative to regional analgesia in some obstetric units and although inferior to epidural analgesia, it provides satisfactory labour analgesia. There have been case reports of respiratory depression, and even cardiorespiratory arrest associated with remifentanil PCA; parturients require close monitoring and supplemental oxygen administration.

Neuraxial Analgesia

A neuraxial analgesia technique is an extremely popular and effective method of providing labour analgesia in the labour ward.

Before a neuraxial analgesia technique is performed, a full history including any relevant obstetric information should be taken. A discussion should follow including the risks and benefits of the procedure before obtaining consent from the patient. Risks that should be discussed include:

- Failure (unilateral, unblocked segment, epidural catheter migration) requiring resiting of the epidural catheter
- Side effects of opioids
- Hypotension
- Motor blockade preventing ambulation and loss of sensation to bladder distension
- Accidental dural puncture (ADP) and postdural puncture headache
- Nerve injury
- Infection

Side-effects of neuraxial opioids may be troublesome. Pruritus is common and is treated either with an opioid antagonist titrated to effect or chlorpheniramine. Gastric stasis, nausea and vomiting are also common.

Nerve damage is far more common from pressure effects from the fetal head or obstetric interventions (lithotomy position, forceps or ventouse delivery) than related to epidural nerve block (Box 5.8.1).

Neuraxial Analgesia Techniques for Labour

All neuraxial analgesia techniques should be performed under strict aseptic conditions, with intravenous access in place, resuscitation drugs and appropriate trained staff immediately available.

Neuraxial techniques for labour analgesia are as follows:

- Epidural analgesia
- Combined spinal-epidural (CSE) analgesia

The advantage of the CSE technique compared with the epidural technique is its faster (spinal) onset of effective analgesia, making it particularly useful in the later stages of labour (e.g. prolonged second stage), and when resiting an epidural catheter for a failed block with epidural analgesia during labour. The time to effective analgesia with an epidural technique is variable, taking at least 20–30 min.

It may be necessary for fetal monitoring to continue throughout the neuraxial technique. Insertion of the epidural with patient lying on her side better preserves the uteroplacental circulation.

BOX 5.8.1 Relative Risks of Neuraxial Analgesia; Ranked from Common to Rare

Common	Itching, nonambulation
↓	Failure of technique
	Headache, transient numbness, reactions to skin preparation
Rare	Nerve palsy, accidental intravenous injection (life-threatening)

The most common space used for lumbar neuraxial analgesia is L3/4. Once inserted, the catheter should be aspirated to check that it is not intravenous or intrathecal. If there is any doubt, the catheter should be removed and the procedure should be repeated. A length of 4–5 cm of catheter should be left in the epidural space.

If an epidural technique has been used to initiate labour analgesia, up to 20 mL of a low-concentration solution, usually in divided doses, is administered via the epidural catheter. The level of nerve blockade should be checked after 20 min.

For CSE, a needle-through-needle technique (fine-bore spinal needle passed through the epidural needle) is usually employed in which 3–5 mL of the low-dose mixture is administered via the spinal needle to initiate analgesia. Once the initial spinal injection has worn off (usually 1–2 h later), subsequent doses of the mixture are given via the epidural catheter. A 10 mL dose of low-concentration local anaesthetic solution should be administered via the epidural catheter immediately after completing the CSE technique, to confirm catheter placement in the epidural space.

Monitoring of maternal blood pressure, pulse and fetal heart rate is essential following the initial dose.

Subsequent doses are administered by the midwife, or by the patients themselves in the case of patient-controlled epidural analgesia (PCEA).

Following all neuraxial nerve blocks in labour, a postnatal review to check for satisfaction and complications should be part of normal patient care. A patient should not be discharged home until her motor and sensory functions have returned to normal, she is fully mobile and has passed urine.

Drugs Used for Regional Pain Relief in Labour

Ambulatory epidurals are associated with high maternal satisfaction, but not necessarily a reduction in instrumental or operative delivery rates.

The concentration of local anaesthetic is more important than the choice of drug to use. The aim is to use very low concentration local anaesthetic solutions (bupivacaine and L-bupivacaine 0.0625%–0.125% or ropivacaine 0.07%) in combination with a lipophilic opioid drug (such as fentanyl or sufentanil), as this is associated with greater preservation of lower limb function. Premixed solutions are preferred to reduce drug administration errors.

L-bupivacaine and ropivacaine provide excellent labour analgesia, but with less cardiotoxicity than bupivacaine and a reduced incidence of motor block. It has been suggested that ropivacaine produces less motor block than both bupivacaine and L-bupivacaine.

Epidural Drug-Delivery Systems

The use of new epidural delivery systems, such as PCEAs and PIEB (programmed intermittent epidural bolus) in combination with PCEA, is associated with a reduction in both the hourly dose and total dose of local anaesthetic required, and an increase in patient satisfaction.

PCEA allows the parturient to deliver a small dose of the low-concentration epidural mixture when it is needed. PIEB in combination with a PCEA delivers a regularly timed automatic bolus of local anaesthetic, which can be supplemented by PCEA bolus doses by the parturient if required. No additional monitoring, other than those that are usually performed during labour, is required as long as the dose of bupivacaine in the bolus does not exceed 10 mg.

Contraindications to Neuraxial Analgesia

These may be absolute or relative. In all cases, the risk:benefit profile of performing neuraxial analgesia should be considered.

Absolute contraindications to regional analgesia are few, but relate to serious complications, including:

● Patient refusal
● Infection (e.g. local sepsis)
● Coagulopathy, recent anticoagulant therapy or thrombocytopaenia
● Potential for hypovolaemia and hypotension (e.g. antepartum haemorrhage)

The relative contraindications for which a risk:benefit ratio has to be determined and optimized are best approached electively through referrals to an anaesthetic antenatal clinic.

A recent (within 4 h of performing neuraxial block) coagulation screen and full blood count may be required to aid decision-making in certain situations such as antepartum haemorrhage, placental abruption, anticoagulant therapy, major sepsis, liver disease, severe pre-eclampsia and HELLP (Haemolysis, Elevated Liver enzymes, Low Platelet count) syndrome. A coagulation screen is not required if aspirin or nonsteroidal anti-inflammatory drugs (NSAIDs) have been taken.

Failed/Inadequate Neuraxial Block

A failed or inadequate neuraxial block is common, occurring in 1:10 regional techniques performed in the labour ward. In some of these cases, it may be necessary to resite the epidural catheter. A CSE technique should be considered as the time to effective analgesia is reduced.

If the pain is unilateral, an additional top-up dose (usually 10–20 mL) of the low-dose epidural mixture should be administered. If this fails, resiting the epidural catheter should be discussed with the patient. There is no evidence that pulling back the epidural catheter or administration of higher concentration local anaesthetic drugs is helpful.

If there is no detectable block, a further top-up may be required, or the catheter may need to be resited. In the case where there is no detectable block, it is imperative to ensure that the catheter is not intravenous, by aspirating prior to any injection. If there is no detectable block after this additional top-up, the epidural catheter should be removed and resited.

Accidental Dural Puncture

An ADP occurs when the dura is inadvertently breeched by the epidural needle. This is in contrast to a deliberate dural punture (DP) during an intrathecal/spinal nerve block. Any accidental (or indeed deliberate) dural puncture can result in headache, and the likelihood and severity of the pain is influenced by the size of the hole in the dura, which in turn depends on the needle size that pierced the dura and the number of punctures.

If there is doubt, confirmation of CSF can be made by testing the fluid aspirated from needle or catheter, which will be:

● Positive for glucose
● Warm
● Positive for protein
● Turbid when thiopental is mixed with CSF (a pH test)

If the technique had been otherwise uncomplicated, the epidural should be resited. If the technique has been extremely difficult, or the situation is urgent, an intrathecal catheter might be indicated.

Conversion to Intrathecal Analgesia

If an ADP is diagnosed during epidural insertion, conversion to intrathecal analgesia may be considered by passing the epidural catheter into the intrathecal space. However, the extradural catheter is firm and has the potential to damage the spinal cord as it passes into the intrathecal space.

No more than 2–3 cm of the catheter should be passed into the CSF. The catheter should be clearly marked as being intrathecal. Both the patient and the attending midwife should be informed.

A standard dose, 3–5 mL of low-concentration epidural solution should be given via the intrathecal catheter to initiate analgesia. Further top-up doses of 3–5 mL must be administered only by the anaesthetist. Epidural delivery systems cannot be used.

Managing an intrathecal catheter on the labour ward is not without problems and can be hazardous. Potential problems with an intrathecal catheter include maternal hypotension and a high block which may result in maternal cardiorespiratory collapse. This may occur if the intrathecal catheter is mistaken for an epidural catheter.

Resiting the Epidural

The more common approach is to site an epidural catheter in another interspace; explain what has happened to the patient and midwife, with discussion about subsequent management.

An anaesthetist should give further doses of local anaesthetic through a resited epidural catheter. If there is no evidence of intrathecal spread, it may be appropriate to continue with midwife top-up boluses or other epidural delivery systems.

There is no restriction on the mode of delivery after ADP with an epidural needle because there is no evidence of increasing adverse effects with pushing during the second stage. Extra care should be taken when topping up an epidural with high concentration local anaesthetic, such as that required for emergency caesarean delivery, when there has been a previous ADP.

Postdural Puncture Headache and Epidural Blood Patch

Postdural puncture headache (PDPH) occurs in about 80% of patients. PDPH is postural (worse on standing, relieved on lying flat), can be frontal or occipital, and can be associated with visual symptoms (photophobia), hearing loss and tinnitus. It is usually self-limiting, but can be very debilitating and can affect bonding between mother and baby.

Treatment of PDPH include adequate fluids (oral, intravenous) and simple oral analgesia.

Caffeine has not been shown to be effective and simple, longer acting analgesics are preferable.

An epidural blood patch (EBP) is indicated if the headache is severe, preventing normal function, and other diagnoses have been excluded. EBP is contraindicated if the woman is systemically septic. EBP is typically performed about 48 h after the ADP in women who develop a PDPH, to achieve the maximum chance of success. If the EBP is performed too early, there is a higher risk of failure. Prophylactic EBP (performed at the time of the ADP) has not been shown to be effective at either preventing the onset or the severity of PDPH. The success rate is about 70% with the first EBP whereas up to 90% of patients report relief of symptoms with a subsequent EBP.

EBP requires two anaesthetists, the first to access the epidural space at or close to the site of the original dural puncture, the second to obtain fresh maternal blood aseptically once the epidural space has been identified. The first anaesthetist immediately injects up to 30 mL of the collected maternal blood through a Tuohy needle. The injection should stop immediately if the patient complains of severe backache or worsening headache. Once the decision to stop injecting has been made, the needle should be flushed with saline to avoid spilling the blood into other tissues as it is withdrawn and initiating a painful inflammatory response, or acting as a conduit for infection. Blood cultures taken at the time of the blood patch can be useful if the woman develops pyrexia, although this is not performed routinely.

The patient should lie flat for 2 h after the EBP procedure, then, if she is feeling well enough she can be discharged home, once follow-up has been arranged.

If there is no relief of symptoms, a second EBP may be performed (usually not within 24 h of the first EBP), as long as there are no other signs or symptoms suggesting a more serious pathology.

It is advisable to perform imaging of the head and/or lumbar spine prior to considering a third EBP, to exclude other differential diagnoses.

About half of patients who present with headache have had no identifiable ADP and an alternative diagnosis should be considered, especially if the headache is not typical of a PDPH.

The most common cause of non-ADP headache is migraine. Fever may indicate a febrile origin (e.g. meningitis). Cerebral thromboses are more common in pregnancy than in the nonpregnant state, and other cerebral pathology may be more frequent in obstetrics with conditions such as pre-eclampsia.

OPERATIVE OBSTETRICS

All patients for operative obstetric procedures, whether under general or regional anaesthesia, should undergo routine pre-anaesthetic assessment with specific questions relating to the obstetric emergency if indicated. At this time, information can be given to the patient about any intended procedure and its associated risks. Examination of the airway should be performed as well as examination of the back if neuraxia nerve block is contemplated. During the preoperative assessment, the particular risks of surgery should be assessed, in case further investigations or treatments are appropriate (e.g. cross-matched blood ordered or a coagulation screen).

For all operative delivery procedures, a left lateral tilt is employed to protect the mother from aortocaval occlusion and subsequent hypotension (discussed earlier).

Routine monitoring (pulse, ECG, arterial BP and oxygen saturation) should be commenced.

Any obstetric procedure where a concentrated solution of local anaesthetic is used should be performed in an operating theatre with an anaesthetist present.

The Lithotomy Position

The lithotomy position is a common position for surgical procedures and medical examination involving the pelvis and lower abdomen. General anaesthesia should not be induced in the lithotomy position because the increase in pressure on the stomach can force gastric contents into the pharynx and subsequently into the lungs; in addition, it can make access to the airway more difficult.

When a patient under general or regional anaesthesia is put into this position, the following risks should be minimized:

● Pressure on calf muscles inducing deep vein thrombosis – use correct position, thromboembolic deterrent (TED) stockings, pneumatic compressions devices

- Pressure on peripheral nerves (sciatic, femoral, common fibular, posterior tibia, saphenous, brachial plexus) – avoid with careful positioning and padding
- Backache from moving legs independently – always move legs together

When a patient under general anaesthesia is put into this position, the following additional risks should be minimized:

- Regurgitation and aspiration of stomach contents – use of a cuffed oral tracheal tube
- Limited respiratory muscle excursion – ventilate if necessary

Instrumental and Complex Vaginal Delivery

Anaesthesia may be required for instrumental and for complex vaginal (breech/twin) delivery. Where an epidural catheter is in situ, the existing nerve block should be assessed and if working well, should be extended with a top-up using a high-concentration local anaesthestic solution, to T4 (cold) or T5 (touch) in order to be prepared for a possible caesarean delivery.

In the absence of an existing epidural block, or when an existing epidural has not been effective, consider either a CSE or single-shot spinal technique. The clinical situation and time available will determine which of these techniques would be the most appropriate.

General anaesthesia is not usually appropriate for either instrumental or complex vaginal deliveries, as expulsive effort by the parturient is usually required for their success.

Retained Placenta

A retained placenta is when all or part of the placenta or membranes remain inside the uterus for more than 30 min after the birth of the baby, where the third stage of labour has been managed actively. In some patients, there may be associated shock and hypovolaemia associated with severe blood loss requiring activation of the major obstetric haemorrhage call, maternal resuscitation and critical. Tocolytics (such as glyceryl trinitrate (GTN) or volatile anaesthetics) may be required to reverse smooth muscle spasm; however, this can increase the likelihood of bleeding from the placental bed.

In all cases (from minor to major blood loss), the estimated and expected blood loss needs careful assessment. Maternal resuscitation with oxygen, intravenous fluids and blood products may be required. Full monitoring, including urine output and coagulation, should be initiated.

If resuscitation is incomplete prior to arrival in the operating theatre, a general anaesthetic with precautions against aspiration is the method of choice.

If the patient is stable and there are no contraindications, a regional anaesthetic technique is appropriate. Either an existing epidural block sited for labour can be extended or spinal anaesthesia can be performed. A block to cold to T6 (lower sternum) is sufficient for manual removal of a placenta (MROP).

Cervical Suture

Cervical incompetence complicates about 1 in 500 pregnancies and is the most common cause of miscarriage. Cervical cerclage involves placing a suture around the cervical os of the uterus in order to prevent premature opening of the cervix.

Regional and general anaesthesia can be used safely for the procedure. One advantage of general anaesthesia is the shorter recovery time.

If general anaesthesia is chosen, nitrous oxide should be avoided. Choice of airway (SAD or cuffed tracheal tube) depends on the gestation of the woman undergoing the procedure. General anaesthesia is associated with greater demand for opioid and nonopioid analgesics in the immediate postoperative period, as well as with more nausea and vomiting.

Regional anaesthesia provides superior postoperative analgesia and less nausea and vomiting, but it can delay discharge due to motor weakness and inability to pass urine.

Nonsteroidal anti-infammatory drugs should be avoided in pregnancy.

Caesarean Delivery

CS is the most common operation performed in the labour ward. In 1985, the World Health Organization recommended a rate of up to 15%, but the relevance of this figure to modern obstetric practice is debatable. In developed countries, the CS rate now exceeds 25% and in larger obstetric units that serve a high-risk population, CS rates exceed 30%.

Delivery by CS is considered to be safe. There are certain circumstances where a caesarean delivery may be safer and is therefore the preferred mode of delivery, e.g. breech presentation, multiple pregnancy when the first twin is not cephalic, preterm birth, placenta praevia, morbidly adherent placenta, mother-to-child transmission of maternal infection.

The overall risk of maternal mortality from CS is although very low, it is still higher than that of a vaginal delivery. The risks of an emergency CS are related to previous CS, trial of labour, abnormal fetal presentation, multiple pregnancy, haemorrhage, pre-eclampsia, premature labour, intrauterine fetal growth retardation, augmented labour and coexisting medical diseases.

In the vast majority of cases, a transverse incision is made in the lower uterine segment to gain access and deliver the baby. In certain clinical situations, or if the baby is very premature and the lower segment is not formed, the main body of the uterus may be incised. This classical incision results in greater blood loss, more postoperative pain, and in future pregnancies the scar formed is at greater risk of dehiscence than with a transverse incision.

Grades of Urgency for Caesarean Section

Discussion between the obstetrician and anaesthetist determines to some extent the type of anaesthesia required. Outcome may be influenced by the grade of urgency, and the following definitions without a time base have been agreed upon:

- Grade 1 – immediate threat to life of mother or fetus
- Grade 2 – maternal or fetal compromise that is not immediately life-threatening
- Grade 3 – needing early delivery, but no maternal or fetal compromise
- Grade 4 – at a time to suit the patient and maternity team

Anaesthetic Technique

For all types of anaesthesia for CS, the preparation for surgery should include:

- Prophylaxis to prevent aspiration of stomach contents
- Blood group to save or to perform cross-match, if indicated
- Trained anaesthetic assistant in attendance
- Intravenous access
- Left lateral tilt
- Vasopressor and anticholinergic drugs immediately available
- Oxygen (not mandatory for neuraxial nerve block, but should be given if indicated, e.g. CS for fetal distress or major obstetric haemorrhage)
- Oxytocin available for administration after delivery (given by slow intravenous bolus (dose 5 units) or by infusion (10 units/h) to prevent hypotension)
- Antibiotic administration as prophylaxis for sepsis prior to skin incision
- Admission to a dedicated recovery/high-dependency area for at least 1 h after delivery
- Adequate pain relief
- Adherence to thromboembolism guidelines after surgery

General Anaesthesia for Caesarean Delivery

Despite comprising only 0.8% of all general anaesthetics performed, obstetric cases account for 10% of reports of accidental awareness under general anaesthesia (AAGA), making it the most markedly overrepresented of all the surgical specialties studied. Most of these cases occur during CS.[3]

Traditionally, a rapid sequence induction has been employed for CS using thiopental and suxamethonium, cricoid pressure, functioning suction and equipment at hand for a difficult intubation. A smaller cuffed tube tracheal tube may be required if there is associated airway swelling complicating pregnancy. However, there has been a move recently towards the use of propofol and rocuronium (reversible with sugammadex) in place of thiopental and suxamethonium for rapid sequence induction for CS.

Anaesthesia should be monitored and maintained with an adequate amount of anaesthesic agent to prevent awareness. Depth of anaesthesia monitors are now widely available, and can be used to aid the anaesthetist. Nitrous oxide or alternatively total intravenous anaesthesia with propofol can be used with isoflurane, sevoflurane or desflurane to provide maintenance of anaesthesia. Atracurium or vecuronium can be given, if suxamethonium was the initial neuromuscular blocking drug administered. The effects of the neuromuscular blocking drug should be assessed with a nerve stimulator, and reversal of paralysis should be confirmed prior to waking the patient.

Analgesia should be administered intraoperatively and continued postoperatively. Opioids such as morphine are usually administered intraoperatively, and postoperatively by intravenous patient-controlled analgesia (PCA). Ultrasound guided bilateral transverse abdominis plane (TAP) block with a local anaesthetic such as bupivacaine, followed by oral morphine is an acceptable alternative.

On completion of surgery, the mother should be extubated on her side, once fully awake and responding to commands, to prevent aspiration of gastric contents. In the case of emergency surgery with a full stomach, an orogastric or nasogastric tube should be passed prior to waking and gastric contents should be aspirated.

Regional Anaesthesia for Caesarean Delivery

An epidural, spinal or a CSE technique may be used.

Epidural anaesthesia is commonly used to provide anaesthesia for emergency CS, when an epidural catheter had been previously placed for labour analgesia. Up to 20 mL (usually in divided doses) of 0.5% bupivacaine or *L*-bupivacaine is administered via the epidural catheter in combination with an opioid, e.g. up to 100 µg fentanyl. Effective surgical anaesthesia is achieved in 7–15 min. If time to surgical anaesthesia is critical, 20 mL of 2% lidocaine with 1:200,0000 adrenaline (epinephrine) in combination with up to 100 µg fentanyl will achieve effective surgical anaesthesia in 7–11 min. Adding 2 mL 8.4% bicarbonate to this mixture will result in effective surgical anaesthesia in 5–7 min.

A single-shot spinal is a popular method for both elective and emergency cases, as the procedure is quick to perform and onset of surgical anaesthesia is fast. The disadvantage is that it is effective for a finite length of time. As the ED_{95} of bupivacaine is 11–13 mg, the recommended spinal dose of 0.5% 'heavy' bupivacaine is 2.2–2.6 mL. Intrathecal bupivacaine is usually administered in combination with an opioid such as morphine 100–200 µg, or (if available) diamorphine 300–400 µg.

A CSE technique is also popular for both elective and emergency cases. It takes longer to perform and so may not be appropriate for very urgent time-critical cases. Onset of surgical anaesthesia is fast due to the spinal component, with the advantage of prolonged nerve block due to the epidural component in case surgery is prolonged. It can also provide postoperative pain relief. A similar dose of local anaesthetic to a single-shot spinal can be administered.

Alternatively, a much smaller dose may be used followed by sequential topping-up of the epidural with high concentration local anaesthetic to achieve surgical anaesthesia. This technique is particularly useful in high-risk cases, e.g. in patients with cardiac disease.

With all three techniques, arterial BP should be measured up to every minute while the nerve block is developing. Maternal hypotension should be promptly treated. Nausea often precedes hypotension, and its presence should alert the anaesthetist to check and treat the blood pressure.

The extent of the nerve block (both upper and lower limits) should be measured and documented. A block to T4 (nipples) and S5 (anal canal) to cold is required. A block to touch to T5 is also widely quoted as acceptable. It is not possible to completely block the sensation of touch; therefore, the mother should be warned about the type of feelings she may experience.

If the mother complains of pain, she should be reassured and treated immediately. Various strategies are available to relieve the pain, but until these are effective it may be necessary to temporarily stop the surgery. Strategies include:

- Epidural top-up of local anaesthetic
- Epidural opioid
- Entonox
- Intravenous boluses of fentanyl or alfentanil
- Local anaesthetic infiltration by the surgeon if surgery is close to completion
- Intravenous ketamine (rarely)

The choice of agent and likelihood of success will depend on the stage of surgery, whether the fetus has been delivered and any surgical complications encountered. General anaesthesia may be the best option if pain occurs prior to delivery of the fetus and when surgery has only recently started. A maternal request for general anaesthesia should not go unheeded. All episodes of pain, treatment and explanation given should be recorded in the patient's notes. The patients should be followed-up postoperatively.

Postoperatively, combinations of analgesics can be very effective. If intrathecal fentanyl has been used and an epidural catheter is in place, morphine 5 mg or diamorphine 3 mg can be injected epidurally to provide long-lasting pain relief. Oral morphine is preferable to intravenous or intramuscular preparations. Codeine use is controversial because of concerns about fetal toxicity in mothers who are abnormal metabolizers of the drug. Oral or intravenous paracetamol in combination with a NSAID, if not contraindicated, should be prescribed. Regular antiemetics and laxatives are prescribed.

Management of hypotension: Hypotension is common after a spinal nerve block, occurring in up to 80% patients. It is due to a combination of loss of sympathetic tone and aorto-caval compression. Maternal hypotension results in unpleasant symptoms in the mother and reduced uterine blood flow, which could potentially be harmful for the fetus. Phenylephrine has replaced ephedrine as the vasopressor of choice, due to concerns about an association between ephedrine use and fetal acidosis. A phenylephrine infusion at 25–50 μg/min should be commenced at the start of spinal injection and titrated to maintain maternal systolic BP at ≥80% of baseline. If the arterial BP falls despite the infusion, a bolus dose of phenylephrine should be administered and the infusion rate should be increased. If maternal heart rate also decreases, an anticholinergic drug should be administered.

The use of alternative vasopressor drugs (such as dilute norepinephrine solutions) to treat spinal hypotension are being explored.

New automated closed-loop vasopressor systems have been developed to deliver vasopressor drugs and maintain good blood pressure control during elective CS, with minimal interventions required from the attending anaesthetist.

Fluid administration: Crystalloid preloading (administration prior to spinal injection) is no longer recommended, as it neither reduces the incidence of maternal hypotension nor vasopressor requirements. In contrast, crystalloid co-loading (administration at the time of spinal injection) with 1 L crystalloid has been shown to reduce both the incidence of spinal hypotension and the amount of total vasopressor required. Colloid administration is also effective but confers no advantage over crystalloid co-loading, and it is more expensive and has been associated with a higher incidence of side effects and complications.

Anaesthetic Complications

Life-threatening complications from regional anaesthesia include local anaesthetic toxicity and total spinal.

Local anaesthetic systemic toxicity: This can occur when a high-concentration local anaesthetic (or a large volume of dilute local anaesthetic) is inadvertently administered intravenously. Toxicity manifests as central nervous system (CNS) excitement, such as circumoral tingling, visual and auditory disturbance, followed by CNS depression and cardiovascular collapse. Management should follow the basic principles of airway, breathing and circulation. If cardiorespiratory arrest occurs, basic and advanced life support should be performed, with special attention to specific requirements of the pregnant patient. Seizures should be controlled with benzodiazepines, thiopenal or propofol in small doses. Manage arrythmias using standard protocols, although avoid giving further doses of lidocaine. Lipid emulsion therapy is recommended for severe systemic toxicity, and should be considered when CNS depression occurs or there is cardiovascular compromise. Lipid emulsion is initially given as a bolus, and then by intravenous infusion. If the patient is in cardiopulmonary arrest, CPR should continue throughout treatment with lipid emulsion.[4]

Complete spinal block following spinal anaesthesia: A high or complete spinal block is a recognized complication of spinal anaesthesia. Clinical manifestations can be divided into cardiorespiratory or neurological:
● Cardiorespiratory: hypotension, bradycardia, apnoea, hypoxia and cardiac arrest

- Neurological: rapidly ascending block, nausea, anxiety and loss of consciousness

Management is supportive and depends on the degree and height of block. Early recognition is vital. Bradycardia should be treated with vagolytics such as atropine; hypotension needs prompt management with vasopressor agents and intravenous fluid boluses. Phenylephrine should be avoided in the presence of bradycardia. Atropine and ephedrine are preferable. Apnoea and hypoxia should be treated by oxygenation, intubation and ventilation. A small amount of sedation and muscle relaxation should be given prior to intubation to protect against awareness. The airway should be secured, and ongoing treatment should be supportive.

Fetal distress is likely due to profound hypotension and hypoxia, and urgent delivery of the fetus may be required once the mother's airway has been secured. Analgesia will not be needed. General anaesthesia will be necessary to avoid awareness. Transfer to critical care may be required until there is evidence of adequate spontaneous respiratory effort.

Enhanced Recovery in Obstetrics

Enhanced recovery programmes (ERP) following CS have been implemented successfully enabling next day discharge. Other benefits include reduced morbidity and earlier return to normal activities. Key features of any ERP include:

- Correct &/or optimize pre-existing anaemia or comorbidities
- Patient information
- Reduced starvation times
- Optimization of fluid balance intra-operatively
- Pain management
- Minimize postoperative nausea and vomiting
- Early oral intake postoperatively
- Avoidance of systemic opioids
- Early removal of urinary catheter and drains
- Early mobilization
- Venous thromboprophylaxis

OBSTETRIC COMPLICATIONS

Sepsis

Deaths from genital tract sepsis have risen over recent years despite an overall reduction in maternal mortality. Many of the cases of maternal death were from community acquired Group A streptococci. Delays in recognizing sepsis, prescribing antibiotics and seeking consultant help have all been implicated as contributing to maternal deaths from sepsis. Immediate aggressive treatment

BOX 5.8.2 **Principles of Sepsis Management**

Think sepsis at an early stage
Timely recognition
Rapid administration of intravenous antibiotics
Senior review
Early advice from an infectious diseases physician, microbiologist and critical care
Influenza vaccine recommended for all pregnant women

offers the best hope of recovery. Each hour of delay in achieving administration of effective antibiotics is associated with an increase in mortality. The principles of management are outlined in Box 5.8.2.

Pre-Eclampsia and Eclampsia

Pre-eclamptic toxaemia (PET) is a multisystem disorder of pregnancy characterized by pregnancy-induced hypertension in association with proteinuria (>0.3 g in 24 h) with or without oedema.

The following constitutes severe pre-eclampsia:

- Severe hypertension – a diastolic BP (dBP) ≥ 110 mm Hg on two occasions, or a systolic BP (sBP) ≥ 170 mm Hg on two occasions, together with significant proteinuria (at least 1 g/L).
- Moderate hypertension – dBP ≥ 100 mm Hg together with other symptoms or signs.

Clinical features of severe pre-eclampsia are as follows:

- Headache
- Visual disturbance
- Epigastric pain/vomiting
- Clonus
- Papilloedema
- Liver tenderness or right upper quadrant pain
- Reduced platelet count ($<100 \times 10^6$/L)
- Abnormal liver function tests
- HELPP syndrome

HELLP syndrome is an important variant of severe PET.

Management of severe pre-eclampsia involves:

- Controlling maternal blood pressure
- Preventing and controlling maternal seizures
- Fluid management
- Optimal timing of delivery for both mother and baby

Blood Pressure Control

Systolic BP >170 mm Hg or dBP >110 mm Hg should be treated. Treatment can be considered at lower degrees of hypertension if there are other symptoms and signs of severe disease. Intravenous labetalol or intravenous hydralazine can be used for the acute management of severe hypertension; these are usually initially given as a bolus dose, and then by an infusion. Drugs containing ergot alkaloids should be avoided, because of the risk of precipitating a hypertensive crisis (e.g. syntometrine, ergometrine).

Seizure Prevention and Control

Seizure control should follow the basic principles of airway, breathing and circulation. Magnesium sulphate reduces the risk of an eclamptic seizure and is the drug of choice to prevent and control seizures. It is given as an initial bolus dose of 4 g over 5–10 min followed by an infusion of 1 g/h. Recurrent seizures can be treated with a further bolus dose of 2 g or by increasing the infusion rate to 1.5–2 g/h.

Seizures are typically short and self-limiting. However, if convulsions persist, intubation may be required to protect the airway and maintain oxygenation. Once magnesium sulphate has been given, the infusion should continue for 24 h after delivery, or until 24 h from the last eclamptic seizure. Women receiving magnesium infusions should have regular assessment including urine output, maternal reflexes, conscious level, respiratory rate and oxygen saturations, as magnesium when given at high doses can cause CNS and respiratory depression. The therapeutic range is 2–4 mmol/L measured 4–6 h after the loading dose. Levels should be checked if toxic effects or a convulsion occurs. The antidote for magnesium toxicity is 10 mL calcium gluconate 10%. Magnesium is contraindicated in acute renal or cardiac failure.

Fluid Management

Pulmonary oedema is a significant cause of death complicating pre-eclampsia. Fluid restriction is therefore advisable to reduce the risk of fluid overload in the intrapartum and postpartum periods. Total fluid input (including any ongoing infusions) should be limited to 80 mL/h or 1 mg/kg/h.

Specific Anaesthetic Management

Severe pre-eclampsia and eclampsia are obstetric emergencies. Urgent delivery of the fetus is often required. Blood pressure and seizure control should be optimized prior to induction of anaesthesia, because of the risk of intracerebral haemorrhage in the mother. Regional or general anaesthesia can be used, depending on the urgency of the situation, the platelet count and recent clotting results. For these reasons, general anaesthesia is often preferred. An arterial line should be sited prior to induction of anaesthesia. Large swings in blood pressure should be avoided to reduce the risk of intracerebral haemorrhage. An infusion of labetalol or hydralazine may be required, but an infusion of phenylephrine may be needed following induction of anaesthesia.

Specific investigations within the immediate 4-h period prior to performing regional blockade include a full blood count, electrolytes, liver function tests and coagulation screen (if the recent platelet count is $>100 \times 10^9$/L, a coagulation screen is not essential).

All obstetric units should have guidelines for the management of pre-eclampsia and eclampsia. The anaesthetic problems associated with severe eclampsia are outlined in Box 5.8.3.

Amniotic Fluid Embolism

A dramatic change in cardiorespiratory status at the time of membrane rupture (e.g. at CS or spontaneous vaginal delivery) may indicate the passage of amniotic fluid into the general circulation. Collapse, desaturation, respiratory distress and coma suddenly present and death is common. Management should follow the basic principles of airway, breathing and circulation. If cardiorespiratory collapse occurs, basic, and then advanced life support algorithms for the pregnant patient should be followed. The resultant haematological effects of the amniotic fluid are disseminated intravascular coagulation (DIC) with hypofibrinaemia and excessive bleeding. The diagnosis can be difficult, but may be confirmed by the presence of fetal squames in the maternal circulation or tissues. If the mother is successfully resuscitated, her ECG may show signs of right heart strain, due to deposits of fibrin in the pulmonary circulation.

BOX 5.8.3 Anaesthetic-Related Problems Associated with Severe Pre-eclampsia

Laryngeal oedema
Coagulation abnormalities/low platelets contraindicating regional anaesthesia (platelet count $< 80 \times 10^9$/L)
Pulmonary oedema
Risk of convulsions
Exaggerated hypertensive response to laryngoscopy (obtund with intravenous opioids)
Magnesium sulphate can prolong neuromuscular block and cause dysrrhythmias
Renal impairment
Risk of placental abruption and massive obstetric haemorrhage

Disseminated Intravascular Coagulation

The diagnosis of DIC is made by a coagulation screen, revealing widespread abnormalities, including fibrin degradation products. DIC can complicate major haemorrhage, intrauterine fetal death, amniotic fluid embolism (AFE) and hydatidiform molar pregnancy. Continuing bleeding may be the first sign of DIC, as fibrin and fibrinogen are destroyed by fibrinolysins, or products in the amniotic fluid stop the conversion of prothrombin to thrombin. A fibrinogen level less than 1 g/L is characteristic. Specialist advice from haematology should be sought and products such as fresh frozen plasma, cryoprecipitate and fibrinogen concentrate may be required.

Convulsions

Differential diagnosis for convulsions:

- Local anaesthetic systemic toxicity
- Eclampsia
- Amniotic fluid embolism
- Total spinal anaesthesia
- Hypoxia (e.g. from pulmonary embolism)
- Epilepsy

Management should follow the basic principles of airway, breathing and circulation.

Maternal Collapse

Although the maternal death rates are low in developed countries, complications do arise requiring prompt assessment, resuscitation and critical care. Causes of maternal collapse are outlined in Box 5.8.4.

The latest advanced life support algorithms should be followed.[5] A maternal cardiac arrest call should be put out. Other specific consideration in the preg-

---

BOX 5.8.4 Causes of Maternal Collapse

Haemorrhage
Sepsis
Aortocaval occlusion
Anaphylaxis
Shock from acute inversion of the uterus (with associated bradycardia from autonomic activity)
Amniotic fluid embolism
Cerebrovascular event

nant patient include positioning to avoid IVC occlusion (with manual displacement of the uterus),[5] early intubation to avoid aspiration, perimortem CS (from 20 weeks gestation) to aid effectiveness of chest compression and resuscitation attempts. Cardiopulmonary resuscitation is unlikely to be successful with a gravid uterus. In situations such as nonsurvivable maternal trauma or prolonged maternal pulselessness, there is no reason to delay performing perimortem CS (see also Chapter 2.10).

Haemorrhage

Blood loss is common during delivery. Blood loss is initially tolerated well during delivery, as uterine contraction releases blood into the maternal systemic circulation, providing an autotransfusion of about 500 mL. Haemorrhage when it occurs can be concealed (not visible) or revealed (apparent). Antenatal blood loss can compromise the fetus either through a poor maternal blood supply or from direct loss of blood (e.g. placental abruption). Antepartum haemorrhage occurs from placenta praevia, placental abruption (associated with pre-eclampsia, cocaine use) or other causes. Postpartum blood loss can come from anywhere along the reproductive tract and the source of bleeding can be hard to locate without surgery. One of the fist sign of an antepartum haemorrhage in the mother is fetal distress, as the splanchnic vasoconstriction that occurs reduces uterine blood flow. Therefore, monitoring of the fetus can be a valuable tool in early haemorrhage.

A protocol for major obstetric haemorrhage and drills are recommended to aid familiarity and assess their effectiveness. Group O rhesus-negative blood should be available for immediate use in an emergency. If the situation is less urgent, group-specific blood or cross-matched blood is preferred.

A major obstetric haemorrhage should be declared if blood loss exceeds, or is expected to exceed, 1500 mL. The principles of management of a major obstetric haemorrhage include:

- Blood packs ordered – usually 6 units packed red cells, 4 units FFP (cryoprecipitate and platelets are required)
- Two large-bore intravenous cannulae (blood taken for FBC, coagulation, fibrinogen and cross-match)
- Rapid administration of warmed i.v. crystalloid
- Monitoring of blood pressure, heart rate, respiration rate, urine output, temperature and fetal heart rate if antenatal
- Arterial cannulation
- Pharmacological – consider uterotonic drugs if postnatal
- Surgical management: bimanual compression, brace sutures, intrauterine tamponade with a balloon
- Radiological embolization of internal iliac arteries
- Critcal care once bleeding has stopped

Placenta Praevia

Placenta praevia is usually diagnosed by ultrasound near to term because the placental site can move during the last trimester, when the lower segment is formed. A placenta partially or completely covering the internal os is a major placenta praevia. A placenta in the lower uterine segment, but not encroaching on the internal os is a minor placenta praevia. Delivery will need to be by CS. If the placenta lies in the path of the surgeon at CS, blood loss before delivery of the baby is expected. Women with a previous CS or a uterine scar from previous uterine surgery (such as uterine myotomy or myomectomy) have an increased risk of having a morbidly adherent placenta (placenta accreta). These women must have their placental site imaged during pregnancy by ultrasound and if necessary MRI investigation may be required to assess the extent of the placenta accreta.

Deliveries of women with placenta praevia, especially those with morbidly adherent placentae, require careful planning involving a large multidisciplinary team of obstetricians, anaesthetists, haematologists, radiologists and critical care. The woman should be counselled about the risks of large blood loss, the need for blood transfusion and the possibility of a hysterectomy, should the bleeding be life-threatening.

The type of anaesthetic selected will depend on the experience of the anaesthetist, the mother's preferences and the expected pathology. In all cases where massive blood loss is expected, two large-bore intravenous cannulae and an arterial line should be sited prior to surgery. Other precautions will include the use of cell salvage and a pressurized and warmed system for delivering fluids and blood products.

THROMBOEMBOLISM RISK MANAGEMENT IN PREGNANCY AND DELIVERY

Thromboembolism prophylaxis for CS depends on the risk category of the woman. In the low-risk category (i.e. patients without additional risks), TED stockings and low–molecular-weight heparins (LMWH) such as enoxaparin or dalteparin are given subcutaneously once daily The dose of the LMWH will depend on the weight of the parturient.

High-risk patients, such as those with a history of thromboembolic disease, thrombophilia or a high body mass index, should be risk assessed and an LMWH may need to be given antenatally, as well as for a prolonged period postpartum. This is typically 10 days for those with a high body mass index, but can be up to 6 weeks for those who have a history of previous venous thromboembolism.[6] Very high risk women, such as those with a metallic prosthetic heart valve, require an individually tailored regimen. The window in which the LMWH is stopped is kept as narrow as possible. If the delivery plan is for a vaginal delivery, the LMWH is stopped at the onset of spontaneous labour. If the plan for delivery is an elective CS,

> **BOX 5.8.5 Principles of In Utero Fetal Resuscitation: SPOILT Acronym**
>
> S: stop syntocinon
> P: position change (full left lateral or tilt)
> O: oxygen administration to the mother
> I: intravenous fluid administration
> L: low blood pressure (treat with phenylephrine)
> T: tocolysis to relax the uterus (GTN/terbutaline)

Source: Adapted from Thurlow JA, Kinsella SM. Intrauterine resuscitation: active management of fetal distress. Int J Obstet. Anesth 2002;11:105.

the LMWH will be stopped 24 h prior to surgery. If the appropriate length of time since the last dose of LMWH has not elapsed, alternatives to regional analgesia need to be considered, and if an operative delivery is required, general anaesthetic will be needed.

An epidural or spinal nerve block should not be sited within 12 h of a prophylactic dose of LMWH or within 24 h of a treatment dose, unless there are special circumstances. A prophylactic dose of LMWH can be administered 6 h following spinal injection or removal of the epidural catheter. A treatment dose of an LMWH should not be commenced until 12 h after spinal injection or removal of an epidural catheter.

Severe Fetal Distress

In severe fetal distress, in utero fetal resuscitation should be considered to improve fetal outcome. It may convert a category 1 CS into a category 2 CS, allowing surgery to be performed in a more controlled manner, and potentially allow more time for a regional anaesthetic to be performed or extended. The principles of fetal resuscitation are outlined in Box 5.8.5.

Prepare for emergency CS in theatre. If an epidural catheter is present, commence the top-up using a fast-acting epidural mix. If no epidural catheter is present, discuss with the surgeon if there is time to perform a single-shot spinal anaesthetic. If attempts at in utero fetal resuscitation fail and there is continuing fetal distress, a general anaesthetic should be performed, to enable immediate delivery of the fetus.

REFERENCES

1. Knight M, Tuffnell D, Kenyon S, Shakespeare J, Gray R, Kurinczuk JJ, editors. On behalf of MBRRACE UK. Saving Lives, Improving Mothers' Care – Surveillance of maternal deaths in the UK 2011-2013 and lessons learned to inform maternity care from the UK and Ireland Confidential Enquiries into Maternal Deaths and Morbidity 2009-2013. Oxford: National Perinatal Epidemiology Unit, University of Oxford; 2015.

2. Mushambi MC, Kinsella SM, Popat M, Swales H, Ramaswamy KK, Winton AL, et al. Obstetric Anaesthetists' Association and Difficult Airway Society Guidelines for the management of difficult and failed tracheal intubation in obstetrics. Anaesthesia 2015;70:1286–06.
3. Pandit JJ, Andrade J, Bogod DG, Hitchman JM, Jonker WR, Lucas N, et al. The 5th National Audit Project (NAP 5) on accidental awareness during general anaesthesia: summary of main findings and risk factors. Br J Anaesth 2014;113:549–59.
4. Association of Anaesthetists of Great Britain and Ireland. Management of severe local anaesthetic toxicity. AAGBI Safety Guideline. London: AAGBI; 2010.
5. American Heart Association. Highlights of the 2015 American Heart Association guidelines update for CPR and ECC. Available at https://eccguidelines. heart. org/index. php/circulation/cpr-ecc-guidelines-2/
6. Royal College of Obstetricians and Gynaecologists. Reducing the risk of venous thromboembolism during pregnancy and the puerperium. Green-top Guideline No. 37a. London: RCOG; 2015.

FURTHER READING

Clark V, van de Velde M, Fernando R. Oxford Textbook of Obstetric Anaesthesia. Oxford: OUP; 2016.

Chapter 5.9

Ophthalmic Surgery

Andrew Presland

GENERAL CONSIDERATIONS

A vast majority of ophthalmic procedures are now performed as day cases, a situation facilitated by the continuous development of minimally invasive microsurgical techniques. Most procedures are amenable to local anaesthesia. General anaesthesia is required for children, adults unable to cooperate or lie still, squint surgery, orbital surgery and to satisfy patient choice. Anxiety surrounding eye operations is disproportionate, so it is essential to offer empathy and reassurance when preparing the patient.

ANATOMY OF THE EYE AND ORBIT

The sclera is the tough outer coat of the eye, with the transparent cornea at the front. The sclera is surrounded by Tenon's capsule, an avascular membrane. The cornea is oxygenated through both surfaces – from aqueous humour and air. Aqueous humour fills the space between the cornea and the lens, which is divided by the iris into anterior and posterior chambers.

The lens is attached to the ciliary body by the suspensory ligament, the filaments of which are frequently referred to as zonules. Between the ciliary body and the front edge of the retina is the pars plana, the entry point for vitreoretinal surgery and intravitreal injections. The retina and the choroid behind it are very vascular.

Six extraocular muscles move the eye (Fig. 5.9.1): two oblique (superior and inferior) and four rectus muscles (lateral, medial, superior and inferior) which form a cone behind the eye containing all the sensory nerves to the eye, the motor nerves and the ciliary ganglion. Extraocular muscles are extremely sensitive to muscle relaxants.

The eye is not in the centre of the orbit, being more superior than inferior. The inferior margin of the orbit is an obvious and easily palpable landmark and drops away from the eye as it goes laterally.

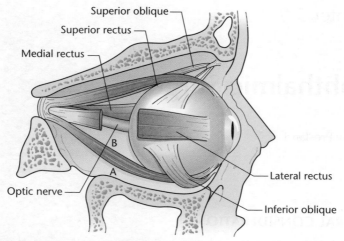

FIGURE 5.9.1 Diagram of the lateral aspect of the right eye. The extraocular muscle cone is shown surrounding the optic nerve. The lateral rectus is partially excised for clarity. The intraconal structures (not shown) include the third, fourth and sixth cranial nerves supplying the extraocular muscles, the ophthalmic branch of the fifth cranial nerve (V1, sensory to the sclera and cornea), ciliary ganglion (transmitting sensory fibres to V1 and both sympathetic and parasympathetic fibres to the eye) and the retinal vessels (from the ophthalmic vessels). A and B represent the extra- and intra-conal spaces, respectively. Local anaesthetic injected extra-conally must diffuse from site A into the cone to reach the sensory and motor neurones. B indicates the target site for a true retrobulbar injection.

Innervation

Motor Innervation

- Superior oblique muscle from the fourth cranial nerve (trochlear nerve)
- Lateral rectus from the sixth cranial nerve (abducens nerve)
- All other extraocular muscles, including levator palpebrae superioris, from the third cranial nerve (oculomotor nerve)
- Orbicularis oculis by the seventh cranial nerve (facial nerve)

Sensory Innervation

- The optic nerve conveys vision only.
- The conjunctiva is innervated superiorly by the supraorbital, supratrochlear and infratrochlear nerves, laterally by the lacrimal nerve, and the circumcorneal area from the long ciliary nerves; inferiorly innervation is by the infraorbital nerve – the terminal branch of the maxillary division of the fifth cranial nerve.
- The sclera and cornea are innervated by the long and short ciliary nerves – all derived from the ophthalmic division of the fifth cranial nerve (trigeminal nerve).

Parasympathetic Innervation

- Fibres from the Edinger–Westphal nucleus (parasympathetic part of the third nerve nucleus in the midbrain) run with the third cranial nerve, synapse in the ciliary ganglion, then pass via the short ciliary nerves.
- Stimulation causes constriction of the pupil and contraction of the ciliary muscle.

Sympathetic Innervation

- Fibres from T1 synapse in the superior cervical ganglion and pass via the carotid plexus to join the long ciliary nerves.
- Stimulation causes dilatation of the pupil.

Intraocular Pressure

Normal intraocular pressure (IOP) is 10–20 mmHg. It is determined by the production of aqueous humour in the ciliary body and its absorption at the canal of Schlemm, venous sinuses at the junction of the iris and sclera. Transient changes are common (Table 5.9.1) but have little bearing on an intact eye. During surgery with an open globe, pressure changes can have devastating consequences.

LOCAL ANAESTHETIC TECHNIQUES

Anaesthetic practice varies throughout the world, and even within departments. A variety of local anaesthetic techniques are available for most procedures, and each case should be considered individually before a suitable approach is selected. Anyone with a regular ophthalmic anaesthetic practice would be wise to master more than one technique.

TABLE 5.9.1 Factors Influencing IOP

IOP May Be Increased by	IOP May Be Decreased by
• Hypertension	• Hypotension
• Hypercapnia	• Hypocapnia
• ↑Venous pressure, e.g. head down tilt or tight tracheal tube ties	• ↓Venous pressure, e.g. head up tilt
• Suxamethonium (transient ~ 5 min)	• Inhalational anaesthetics
• Local anaesthetic block (trivial)	• Mannitol and acetazolamide
• Ketamine (transient ~ 1 min following i.v. bolus)	• All other intravenous anaesthetic agents
• Coughing, straining, retching	• Mechanical pressure on the eye

Topical

Topical anaesthetic techniques are popular for cataract surgery; they require no special equipment or expertise and the effects are instant. The drops have no effect on the optic nerve so the vision is preserved, allowing for optimal postoperative visual recovery. Proxymetacaine 0.5%, oxybuprocaine 0.4% or tetracaine 0.5% or 1% are commonly used. Oxybuprocaine and proxymetacaine do not sting on insertion; tetracaine stings initially and, in awake patients, is often preceded by one of the other agents. There is no akinesia. The iris remains sensitive. All topical anaesthetic drops can result in damage to the cornea if used repeatedly.

Intracameral anaesthesia may be used to supplement topical anaesthesia for cataract surgery. The surgeon injects a small volume of local anaesthetic into the anterior segment to desensitize the iris. The eye is a biological camera, hence 'intracameral'.

Sub-Tenon Block

Sub-Tenon block (STB) is used for a wide range of ophthalmic procedures. After topical anaesthesia and tissue dissection, a blunt cannula is passed into the plane between Tenon's capsule and the sclera, and local anaesthetic injected into the potential space. A single injection in the inferonasal quadrant is the most common approach. Choice and volume of injectate will depend on the nature and anticipated length of surgery but can be topped up by the surgeon if necessary.

STB has become increasingly popular in recent years, owing to its improved safety profile compared to sharp needle blocks (SNBs). However, it may be difficult or impossible to perform the block if the conjunctiva is very scarred, or in the presence of explants – silicone bands known as scleral buckles sometimes used to treat retinal detachment.

Retrobulbar Block

Retrobulbar block is achieved by injection into the muscle cone behind the eye. It has been used since the mid-1930s, but is increasingly regarded as outdated and unsafe because of a small, but significant, incidence of globe perforation, periocular haemorrhage, and subarachnoid injection through the sheath of the optic nerve.

Peribulbar Block

Peribulbar block is achieved by using a sharp needle to deliver local anaesthetic within the orbit, but outside the muscle cone. The preferred injection sites are inferolaterally, either directly through the skin or through the conjunctiva, and medially through the canthus. Transconjunctival injection is preceded by topical local anaesthetic drops.

Anaesthesia is achieved by diffusion and mass spread throughout the orbit. Compared to retrobulbar block a larger volume of injectate is needed, and a little extra time is required before anaesthesia is established. Although the risks are less than with retrobulbar block, a misdirected needle can result in the same complications.

For SNBs such as peribulbar and retrobulbar blocks, a good understanding of orbital anatomy is essential. The lateral orbital wall is at 45° to the saggital plane, and the orbital floor rises gently moving towards the apex at the back. The inferolateral approach must account for these anatomical features, but must be balanced by the need to avoid globe perforation.

A myopic patient (someone who needs glasses for distance) will have a long eye. SNBs are contraindicated if the axial length (A-P dimension) is ≥26 mm as the incidence of globe perforation rises rapidly. Staphylomas, outpouchings of choroid and retina that protrude through thin sclera, are more common in myopes. The presence of a staphyloma is also a contraindication to SNBs.

Advantages and disadvantages of different blocks are shown in Table 5.9.2.

TABLE 5.9.2 Advantages and Disadvantages of Commonly Used Local Anaesthetic Blocks

Type of Local Anaesthetic Block	Advantages	Disadvantages
Topical	Simple, fast, no skill required, minimal risk of complications related to the drops except drug error	Only suitable for very simple, minimally invasive surgery
Sub-Tenon (STB)	Excellent safety profile, excellent quality of anaesthesia for most types of eye surgery, easy for surgeon to top up on table if required	Requires some sterile equipment for dissection, may be difficult or impossible if tissues are very scarred or explants are present
Peribulbar	No special equipment needed (needles and syringes are available worldwide), improved safety profile compared to retrobulbar, best akinesia	Sight and life-threatening complications more common than STB, onset may be slow
Retrobulbar	Rapid, profound anaesthesia, no special equipment needed	Highest risk of sight and life-threatening complications in this group

Drugs

Drugs commonly used for nerve blocks include:

- Lidocaine, usually 2%.
- Bupivacaine, 0.5% or 0.75%.
- Hyaluronidase, 7.5–15 U/mL – This enzyme breaks down the extracellular matrix, improving spread of local anaesthetic solutions; higher concentrations offer no benefit, and it is debatable that there is any discernable difference with larger injectate volumes (>8 mL).
- Sodium bicarbonate, 8.4% – Increasing the pH of the local anaesthetic solution reduces discomfort on injection and increases hyaluronidase activity (most effective at a neutral pH).
- Epinephrine (adrenaline), 1:200,000 solution – This is sometimes used to extend block duration; however, retinal arteries are end-arteries, adding unnecessary risk for minimal gain (similar effects can be achieved by using longer acting drugs or topping up the anaesthetic).

Mixtures of local anaesthetic drugs are popular, but there is no evidence of their superiority over an appropriately selected single agent in the correct dose.

Complications

Globe Perforation

Signs of globe perforation are a soft eye, blood in the eye and loss of red reflex. If suspected, the patient should be referred to a vitreoretinal unit without delay.

Retrobulbar Haemorrhage

Retrobulbar haemorrhage is an acute haemorrhage caused by an arterial puncture. The bleeding will not stop until the area is tamponaded and so pressure should be applied as soon as possible. The principal problem is the inability of the eyelids to close, leading to corneal dehydration. A surgical canthotomy or drugs may be required to reduce IOP.

Subarachnoid Injection

Injection into the cerebral spinal fluid (CSF) is a potential complication if sharp needles are used. Brainstem anaesthesia may cause respiratory arrest.

Extraocular Muscle Damage

Laceration by sharp instruments, or direct myotoxicity from intramuscular drug injection can cause scarring and shortening of extraocular muscles. This results in permanent double vision and squint, requiring surgical correction.

Minor Complications

Minor complications include venous bleeding, which leads to bruising but no rise in pressure, chemosis and muscle weakness after return of sensation.

Any temporary reduction in visual acuity is dependant on the mode of block and dose of local anaesthetic used but is unpredictable. The patients should be warned about possible temporary loss of vision (unless topical).

GENERAL ANAESTHESIA

Indications for general anaesthesia include:

● Patients unable to cooperate, e.g. those with learning difficulties or dementia
● Patient phobias, especially severe claustrophobia
● Children
● Lengthy operations – it is unreasonable to expect patients to lie still for very long periods
● Surgery on the bony orbit
● Squint surgery, although some procedures are now being performed under local anaesthetic
● Patient choice – it is reasonable to discuss alternatives, but not to pressurize patients into local anaesthesia if they are making an informed decision

Drugs Used in General Anaesthesia

Premedication

Premedication is rarely necessary; high turnover day-case lists make the logistics of premedication and possible hangover effects unattractive. However, anxiolysis is indicated for selected patients, and is often used for children. Benzodiazepines are safe and effective. Glycopyrrolate is useful to prevent pooling of saliva and may reduce the incidence of the oculocardiac reflex.

Intravenous Agents

Propofol, thiopental and etomidate all reduce IOP. Ketamine causes a small, transient rise in IOP; it is sometimes used for glaucoma surveillance in children when an accurate IOP measurement under anaesthesia is required.

Neuromuscular Blocking Drugs

Suxamethonium causes a small and transient rise in IOP (7–8 mmHg, maximal at 2 min); there is no reason to avoid it when deemed necessary for a rapid sequence induction (RSI). The mechanism of this is still not fully understood. Contraction of the extraocular muscles may account for 20% of the rise, but 80% will still occur in the curarized patient. The effect can be reduced by a prior injection of a small dose of a nondepolarizing agent or acetazolamide 500 mg.

Nondepolarizing muscle relaxants may be used to facilitate controlled ventilation. This has the advantage that PCO_2 (and therefore IOP) can be controlled. Rocuronium can be used for a modified RSI with sugammadex in reserve.

Volatile Anaesthetic Agents

All volatile agents lower IOP. They are widely used for induction of anaesthesia in children and for maintenance of anaesthesia in both adults and children.

Nitrous Oxide

Nitrous oxide (N_2O) should be avoided if the use of intraocular gases such as sulphur hexafluoride (SF_6) or perfluoropropane (C_3F_8) is planned – usually the preserve of retinal detachment surgery. Check with the surgeon in advance.

Nonsteroidal Anti-Inflammatory Drugs

Nonsteroidal anti-inflammatory drugs (NSAIDs), along with paracetamol, provide excellent postoperative analgesia and have opioid sparing activity. Some advise avoiding NSAIDs for surgery on the bony orbit as they may contribute to an increased bleeding.

General Anaesthetic Techniques

The aim of anaesthesia is to provide smooth induction, maintenance and emergence from anaesthesia, minimizing increases in IOP while maintaining cardiovascular stability. Control of IOP will prevent herniation of ocular contents when the eye is open. There are many ways to achieve these goals.

Supraglottic airway devices (SADs) are suitable for most cases, both spontaneously breathing and ventilated patients and they enable a smooth emergence. Reinforced or flexible SADs can be optimally positioned away from the surgical field. Tracheal tubes may be used for those in whom there are contraindications to SADs, or may be preferred if blood is expected in the airway e.g. lacrimal or orbital surgery, where a throat pack is also advisable. The routine use of a nerve stimulator is recommended.

Total intravenous anaesthesia (TIVA) provides excellent conditions for ophthalmic anaesthesia and may be preferred. It is also associated with a lower incidence of postoperative nausea and vomiting (PONV), common after some ophthalmic procedures.

Patients are often at the extremes of age and frequently have comorbidities. Common problems encountered in ophthalmic patients include:

- Diabetes – Diabetic patients frequently present for ophthalmic surgery; many will have had very poor control over many years with associated complications, e.g. renal and cardiac disease. Optimizing both diabetic control and comorbid conditions can be extremely challenging.
- Old age – The majority of patients are elderly with variably managed comorbidities; hypertension, ischaemic heart disease and respiratory disease are common.
- Inherited conditions or syndromes – Down's syndrome and other rarer congenital conditions have ocular manifestations.

- Trauma – In cases of perforating eye injury, there may be associated trauma.
- Positioning – Arthritis, cardiorespiratory disease and frailty can make optimal positioning difficult and may preclude local anaesthesia.
- Anticoagulants – These are frequently encountered and are a relative contraindication to SNBs; a STB is considered safe as the risk of arterial puncture is minimal. Some surgeons prefer to stop anticoagulants before surgery but this should only be done after discussion with the prescribing physician.

SPECIFIC OPERATIONS

Cataracts

Local techniques are preferred; there is some evidence that there is higher satisfaction (both patients and surgeons) using an STB compared to topical (with or without intracameral anaesthesia).[1]

Vitrectomy (Including Retinal Detachment)

Nitrous oxide should be avoided if either SF_6 or C_3F_8 gas is to be used. N_2O diffuses into the gas in the vitreous, causing a rise in pressure. If used, it must be discontinued 15 min before intravitreal gas is used. Regional orbital blocks are increasingly popular for vitreoretinal cases; advances in equipment and surgical techniques have reduced the duration of all but a few of these cases.

It is particularly important to minimize PONV after retinal detachment surgery, as it may cause further detachment. Posturing of the patient may be required immediately upon completion of surgery. This is easier if local anaesthesia has been used.

The addition of a scleral buckle for repair of retinal detachment is much more traumatic and may be an indication for general anaesthesia.

Perforating Eye Injury

A careful history should be taken with attention to other injuries; unsurprisingly head injury is often associated with ocular trauma. Any rise in IOP risks expulsive haemorrhage and consequently a smooth induction without coughing or straining is essential. It is usually possible to delay surgery; optimal timing should be discussed with the surgeon taking into account fasting status and the relative urgency of surgery. If necessary either a RSI or modified RSI can be used.

General anaesthesia is used in almost all cases; integrity of the globe is required for predictable spread of local anaesthetics.

Squint (Strabismus) Surgery

Preoperative assessment is important as strabismus may be associated with certain diseases or syndromes such as neuromuscular or metabolic disorders or congenital heart disease. Malignant hyperthermia is no longer considered to be an issue associated with strabismus. There is a particularly high incidence of the oculocardiac reflex; stimuli arising in or near the eye, especially traction on the rectus muscles or pressure on the globe, may cause bradycardia, arrhythmias and rarely cardiac arrest. The afferent pathways are via the ophthalmic division of the trigeminal nerve, via the trigeminal ganglion on the floor of the fourth ventricle. Efferents are via the vagus. Cardiac monitoring is essential and prophylactic use of vagolytics is recommended. If severe bradycardia occurs, the surgeon should immediately release traction on the muscle. Atropine or glycopyrrolate can be given to attenuate the oculocardiac reflex.

There is a high incidence of PONV; prophylactic antiemetics are recommended.

Dacryocystorhinostomy

Even small amounts of blood can completely obscure surgical field. Nasal cocaine or adrenaline-containing solutions may be used to provide vasoconstriction of the adjacent nasal mucosa. Moderate hypotension and head-up position are helpful.

The procedure can be performed under local anaesthesia and sedation.

REFERENCES

1. Guay J, Sales K. Sub-Tenon's anaesthesia versus topical anaesthesia for cataract surgery. Cochrane Database Syst Rev 2015;27(8):CD006291.

Anaesthesia for Dental and Maxillofacial Surgery

Miriam V. Chapman, Suyogi V. Jigajinni

Dental and maxillofacial anaesthesia is a challenging and diverse specialty. The anaesthetist must be experienced in the management of the shared, distant and potentially difficult airway and must have an understanding of the need to provide surgical access. There should also be awareness of the perioperative requirements relating to the many different procedures performed for a wide range of pathologies. Excellent care requires careful assessment, planning and coordination throughout the perioperative period.

GENERAL CONSIDERATIONS

Preoperative Assessment

A detailed and thorough preoperative cardiorespiratory and airway assessment is essential; more complex patients or those with a potentially difficult airway should have an anaesthetic review in a preoperative assessment clinic. A thorough history should be tailored to the specific type of procedure planned, accompanied by a detailed examination of the patient, review and discussion of available imaging with the teams involved. Valuable information (i.e. ability to bag mask ventilate, best direct laryngoscopy grade and endotracheal tube size used) is also available from previous anaesthetic charts.[1]

Dental Surgery

Patients having general anaesthesia for dental surgery include children and adults with learning disability, psychological problems or physical conditions that prevent treatment under local anaesthesia (LA).

Complex Surgery

Patients undergoing more complex or cancer surgery may be elderly, have multiple comorbidities or a history of smoking or alcohol excess. Oncology patients may have undergone chemo- and radiotherapy resulting in frailty and malnutrition or may have had previous airway surgery including tracheostomies resulting in airway distortion.

Orthognathic Surgery

Patients presenting for orthognathic surgery may have syndromes associated with anatomical, airway or medical implications, e.g. Down's, Goldenhar, Pierre–Robin and Treacher Collins syndrome (see Appendix 2).

AIRWAY

Airway Assessment

A thorough airway assessment is essential including a detailed history, examination and review of any radiological scans and previous anaesthetic charts.

Red-flag symptoms should be identified; these may suggest supraglottic or upper airway obstruction: a change in voice, hoarseness or hot potato voice (indicative of peritonsillar abscess), stridor, inability to lie flat or a feeling of suffocation.

Trismus can be caused by pain, airway or dental infections, fractures involving the temporomandibular joints (TMJ) or squamous cell carcinoma of the head and neck. It may or may not be reduced by induction of anaesthesia; this must be carefully considered preoperatively. Trismus resulting from dental infections is unlikely to resolve postinduction and an awake fibreoptic intubation (AFOI) should be considered. Any type of airway infection must be taken extremely seriously as progression to airway compromise may be very rapid.

In the emergency setting, trauma patients must be assessed for associated injury and exact location of maxillofacial fractures: those involving the TMJ may prevent mouth opening postinduction, Le Fort III fractures place the airway at risk of complete obstruction and preclude the nasal route for securing the airway.

After preoperative assessment and following discussion with the surgeon, a detailed anaesthetic management plan should be formulated. This should include a detailed airway management plan to ensure a safely secured airway that will also allow adequate surgical access. Factors to be considered include type and duration of surgery, patient position, anticipated blood loss, need for invasive monitoring and vascular access, extubation plan and postoperative destination.

Choice of Airway

The correct choice of airway is paramount. The decision is made jointly with the surgeon depending on surgical, anaesthetic and patient factors to provide a safe and secure airway that enables surgical access. See also Chapter 2.6.

Supraglottic Airway Devices

A reinforced supraglottic airway device (SAD) with a throat pack is increasingly the airway of choice for dental surgery and for some types of less complex oral surgeries. SADs are not appropriate for procedures requiring dental occlusion or where there is a high risk of aspiration. Fixing the device in a northward direction optimizes the surgical access. It must be safely secured, as it can be displaced. Extreme vigilance is needed perioperatively; obstruction commonly occurs from the posterior mandibular forces applied by the operator, especially during dental extractions. This can be counter-pressured by a jaw thrust applied by either the second surgeon or anaesthetist.

Tracheal Tubes – Nasal or Oral

A cuffed nasal tracheal tube (TT), secured flush on the forehead, provides excellent surgical access and a protected airway and remains the airway of choice for most maxillofacial operations. However, there are contraindications to (coagulopathy, midface instability, basal skull fracture) and recognized complications from (epistaxis, meningitis, sinusitis) nasal intubation. Nasal TTs can be inserted using direct laryngoscopy facilitated with Magill's forceps, or using a 'blind' technique, with a fibrescope. More recently, videolaryngoscopy has been used.[2]

Surgery not involving the oral cavity or requiring dental occlusion may be performed with a south-facing oral TT, but should be discussed with the surgeon.

Submental Intubation

Certain procedures necessitating dental occlusion cannot be performed with a nasal TT, e.g. choanal atresia and craniofacial trauma. In these cases, submental intubation is indicated – it is much less invasive with fewer complications than a tracheostomy, but provides similar operating conditions.[3]

An oral TT which can be disconnected from its connector (as with the intubating LMA tracheal tube, Intavent®) is placed. The surgeon forms a passage between the floor of the mouth and the skin at the lower border of the mandible; the TT is disconnected from its connector, the proximal end passed through the passage externally and then, reconnected to the breathing circuit. This is sutured in place allowing surgery, dental occlusion and ventilation to take place. Once surgery has finished, the whole process is reversed allowing extubation as usual.

Front of Neck Access

Elective surgical tracheostomies form part of the airway management plan for major complex maxillofacial surgery where postoperative airway swelling and airway distortion is anticipated. In the critical airway setting, surgical tracheostomies can be performed under LA prior to induction. Access via the cricothyroid membrane may be necessary in the emergency 'cannot intubate, cannot oxygenate (CICO)' scenario or for patients presenting with upper airway obstruction.

Videolaryngoscopes (VL)

The introduction of VLs has radically transformed airway management options. In 2001, the GlideScope® was introduced: a high-resolution digital camera placed at the tip of an improved Macintosh laryngoscope blade, attached to a high-definition screen which enabled airway structures to be easily visualized. Many new types of VL have been developed since then. They are increasingly popular in a variety of clinical scenarios including the passage of nasal TTs where tissue structures are aligned such that a nasal TT can be easily passed without the use of Magill's forceps.

Throat Packs

Throat packs are commonly used in dental and maxillofacial surgery to absorb debris, blood and secretions and prevent soiling of the lower respiratory tract. However, throat pack retention can result in postprocedural airway obstruction. National and local policies should be in place to prevent this. Throat packs can also be a cause of postoperative sore throat.

SURGICAL PROCEDURES AND CLASSIFICATION

There are a wide range of maxillofacial and dental surgical procedures broadly classified as shown in Table 5.10.1.

TABLE 5.10.1 Range of Dental and Maxillofacial Procedures[1]

Dental surgery	Exodontia (extractions) Conservations (preservation of decayed teeth)
Oral surgery	Bony cysts Salivary gland disease Bone grafting Laser procedures
Trauma surgery	Mandibular, zygomatic and nasal fractures – fixation with plating Closed reduction and splinting of nasal fractures
Craniofacial surgery	Orthodontic and aesthetic procedures for facial bone deformities Le Fort (maxillary), mandibular (Obwegeser/saggital ramus split) osteotomies Advancement genioplasty
Cancer surgery	Resection of head and neck cancers reconstructions with rotational or free flaps and bone grafting
Surgery for toxic airways/infection	Incision and drainage of dental abscesses and soft tissue infections of neck, oropharynx and submandibular space Ludwig angina (spreading submandibular cellulitis)

TECHNICAL CONSIDERATIONS

Airway Management Plan

The technique chosen to secure the airway depends upon fundamental anaesthetic judgements:

- Will it be possible to bag/mask ventilate postinduction of general anaesthesia?
- Will it be possible to insert airway adjuncts or SADs to aid ventilation?
- Is the exact size and location of the lesion clear? Will it affect the ability to get a good seal when manually ventilating and will it be possible to bypass it with a fibrescope?
- Is there the risk of bleeding from airway instrumentation?
- Will it be possible to perform direct laryngoscopy?
- Will a videolaryngoscope aid airway management?
- Is the cricothyroid membrane palpable? Will ultrasound of the airway help its location?

Securing the Airway

Asleep

The majority of cases allow conventional intravenous induction, manual ventilation, muscle paralysis and placement of a TT using direct laryngoscopy, a fibreoptic technique or a videolaryngoscope. However, the operator may opt for spontaneous ventilation to maintain airway tone and allow rapid reversal of anaesthesia using either inhalational or an incremental total intravenous anaesthesia (TIVA) technique. If difficulty is anticipated, airway equipment – bougies, introducer stylets, oral and nasopharyngeal airways, a videolaryngoscope and fibreoptic scope (focussed and orientated correctly) should be immediately available.

To reduce bleeding during nasal intubation, nostrils should be sprayed with a local anaesthetic and vasoconstrictor solution, e.g. co-phenylcaine (5% lidocaine and 0.5% phenylephrine). Before a fibreoptic technique, intravenous glycopyrrolate 20 min preprocedure is useful to reduce secretions.

Awake

The decision to proceed with an awake technique is critical to the safe management of dental and maxillofacial patients. An awake technique should be performed if it is anticipated that induction of anaesthesia might result in the inability to perform mask ventilation or use airway rescue techniques. For the majority of cases an AFOI will be employed; in scenarios where this is not possible (impending airway obstruction from glottic tumours, bleeding into upper airway) an awake tracheostomy should be considered.

Different centres have their own methods of airway topicalization (Chapter 2.6). The administration of sedation enhances acceptability, patient cooperation and provides some amnesia (important for patients needing repeated AFOI). Useful agents include propofol, an opioid (remifentanil) or benzodiazepines.

However, sedation requires careful titration and monitoring for apnoea and airway obstruction.

Intraoperative

Considerations common to many maxillofacial operations include:

- Patient positioning – The patient's head will be positioned away from the anaesthetic machine; access for several surgeons should be allowed. A head ring or Reuben's pillow with a sandbag beneath the shoulders stabilizes the head and extends the neck. The breathing system and gas sampling tubing must be extended, as must intravenous lines. Pressure point protection is especially important when surgery is prolonged.
- Eye care – Extra care is needed to prevent damage to the eyes from pressure or abrasions. Ointment is applied to the eyes, which are taped shut and carefully padded.
- Airway fixation – Particularly important for the distant airway that can become disconnected or obstructed by operating surgeons. North-facing nasal TTs should have padding placed underneath and should be secured without pressure at the nasal rim, which can cause ischaemic injury during prolonged surgery.
- Optimizing surgical field – Head up tilt and hypotension can improve the surgical field and reduce blood loss.[4] This can be achieved by using a variety of pharmacological agents including remifentanil, β-blockade and clonidine.
- General – Temperature should be monitored and patients actively warmed with forced air warming blankets, warm fluids and warming mattresses for longer procedures. Venous thromboembolism (VTE) prophylaxis (elastic compression stockings, pneumatic compression boots and subcutaneous heparin) is essential especially for high risk cancer patients having prolonged surgery.
- Postoperative nausea and vomiting (PONV) can result in haematoma formation and airway compromise. Regular antiemetics, e.g. ondansetron, cyclizine and dexamethasone can address this. The use of a TIVA technique also has a role. Dexamethasone will reduce postoperative airway swelling.

Postoperative

- Emergence and extubation – These are of equal importance to intubation and require similar planning. An extubation strategy should be formulated following a risk assessment dependent on anaesthetic and surgical skill sets, possible airway swelling and aspiration risk from debris. Techniques include awake extubation sitting up, or spontaneously breathing deep extubation. Following careful laryngoscopy and suction, throat packs are removed and documented, according to local protocols.
- Delayed extubation – This may be required, e.g. in case of serious airway infections or complex cancer surgery. Formal tracheostomy is an option in cases where airway compromise may be prolonged.
- Postoperative destination – This should be considered preoperatively and finalized depending on the extubation strategy: extended recovery, high

dependency or intensive care may be appropriate depending on patient and surgical factors.

- Analgesia – A balanced analgesic regimen including paracetamol, nonsteroidal anti-inflammatory drugs (NSAIDs), codeine or tramadol should be prescribed. Patient-controlled analgesia (PCA) is rarely needed and best avoided unless patients are undergoing prolonged cancer surgery or suffering form chronic pain issues.

ANAESTHESIA FOR DENTAL SURGERY

The first general anaesthetic (GA) performed in England was for the extraction of a molar tooth in 1846. James Robinson, a dentist, gave the anaesthetic and performed the procedure in his dental surgery. The practice of the dentist acting as both surgeon and anaesthetist gained popularity and the number of GAs performed in dental surgeries rose exponentially with a recognized risk profile. In the UK, things began to change with the 1990 'Poswillo Report' which recommended that standards of staffing and equipment for anaesthesia should be the same whether in hospital, dental clinic or dental surgery. In 1998, the General Dental Council mandated that only accredited anaesthetists should perform dental anaesthetics and then, in 2002, the Department of Health effectively restricted dental anaesthesia to hospitals, thus bringing it into line with anaesthesia for other surgical specialties.

General Considerations

Despite recommendations that GA should only be used where no alternatives exist, there has been a marked increase in patient demand for GA to facilitate dentistry and dental surgery. This must be addressed with careful risk versus benefit counselling discussions.

Indications for use of general anaesthesia in dentistry include:

- Inability to provide adequate LA (acute infections)
- Inability to cooperate or tolerate LA (children, adults with learning disabilities, adults with psychological problems, e.g. needle-phobic patients)
- Inability to cooperate physically with dental surgery under LA (movement disorders, contractures, inability to open the mouth or keep it open for a length of time)

Dental surgery patient groups include:

- Children – Presenting for exodontia, often their first hospital visit. Poor dental health is associated with poor diet, increased weight and obesity and lower socioeconomic status.
- Adults with learning difficulties – Physical or psychological; this requires a carefully planned team approach involving patients, parents, carers, guardians, surgeons and anaesthetists. Planning begins well in advance with

pre-assessment and should address medical and consent issues and enable a strategy to be formulated to enable these vulnerable patients to undergo a successful dental treatment. A full explanation of the plan with risks and benefits should be given to the parents or carers.

● Adult dental-phobic patients – An increasing number of patients refuse surgery due to fear of dentistry. It is often possible to enable procedures with LA block, sedation and reassurance, nonetheless some will require a GA.

Pre-Assessment

This should address whether a GA for dental treatment presents an acceptable risk/benefit profile. These patients have a higher incidence of comorbidities which may be untreated as access to health care is unpredictable. Comorbidities include epilepsy, obesity, deafness, visual loss, emotional and psychiatric problems (autism) making communication and cooperation challenging.

Airway difficulties are more common due to orthopaedic and neuromuscular problems and airway examination is also difficult due to a lack of cooperation. Orthopaedic contractures make venous access and patient positioning difficult.

Down's Syndrome

Patients may have cardiac disease, e.g. atrial septal defects, and are also at risk of cervical spine instability. Care must be taken while manipulating the head and neck during anaesthesia.

Cardiac Pathology

The presence of congenital heart disease should always be considered when dealing with patients with learning disabilities, as it forms part of certain congenital syndromes. Antibiotic prophylaxis has been advocated in patients with valve lesions, a history of infective endocarditis and most congenital heart defects. In the UK, the National Institute for Clinical Excellence no longer considers this necessary for routine dental treatment. Local guidance should be followed.

Technical Considerations

Premedication

Premedication may be useful in children with challenging behaviour. Midazolam orally (0.25–0.75 mg/kg), intranasally (0.2–0.3 mg/kg) or buccally (0.2–0.5 mg/kg) has been used (maximum dose 20 mg). For adults with learning difficulties oral midazolam (10–40 mg disguised in clear juice or intranasally) can be given on arrival in the day-surgery unit. The patient should be placed in a suitable environment to become sleepy, and then safely moved into the anaesthetic room. As the patients present repeatedly for treatment, the optimum plan for their particular needs can be developed.

Airway Management Plan

The choice of airway will depend on the patient and the surgical and anaesthetic factors. It is vital to liaise and communicate with the operating surgeon.

Nasal Mask

Traditionally, nasal dental masks (Goldman or McKesson) were used with a purely inhalational anaesthetic technique. It is still used for short procedures in children when both the dentist and anaesthetist are familiar with its use. The mouth is kept open with a prop and the anaesthetist holds the mask over the nose while supporting the jaw in order to maintain the airway and provide counter-pressure. This technique demands an exceptional degree of vigilance as adequate spontaneous ventilation can be detected only by a combination of looking at chest movement, observing the reservoir bag and listening to the airway. It is not a technique to be used by the occasional dental anaesthetist or in difficult airways, and has been largely superseded by SADs.

SAD or Tracheal Tube

A reinforced SAD, with a throat pack, is increasingly the airway of choice for shorter dental surgery. For longer surgery, procedures requiring irrigation or better surgical access a cuffed TT, in combination with a throat pack, is required. Small children (under 5 years) or patients with a contraindication to nasal intubation may be intubated orally. Even with a cuffed tube, a throat pack is recommended: many dental drills spray large volumes of water into the mouth.

Intraoperative

- The general principles of day care surgery should be followed (Chapter 5.3). Standards of monitoring and the operating theatre environment should be as for any other type of surgery.
- The choice between an inhalation and intravenous induction will depend on the patient age and cooperation.
- Induction for patients with learning difficulties may involve gaseous induction by stealth or an intravenous technique where feasible. Parents or carers should be involved in these choices and assist in keeping the patient calm; success depends on careful planning and patience. Attention must be paid to specific stressors for individual patients – minimizing noise and light in the anaesthetic room. Induction may have to take place in a wheelchair or reclining chair; it may be necessary to secure the airway in the sitting position before using a hoist to transfer the patient onto the operating table or trolley.
- Anaesthetic techniques permitting rapid return of consciousness are suitable. For extensive and complicated restorations, it may be better to manage the airway with a TT and controlled ventilation. Antiemetics and dexamethasone should be prescribed to address PONV and swelling.

Postoperative

- Recovery – Oxygen is given and saturations are closely monitored; 30% of dental deaths occur in the recovery phase, probably because of unrecognized respiratory obstruction. SADs or TTs should be removed after vital reflexes have returned. The patient is placed in the lateral position either without a pillow (head down) or sitting up. They should not be left alone until conscious, maintaining and protecting their airway.
- Analgesia – A balanced regimen, e.g. paracetamol and NSAIDs should be prescribed. Opioids are seldom necessary. Local blocks performed under GA are effective in older children, but the younger children (under 5 years) tend to find numbness more distressing than pain.

SPECIFIC MAXILLOFACIAL AND DENTAL PROCEDURES

Open Reduction Internal Fixation of Mandibular Fracture

- The patient is supine, head up, with the head in a soft, padded head ring.
- Duration of surgery varies depending on fracture position and complexity but is typically between 1 to 3 h.
- Blood loss is usually minimal but can be more if the fracture is complex.
- Postoperative pain can be moderate; the mainstay of treatment will be oral analgesics and opioids.
- Airway management usually involves placement of a nasal TT and throat pack.
- Simple mandibular fractures do not usually cause airway problems. Reduced mouth opening may be caused by pain, muscular spasm or haematoma; this usually resolves following induction of anaesthesia and muscle relaxation. However, this should be discussed with the surgeon and if considered unlikely to improve, an AFOI may be necessary. Suspicion should be high in cases with significant swelling, condylar fractures, TMJ involvement or delayed presentation.
- Le Fort III maxillary fractures risk impending airway compromise due to the posterior displacement of the midface obstructing the oropharynx. Oral and nasal intubation may not be possible and awake tracheostomy or emergent cricothyroidotomy may be required.
- Traumatic facial injuries may be associated with other injuries or burns; a full trauma survey is needed prior to anaesthesia with particular attention to the risk of head injury, cervical spine instability, airway oedema (burns), thoracic injury and blood loss.
- Alcohol or drug intoxication often contributes to trauma – if intoxication is suspected, surgery should be delayed; if not possible, the anaesthetic technique should be modified accordingly.

Mandibular and Maxillary Osteotomies

- These procedures aim to realign the facial skeleton in order to correct any deformity or malocclusion.

- The patient is positioned supine, head up with the head in a soft, padded head ring.
- The duration of these procedures range from 2 to 6 h.
- Blood loss can be extensive if the surgeon plans a down fracture of the maxilla and segment disimpaction; consider blood cross-match and tranexamic acid 1 g.
- Postoperative pain can be moderate – oral analgesics and oral opioids are indicated; PCA may be required in certain cases.
- Airway management requires a nasal TT and throat pack. Patients may be syndromic, with conditions such as Pierre Robin, Treacher Collins or Goldenhar syndrome. These require careful airway assessment and planning and may have had several staged procedures already. Access to previous documentation of the airway anatomy and management is useful. Wire mandibular fixation may be required postoperatively, if so, liaison with the surgical team is important to plan for emergence and extubation. Wire cutters must be immediately available in the recovery and postoperative period in the case of airway compromise.
- Patients are usually relatively young and fit but if the deformity is syndromic, other features of the condition should be identified, particularly cardiac involvement, which might have anaesthetic implications.
- The use of mild hypotensive anaesthesia to minimize blood loss and optimize the surgical field should be considered. Invasive arterial monitoring, urinary catheter insertion and intraoperative warming may be indicated for longer procedures.

Head and Neck Cancer Surgery

Surgical management depends upon the size, location and type of tumour; extensive disease will require tumour resection, selective neck dissection and reconstruction. Pedicled or free-flap tissue transfer is needed to improve cosmetic appearance and restore the ability to swallow and speak. The flap harvest site selection is dependent on surgical site, bony involvement as well as patient comorbidities and functional status.

- Free tissue transfer flaps are ideal for large soft tissue intraoral defects. Radial forearm and anterolateral thigh free flaps are thin and pliable and can be folded or tubed to compensate for palatal and pharyngeal defects. The flap can be harvested at the same time as tumour resection with minimal donor site morbidity. Elderly patients or with significant comorbidities, e.g. peripheral vascular disease or diabetes are not ideal candidates for transfer flaps due to the length of surgery and risk of graft failure.
- Pedicled flaps consist of skin and muscle raised and rotated to cover the defect. The vascular pedicle remains intact so there is no interruption of flap blood supply. Commonly used flaps are pectoralis major, deltopectoral and temporalis. As a one team, one-stage reconstruction with

no microvascular anastomosis, the duration of surgery is significantly reduced making pedicled flaps suitable for high-risk patients.
- Major reconstructive surgery with bony involvement is best managed with an osteocutaneous free flap (fibula, iliac crest, scapula) and may be in combination with regional tissue transfer.

Positioning usually commences in the supine, head up position with head in a head ring. However, further repositioning may be required depending upon the site for flap harvest – both scapular and latissimus dorsi sites require the lateral position for harvest with subsequent return to the supine position for anastomosis. Procedures are prolonged and care must be ensured to protect pressure areas.

Careful airway assessment is required – tumour size and site, and previous radiotherapy may necessitate an AFOI. Patients often have comorbidities such as cardiorespiratory disease needing thorough preoperative assessment and risk stratification. Recent chemotherapy risks immunosuppression and may exacerbate an already poor nutritional state caused as a consequence of the tumour position itself.

Airway management depends on the surgical site and whether surgical tracheostomy will take place at the beginning or end of the operation. If planned from the outset, an oral TT can be placed, if planned for the end, a nasal TT is passed. For resections not expected to cause significant postoperative airway distortion or swelling a tracheostomy may be avoided, the patient being kept sedated for a period of time and extubated on critical care following careful assessment.[5]

Intraoperative monitoring should include invasive arterial monitoring, central venous access, urinary catheterization. Haemodynamic targets alter throughout the course of the procedure with relative hypotension during dissection and resection but a hyperdynamic circulation and increased blood pressure for microvascular anastomoses and to maintain flap perfusion postoperatively. The choice of inotropic and vasoactive agents used to achieve these goals varies. Increasingly fluid management regimes are becoming more conservative and may be guided with cardiac output monitoring.[6]

Temperature management and VTE prophylaxis are essential.

Postoperative pain is moderate and PCA techniques or opioid infusions are needed. Postoperative critical care is essential for these patients and flap success. Meticulous haemodynamic monitoring and flap observations are required. Although the usual aim is to transfer patients to the critical care environment awake and spontaneously breathing, if the surgery is particularly prolonged or complicated, there may be a preference to maintain sedation and ventilation for a period of time. Many units are introducing the principles of enhanced recovery to this group of high-risk patients.

REFERENCES

1. Pavlakovic L, Lee G. Anaesthesia for maxillofacial surgery. Anaesth Intensive Care Med 2014;15:379–84.
2. Florian Heuer J, Heitmann S, Crozier T, BleckmannA, Quintel M, Russo S. A comparison between the GlideScope® classic and GlideScope® direct video laryngoscopes and direct laryngoscopy for nasotracheal intubation. J Clinical Anesth 2016;33:330–6.
3. Prakash VJ, Chakravarthy C, Attar A. Submental/transmylohyoid route for endotracheal intubation in maxillofacial surgical procedures: A review. J Int Oral Health 2014;6:125–8.
4. Lin S, McKenna SJ, Chuan-Fong Y, Chen YR, Chen C. Effects of hypotensive anesthesia on reducing intraoperative blood loss, duration of operation and quality of surgical field during orthognathic surgery- a systematic review and meta-analysis of randomized controlled trials. J Oral Maxillofac Surg 2017;75:73–86.
5. Coyle M, Tyrrell R, Goddenc A, Hughes C, Perkins C, Thomasd S, et al. Replacing tracheostomy with overnight intubation to manage the airway in head and neck oncology patients: towards an improved recovery. British J Oral Maxillofac Surg 2013;51:493–6.
6. Chalmers A, Turner M, Anand R, Puxeddu R, Brennan P. Cardiac output monitoring to guide fluid replacement in head and neck microvascular free flap surgery – what is current practice in the UK? British J Oral Maxillofac Surg 2012;50:500–3.

Chapter 5.11

Orthopaedic and Trauma Surgery

Richard Griffiths, Fiona Faulds

This is a huge and varied area of practice. Around 160,000 primary hip and knee replacements are carried out in England and Wales alone every year.[1] These procedures have the ability to be life changing for a majority of patients. They reduce pain, reduce reliance on analgesic medications and improve mobility.

GENERAL CONSIDERATIONS

Pre-assessment

Pre-assessment clinics are particularly valuable in orthopaedics. Major elective surgery is increasingly offered to a population with considerable comorbidities and rising obesity levels. Not only can the anaesthetist assess fitness but also the patients benefit from a full discussion of the potential and recommended anaesthetic techniques. Where there are several anaesthetic options, as in lower limb surgery, it gives both parties time to discuss all options.

Blood Conservation

Donor blood is increasing in cost and the supply is declining. Modern transfusion practice should focus on blood conservation. In addition, blood transfusion is immunosuppressive and may increase the infection rate, an important consideration when implants are to be used. The following points should be noted:

- Preoperative anaemia has been shown to be associated with increased mortality, acute kidney injury and infection.[1] Optimization of the haemoglobin level should be considered, using iron supplementation and erythropoietin where indicated, but is only possible if pre-assessment occurs at least 4 weeks before planned surgery.
- Strict application of transfusion thresholds is important to conserve blood supply and to reduce complications. A 2012 Cochrane review established

682

that, for most patients, it is safe to avoid transfusion until haemoglobin levels drop below 7–8 g/dL.[2]
- Anaesthetic technique influences blood loss, being less with regional anaesthesia. Other techniques used include isovolaemic haemodilution, autologous predonation and cell salvage.

Tourniquets

Upper or lower limb arterial tourniquets are valuable in achieving a bloodless surgical field. They also have the potential to cause direct skin, tissue, muscle and nerve damage if used incorrectly.[3]

General Points

The tourniquet should be:

- Wider than half the limbs diameter – the wider tourniquets reduce direct pressure under the cuff while maintaining occlusion
- Placed over the widest part of the limb
- Padded carefully and not twisted after application
- Free from cleaning solutions that might damage the skin under the tourniquet
- Inflated to a maximum pressure of 250 mmHg and 300 mmHg for the upper limb and lower limbs, respectively, or 100 mmHg above systolic arterial pressure
- Ischaemic time should be kept to a minimum and not exceed 2 h. During longer procedures it may be necessary to deflate the tourniquet for 10 min before re-inflation
- Attached to an automated gas control system to minimize the chances of over-pressurization

Exsanguination

- This is contraindicated if there is tumour, deep vein thrombosis (DVT) or frank sepsis in the limb.
- The use of Esmarch bandages is not recommended, as it gives uncontrolled and occasionally very high pressures. The Rhys-Davies exsanguinator is safe on normal sized limbs. When rolled onto the limb, it gives a controlled and evenly spread pressure.
- Maximum exsanguination can also be achieved by elevating the arm to 90° or the leg to 45° for 5 min.
- Approximately 800 mL may pass into the remaining circulation from exsanguination of the leg. This may be poorly tolerated in patients with cardiac failure.

Tourniquet Inflation

- Antibiotics, if required, should be administered at least 5 min before inflation to allow tissue penetration.

- Inflation causes a sudden rise in systemic vascular resistance (SVR) and circulating volume usually resulting in a transient increase in blood pressure.
- Tourniquet pain develops over time and is variable between patients. It causes a rise in heart rate and systolic blood pressure, which can be difficult to control with opioids or increased depth of anaesthesia. This can be attenuated with the inclusion of low-dose ketamine in the order of 0.25 mg/kg, preferably before tourniquet inflation.[3]
- Tourniquet use leads to a hypercoagulable state mostly due to an increase in platelet aggregation.

Tourniquet Deflation

- This may lead to an increase in PCO_2 in the order of 2.5 kPa. This may be detrimental, particularly in those with a head injury. Ventilation may need to be adjusted to account for the increased CO_2.
- Reduction in core body temperature is seen due to redistribution of body heat and the return of a small volume of cold blood from the limb.
- Potassium may rise by 0.3 mmol/L and lactate to 2.3 mmol/L – the resulting acidosis causes a fall in SVR and blood pressure. In addition, the effective circulating volume is reduced as the limb is refilled with blood.
- Following deflation, there is a period of increased fibrinolytic activity and this may increase surgical bleeding for a short period.

Contraindications

- Sickle cell disease is a relative contraindication – use may precipitate a sickle cell crisis.
- Peripheral vascular disease is a relative contraindication due to the potential for direct vascular injury.
- Exsanguination should be avoided in the presence of DVTs, due to the risk of massive and/or fatal pulmonary embolism.

Cement

Cement is commonly used in joint replacement surgery. The quality of the bone–cement interface is important to prevent future loosening, more likely to occur here than at the cement–prosthesis interface. The technique involves pressurized cementing, forcing cement into bone canaliculi. This has been particularly important in total hip replacement (THR) surgery but its use is decreasing; from 60% of all hip replacements in the UK in 2003, to only 31% in 2014.

Bone cementing implantation syndrome (BCIS) can occur. The incidence varies but can be 25%–30% in high-risk groups, e.g. fractured neck of femur. It results in hypotension, hypoxia, loss of consciousness and rarely fatal arrhythmias. Other high-risk groups include ASA 3–4 patients, patients with chronic obstructive pulmonary disease (COPD), taking diuretics or warfarin.[4]

The surgeon should warn the anaesthetist when cementing begins; significant hypovolaemia must be avoided as this also predisposes to an adverse reaction to cementing. Existing guidelines outline the role of staff during cementing to minimize morbidity and mortality.[5]

Intravenous fluids, vasopressors, increased inspired oxygen concentration and occasionally inotropic support may be required.

Thromboembolic Disease

DVT is very common following major lower limb joint surgery, with approximate incidences of 55% for THR, 65% for total knee replacement (TKR) and 65% for fractured neck of femur. National Institute of Clinical Excellence (NICE), 2015 guidelines include advice for prevention of venous thromboembolism – mechanical and pharmacological methods, including anti-embolism stockings, foot impulse devices or intermittent pneumatic compression devices should be started at admission unless contraindicated, and continued until mobility is no longer significantly reduced. It also recommends adding pharmacological prophylaxis after surgery.[6] Agents licensed following THR and TKR surgery include:

- Dabigatran etexilate – orally administered direct thrombin inhibitor
- Fondaparinux sodium
- LMWH – low-molecular-weight heparin
- Rivaroxaban – orally administered factor Xa inhibitor
- UFH – unfractionated heparin

More recently, agents have been developed – specifically designed as antidotes for some of the newer orally administered prophylactic agents. Idarucizumab (Pradaxa) is newly licensed in the UK for the specific reversal of dabigatran when rapid reversal is required. Andexanet is currently going through trials and is designed to be a specific antidote to factor Xa inhibitors including rivaroxaban.

Other Emboli

Air Embolism

Air embolism can occur when large veins are open to air, particularly when venous pressure is low. Classically, during shoulder surgery in the sitting position when open veins are higher than the right atrium but it can also occur during pelvic surgery. A large air bolus in the right heart prevents forward blood flow; if it breaks up and moves to the lungs it results in severe ventilation–perfusion mismatch. Clinical features include an abrupt reduction in $EtCO_2$, loss of blood pressure, hypoxaemia and possibly cardiac arrest.

The surgical site should be flooded with saline to prevent further air entry. Nitrous oxide, if in use, should be discontinued to prevent enlargement of air bubbles. The patient should be laid flat or tilted head-down to reduce air entry.

686 SECTION | 5 Anaesthesia for Various Procedures

If a central venous line is in place, air may be aspirated from the right atrium. External cardiac massage may help break up the air bolus in the heart.

Fat Embolism

Fat emboli are a frequent occurrence with fractures of the femur, tibia and pelvis. However, the incidence of the fat embolism syndrome is <1% of such fractures. The syndrome may arise spontaneously if high-risk fractures are not fixed; fixation should occur within 24 h, unless other injuries prevent this. The syndrome can also be seen in major soft tissue injury, bone marrow harvesting, liposuction, hepatic failure, acute pancreatitis and severe burns. The principal features are as follows:

- Respiratory – tachypnoea, haemoptysis, crepitations, hypoxaemia and patchy shadows or 'snowstorm' on chest X-ray
- Petechial rash – classically over the upper body and mucous membranes
- Neurological – confusion, decreased conscious level, coma, decerebrate posturing
- Thrombocytopenia – probably due to platelet consumption
- Cardiovascular – tachycardia
- Pyrexia – >39°C
- Jaundice, acute renal failure and unexplained anaemia

Fat emboli will occur to some extent during reaming of long bones before nailing; surgeons will avoid intramedullary fixation when other modes of fixation are feasible. The clinical signs may be noted during or after surgery. Treatment is supportive and usually in the intensive care unit (ICU).

Tumour Embolism

A patient with disseminated malignancy may present with pathological fractures. Fixation may improve the quality of life; however, reaming a long bone full of tumour carries a high risk of significant or fatal tumour embolism. Massive pulmonary embolism may occur. Prolonged resuscitation may not be appropriate, although advanced life support should be instituted at first. These discussions should take place with the patient in advance so that they are able to make an informed choice about their care.

Anti-Inflammatory Drugs in Orthopaedics

Nonsteroidal anti-inflammatory drugs (NSAIDs) are very useful for bony pain. Patients frequently use them to control arthritic symptoms and they are often well tolerated, with few side effects. However, in the perioperative setting of starvation, possible dehydration and general anaesthesia, their tolerance may be different. For this reason, along with their antiplatelet effects, few are licensed for acute postoperative pain, although they are effective and widely used.

NSAIDs inhibit osteocyte activity, reducing the formation of new bone. Where bone healing is critical or delayed, the surgeon may wish to avoid or restrict the use of the agents. Conversely, where there is a risk of heterotopic ossification, NSAIDs may be used to prevent this.

Infection in Orthopaedics

Infection around a prosthesis is a disastrous complication – removal of the prosthesis and staged revision surgery may be required. A Girdlestone hip or fused knee joint may be the final outcome. Prophylactic antibiotics are used for all operations involving prostheses and hospitals will have local guidelines compiled in combination with microbiologists.

Urinary catheters may introduce infection. Common practice has been to avoid them where possible. However, if required, it is preferable to site this in the clean theatre environment before the prosthesis is inserted, rather than postoperatively on the ward. In some centres, a catheter is routinely placed before all lower limb joint replacement surgery.

Orthopaedic theatres should be equipped with filtered laminar airflow systems providing up to 500 air changes/h. Strategies to maximize the benefits of these systems are as follows:

- Some systems focus laminar airflow onto a central square containing the operating table. A screen of sterile drapes inline with the border of this square optimizes airflow past the patient
- The anaesthetist should avoid leaving the anaesthetic room door open as this disturbs airflow
- The number of people in the theatre should be kept to a minimum because each person introduces a fresh load of organisms to the air
- Extra strategies to conserve heat and warm the patient are required

There is no evidence that wearing a surgical mask reduces wound infection. More bacteria are shed from the skin and clothing than expelled from the nose and mouth. Masks increase the shedding of squames due to friction on the skin of the face and neck; orthopaedic surgeons often wear hoods tucked in around the neck. However, bacterial counts are increased on surfaces directly opposite the face and reduced, for a short period of time, by a suitable surgical mask. It remains common practice for the theatre team to wear facemasks despite the lack of good evidence.

TECHNICAL CONSIDERATIONS

Orthopaedic surgery provides many opportunities for regional and peripheral nerve blocks. There is evidence that mortality is lower for primary hip replacements with spinal anaesthesia compared to general anaesthesia. In addition, a study of over 14,000 primary knee replacements found lower frequencies of superficial wound infections, blood transfusions and overall complication rate when performed under spinal anaesthesia compared to general anaesthesia.

The following should be considered when considering regional techniques:

- Is there a clinical reason to offer a regional block as above, or any contraindications, for example, coagulation or anatomical defect?
- Would a regional block provide helpful postoperative analgesia, for example, interscalene block for shoulder surgery?
- Could the patient be managed satisfactorily without the nerve block? Any tendency to offer a block because it provides an opportunity to acquire new skills rather than for the benefit of the patient should be resisted.
- Would a catheter placed for continuous nerve blockade be helpful? This is increasingly popular, but requires experience, skill and regular practice – should the assistance of a more experienced anaesthetist be sought?
- Will a numb limb be a hazard to the patient postoperatively or interfere with rehabilitation, e.g. patients after knee hemiarthroplasty may wish to walk on the first day? This has been addressed in some areas, e.g. adductor canal blocks over femoral blocks to spare quadriceps function and reduce interference with rehabilitation.
- Can the patient look after a numb and weak limb? With careful selection and instruction, the patients may be discharged home in this state; however, disastrous complications have been reported, e.g. severe burns after falling asleep against a hot radiator.
- Will the block be sufficient? Will sedation or a general anaesthetic be necessary?
- Finally, but importantly, is the patient willing to receive the block either awake or asleep? The anaesthetist should explain the risks, benefits and alternatives. If a patient declines a nerve block without an apparently sound reason, their wishes must be respected.

Regional Blocks

The following regional blocks are useful for orthopaedic surgery:

- Spinal anaesthesia – The addition of opioids improves analgesia but increases postoperative nausea and vomiting (PONV), itch and urinary retention. There is a risk of delayed respiratory depression, especially if parenteral opioids are used in addition.
- Femoral and sciatic nerve blocks are useful, but are being superceded by more targeted nerve blocks, reducing the amount of motor blockade.
- Adductor canal blocks are simple to perform – These target the femoral nerve more distally after the motor component has left it, providing sensory blockade with almost intact motor function.
- Femoral 3-in-1 block, as described by Alon Winnie in 1973, is useful as an adjunct to general anaesthesia for hip surgery, including fractured neck of

femur and THR. This blocks the lumbar plexus as local anaesthetic injected into the femoral sheath in the inguinal region tracks proximally, by means of distal digital pressure and massage. Large volumes of solution are required. The nerves blocked are femoral nerve, lateral cutaneous nerve of the thigh and obturator nerve. Obturator nerve blockade is least reliable; it supplies sensory fibres to the hip joint.

- Fascia iliaca block is more reliable than a 3-in-1 for blocking femoral, lateral cutaneous nerve of the thigh and obturator. It is widely used for analgesia in hip fractures and postoperative analgesia for hip hemiarthroplasty. It is easily performed by anatomical landmarks and has largely replaced lumbar plexus block.
- Popliteal nerve block is useful for foot or ankle surgery. Posterior and lateral approaches are described. The lateral approach is useful in trauma patients when raising the leg in a plaster cast or turning prone may be difficult. The saphenous nerve (from the femoral nerve) may supply part of the great toe; popliteal block alone is not reliable for surgery in this area.
- Ankle block is useful for postoperative analgesia in the foot. Five separate nerves are blocked and only the injections appropriate for the operation need be done. In skilled hands it can be effective, but occasional practitioners have a lower success rate.
- Brachial plexus block – The interscalene approach is commonly used for postoperative analgesia in shoulder surgery. The axillary approach, used for elbow, forearm and hand surgery, gives less reliable cover of the lateral aspect of the arm and supplementary distal blocks may be required for full anaesthesia. The supra- and infraclavicular approaches are reliable blocks for forearm and hand surgery, but carry a risk of pneumothorax.
- Peripheral nerve blocks in the forearm or wrist can be useful for minor procedures or adjuncts to partially effective brachial plexus blocks. The tourniquet area is not covered, which limits their usefulness.
- Bier's block is occasionally used in patients considered unfit for general anaesthesia when brachial plexus blockade has failed. Hand surgeons notice an excessive ooze of blood. A double cuff must be used to allow anaesthesia of the tourniquet area.
- Continuous infusion catheters are gaining popularity and are mainly used for brachial plexus blocks.

Before or after Induction of General Anaesthesia

Orthopaedic patients may present particular difficulties when performing blocks awake. Arthritis or injury may prevent optimal positioning and patients with fractures poorly tolerate twitches from nerve stimulation. The anaesthetist should discuss the risks, benefits and alternatives with the patient before deciding whether to perform the block with the patient awake or anaesthetized. There is a body of established opinion that peripheral nerve blocks may be conducted in anaesthetized patients, assuming a meticulous technique.[7] Ultrasound is often used for guidance – for identification of vessels and other hazards, to guide needle tip position and to check the spread and distribution of local anaesthetic. It has not been shown to reduce the rates of nerve damage but has reduced the rates of local anaesthetic toxicity.[8] Whether done awake, sedated or anaesthetized, the guidelines from the 'Stop Before You Block' campaign should be followed to minimize the chances of wrong sided or site block.[9]

Sedation Techniques

For many patients, fear of being awake in the operating theatre is a barrier to accepting a regional technique for orthopaedic surgery. Drilling into bone is noisy, and can be distressing, simple distraction strategies such as conversation may be ineffective. Sedation can sometimes result in a confused and uncooperative patient. There should always be a plan for airway management, in case control is lost or the procedure lasts longer than unexpectedly for the duration of the regional block. This can happen in any major joint surgery. Placing a supraglottic airway device (SAD) may be easy, but intubation of a patient in the lateral position under a sterile screen may be difficult. Unless intubation is likely to be straightforward, definitive airway control from the outset should be considered.

A range of sedation techniques can be offered. The following are commonly used:

- Intermittent boluses of 0.5–1 mg midazolam: The level of consciousness is likely to fluctuate with this technique. It is useful where the aim is anxiolysis rather than sedation. Disinhibition may also occur. Additional oxygen is usually needed.
- Continuous infusion of propofol, using a standard syringe driver (1–3 mg/kg/h titrated to effect) or a target-controlled infusion (1–2 μg/mL): Stable sedation is usually achieved; amnesia is usual, but not guaranteed. Airway control may be a problem, especially if the patient is supine. Additional oxygen should be given as required and respiration monitored with capnography. The target is light sedation, with the patient responsive to voice, to minimize chances of postoperative delirium particularly in the hip fracture population.

SPECIFIC OPERATIONS

Hip Replacement and Revision Hip Surgery

Hip replacement surgery is common and the impact on quality of life profound. However, an increasingly frail patient population, combined with rising obesity rates make these cases challenging. Revision surgery is a major procedure; patients tend to be older and with more comorbidities than for primary hip surgery. The anaesthetist, surgeon, patient and patient's family must consider, whether the risk–benefit analysis is in the patient's favour.

The 30-day mortality rate after hip replacement is 0.3% and the incidence of significant complications approximately 4%–5%. These include dislocation, infection, DVT and nonfatal pulmonary embolus. Many patients say that they would 'rather be dead' than live in pain. If the anaesthetist believes that the patient is adequately informed, the decision to proceed should be made by the patient.

Regional Techniques

Regional anaesthesia is the technique of choice recommended by the British Orthopaedic Association. It has the following benefits:

- Reduced risk of DVT and pulmonary embolus
- Reduced blood loss and need for blood transfusions
- Drier surgical field – may give better conditions for cementing
- There may be less confusion in recovery – lack of cooperation can lead to early dislocation
- Reduced superficial wound infection
- Reduced mortality

Sedation may be offered in addition to a regional technique, according to patient preference. A common dose for spinal anaesthesia is 2.5–3 mL 0.5% bupivacaine with or without an opioid such as 250–300 µg diamorphine in 0.5 mL normal saline or sufentanil 2.5–5 µg.

Patients may not tolerate the lateral position for longer procedures. Many will have arthritis in other joints and become very uncomfortable, particularly with dependent arm and shoulder pain. A general anaesthetic may become necessary but this is difficult in the lateral position during surgery and should not be undertaken lightly. Combined regional and general anaesthesia from the outset is often used. More hypotension is expected with this combination, which can be managed with vasopressors and fluids.

Specific Hip Procedures

There are several different kinds of hip prosthesis and the acetabular and femoral components may be cemented or uncemented. If an uncemented component is used, there is less benefit from a dry field during the period of insertion. Complex primary hip replacement and revision hip surgery are becoming more common. The anaesthetist should determine an estimated surgical time and blood loss in advance. Bone grafting, using donor or native femoral head, will add an additional 2 h. The surgeon may change the planned procedure if difficulties arise. Invasive monitoring should be considered.

Practical Points

The lateral position is the most common, although sometimes the supine position with a sandbag under the hip is used. There must always be good venous access and warming devices. Many centres place a urinary catheter in all patients, with antibiotic cover, e.g. 120–160 mg gentamicin. Blood loss is usually about 300–500 mL, but a similar amount is lost postoperatively into the tissues and the drain, if used. Blood transfusion should not be routine. Tranexamic acid is commonly used for its antifibrinolytic activity. In revision, surgery blood loss may be 1–2 L and cell salvage should be considered. If the hip is infected, blood loss is even greater and may be brisk.

Postoperatively great care should be taken to avoid early dislocation – the surgeon should personally supervise the hip when the patient is moved or turned. Internal rotation must be avoided and the legs kept abducted using a wedge-shaped pillow between the ankles.

A range of options exist for postoperative analgesia. Intrathecal diamorphine provides useful analgesia but may cause nausea, itch and urinary retention. Common regimes involve synthetic long-acting opioids such as oxycodone-modified release combined with rescue preparations such as oxycodone immediate release or patient-controlled analgesia (PCA) with intravenous morphine. Constipation should be anticipated and actively prevented. NSAIDs and regular paracetamol are helpful. Gabapentin, an anticonvulsant agent is gaining popularity in the treatment of acute surgical pain. It has been shown to have a useful role in a multimodal analgesic approach.

Knee Replacement Surgery

TKR is a markedly painful operation, much more so than hip replacement. Revision knee surgery is variable and the procedure should be discussed with the surgeon beforehand. Hemiarthroplasty or unicompartmental replacement is sometimes performed in patients with single-compartment arthritic changes. This occurs when a varus or valgus knee develops arthritic changes confined to the compartment taking the main load. A small anterior incision is used, making it quicker than a TKR, and blood loss is less. It is considerably less painful afterwards; patients can be mobilized on the day of surgery and discharged after 3 days. Adductor canal block is helpful as it provides quality analgesia without affecting mobilization.

Use of Regional Techniques

A variety of anaesthetic techniques are used with postoperative pain management a prime consideration. Early mobilization may be planned using a passive movement machine, which flexes the knee to a prescribed degree; this is painful without nerve blockade. Anaesthetic and analgesic techniques available include the following:

- Spinal anaesthesia – plain or combined with long-acting intrathecal opioids is a popular technique.
- Adductor canal block – with or without popliteal block is commonly used following spinal or general anaesthesia.
- Intracapsular bupivacaine 0.125% – Its use by surgeons is increasing.

- Epidural analgesia – is now rarely used due to hypotension, motor blockade and potential interference with physiotherapy
- Opioid analgesia is an option after general anaesthesia, but significant doses are needed; PCA gives greater patient satisfaction. NSAIDs are a useful supplement, but some surgeons object to their use in the perioperative period because of their effect on bone growth and healing. Gabapentin is gaining popularity for treatment of acute surgical pain. It has been shown to have a useful role in a multimodal analgesic approach.

Patient preference and comorbities should play their part in determining the choice of technique. Blood loss is controlled by the tourniquet during surgery; regional anaesthesia will help to control blood pressure during the early recovery phase and reduce bleeding. It also reduces the incidence of DVT.

Practical Points

The patient is supine for these procedures; airway control can be a problem under sedation. The operation takes 60–90 min. The tourniquet is released after application of a firm compression bandage and there may be 500–700 mL blood loss in the first few minutes; the surgeon may wish to clamp the drain for a period. A reperfusion drainage system, where drained blood is transfused back into the patient, is well established. However, returning unwashed blood to the patient in this way is associated with febrile episodes and is not universally recommended. Hidden loss in the tissues may equal the visible loss. Regular haemoglobin checks are advised, but strict transfusion thresholds should be observed. Blood transfusion is required infrequently. Tranexamic acid is commonly used to minimize fibrinolysis.

Other Knee Operations

Knee arthroscopy is commonly performed as a day case under tourniquet. It is a short procedure (15–60 min). NSAIDs provide adequate postoperative analgesia, and the surgeon may place local anaesthetic into the knee joint and portal sites (20 mL 0.5% bupivacaine).

Cruciate ligament reconstruction is a 2-h, mainly arthroscopic, procedure performed in the supine position. There is a small incision below the knee to secure the reconstructed tendon. Postoperative pain is variable, but generally moderate. Patients are usually sent home on the day of the procedure. Pain is well controlled with an adductor canal block and NSAIDs, where tolerated. Low-dose ketamine at the beginning of the procedure can help with tourniquet pain as described earlier. Occasionally, stronger analgesia is required in recovery.

Ankle and Foot Surgery

Operations on the metatarsals and toes are common. Other procedures include ankle arthrodesis, tendon transfers, ankle arthroscopy or ankle replacement in specialist centres. Patients often suffer from diabetes mellitus, vasculopathy and peripheral neuropathy and need careful preoperative assessment.

Postoperative pain is significant. Osteotomy, bunion surgery, ankle arthrodesis and replacement are particularly painful. A nerve block, such as ankle, popliteal or sciatic block, is desirable. Compartment syndrome of the foot is an important consideration – it is wise to discuss this possibility with the surgeon before any nerve block. PCA with morphine may be needed after the block wears off and may prevent same-day discharge, even after limited surgery. NSAIDs should be used with care due to impaired bone healing. Wound healing is a particular problem in the foot, owing to the lack of soft tissue volume to accommodate swelling and possible vascular compromise.

Shoulder Surgery

The patients requiring shoulder surgery range from fit sportsmen with recurrent injuries to patients with severe rheumatoid arthritis with multiple comorbidities. All shoulder surgery, with the exception of diagnostic arthroscopy, is extremely painful and a postoperative pain management plan is a high priority.

Specific Procedures

The commonest procedures are rotator cuff repairs and operations on the acromioclavicular joint. These take 1–2 h and can be arthroscopic or open. Blood loss is minimal. Shoulder replacement is a 2–3 h procedure and blood loss is usually less than 500 mL.

Practical Points

For shoulder surgery, the patient is usually placed in the 'deckchair' position with the feet adjacent to the anaesthetic machine. Practical considerations include the following:

● There is restricted or no access to the head – a safe airway is essential. Patients with rheumatoid arthritis and an unstable neck may need an awake fibreoptic intubation (AFOI). A south-facing preformed or armoured tube is most convenient.
● Long ventilator tubes and intravenous connecting lines are needed; alternatively, a venous cannula is placed in the foot.
● The head must be carefully secured to the support.
● Optimal head-up positioning should be achieved slowly, checking blood pressure as the tilt is increased; vasopressors may be needed in addition to fluids.
● The brain is significantly above the arm; this must be taken into account when deciding the target blood pressure.
● Longer procedures require warming devices and the temperature monitored; if the patient is completely covered by a waterproof sterile drape, heat loss may be minimal.

- Air embolism can occur.
- At the end of surgery, anaesthesia should be maintained until the patient is safely placed on a trolley or bed. The head support may be inadequate as the patient starts to move about.
- Postoperative analgesia usually includes an interscalene brachial plexus block – if a single injection is given, there must be an analgesic plan for when it wears off. Inpatients can receive PCA opioid, although there may be a delay until this provides adequate analgesia. Patients discharged with a working block often have severe pain at home. Instructions on the use of multiple oral analgesics are often misunderstood. Some centres now provide patient-controlled regional analgesia via an interscalene catheter, even allowing this at home in selected patients.

Elbow Surgery

Elbow Replacement

Elbow replacement is most commonly performed in patients with rheumatoid arthritis, who often have significant comorbidity. The procedure takes about 2 h and a tourniquet is used. The procedure is as follows:

- The usual positioning is lateral, with the operated arm uppermost and 'draped' over a padded support, with the hand hanging down. The prone position is also used, with the arm over the edge of the table, but this presents difficulties, especially in patients with unstable necks.
- A tracheal tube or an SAD may be used. Patients with rheumatoid arthritis affecting the neck will require careful airway management; AFOI should be considered.
- Brachial plexus block is not adequate as the sole anaesthetic, but is extremely useful for postoperative pain – the axillary approach is the route of choice.
- Early mobilization is important, and a continuous passive movement machine may be used, which is greatly facilitated by brachial plexus block. A single injection of local anaesthetic may provide analgesia for up to 24 h, but this may be prolonged by the use of an axillary catheter.

Elbow Arthrolysis

Elbow arthrolysis is performed to correct stiffness in the elbow. An axillary block with a catheter is ideal and can be used to facilitate postoperative continuous passive movement, if required.

Hand Surgery

Operations on the hand are usually suitable for local or regional analgesia, which must extend to the tourniquet area unless the operation lasts less than 10 min (e.g. carpal tunnel release). Brachial plexus blocks and more distal blocks are useful. Operating conditions may be poor with a Bier's block hand surgery, owing to venous engorgement, but this can be useful when everything else fails. A supraclavicular brachial plexus block is useful where sympathectomy is required, as for finger reimplantation or free flap surgery, and may be prolonged by the use of a catheter.

Spinal Surgery

Spinal operations range from relatively short operations such as microdiscectomy to major procedures with massive blood loss and the possible requirement for access through the chest or abdomen. These major procedures require anaesthetists experienced in this area; successful results depend on close cooperation between surgeon and anaesthetist.

Pre-Assessment

Five principal pathologies present for spinal surgery:

- Trauma
- Infection
- Malignancy with vertebral collapse
- Idiopathic or congenital problems, usually scoliosis
- Degenerative disease of the bones or the discs

Pre-existing neurological deficit should be documented and the stability of the spine should be discussed with the surgeon. A full range of aids to intubation, including equipment for awake intubation, may be needed. Radiographic screening time is sometimes prolonged; pregnancy should be excluded in women of childbearing age. Particular care with pre-assessment is needed for scoliosis and extensive malignancy.

Scoliosis

Patients with scoliosis usually now undergo a single major procedure instead of the multiple procedures of the past. Untreated idiopathic scoliosis may progress rapidly, causing a restrictive respiratory defect, pulmonary hypertension, right heart failure, respiratory failure and death in the fourth or fifth decade. Duchenne muscular dystrophy, cerebral palsy and von Recklinghausen disease (neurofibromatosis) are important causes of scoliosis and these patients may have other associated pathologies. Respiratory and cardiac function must be carefully assessed and the risks of surgery must be fully discussed with the patient and family. Postoperative high-dependency or intensive care should be considered. Scoliosis surgery improves respiratory function, quality of life and life expectancy.

Duchenne Muscular Dystrophy

Patients with Duchenne muscular dystrophy are an exceptionally high-risk group. The mortality is especially high over the age of 12 years. Difficulties include lack of venous access, higher blood loss, cardiac involvement and severe respiratory compromise.

Malignancy

Patients with metastatic cancer are increasingly being offered surgery to stabilize the spine. They may have respiratory or circulatory complications of their disease or its treatment, and be poorly nourished with acute and chronic pain.

Positioning

Correct positioning for spinal surgery is vital and helps lower venous pressure, reducing blood loss and improving the operative field. If prone, the abdomen should hang freely to avoid raised pressure in the inferior vena cava. This can be achieved by using a Montreal mattress, (a full-length curved mattress with a hole in the middle for the abdomen) or a Wilson frame. Some surgeons use a knee–chest position with special supports. This gives a horizontal lumbar spine. Face and head supports designed to protect pressure points are available. Alternatively, a Mayfield® skull clamp (with pins into bone) will avoid pressure on the face and particularly the eyes.

   If the spine is unstable, positioning should be supervised by the surgeon. At least five people are needed, who all understand the principles of a log roll. The anaesthetist should ensure that the brachial plexus is not stretched or compressed in the axilla by the spinal mattress, which may occur if the arms are placed on supports beside the head. Alternatively, the arms can be placed by the patient's sides. However, this can interfere with X-ray screening and limit access to the arms – reliable venous access and extension tubing will be needed. The neck should not be extended and the eyes clear of pressure. A checklist for prone positioning has been suggested to aid the checking of all important areas.

Conduct of Anaesthesia

Requirements for spinal surgery may include slight hypotension with low venous pressures. A mean arterial pressure of 60 mmHg is necessary to maintain spinal cord perfusion in normotensive patients. There is no evidence to support any particular anaesthetic technique. Invasive monitoring may be appropriate.

   An armoured tracheal tube is useful; access to the airway is very poor and fixation of the tube must be totally secure. If an anterior approach is used to the thoracic spine, a double-lumen tube or bronchial blocker allows collapse of one lung; although, simple lung retraction may achieve satisfactory operating conditions if using a standard tube. Discussion with the surgeon is needed.

Blood Loss

Blood conservation should be a priority; complete avoidance of blood transfusion is possible even in major spinal surgery. Simple measures include preoperative optimization of the haemoglobin, modest hypotension and control of coagulation. Point of care testing such as thromboelastography can give rapid information about clotting. Cell salvage may be beneficial. There may be additional benefit from antifibrinolytic agents such as tranexamic acid. Warming devices for fluids and the whole patient should be used, and the body temperature should be monitored.

Spinal Cord Monitoring

Spinal cord monitoring may be used when significant alterations to spinal alignment are made or spinal instrumentation is used as direct cord injury or interruption of its blood supply may occur. Spinal cord monitoring may reduce the incidence of neurological damage from 3.7–6.9% to 0.5%. Historically, cord function was checked by intraoperative wake-up tests. This required considerable anaesthetic skill and did not provide continuous monitoring of spinal cord integrity. Somatosensory evoked potential (SSEP) monitoring is now used – a sensory nerve in the leg (e.g. posterior tibial) is stimulated and the response is detected by an epidural electrode placed above the level of surgery by the surgeon. Data are interpreted by a neurophysiologist during the procedure. Neural transmission is affected by anaesthesia. Nitrous oxide 60% with isoflurane 0.5 MAC has little effect, but higher levels of volatile can abolish the SSEP altogether. Intravenous agents and opioids also affect the SSEP. A constant depth of anaesthesia allows interpretation of subtle changes in the SSEP. Some centres also use motor evoked potentials, where the stimulus is applied to the cord above the level of surgery and electrical activity sensed in the appropriate muscles. Muscle relaxant is avoided and a total intravenous anaesthesia (TIVA) technique is usually employed.

Postoperative Considerations

Pain can be severe for several days after major spinal surgery. Intravenous opioids are most useful, either continuous infusion or PCA, but ileus may occur. Respiratory depression is a particular hazard, especially where there may already be respiratory compromise. High-dependency care should be considered. Intrathecal opioids given by the surgeon may be useful. Epidural analgesia, via a catheter placed by the surgeon, has been successful, but it risks masking neurological sequelae of the surgery. The risk of abscess or haematoma is very low. Extrapleural catheters and paravertebral blocks are also used.

Thromboembolism is common; without prophylaxis the incidence of DVT is 15% and of symptomatic pulmonary embolus is 2.2%. Compression stockings or pneumatic leg pumps should be used, but the use of heparin or warfarin is controversial because of the risk of bleeding.

Paediatric Orthopaedic Surgery

Children presenting for elective orthopaedic surgery commonly have conditions such as cerebral palsy, muscular dystrophy or arthrogryposis (a group of congenital conditions characterized by multiple joint contractures). Staged or multiple procedures are common, and every effort should be made, especially at the first anaesthetic, to make it free of stress for the child. If fear of the anaesthetic room can be avoided, this will greatly ease the difficulties at subsequent – sometimes dozens return visits.

ANAESTHESIA FOR TRAUMA SURGERY

Trauma is the leading cause of death in the first four decades of life in the UK and the USA. Significant disability after trauma is about three times the death rate. Death within minutes of injury is mostly as a result of trauma to the head, high spinal cord, or heart and great vessels. Deaths within hours of injury may be preventable with prompt assessment and an early management process to accurately identify all significant injuries.

In many countries, there has been reorganization and centralization of major trauma care with the development of major trauma centres, which operate 24 h a day and 7 days a week. These are staffed by consultant-led trauma teams that meet the patient on arrival at the hospital and have immediate access to diagnostic and treatment facilities, including blood transfusion, CT scans and emergency operating theatres. In the UK, these major trauma centres are hubs and work closely with local trauma units in the surrounding areas.

Assessment of the Multiply Injured Patient

In February 1976, a plane carrying a trauma surgeon and his family crashed in rural Nebraska, USA. Although he survived the crash, some of his family did not, and he witnessed the deficiencies of a nonspecialized remote hospital dealing with multiply injured patients. On his recovery, he set up a scheme to care for trauma patients, now practised in more than 50 countries. The Advanced Trauma Life Support (ATLS) programme describes a simple protocol for rapid assessment and early management of patients with multiple injuries.[10] All anaesthetists should be familiar with its basic elements. The first three steps are as follows:

1. Establish an adequate airway with cervical spine control.
2. Breathing – Is it adequate?
3. Circulation – Is it adequate?

Emergency treatment of these three components is instituted as necessary, a rapid assessment of disability (neurological status) performed, together with three basic X-rays of the chest, lateral cervical spine and pelvis. This whole sequence is the primary survey and should identify all immediately life-threatening injuries. Treatment or resuscitation is established simultaneously, which may include transferring the patient to theatre for laparotomy or thoracotomy. When circumstances permit, the secondary survey is performed – a full head-to-toe assessment to identify all remaining injuries. This includes a log roll to assess the posterior surface of the patient, look for evidence of spinal injury and assess anal tone or injury. Many centres include a trauma CT scan in their protocol, which replaces diagnostic peritoneal lavage – detecting significant intra-abdominal injury more reliably. CT assessment can also include the spine, brain and thoracic structures as indicated. Definitive management of all injuries is then planned. The ATLS manual gives details of the full assessment process, management of specific injuries and guidelines for fluid resuscitation.

Further points to consider are as follows:

● The mechanism of injury predicts likely injuries and should be established, e.g. a high-velocity impact in a restrained patient may lead to injuries of the great vessels, including those not immediately apparent.
● Certain injuries indicate the degree of the impact: first rib fracture (a high-impact injury) is suggestive of other intrathoracic injuries, such as significant lung contusion.
● Certain physical signs suggest underlying injury: seat belt marks may indicate injury to the spleen or pancreas
● Hypothermia occurs as a result of exposure both before hospital and during initial assessment. Temperature should be monitored and the patient should be kept covered as much as possible; active warming devices should be used.
● Major trauma causes coagulopathy, which must be monitored and aggressively treated – tranexamic acid, given within 3 h of injury, reduces death from bleeding in trauma patients. Best results are achieved when given within 1 h. It appears to increase risk if given after 3 h following injury.[11]

General Considerations for Trauma Anaesthesia

● Secure intravenous access; ensure cross-matched blood and efficient warming devices for blood and the whole patient.
● Patients with significant trauma have delayed gastric emptying caused by pain, fear, anxiety, shock, disgust (e.g. amputated finger) and opioids. The individual status of each patient should be assessed and rapid sequence induction (RSI) should be planned as needed.
● Nerve blocks provide useful analgesia in certain circumstances – femoral nerve blocks are widely used for fractures of the proximal femur (distal third fractures are innervated by the sciatic nerve); ring blocks are useful for fractured digits. Positioning may be difficult in patients with fractures. They tolerate poorly the use of a nerve stimulator while awake and blocks should be performed under ultrasound guidance where possible. If nerve damage already exists, this must be documented and a nerve block should be used only with caution after careful discussion with trauma surgeons.

Compartment Syndrome

Compartment syndrome may occur in any limb injury, not only in fractures. Haemorrhage and oedema within a restricted fascial compartment cause a rise in pressure, preventing normal perfusion of the muscles and other structures. Untreated, muscle necrosis may occur progressing to nerve and vessel damage, contractures, and sometimes loss of the limb.

There should be a high index of suspicion in tibial shaft fractures, displaced tibial plateau fractures and forearm fractures. When planning anaesthesia for these injuries, nerve blockade and epidural analgesia are relatively contraindicated. If in doubt, discuss with the surgeon. If anaesthetic factors strongly indicate regional analgesia, compartment pressure monitoring should be established. Compartment syndrome can also occur in the foot, particularly after crush injury or a fall causing calcaneal fracture.

Signs and symptoms of compartment syndrome are as follows:

● Pain worsened by passive stretching – the earliest sign. Classically, pain is disproportionate to the degree of injury or surgery.
● Limb is pale and cool.
● Paraesthesia in the distribution of nerves that cross the compartment.
● Distal pulses may be preserved and this does not exclude compartment syndrome – loss of the distal pulse is a late sign.
● Muscle weakness – also a late finding.

Wherever there is clinical suspicion, compartment pressure should be measured by inserting a needle attached to a pressure monitoring line. The diagnosis is confirmed if the pressure is within 30 mmHg of diastolic blood pressure.

Management of compartment syndrome includes the following:

● Release tight bandages or plaster.
● Avoid elevation, as it reduces perfusion still further.
● Urgent surgical decompression and debridement of necrotic muscle within 6 h of injury to ensure complete recovery.
● Splinting of the limb to prevent contracture.

SPECIFIC FRACTURES AND THEIR MANAGEMENT

Head and chest injury are discussed elsewhere (Chapters 5.7 and 5.14, respectively).

Pelvic Fractures

Bleeding from pelvic fractures can be massive and unrecognized. Anterior–posterior fracture dislocation of the ilium on the sacrum may occur, often bilaterally, after compression injury. This 'open book' injury tears posteriorly placed veins within the pelvis. It also increases the capacity of the pelvis considerably, which delays tamponade. Vertical shear pattern fractures, where the ilium moves superiorly on the sacrum, are also associated with massive blood loss. In these cases, application of a pelvic binder may aid resuscitation, but it may be necessary to replace this with an external fixator if there is a delay in transfer to theatre. Laparotomy remains possible working around an external fixator; injuries of the urethra, bladder, vagina and rectum should be considered with any fractured pelvis. Definitive fixation of the pelvic fracture can occur later, and may require transfer to a specialist trauma centre.

Anaesthetic considerations are as follows:

- Fixation may require plating via several different approaches. Prior discussion with the surgeon is required.
- Postoperative pain may be considerable due to extensive muscle stripping and multiple incisions. Epidural analgesia may be useful but is of high risk in the presence of major bleeding and has the potential for coagulopathy.
- Blood loss varies with the approach but can be considerable. The posterior approach risks injury to the superior gluteal artery, which may be very difficult to control. Both anterior and posterior approaches may involve considerable dissection and muscle stripping, often associated with prolonged ooze. Cell salvage should be considered. Rapid massive blood loss is also possible; at least two large cannulae and efficient blood warming should be used.
- With associated comorbidities or extensive blood loss, invasive monitoring is essential but not in a healthy patient with an isolated injury.
- Air embolism may occur.

Spinal Fractures

Where paramedics consider spinal injury a possibility, the patient is transferred to hospital, usually a major trauma centre, on a spinal board with 'triple immobilization' of the neck – a cervical collar, sandbags and tape to prevent turning of the head. The patient should be moved from the board within 1 h of arrival to protect pressure areas. Spinal injury precautions require log rolling by at least five trained personnel and is described in detail in the ATLS manual. Full precautions must continue until the whole spine is cleared – both radiologically and clinically. To make this assessment, the patient must be conscious and have no neurological injury without the influence of alcohol, drugs or severe pain elsewhere. In practice, this may be difficult to achieve.

Nursing care is greatly complicated if the spine cannot be cleared. However, spinal cord injury is so serious that only a senior clinician should authorize discontinuation of spinal injury precautions.

Other considerations include the following:

- 'Spinal shock' can occur if there is cord transection; hypotension responds to fluid and vasopressor therapy. Even with significant cord injury, without transection, some recovery is possible. Perfusion pressures must be maintained and hypoxia should be avoided.

- The neck must be stabilized in-line during intubation; AFOI may be necessary.
- Suxamethonium should not be given to patients with spinal cord injuries after the first 12 h. After this, it may cause massive and fatal potassium efflux from denervated muscle cells. If RSI is required, a modified technique using rocuronium should be used.

Fractured Neck of Femur

There are about 65,000 isolated fractured necks of femur each year in England, the details of which are entered into the National Hip Fracture Database (NHFD). Patients are usually elderly (average age 83 years), often with significant comorbidities and high mortality rates (8.2% died within 30 days). These patients require multidisciplinary team input. Various guidelines outline standards of care for these patients – encompassing timing of surgery (within 48 h of admission), personnel (on dedicated trauma lists with senior medical and theatre staff), modes of anaesthesia, supplemental nerve blockade, avoidance of hypotension and assessment for Bone Cement Implantation Syndrome (BCIS).[12] The Anaesthetic Sprint Audit of Practice (ASAP) in 2014 collected data regarding conduct of anaesthesia in over 16,900 patients since the guidelines were published and found wide variation in adherence.[13] On the basis of these findings, further recommendations were made.

- Perioperative nerve blocks should be offered to all patients who suffer hip fractures.
- Spinal anaesthesia should be considered for all cases due to the reduced incidence of hypotension.
- Departments of Anaesthesia should develop evidence-based standardized approaches to spinal anaesthesia.
- Departments of Anaesthesia should develop protocols to raise awareness of BCIS and specific training for its recognition, avoidance and management.

The incidence of BCIS in these patients can be up to 19%; identification and management of those at risk has been discussed earlier.

Best care for these patients involves fast-tracking immediately following admission, good analgesia, fast essential investigations, minimal delay to operation while awaiting specific investigation and early mobilization after fixation.

There are two types of operation for fixation of fracture of the neck of femur. If the fracture is extracapsular (intertrochanteric), the blood supply to the femoral head is preserved. Screw fixation is performed, most commonly a dynamic hip screw, with the patient supine and raised on a high table to facilitate X-ray screening. If the fracture is intracapsular (subcapital), avascular necrosis of the femoral head occurs in about 6% of cases, particularly if the fracture is displaced, and a cemented hemiarthroplasty is usually performed. If there is concern over the cardiovascular stability of the patient, the surgeon may be willing to consider an uncemented prosthesis. However, these are associated with an increased incidence of early thigh pain, even with minimal activity, and a cemented prosthesis is recommended where feasible. Operating time is about 1 h and blood loss is 200–400 mL. There is no evidence to show that a haemoglobin transfusion trigger of 10 g/dL produces better outcomes compared to a trigger of 8 g/dL, but in those patients with significant cardiac disease, a higher trigger of 10 g/dL may be beneficial.

Amputation

Amputation may need to be considered as an option in the early management of severe crush or impact injuries, or may follow a long series of interventions aimed at saving the limb. General anaesthesia and spinal anaesthesia are commonly used; many of those having spinal anaesthesia request sedation in addition. In orthopaedics and trauma, unlike vascular surgery, the circulation is usually excellent and blood loss may be massive. A tourniquet should be used where possible. Regional techniques exacerbate the effects of hypovolaemia, which must be managed aggressively. There is no evidence that pre-emptive epidural analgesia started 24 h beforehand reduces the incidence of phantom limb pain.

Paediatric Trauma

Trauma is the leading cause of death in children younger than 14 years in the Western world. In the UK, the Trauma Audit and Research Network analysed the children admitted with an Injury Severity Score of >15; 68% were male, with a bimodal age distribution, a first peak for those younger than 1 year and a second peak for those older than 6 years. Most traumas were the result of road traffic collisions (as pedestrians or cyclists) or falls, but a significant number resulted from nonaccidental injury. Seventy-five per cent of injuries were head injuries, but often combined with accompanying injuries. Injuries highly associated with death were head injuries, chest injuries, polytrauma and asphyxia.[14]

Over a quarter of cases will arrive at their nearest hospital, not necessarily a designated trauma unit. Staff at the receiving hospital may not be fully experienced in paediatric trauma, but all anaesthetists should be competent in the initial management and stabilization of an injured child, before transfer to a paediatric centre if necessary.

Some key principles are as follows:

● Initial management follows the same pattern as in adults: airway with cervical spine control, breathing, circulation, rapid assessment of disability, primary radiographs and secondary survey. Knowledge of the normal range of vital signs in young children is essential.

- The cervical spine of children is highly mobile and the head is relatively large: this makes serious neck injury more likely. Spinal cord damage without bony injury is more likely to occur in children than in adults. Imaging needs expert interpretation because 'pseudo-subluxation' (a normal variant) may occur.

- Blood pressure is a poor indicator of hypovolaemia in children; peripheral vasoconstriction, tachycardia and drowsiness are better indicators. If hypovolaemia is suspected, 20 mL/kg of intravenous fluid should be given initially, repeated if necessary, after which blood should be considered. Intraosseous access is useful in young children. Brain injury is not a reason to withhold intravenous fluid. More damage will be done by failing to restore blood volume than by giving excess fluid.

- Children are more likely to have diffuse brain injury with cerebral oedema after trauma, and less likely to have intracerebral haemorrhage requiring surgical treatment. They are also more likely than adults to have a fit after relatively minor head injury.

- The ribs are incompletely ossified in children and cartilaginous joints are more elastic, consequently the thoracic cage is much more flexible than in adults. Rib fractures are rare, but severe underlying thoracic trauma may still be present.

- The abdomen is also poorly protected as the thoracic cage is short and flexible leaving the liver, spleen and kidneys at risk from minor impacts. Paediatric surgeons are more likely to attempt conservative management of injured solid organs than in adults, but possible perforation of the bowel will always be explored. It is especially important to try to conserve the spleen because of the lifelong risk of sepsis.

- Children are prone to aerophagia (air swallowing) when distressed; extreme gastric distension may occur, which gives a risk of vomiting and may confuse clinical findings in the abdomen. A gastric tube should be used to decompress the stomach.

- Parents and other family members may require the care of the admitting trauma team: there will be anxiety and fear, and possibly overwhelming guilt, even if the accident was not predictable or preventable. Parental presence with the child should be considered at all stages, and the family should be cared for by expert personnel.

REFERENCES

1. Fowler AJ, Ahmad T, Phull MK, Allard S, Gillies MA, Pearse RM. Meta-analysis of the association between preoperative anaemia and mortality after surgery. Br J Surgery 2015;102:1314–24.
2. Carson JL, Carless PA, Hebert PC. Transfusion thresholds and other strategies for guiding allogeneic red blood cell transfusion. Cochrane Database of Systematic Rev Issue 4. Art. No. CD002042 https://www.ncbi.nlm.nih.gov/pubmed/22513904; 2012 [accessed 15.10.16].

3. Deloughry JL, Griffiths R. Arterial tourniquets. Contin Educ Anaesth Crit Care Pain 2009;9: 56–60.
4. Olsen F, Kotyra M, Houltz E, Ricksten S-E. Bone cement implantation syndrome in cemented hemiarthroplasty for femoral neck fracture: incidence, risk factors, and effect on outcome. Br J Anaesth 2014;113:800–6.
5. Membership of the Working Party, Griffiths R, White SM, Moppett IK, Parker MJ, Chesser TJ, et al. Safety guideline: reducing the risk from cemented hemiarthroplasty for hip fracture. Anaesthesia 2015;70:623–26. doi: 10.1111/anae. 1303.
6. NICE Clinical Guideline [CG92] Venous thromboembolism: reducing the risk for patients in hospital. https://www.nice.org.uk/Guidance/cg92; 2015 [accessed 15.10.16].
7. Fischer HBJ. Regional anaesthesia- before or after general anaesthesia? Anaesthesia 1998;53:727–9.
8. Orebaugh SL, Kentor ML, Williams BA. Adverse outcomes associated with nerve stimulator-guided and ultrasound-guided peripheral nerve blocks by supervised trainees: update of a single-site database. Reg Anesth Pain Med 2012;37:577–82.
9. NHS England, SALG, RAUK. Stop before you Block. https://www.rcoa.ac.uk/sites/default/files/CSQ-PS-sbyb-supporting.pdf; 2011 [accessed 15.10.16].
10. American College of Surgeons. ATLS student course manual: advanced trauma life support. https://www.facs.org/quality-programs/trauma/atls [accessed 15.10.16].
11. The CRASH-2 collaborators. The importance of early treatment with tranexamic acid in bleeding trauma patients: an exploratory analysis of the CRASH-2 randomised controlled trial. The Lancet 2011;377:p1096–1101. No. 9771.
12. Association of Anaesthetists of Great Britain and Ireland, Griffiths R, Alper J, Beckingsale A, Goldhill D, Heyburn G, et al. Management of proximal femoral fractures. Anaesthesia 2012;67: 85–98.
13. Royal College of Physicians. National Hip Fracture Database. http://www.nhfd.co.uk/20/hipfractureR.nsf/4e9601565a8ebbaa802579ea0035b25d/f085c664881d370c80257cac00266845/$FILE/onlineASAP.pdf; 2014. [accessed 15.10.16].
14. The Trauma Audit and Research Network TARN. 2 years of severe injury in children. 2013–14 Report. https://www.tarn.ac.uk/Content/ChildrensReport2/index.html [accessed 15.10.16].

Chapter 5.12

Otorhinolaryngology

Ravi Bhagrath

GENERAL CONSIDERATIONS

Otorhinolaryngology or ENT surgery ranges from short day-case procedures, such as grommet insertion and endoscopy, to complex head and neck resections lasting many hours. Patient age ranges from the neonate to the elderly.

The surgeon and anaesthetist desire simultaneous access to the airway; good communication and team working before, during and immediately after surgery are vital. If surgery is carried out in the nose or throat, the anaesthetist must preserve a clear airway while optimizing surgical access, and prevent soiling of the trachea and bronchi with blood and debris. Preparations should be made to deal with failure of any of these. Although general anaesthesia is commonly employed, it should be remembered that some operations can be undertaken under local anaesthesia with or without sedation.

LOCAL ANAESTHESIA

Some procedures may be carried out under local anaesthesia. The ability to perform these blocks can be crucial when faced with difficulty in securing an airway. The decision may be made as a result of a lack of anaesthetic equipment or expertise, or due to patient or surgical preference, or patient co-morbidity. However, this should be balanced against the potential drawbacks of an awake patient; vestibular activation during middle ear surgery may produce nausea and patients find it difficult to remain immobile for most types of airway surgery.

Nasal Mucosa

Oral or nasal mucosa may be anaesthetized with topical 4%–10% lidocaine, supplemented by further injection. Dental cartridges are commonly used, containing 2% lidocaine with 1:80,000 epinephrine (adrenaline) (12.5 g/mL). 10% Cocaine solution is a useful analgesic and vasoconstrictor, but subject to legal restrictions. Idiosyncratic reactions have been reported and it should not be used in those with cardiovascular disease. Chlorphenylcaine is a useful ready mix of 5% lidocaine and 2.5% phenylephrine with a mucosal atomizer for nasal anaesthesia and vasoconstriction. Otrovine (xylometazoline) spray is another commonly available vasoconstrictor.

Trigeminal Nerve

The trigeminal nerve supplies sensation to the face through its mandibular, maxillary and ophthalmic divisions. Each division, or the terminal branches, may be blocked.

Opthalmic Division of the Trigeminal Nerve

The supraorbital nerve is a terminal branch of the frontal nerve. It supplies sensation to the ipsilateral forehead and scalp up to the vertex. It may be blocked at the supraorbital notch.

Maxillary Division of the Trigeminal Nerve

The maxillary branch of the trigeminal nerve passes through the foramen rotundum and may be blocked at the sphenopalatine ganglion at the back of the nasal cavity by local anaesthetic instilled into the nose.

The traditional Moffett's solution has been modified and now contains 1 mL 1:1000 epinephrine (adrenaline) (1 mg), 2 mL 5% cocaine (100 mg) and 1–2 mL 8.4% sodium bicarbonate diluted to 10 mL with 0.9% saline.

The patient is positioned supine with the head and neck extended over a shoulder roll. The anaesthetic solution is dribbled into the dependent roof of the nasal cavity. The patient should spit out excess solution rather than swallow it. Cotton wool buds dipped in solution may be passed into the nasal cavity, or the cavity packed with gauze soaked in solution or the solution may be sprayed into the nasal cavity with a mucosal atomizer device.

Greater Auricular Nerve

The greater auricular nerve (C2, C3), a branch of the superficial cervical plexus, is blocked to provide analgesia after tympanomastoid surgery through a postauricular incision. A needle is inserted in front of the lower anterior border of the mastoid process, and advanced first between the mastoid process and meatus, infiltrating 3–5 mL local anaesthetic. The needle is then withdrawn and redirected subcutaneously posterior to the meatus and ear canal until the needle tip is cranial to the canal, infiltrating 4–6 mL of anaesthetic solution.

Cervical Plexus Block

Cervical plexus block is useful for operations in the neck (see Chapter 4.2).

Tympanic Membrane

The tympanic membrane may be anaesthetized for myringotomy with 0.1–0.2 mL of lidocaine/prilocaine cream (EMLA®) or AMETOP® (4% tetracaine) applied for 15 min. It may be toxic to the middle ear and should be used sparingly.

GENERAL ANAESTHESIA

Preoperative Preparation

A history examination and investigations should be performed to determine the degree of risk; useful scoring systems include SORT and P-POSSUM (see chapter 1.1). In the history, symptoms of dypsnoea (positional, exertional, timescale), dysphagia, dysphonia, pain or any symptoms of obstructive sleep apnoea (OSA) should be elicited. A thorough airway examination including Mallampati, jaw subluxation, dentition and cervical spine mobility is done; palpation of the neck is prudent. Patients undergoing head and neck surgery are at increased risk of morbidity and mortality secondary to airway difficulties.[1] Such cases require careful assessment and coordinated planning by skilled anaesthetists and surgeons. Teamwork is crucial as the risk of adverse outcomes is high when any part of this process fails.

Investigations may include a flexible nasendoscopy, spirometry, MRI, PET and CT scan. Flow-volume loops can aid in the diagnosis and location of airway obstruction (Fig. 5.12.1). Flexible nasendoscopy is particularly useful for assessing the nasopharyngeal and oropharyngeal spaces when determining ease of intubation. A measure of the patient's cardiovascular reserve (cardiopulmonary exercise testing [CPET], stress echocardiogram) can be made if major surgery is being considered.

The patient's medication should be reviewed especially with regard to antihypertensives (which should be continued) and antiplatelet or other anticoagulants (e.g. factor Xa inhibitors). In closed-space surgery, middle, inner ear and skullbase surgery, a discussion with the surgeon must be made to determine whether

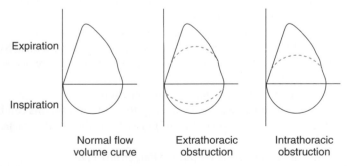

FIGURE 5.12.1 Flow–volume loops demonstrating extrathoracic and intrathoracic obstruction.

drugs such as aspirin and clopidogrel should be discontinued. Patients on warfarin may require bridging therapy with low-molecular-weight heparins (LMWH).

An assessment as to the risk of aspiration is a key component of airway pre-assessment. Manoeuvres such as ensuring preoperative starvation, gastric prokinetics and oro- and nasogastric tubes should be considered.

A discussion regarding the anaesthetic should take place with the patient, potentially including a description of awake fibreoptic intubation (AFOI), preoxygenation and any preoperative vascular access. The patient should be warned of the manner in which they wake-up, i.e. in theatre, recovery or intensive care unit (ICU) but also whether they will wake with an oropharyngeal or a supraglottic airway device (SAD) in-situ, nasogastric tube (NG), nasal or dental packs and the presence of a urinary catheter for longer procedures. The possibility of a sore throat and the analgesia plan should be discussed. This may range from simple analgesia to opioid patient-controlled analgesia (PCA).

Most operations are suitable for day surgery but major cases may need overnight stays if, for example, drains have been placed. High-dependency (HDU) or ICU may be required for major surgery (laryngectomy, neck dissection, retrosternal thyroidectomy).

Premedication

Premedication is rarely required for short or day-case procedures. However, in children or anxious adults, EMLA® cream or AMETOP® gel over marked veins may be advantageous. For children, an anxiolytic agent such as oral midazolam (up to 0.5 mg/kg, maximum 20 mg), paracetamol 15 mg/kg for analgesia can also be useful.

Monitoring

In addition to the recommendations for standards of monitoring during anaesthesia, the following may also be required:

- Arterial cannula – to monitor blood pressure and assess acid–base status in procedures with controlled hypotension, surgery around the vagus or carotid sinus, the internal carotid artery or internal jugular vein, and extensive head and neck resections with flaps or free grafts
- Cardiac output monitoring – for cardiac disease or expected blood loss (usually LiDCO (LiDCO, Cambridge, UK) or PICCO (Pulsion Medical Systems, Munich, Germany) rather than an oesophageal Doppler where access to the head is required)
- Facial nerve monitoring, e.g. parotid tumour excision
- Recurrent laryngeal nerve monitoring, e.g. thyroid surgery; this can be integral to the tracheal tube (NIM™ EMG) or self-attached to the tracheal tube (TT)
- Body temperature and urine output for longer procedures

Principles of Anaesthesia

All patients should be preoxygenated, in a slightly head-up position, to an EtO_2 of 0.87–0.9. Oxygenation via nasal cannulae has been shown to aid this process: Nasal Oxygenation During Efforts of Securing A Tube (NODESAT) and transnasal humidified high-flow oxygen up to 70 L/min techniques, e.g. transnasal humidified rapid insufflation ventilatory exchange (THRIVE) have been shown to extend the apnoeic time in the obese and difficult airways.[2]

Conventional agents such as propofol are used for induction, followed by maintenance with a target-controlled infusion (TCI) of propofol (4–8 µg/mL) or volatile agent (desflurane, sevoflurane, isoflurane) in an oxygen/air mixture. Analgesia is provided with an opioid bolus (fentanyl 1–2 µg/kg, alfentanil 10–20 µg/kg) or remifentanil infusion (TCI at 1–4 ng/mL). Muscle relaxation is achieved with nondepolarizing neuromuscular blocking drugs (NMBs) such as vecuronium, rocuronium or atracurium; peripheral nerve monitoring provides the optimum intubating conditions.

If an oral or nasal TT is required, the operator should be experienced with direct or videolaryngoscopy. In the event of an unexpected difficult intubation, the number of attempts at laryngoscopy should be limited to four.[3] When use of a SAD is planned for airway maintenance, a reinforced device should be considered where there may be manipulation of the head position, e.g. ear surgery. Second-generation SADs (those with high seal pressures, gastric ports, bite blocks, ability to pass a fibreoptic scope) have been shown to be safer and more efficacious in comparison to first-generation devices. Bougies, stylets and external laryngeal manipulation can all aid the intubation process. A continuous capnography waveform with appropriate values of $EtCO_2$ is the best method for confirmation of correct TT placement.

An AFOI may be required to place a nasal or oral TT. This is a core skill, which should be practised. Correct positioning of both the patient and operator along with good airway topicalization are key; many methods have been described in Chapter 2.6.[4]

A throat pack may be required for oral, nasal or sinus surgery to prevent airway soiling. This must be noted at the World Health Organization (WHO) safety check and the patient should be labelled accordingly. Protect the eyes with tape and pads. A head ring, shoulder roll and head-up tilt are often required. Active warming should be used for procedures lasting over 30–45 min and adequate deep venous thrombosis (DVT) prophylaxis should be ensured, e.g. compression stockings, intermittent pneumatic compression boots. Consider the requirement for LMWH in the postoperative period.

Analgesia may be local infiltration, specific nerve blocks, simple analgesics (regular paracetamol), weak (tramadol, codeine phosphate) to strong opioids either orally (oramorph) or as a PCA (fentanyl, morphine). The use of nonsteroidal anti-inflammatory drugs (NSAIDs) must be judged against the possibility of increased perioperative bleeding and postoperative haematoma formation;

there is however, no definitive evidence to support this. A Cox-2 inhibitor, e.g. parecoxib may be considered.

Postanaesthetic Care

Analgesia should be administered before the end of surgery and extubation plans made. Remove any throat pack and suction the pharynx under direct vision. NMBs should be reversed. Sugammadex is able to rapidly reverse steroid-based drugs (vecuronium and rocuronium) which may be advantageous for shorter procedures.

Determine whether the patient is 'low-risk' or 'at-risk' extubation (see Chapter 2.6).[5] Deep extubation (using remifentanil or deep inhalation anaesthesia) provides a smooth emergence, but where airway control is of prime importance, awake extubation should be considered. An airway exchange technique with an SAD can provide smooth emergence (the Bailey manoeuvre).

EARS

Operations on the middle and inner ear include tympanoplasty, ossiculoplasty, stapedectomy, mastoidectomy, cochlear implants and, commonly in children, myringotomy and grommet insertion. Acoustic neuroma removal may involve neurosurgery.

The main issues of operations on the middle and inner ear are as follows:

- Patients may have preoperative hearing loss.
- Some procedures, e.g. skull base and mastoid surgery may be prolonged; careful positioning and DVT prophylaxis are important.
- Quiet, smooth emergence is desirable.
- Postoperative nausea and vomiting (PONV) is common.
- Nystagmus may be a problem postoperatively.

Specific Operations

Myringotomy

General anaesthesia is usual for children with glue ear. Although facemask anaesthesia is possible, conditions are better with a SAD. Some advocate avoiding nitrous oxide (N_2O), at least until insertion of the grommet. Incision of the tympanic membrane is stimulating; anaesthetic depth must be adequate, usually including a short-acting opioid such as alfentanil or fentanyl.

Bradycardia or cardiac arrest can occur if the area of tympanic membrane supplied by the auricular branch of the vagus nerve is incised, this may be prevented by atropine or glycopyrrolate. Intraoperative NSAIDs and i.v. paracetamol (15 mg/kg) provide adequate postoperative analgesia.

Middle and Inner Ear Surgery

Airway

The airway may be managed by a reinforced SAD. However, access is limited and it is extremely inconvenient to adjust this during surgery; tracheal intubation provides a more secure airway. The TT may be replaced by an SAD at the end of surgery for smooth emergence.

Blood Pressure

All attempts to minimize bleeding will facilitate the surgeon's view through the operating microscope and reduce operating time. Mild hypotension is helpful but blood pressure should be kept within 30% of that measured preoperatively; hypotension should be avoided in patients with ischaemic heart disease, hypertension, carotid artery disease or renal dysfunction. Intra-arterial pressure monitoring should be used whenever potent hypotensive agents are given by infusion.

Additional measures include:

- Head-up tilt
- Taping rather than tying the airway
- Pharmacological methods – increased depth of anaesthesia with inhalation agents, remifentanil infusion or opioid boluses; other agents include β-adrenoceptor antagonists (esmolol, labetolol), α2 agonists (clonidine, dexmedetomidine), nitrates and calcium channel antagonists. Agents should be short acting, as a normotension is required at the end of surgery

Facial Nerve Monitoring

This is used when the facial nerve is considered at risk such as middle ear, mastoid, or parotid surgery or acoustic neuroma resection. Needle electrodes, placed in the muscles around the mouth and eye, monitor the EMG and give an audible and visual alert during mechanical or electrical stimulation of the nerve. The monitor's function should be tested before surgery by tetanic stimulation using a peripheral nerve stimulator placed over the facial nerve, just in front of the ear.

A short-acting NMB (e.g. mivacurium) can be used to facilitate intubation, ensuring it has worn off before surgery. Rocuronium or vecuronium can be reversed with sugammadex if necessary. Alternatively, intubation can be achieved with the aid of intravenous anaesthesia and opioids (alfentanil or remifentanil) and 3 mg/kg topical lidocaine to the larynx.

Nitrous Oxide

Nitrous oxide (N_2O) increases middle ear pressure by diffusion. This may cause stapes disarticulation, tympanic membrane rupture and displacement of tympanic membrane graft and potentially hearing impairment. If used, it should be stopped 10–30 min before grafting. Total intravenous anaesthesia (TIVA) appears to give better conditions than an inhalation anaesthesia.

Nausea and Vomiting

PONV is common as a result of labyrinthine disturbance during middle ear surgery. It is less frequent if N_2O is avoided and opioids minimized. TIVA should be considered for those with additional risk factors for PONV. Patients should be kept hydrated; multiple antiemetics are used including dexamethasone with a combination of cyclizine, dopamine antagonists (metoclopramide, prochlorperazine) and 5-HT_3 receptor antagonists (ondansetron, granisetron, dolasetron).

Acoustic Neuroma Surgery

Some acoustic neuroma can be treated using stereotactic radiosurgery. Surgical excision often requires neurosurgical input possibly via posterior fossa craniotomy and procedures can be long (Chapter 5.7).

NOSE

Operations include manipulation of fractured nasal bones, nasal polyp or tumour removal, septoplasty, rhinoplasty, turbinate surgery and functional endoscopic sinus surgery (FESS).

A reinforced SAD or a cuffed TT may be used, with a throat pack, depending on anaesthetic and surgical preference, anticipated blood loss and the duration of surgery. A flexible SAD or a south-facing preformed TT allows the airway to be secured away from the nose (Fig. 5.12.2).

Topical nasal vasoconstriction is extremely useful applied by the anaesthetist or surgeon. Choices include cocaine, xylometazoline or ephedrine drops or spray, Moffett's solution, or dental cartridge injection of local anaesthetic with epinephrine (adrenaline). Block of the sphenopalatine ganglion, which carries the vasodilator fibres to the nasal blood vessels, has been described. The surgeon may wish the eyes to be uncovered.

Surgery is easier with controlled hypotension; the operation may have to be abandoned if bleeding is profuse. Short-acting opioids such as alfentanil or remifentanil are ideal as postoperative pain is not marked.

After throat pack removal, pharyngeal suction should also remove blood clots from behind the soft palate using a laryngoscope or videolaryngoscope (VL). If an SAD is in place, suction is applied to the upper surface of the device at the back of the pharynx. This usually stays in place until awakening.

Nasal packs are often inserted by the surgeon and may stay in overnight. These may be uncomfortable, and may be hazardous in patients with OSA.

Postoperative analgesia is usually provided by simple oral agents. If opioids are required, patients with OSA will require oxygen and careful observation.

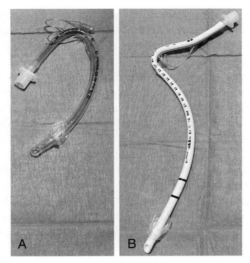

FIGURE 5.12.2 Preformed (RAE) tracheal tubes: (A) oral south-facing tracheal tube and (B) nasal north-facing tracheal tube.

Manipulation of Fractured Nasal Bones

This can be performed under TIVA in the head-down position or using a face-mask. However, older fractures (over 2 weeks), often require vigorous manipulation and an SAD with a throat pack is more common. Occasionally, tracheal intubation may be required.

Anaesthetic agents should permit rapid return of protective reflexes. If plaster of Paris is applied, eyes should be protected.

THROAT

Procedures include removal of foreign bodies (FBs), adenotonsillectomy, tongue-tie surgery, palatal surgery, oesophagoscopy, laryngogoscopy, laryngectomy, thyroidectomy and neck dissection surgery.

Specific Operations

Pharyngoscopy/Oesophagoscopy/Laryngoscopy

Ingested Foreign Bodies

FBs may lodge in the oesophagus at points of physiological or pathological narrowing. Coins, batteries, toys and safety pins are commonly ingested by children. A disc battery must be treated with urgency. Food bolus impaction is common in elderly edentulous adults, often associated with an organic oesophageal narrowing. Ingested FBs may present after many years with a fistula between the oesophagus and respiratory or vascular systems. The nature of the ingested or inhaled FB should be investigated with a PA and lateral chest X-ray (CXR) or CT scan. An ingested FB is unlikely to result in respiratory distress although there may be dysphagia.

A laryngoscopy, pharyngoscopy and oesophagoscopy may be required. This can usually wait until the patient is starved. Premedication with glycopyrrolate can be useful to reduce secretions and prevent episodes of bradycardia. An inhalational induction may be preferred in children. Procedures are often quick and short-acting agents should be used. Occasionally, the FB is seen at laryngoscopy and can be removed. Cricoid pressure should be avoided if the FB is sharp or in the upper oesophagus. Paralysis should be maintained while the rigid endoscope is in the mediastinum.

Oesophageal or pharyngeal perforation may present with mediastinitis: the classic triad of mediastinal pain, pyrexia and surgical emphysema. This is rare but has a high mortality; antibiotics should be started immediately. Surgical repair is rarely required.

Inhaled Foreign Bodies

Inhalation of a FB is a relatively common cause of accidental death in children. Early signs and symptoms include coughing, choking, cyanosis, respiratory distress, noisy or laboured breathing, and unequal chest movement or air entry. The FB is often radiolucent (e.g. coins, plastic, food items), but a CXR may show obstructive emphysema; paired inspiratory and expiratory films show failure of one lung to empty, indicating ball-valve obstruction in that bronchus. Presentation can be delayed, with unresolving pneumonia, consolidation or collapse.

Definitive treatment is removal by rigid bronchoscopy under general anaesthesia or by flexible bronchoscopy under sedation and topical anaesthesia in adults.

Anaesthetic Management of a Child with an Inhaled Foreign Body A senior anaesthetist and surgeon should confirm the diagnosis and assess the urgency and starvation status. Management includes:

- In *extremis*, give 100% oxygen and intubate, consider cricothyrotomy or tracheostomy; a trial of heliox, guided by respiratory effort and oxygen saturation may be useful.
- Inhalational induction is usual, e.g. sevoflurane in oxygen, followed by insertion of i.v. cannula (if not present) and 20 µg/kg atropine.
- Once a deep level of anaesthesia is established, laryngoscopy is performed and the cords and trachea are sprayed with lidocaine 3 mg/kg. Any response to lidocaine administration indicates that anaesthesia is inadequate.
- When ready, a rigid bronchoscope is inserted and a breathing system is attached to its side-arm.

- Anaesthesia is maintained with volatile agent in oxygen or TIVA usually with spontaneous respiration. Alternatively, the child may be paralysed and oxygenated through the bronchoscope.
- Anaesthesia must be adequate to keep the vocal cords relaxed when the FB is withdrawn through them.

Tonsillectomy

The right psychological atmosphere, achieved by whatever means, is of great value in allowing smooth induction of anaesthesia. Preoperative crying and tachycardia increase surgical bleeding. Suitable premedication, especially for fractious children, is 0.5 mg/kg temazepam or 0.2–0.5 mg/kg midazolam syrup. Some advocate oral analgesia preoperatively.

There is greater risk of intraoperative laryngeal spasm, bronchospasm and hypoxia in the presence of a proven upper respiratory tract infection. A higher incidence of profuse bleeding, postoperative chest infection and even cardiac arrest up to 4–6 weeks afterwards has been reported.

Tetracaine (amethocaine) gel or EMLA® cream provides painless venepuncture. Inhalational induction is useful for children who have needle phobia. Parents are warned that either approach may be needed. A south-facing preformed TT is suitable; the Doughty blade on a Boyle–Davis gag keeps it clear of the operative field and it allows access to the adenoids. The anaesthetist must ensure a patent airway when the gag is inserted, by observing and feeling appropriate chest and bag movement and capnography. The tube may kink at the teeth or at the back of the tongue where the gag ends. Either spontaneous breathing or controlled ventilation is acceptable. Removal of the gag can sometimes cause accidental extubation; facilities for re-intubation should be available. In teenagers and adults, a nasal tube can be used. Some anaesthetists use a reinforced SAD for smoother emergence.

Following concerns that the tonsillar bed may contain abnormal prion protein implicated in variant Creutzfeldt–Jakob disease, single-use airway equipment, including the laryngoscope, is recommended, providing patient safety is not compromised.

The patient is placed supine with a shoulder roll. The eyes must be taped. Maintenance intravenous fluid, e.g. Hartmann's, is helpful. Blood loss may approach 10% of blood volume in young children; the haemoglobin should be checked, blood should be grouped and saved or cross-matched if necessary. The cannula should remain in place postoperatively, but fluids are not normally required.

For analgesia paracetamol can be given orally preoperatively (100% bioavailability); intraoperatively either intravenously or by suppository (40 mg/kg). Rectal administration requires parental permission. NSAIDs provide good analgesia and a Cochrane review demonstrated no increase in bleeding, e.g. diclofenac 0.3–1 mg/kg (children older than 6 months) or ibuprofen 5–10 mg/kg. Fentanyl may be administered, if needed, in a dose of 0.25 µg/kg. Dexamethasone (0.1–0.2 mg/kg, up to 8 mg maximum) reduces PONV and may aid analgesia. Topical local anaesthetic in the tonsillar fossae has been described, but is not always beneficial.

Extubation should be deliberately deep or awake; there is no clear consensus and laryngospasm is common. Before extubation, ensure suction of the oropharynx under direct vision. In children, deep extubation is performed in the tonsil position (pillow under the shoulders, semiprone, prevented from rolling onto the face by the pillow and by flexed knees and hips) and this should be maintained until full consciousness is regained. If awake extubation is chosen an oral airway or bite-block should be positioned alongside the TT to prevent occlusion. A 'no-touch' technique, in which no stimulation is given until awakening, appears successful.

Adult tonsillectomy can be performed with a reinforced SAD. These are often painful requiring the use of morphine. If deep extubation is chosen, this can be done in the supine position.

Post-Tonsillectomy Haemorrhage

This has an incidence of 2%–5% in adults but is more common in children. A primary bleed occurs within 24 h; a secondary bleed occurs 5–9 days postoperatively. Surgical intervention is required in only 1%–5% of cases; surgeons may administer diluted 3% hydrogen peroxide gargles and topical epinephrine.

Anaesthesia
- Senior assistance is desirable.
- Ensure the airway is patent; encourage blood to be spat out.
- Ensure good intravenous access: start resuscitation with crystalloid or colloid (20–40 mL/kg initially); obtain cross-matched blood (transfusion is used earlier in children).
- Estimate blood loss: visible blood loss is a fraction of the total; the deficit is at least 20% of blood volume in a shocked child, rising to about 50% if close to circulatory collapse.
- Check the previous anaesthetic chart: note any difficulties, plan for a smaller tube size.
- A reduced dose of induction agent may be required; the blood pressure should be checked frequently.
- The stomach may be full of blood clots: a rapid sequence induction is usual, although some prefer inhalation induction in the lateral position; cricoid pressure and tracheal intubation are used.
- Gastric aspiration before the end of surgery may reduce the risk of postoperative regurgitation.
- Awake extubation is advisable.

Excision of Pharyngeal Pouch

Pharyngeal pouch was first described by Abraham Ludlow of Bristol in 1764; patients may have recurrent chest infections due to aspiration of the contents. The most common operation is endoscopic stapling, but resection through an external neck incision is sometimes necessary.

Tracheal intubation is required with a risk of pouch contents discharging at intubation. Cricoid pressure will not prevent this and handling of the neck should be avoided at this time. If an external approach is necessary, the pouch is packed by the surgeon; a NG will also be placed.

Intravenous fluids are required postoperatively, but recovery after uncomplicated endoscopic stapling is rapid.

Postoperative complications may include oesophageal perforation and rarely mediastinitis.

Thyroidectomy

A total thyroidectomy is performed to treat Graves disease, malignancy or relieve obstructive symptoms from a retrosternal goitre. A hemithyroidectomy may be performed for benign disease or nodules (Chapter 5.4).

Upper Airway Obstruction

Upper airway obstruction may be acute or chronic. Acute obstruction develops over minutes, hours or a few days, whereas chronic obstruction can develop over years. In acute obstruction, symptoms and signs of respiratory difficulty are prominent. In chronic obstruction, when airway narrowing has developed over a period of time, adult patients with a surprisingly narrow airway (about 3.5 mm diameter) may be asymptomatic at rest.

Causes of airway obstruction are seen in Box 5.12.1.

Acute Obstruction

● Acute obstruction – This presents with dyspnoea, anxiety, restlessness, feelings of impending doom and inability to lie flat; these may be associated with a sore throat, dysphagia or dysphonia.
● Signs – There may be swelling of the lips, tongue, floor of the mouth or neck.
● Later signs – Stridor, increased work of breathing: high respiratory rate, dilating alae nasi, rib and intercostal retraction, accessory muscle use,

BOX 5.12.1 Causes of Airway Obstruction	
Outside the tracheal wall	Haematoma, tumour, abscess
Within the tracheal wall	Laryngeal tumour, subglottic stenosis, epiglottitis, vocal cord paralysis, anaphylaxis, angioedema, burns
In the trachea/airway	Foreign body, blood, secretions

upright position, cyanosis, sweating and tachycardia; pyrexia may be present if due to infection.

● Inspiratory stridor indicates extrathoracic pathology; expiratory stridor indicates intrathoracic narrowing.

Management

Patients should be managed in a place of safety: the emergency department, anaesthetic room or HDU. It may be dangerous to send the patient to radiology, especially if they will need to be supine. The surgeons may wish to perform a flexible nasendoscopy. FBs are often radiolucent, but bronchial obstruction is revealed by paired inspiratory and expiratory films where one lung fails to empty in expiration. CT is more commonly performed but this should not delay treatment.

Treatment

● Acute obstruction is treated with 100% inspired oxygen with monitoring.
● Heliox (helium 70%–79%, oxygen 21%) – This reduces work of breathing and improves oxygenation; management must not be delayed to fetch this.
● Nebulized epinephrine (adrenaline) – i.v. in anaphylaxis.
● Dexamethasone 8 mg.
● Chlopheniramine 4 mg i.v. – for anaphylaxis or angioedema.
● Secure the airway by intubation, tracheostomy, emergency cricothyrotomy (needle or surgical) as a final pathway.

Anaesthesia may be needed for removal of an FB or to drain a haematoma or pus. Ludwig's angina is a progressive infection of the submandibular and sublingual spaces, described by Wilhelm von Ludwig in 1836. A senior surgeon and anaesthetist are needed and induction is best performed in theatre with the surgeon scrubbed and ready to perform front of neck access if required.

Anaesthesia options include:

● Preoxygenation (a high-flow technique such as THRIVE works well), i.v. induction with muscle relaxation, videolaryngoscopy and placement of a microlaryngeal tube (MLT)
● AFOI – likely to be very difficult
● Inhalation induction with 100% oxygen and sevoflurane, maintain spontaneous respiration and intubate when deep – really only feasible in children (in adults this can take a long time and be fraught with difficulty)
● Tracheostomy under local anaesthesia
● Where there is no surgeon available for a rapid tracheostomy, consider insertion of a cricothyrotomy needle before induction of anaesthesia or a surgical cricothyrotomy

Chronic Obstruction

Causes of chronic obstruction include benign or malignant tumours, idiopathic subglottic stenosis, inflammatory conditions such as Wegener granulomatosis and progressive scarring secondary to surgery (including previous tracheostomy) or radiotherapy.

There is usually time available to perform CT or MRI of the entire airway and flexible nasendoscopy to identify the degree and site of narrowing. The surgeon and anaesthetist should jointly review the findings, and discuss the management plan for biopsy, debulking or securing the airway.

Airway management options include:

- Intravenous induction, paralysis and direct laryngoscopy (can be followed by placement of a SAD and then jet ventilation (see Microlaryngoscopy)
- AFOI
- Tracheostomy under local anaesthesia

Surgical Tracheostomy

Surgical tracheostomy is indicated for

- Relief of acute upper airway obstruction
- Management of chronic airway obstruction
- Management of airway trauma
- Planned secure airway following head and neck surgery
- In ICU, where prolonged respiratory support is anticipated

Anaesthesia for Surgical Tracheostomy

Percutaneous tracheostomies are frequently performed in ICU; however, if there are anatomical difficulties, a surgical tracheostomy can be done under local or general anaesthesia in theatre. The size of the planned tracheostomy tube and connectors should be checked with the surgeon and scrub team preoperatively. Airway management for general anaesthesia may be challenging due to the underlying condition. Anaesthesia may be intravenous or inhalational, but 100% O_2 should be used before tube changeover. At changeover, the anaesthetist slowly withdraws the TT (guided by the surgeon) until only its tip is visible in the trachea and the surgeon inserts the tracheostomy tube. Correct placement of the tracheostomy tube must be confirmed with capnography before removing of the TT.

Postoperative complications include bleeding, dislodgement, airway obstruction, infection and later trachecutaneous fistula.

Microlaryngoscopy

Microlaryngoscopy involves an examination of the larynx; it may include biopsy or treatment with cauterization or laser to tumours, for subglottic stenosis, glottic webs or vocal cord surgery.

Requirements and issues include:

- Good muscle relaxation of the vocal cords is required.
- Laryngoscopy causes hypertension and tachycardia.
- Lesions can obstruct the airway.

- Airway soiling by blood, debris or smoke must be avoided.
- Topical lidocaine 3 mg/kg on the cords reduces emergence laryngospasm and facilitates extubation; this also requires the patient to be nil by mouth postoperatively for 90 min, postadministration.

Techniques

- Microlaryngeal tube – A cuffed MLT (5.0–6.0 mm) is used through the nose or mouth (consult surgeon). The tube lies posteriorly, so most of the cords can be seen when the surgical suspension laryngoscope is placed. The NMB used depends on the expected duration of surgery but cord immobility is essential; either inhalational or intravenous anaesthesia may be used. This provides good control of the airway, with secure ventilation and prevention of airway soiling.
- Supraglottic jet ventilation – A high-pressure source, connected to a 4 Bar oxygen supply, is attached to a surgical jet needle on the suspension laryngoscope. Ventilation is achieved by an automatic jet ventilator (e.g. Monsoon^{TM}, Mistral^{TM}) or a manual injector (e.g. Manujet III^{TM}). The laryngoscope must be pointed at the larynx and the cords must be paralysed; adequate inspiration and expiration should be confirmed by inspection of chest movement. TIVA is required. This technique provides excellent glottic and tracheal visualization.
- Subglottic jet ventilation – A 4 mm OD uncuffed tube (e.g. Hunsaker®) is placed transglottically and ventilation is achieved by using a high-pressure source (as above). Expiration must be assured to prevent barotrauma; automatic jet ventilators will not provide a positive pressure burst until the tracheal pressure has fallen to baseline reducing the incidence of barotrauma and volutrauma.
- Transtracheal jet ventilation – A transtracheal jet ventilation needle (e.g. Ravussin (VBM GmBh, Sulz, Germany) 13G) is inserted through the cricothyroid membrane or trachea. This technique is used if there is little possibility of supraglottic intubation; there is the risk of bleeding into the airway.

Laser Surgery of the Larynx

Lasers used include carbon dioxide, argon, yttrium–aluminium–garnet (YAG) and potassium-titanyl-phosphate (KTP). The surgeon, using the operating microscope, guides the laser beam to excise laryngeal lesions. Formal protocols ensure safety of the patient and staff.

Anaesthesia is as for microlaryngoscopy, but with the added danger of potentially fatal airway fires. The required triad for an airway fire is:

- Laser energy
- Combustible material, e.g. TT or surgical patty
- Oxygen or nitrous oxide as the oxidant

If fire develops, ventilation should be stopped immediately and the burning tube removed before dousing any remaining burning material with saline.

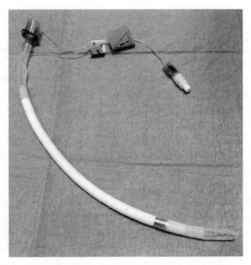

FIGURE 5.12.3   Laser-resistant tracheal tube for laryngeal surgery.

Laser-induced fires are avoided by using a laser-resistant tube (Fig. 5.12.3). Even so, it is wise to reduce the oxidant source by avoiding N_2O and by using a low-inspired oxygen. Alternatively, avoid a tube altogether and use supraglottic ventilation.

Laryngectomy and Neck Dissection

Preoperative Assessment

Coexisting respiratory and cardiovascular disease are common in patients with laryngeal cancer. Assess any narrowing of the laryngeal aperture and signs or symptoms of upper airway obstruction. Review anaesthetic records from any previous biopsy, results of flexible nasendoscopy, and review CT and MRI scans.

Discuss the need for possible blood transfusion, arterial line, nasogastric tube and, if there is concurrent neck dissection prolonging surgery, a urinary catheter. A central venous line should not be placed in the neck and is not needed routinely for simple laryngectomy. The patient must be prepared for a period without speech after surgery. Postoperatively either a specialized ENT ward or HDU bed is usually required.

Anaesthetic Technique

These cases often have a predicted difficult airway. Plan intubation carefully, with a plan B formulated (see chapter 2.6). Good preoxygenation and careful videolaryngoscopy with placement of an MLT or reinforced TT will work if the airway has been carefully assessed. Where there is obstruction to the glottic inlet, an AFOI may be difficult. A tracheostomy under local anaesthesia is rarely required in the elective setting.

Invasive arterial monitoring is indicated for complicated surgery or for radical neck dissection. A large-bore intravenous cannula is useful as blood loss can occasionally be significant; ensure blood is grouped and saved. A shoulder roll and head ring is used; place padded arms by the side, and protect eyes with tape and padding. Protect pressure points, monitor and maintain body temperature and ensure DVT prophylaxis.

Retraction of the carotid sinus during surgery can result in a labile arterial pressure and bradycardia. Atropine and a vasoconstrictor should be readily available. Be aware of the possibility of air embolism.

The airway is interrupted when the larynx is divided from the upper trachea. One-hundred per cent oxygen is given prior to changeover until end-tidal oxygen is about 0.9. Ensure the surgeon has the correct tube and connectors. The oral TT is removed; another is placed directly into the upper trachea and the circuit tubing is moved from the head to the chest. A Laryngectomy (Montandon) tube or an armoured tube should be used avoiding inadvertent endobronchial intubation.

At the end of surgery, a cuffed tracheostomy tube (e.g. Tracoe®, Shiley™ cuffed, unfenestrated) with a standard 15 mm connector is inserted to allow inspired gas to be warmed and humidified and to protect against soiling of the respiratory tract by blood. A fine-bore feeding tube is usually required for nutrition and is placed by the surgeons. Postoperative ventilation is rarely needed. However, a new tracheostomy often causes significant discomfort for the first few days; consider a PCA with regular i.v. paracetamol. Care of the tracheostomy includes humidification and aseptic suction.

More complex procedures including using colon or stomach (gastric pull-up) as pharyngeal replacement operating with general surgery or plastic surgeons may be lengthy and pose additional problems:

- Blood loss is greater, cross-match 4 units of blood; insert arterial and central venous access (usually femoral), urinary catheter and NG tube.
- Bradycardia, hypotension and arrhythmias may occur during mobilization of the oesophagus and transfer of the stomach or colon to the neck.
- N_2O should be avoided.
- Mediastinal contents may be damaged; tracheal rupture can occur which requires immediate endobronchial intubation.
- Analgesic requirements are considerable – consider PCA as well as TAP (transverse abdominis plane) blocks for the abdominal incision.
- Postoperative ventilation may be needed until the patient is warm and stable. Consider a feeding jejunostomy for postoperative nutrition.

Skull Base Surgery

Neurosurgical considerations (Chapter 5.7) apply for these lengthy operations. Facial nerve (VIIth cranial nerve) monitoring may be required. The glossopharyngeal, vagus and accessory nerves (IXth, Xth and XIth) and the hypoglossal nerve (XIIth) may be damaged. Both the jugular vein and carotid artery may be removed at surgery. A lumbar spinal drain may be used. Overnight HDU care is required.

REFERENCES

1. 4th National Audit Project of The Royal College of Anaesthetists and The Difficult Airway Society. Major complications of airway management in the United Kingdom, Report and Findings. London: Royal College of Anaesthetists; 2011.
2. Patel A, Nouraei SA. Transnasal humidified rapid insufflation ventilatory exchange (THRIVE): a physiological method of increasing apnoea time in patients with difficult airways. Anaesthesia 2015;70:323–9.
3. Frerk C, Mitchell VS, McNarry AF, Mendonca C, Bhagrath R, Patel A, et al. Difficult Airway Society 2015 guidelines for management of unanticipated difficult intubation in adults. Br J Anaesth 2015;115:827–48.
4. Leslie D and Stacey M. Awake Intubation. Contin Educ Anaesth Crit Care Pain 2015;15:64–7.
5. Popat M, Mitchell V, Dravid R, Patel A, Swampillai C, Higgs A. Difficult Airway Society Guidelines for the management of tracheal extubation. Anaesthesia 2012;67:318–40

FURTHER READING

Checketts MR, Alladi R, Ferguson K, et al. Recommendations for standards of monitoring during anaesthesia and recovery 2015: Association of Anaesthetists of Great Britain and Ireland. www.aagbi.org/sites/default/files/Standards_of_monitoring_2015_0.pdf; accessed 25.04.2017.
Weingart SD, Levitan RM. Preoxygenation and prevention of desaturation during emergency airway management. Ann Emerg Med 2012;59:165–75.
National Tracheostomy Safety Project www.tracheostomy.org.uk; accessed 24.04.2017.

Chapter 5.13

Plastic Surgery and the Care of Burns

Simon Maguire, Sophie Bishop

ANAESTHESIA FOR BURNS

Burn injuries are an important and preventable global health problem, the World Health Organization estimates that 26,500 people die each year from fire-related burns.[1] The majority are simple burns, which can be managed in the community; however, major burns are systemic injuries requiring specialist multidisciplinary care. Burns requiring hospital admission occur most frequently in the extremes of age, among socio-economically deprived groups, and those with complex medical conditions or psychiatric illness. Burns are usually thermal injuries to the skin and subcutaneous tissue; some important causes of burns and scalds are listed in Table 5.13.1. Burn wound severity is described by percentage of total body surface area (TBSA) burnt and depth. The assessment of burn

TABLE 5.13.1 Some Important Causes of Burns and Scalds

Flame burns
Scalds (hot liquids)
Contact burns (hot solids)
Chemicals (acids or alkalis)
Electrical burns (high and low voltage)
Flash burns
Sunburns
Friction burns
Radiation burns
Burns from lightning strike

TABLE 5.13.2 Depth of Burn

Simple erythema – reversible redness of the skin, typical of sunburn

Superficial dermal – involves only the upper layers of the skin and usually heals within 2 weeks with minimal or no scarring

Deep dermal – involves superficial and deeper layers of skin, without surgery it will usually be associated with delayed healing, usually requires excision and grafting to heal

Full thickness – involves all layers of skin and sometimes underlying tissues; requires excision and grafting to heal

depth will help to determine the need for surgery, guide treatment, and predict outcomes (Table 5.13.2).

Initial Assessment and Resuscitation

Prehospital care starts with stopping the burning process, helping the person to 'drop and roll'. The burnt area should be cooled with tepid water, avoiding hypothermia, and then covered with cling film to reduce both pain and contamination of the wound.

History

The history of injury can provide valuable information about the nature and extent of the burn, probability of inhalation injury and other injuries. A full medical history and drug allergies should be obtained on admission, as this may be the only opportunity. It is important to remember that burns can be associated with other major trauma, if there is a history of an explosion, road traffic accident or jumping from a burning building.

Management

All major burns should be managed initially according to trauma resuscitation guidelines, using a systematic ABCDE approach.

A – Airway with Cervical Spine Control

On arrival, all burn patients should receive 100% oxygen through a nonrebreathing mask. The burnt airway is always at a risk of compromise from airway oedema, which develops with time. Early tracheal intubation should be considered in the presence of any of the following features:

- Stridor
- Hypoxaemia
- Hypercapnia
- Glasgow coma score (GCS) <8

- Deep facial burns
- Full-thickness neck burns

If intubation is done at an early stage, it is usually straightforward, as swelling of the airway has not yet occurred. An uncut tracheal tube (8.0 mm or above) should be used due to the development of orofacial oedema and to allow subsequent bronchoscopy. Suxamethonium is safe in the first 24 h after a burn injury but contraindicated after this due to the risk of hyperkalaemia, which is thought to occur due to the release of potassium from extrajunctional acetylcholine receptors. This risk can persist for up to 1 year. High-dose nondepolarizing relaxants are a safe alternative. If there is any doubt as to airway stability, the airway should be secured earlier rather than later because intubation is likely to become more difficult. Patients who are to be transferred by ambulance to a burns service should have their airway secured before transfer unless there is no risk to the airway.

B – Breathing and Inhalation Injury

Assessment of breathing is important, as there are several ways that a burn injury can compromise respiration.

Inhalational Injury Inhalational injury is defined as the aspiration of superheated gases, steam or noxious products of incomplete combustion. Burns occurring as a result of combustion within a confined space, such as a house or garage, should be assumed to have resulted in an inhalation injury until proven otherwise. Inhalational injury is rarely seen with a flash burn. Signs and symptoms are listed in Table 5.13.3. Inhalational injury significantly increases morbidity and mortality, and resuscitation fluid requirements are increased by up to 50%.

Carbon Monoxide Poisoning Inhalation of the products of combustion may lead to systemic poisoning (CO, cyanide), which can lead to death at the scene. This should be suspected in any unconscious patient, or patients with nausea and

---

TABLE 5.13.3 Signs and Symptoms Suggestive of an Inhalational Injury

- Soot around the face
- Singed nasal hair/eyelashes and eyebrows
- Carbonaceous sputum
- Inspiratory stridor
- Voice changes/hoarseness
- Swollen uvula
- Tachypnoea
- Wheeze
- Carboxyhaemoglobin

vomiting, headache, hypotension and convulsions. Carbon monoxide has 200 times greater affinity for haemoglobin than oxygen; the oxyhaemoglobin dissociation curve is shifted to the left and the cytochrome oxidase system inhibited causing tissue hypoxia and metabolic acidosis. Standard pulse oximeters cannot differentiate between carboxyhaemoglobin and oxyhaemoglobin, giving a falsely reassuring oxygen saturation reading. Poisoning can be detected by measuring carboxyhaemoglobin levels with a reading of more than 15% significant. One hundred per cent oxygen reduces the half-life of carboxyhaemoglobin by a factor of four.

Mechanical Restriction of Breathing Deep dermal or full-thickness circumferential burns of the chest may reduce chest compliance. Escharotomies may be required to allow adequate ventilation, but are rarely needed before admission to a burns centre.

Blast Injury This can result in pneumothoraces, lung contusions, adult respiratory distress syndrome (ARDS).

C – Circulation and Fluid Resuscitation

Wide-bore venous access should be achieved immediately upon arrival at hospital, through unburned skin if possible, and baseline bloods sent. Conventional sites for intravenous access may be unavailable and central venous access is likely to be required. Developing oedema will make intravenous access more difficult with time. If there are signs of immediate hypovolaemic shock, this is unlikely to be the result of the burn and other injuries should be sought. An infusion of warmed Hartmann's solution should be commenced immediately and titrated to cardiovascular signs until the burn calculation is made.

As a general rule, burns of less than 15% TBSA can be managed with oral or intravenous fluid administered at 1.5 times maintenance rate and careful attention to hydration status.

Formal intravenous fluid resuscitation is required for major burns:

- >10% TBSA in children
- >15% BSA or 10% TBSA with inhalation injury in adults

The most commonly used regimen is the Parkland formula (Box 5.13.1).

However, formulae for fluid resuscitation should only serve as a guideline. A urinary catheter should be inserted and hourly urine output used as a guide to

---

BOX 5.13.1 Parkland Formula for Fluid Resuscitation

- 4 mL/kg/(% burn) predicts fluid requirement for the first 24 h after burn injury.
- Half of this volume is given in the first 8 h from the time of injury; the remainder is given over the next 16 h.
- The fluid of choice is currently Hartmann's solution.
- Any delay in beginning fluids should be made up by the end of the first 8 h; fluid already given should be deducted from the calculated requirement.

resuscitation alongside other cardiovascular parameters with the aim to replace intravascular volume in order to preserve tissue perfusion and minimize ischaemia and inflammatory responses.

Example of Fluid Calculation A case of flame burn was admitted at 23:00: male, 56 years old, weighing 70 kg, 45% flame burn. The burn occurred one hour earlier (at 22:00); 1000 mL of crystalloid was already administered by the emergency services.

- *Total fluid requirement for first 24 h:*
  - 4 mL × (70 kg) × (45% TBSA) = 12,600 mL in 24 h.
- *Half to be given in first 8 h, half over next 16 h:*
  - he should receive 6300 mL during 0–8 h and 6300 mL during 8–24 h.
- *Subtract fluid already given and calculate hourly infusion rate for first 8 h:*
  - 6300 mL (fluid for first 8 h) – 1000 mL (fluid already administered) = 5300 mL.
  - Burn injury was at 22:00; therefore, 8-h point is 06:00: 5300 mL needed over next 7 h.
  - 5300/7 = 757 mL/h from 23:00 to 06:00.
- *Calculate hourly infusion rate for next 16 h:*
  - 6300/16 = 393 mL/h from 06:00 to 22:00.

D – Disability

An assessment of the conscious level should be made using the GCS.

E – Exposure Preventing Hypothermia and Burn Estimation

The patient should be examined (including the back, which may require log rolling) to obtain an accurate estimate of the burn area and check for associated injuries. Active warming should be used; patients will lose heat rapidly. Warm airflow blankets and radiant heaters are effective. Ensure jewellery and watches are removed from the burnt limbs. Burns are classified by both the TBSA burnt and depth. The Lund and Browder chart can be used to assess the TBSA. If this is not available, Wallace's 'rule of nines' is useful for estimating the TBSA in adults:

- 18% each for chest, back and legs apiece
- 9% each for heads and arms apiece
- 1% for the perineum

This is quick to apply and easy to remember. Depth assessment is subjective and reassessment in the first 24–72 h will be required, as depth can increase after the injury as a result of inadequate treatment or infection.

Analgesia

Patients are often in significant pain either from burns or additional injuries; analgesia should be provided as soon as possible. Full-thickness burns are painless, but painful partial-thickness burns will also be present; an intravenous opioid such as morphine can be to effect.

Any emergency department may be involved in the initial resuscitation of a burns patient; however, certain injuries should be referred to and managed within a specialist burns unit. Guidance is available (Table 5.13.4) to help decide which burns to refer.[2,3] If in doubt, cases should be discussed with the local burns unit. Transfer of a patient with major burns to a burns unit will require an anaesthetist trained in the transfer of critically ill patients.

Anaesthesia for Burns Surgery

Anaesthesia and surgery for the burns patient should be performed in specialist units with appropriate infrastructure and staff dedicated to, and familiar with the challenges posed by this group of patients. A multidisciplinary approach is necessary with burns surgeons, anaesthetists, intensivists, theatre staff, nurses, physiotherapists, psychologists and pain specialists; the resource use is enormous.

There is a move towards early burn excision (with grafting if possible) to help reduce inflammatory focus and infective risk, but this decision needs careful consideration of the physiologic status of the patient. There are four main reasons for patients with major burns to come to theatre:

- Escharotomy or decompression – typically for circumferential burns or where there is a suspicion of increased compartment pressures (>40 mm Hg)
- Burns excision or skin grafting
- Wound clean and dressing change
- Reconstructive procedures

Preoperative Considerations

This is probably the most important part of the process and will be dictated by the burn area as well as the systemic insult. The main considerations are

---

TABLE 5.13.4 National Burn Care Referral Guidance for Patients with Burn Injuries[2]

TBSA – All burns ≥5% TBSA in children or ≥10% in adults

Depth – Full-thickness burns, circumferential burns

Site – Face, hands, perineum, feet, inhalational injury

Mechanism – Chemical injury, electrical, friction or cold burn

Suspected nonaccidental injury in a child

Other factors – Pre-existing comorbidities which may affect healing of the burn (e.g. immunosuppression and pregnancy), associated injuries (fractures/head injury/crush injuries) and any other burn not healed in 2 weeks

TABLE 5.13.5 Preoperative Considerations

Cardiovascular	Recent trends in heart rate, blood pressure, cardiac output Capillary refill time in nonburned area Inotropic or vasopressor requirements
Respiratory	Airway – facial or laryngeal oedema, exudate or burn on face making facemask ventilation difficult Lung injury, lung compliance, FiO_2 requirement Minute ventilation and PEEP requirements
Haematological	Haemoglobin concentration, assessment of coagulation; ordering of red cells, plasma, platelets or albumin as appropriate
Metabolic	Lactate, base excess; assessment of renal function
Monitoring	Intravenous access (peripheral and central), arterial access, location for ECG electrodes, BP cuff and pulse oximetry
Communication	Discussions with: Patient about postoperative analgesia Surgeons about surgical priorities and to set limits on the procedure, based on blood loss and physiological responses Blood bank regarding the need for products

set out in Table 5.13.5. Discussion with the surgical team should set limits on debridement or grafting in major burns. Particular attention must be paid to the airway, if not intubated, and ventilatory parameters if the patient is ventilated on an intensive care unit (ICU). Many patients often require high levels of PEEP and high minute ventilation, which may have implications for transfer to theatre. Patients will have a systemic inflammatory response to their injury and will often be on vasoactive agents to manage their cardiovascular parameters. It should be noted if these have changed significantly in the previous 6 h in order to gauge how well the patient may tolerate further surgical insult in theatre.

Intraoperative Care

Drugs

Sedative agents used in ICU should be continued in theatre. It is often difficult to assess the depth of anaesthesia in critically ill patients requiring general anaesthesia for surgery, particularly where there are massive fluid shifts or blood loss. We usually continue intravenous sedation (propofol, midazolam, opioid) with the addition of an inhalational agent and further opioids as required. The pharmacokinetics of drugs is altered, partly due to changes in the levels of major drug-handling proteins – albumin (decreases) and α1-acid glycoprotein (increases).

Suxamethonium is considered unsafe, 24 h after any burn, due to the potential for hyperkalaemia. Nondepolarizing neuromuscular blocking drugs are safe but requirements are much greater than in nonburned patients.

Blood Loss

Blood loss can be extensive during major burn excision and grafting but is often difficult to assess as it seeps from a large exposed surface area rather than directly from a blood vessel. A blood loss of 50–100 mL per percentage area excised and grafted should be anticipated. Blood and blood products must be readily available; these patients do not tolerate brisk volume depletion. Regular assessment of haemoglobin concentration and arterial blood gas analysis will aid with the treatment of blood loss and fluid shifts in theatre.

Monitoring

Monitoring can be challenging, as there may be limited skin available for ECG and pulse oximetry. Skin staples can be applied and used as anchors for ECG monitoring with clips attached. Arterial and central venous pressure (CVP) monitoring is usual in major burns and cardiac output monitoring is advisable to guide fluid and inotropic or vasopressor use. Temperature monitoring is essential; all methods to reduce heat loss should be employed, as patients have impaired central temperature control. The theatre temperature should be set at 28–32°C. A loss of more than 1°C should prompt discussions about whether to proceed with surgery, as hypothermia is poorly tolerated.

Analgesia

For less major burns, central neuraxial or major plexus blocks are of benefit for both intraoperative and postoperative analgesia, as well as assisting with physiotherapy in the early postoperative phase.

Postoperative Care

The timing of extubation will depend on many factors including systemic and metabolic injury, the need for further surgery, and any concerns about airway oedema or developing lung injury.

Pain can be a major problem for this group of patients and the input of a multidisciplinary group is required to manage this over the course of what may be several months. Standard opioids are used along with co-analgesics such as anticonvulsants (pregabalin, gabapentin), ketamine, antidepressants (amitriptyline), $\alpha 2$ agonists and benzodiazepines. Nonpharmacological input from pain specialists and psychologists are complementary to this. It must be recognized that all procedures (including dressing changes and line changes) add greatly to ongoing, persistent background pain and distress; procedures should be planned accordingly.

ANAESTHESIA AND FREE TISSUE TRANSFER

Advances in plastic surgical techniques over the last 20 years have enabled surgeons to be more ambitious with reconstructive surgery, now including transplantation of hands and feet. Providing modern anaesthesia for these patients requires an understanding of the physiology of flow and free tissue transfer.

BOX 5.13.2 Flap Classification According to the Type of Tissue Being Transferred

- **Myocutaneous** – lattisimus dorsi (LD), transverse rectus abdominus myocutaneous (TRAM)
- **Fasciocutaneous** – radial forearm, lateral arm, anterolateral thigh (ALT), deep inferior epigastric perforator (DIEP)
- **Osseous** – fibula, forearm, iliac crest

Different types of flaps are used according to the defect that needs repairing and these are classified according to the type of tissue being transferred (Box 5.13.2).

Free tissue transfer involves moving a section of tissue with its blood supply to another location. This free vascularized tissue will have certain important properties: it will be subject to ischaemia (from clamping at its origin until the anastomoses are completed and flowing), it will have no lymphatic drainage (and therefore subject to interstitial oedema), and it is denervated.

Flap failure is devastating for patients and can be due to a number of factors as outlined in Table 5.13.6.

Early recognition of problems and intervention can reduce flap failure. Monitoring the flap is essential and staff caring for these patients must be able to recognise an ischaemic flap postoperatively. This includes flap colour, temperature, capillary refill time, skin turgor and bleeding after skin piercing. If the problem is arterial (inflow) the flap is pale, cool with a slow capillary refill time. If the problem is venous (outflow) the flap is warm, congested with a brisk capillary refill time and rapid bleeding on pinprick. Regular assessments of blood flow can be also be made by using a Doppler probe over the flap.

General Principles

There are general principles which are common to anaesthesia for these procedures. It is essential to ensure good forward flow with adequate cardiac output

TABLE 5.13.6 Factors that May Influence Flap Failure

Factor	Example
Blood supply	Ischaemia or reperfusion injury There is some evidence that remote ischaemic conditioning (RIC) may improve flap survival
Mechanical	There may be tension at the anastomosis or kinking of the vessels due to positioning within the wound
Infection	Local or generalized sepsis
Blood clot	Arterial or venous Anticoagulants have been used to help reduce these

and blood pressure. Flow to the flap should be considered in light of the Hagen–Poiseuille equation as below:

$$Q = \frac{\pi P r^4}{8\eta l}$$

where:
Q = flow in L/s
P = pressure in Pa
r = radius of the tube in m
l = length of the tube in m
η = viscosity in Pa/s

Consequently manipulation of the pressure gradient across transplanted tissue, vessel radius and blood viscosity should improve flow through the flap.

The patient should be kept warm, well hydrated with a low or normal haematocrit and consideration given to avoiding vasoconstriction. There is a relationship between blood viscosity, haematocrit and oxygen transport to the tissues with an optimal haematocrit in this setting of approximately 30%–35% (Fig. 5.13.1).

Preoperative Assessment

A thorough preoperative cardiovascular and respiratory assessment must be performed including an assessment of the patient's ability to tolerate a prolonged procedure. There should be a realistic discussion about surgical and anaesthesia expectations and a plan for postoperative pain management. The patient must be encouraged and supported to stop smoking preoperatively to improve chances

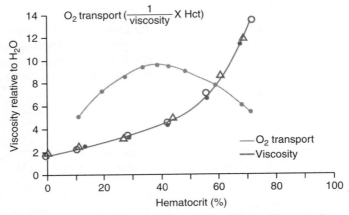

FIGURE 5.13.1   Relationship between blood flow and haematocrit.

of flap survival. They should be on an enhanced recovery pathway with high calorie preoperative drinks and meticulous attention to thromboprophylaxis.

Intraoperative Care

The theatre environment should be warm, including the anaesthetic room with fluid warmers and hot air body warming devices for the nonsurgical areas.

The duration of surgery is often very long. Consequently anaesthesia technique is usually a combination of remifentanil and desflurane or total intravenous anaesthesia (TIVA). Remifentanil provides good intraoperative analgesia, allows rapid control of blood pressure and when combined with desflurane a prompt recovery. Invasive arterial monitoring is recommended; additional monitoring includes a urinary catheter, skin: core temperature gradient measurement and cardiac output monitoring, typically oesophageal Doppler. Central venous access can be useful if peripheral access is limited by the surgical field.

These are often long procedures and diligent fluid management is essential. Fluid overload must be avoided (oedema is not good for a flap) whilst maintaining an adequate preload and an appropriate cardiac ouput. Mean arterial pressure should be considered and maintained in the light of pre-induction level with hourly measurements of urine output. Hypotension should be avoided and can be treated by a combination of fluids and low-dose vasopressors. There has traditionally been a reluctance to use vasopressors due to the theoretical risk of flap vasoconstriction and failure, but their use is common and has been shown to have no effect on the incidence of flap failure.[4]

Careful positioning is essential to avoid pressure sores or peripheral nerve damage. It is worth being fastidious about having an hourly check and documentation of pressure areas. If possible passive movement of the limbs during the procedure should be performed.

Postoperative Care

Postoperative care should continue in a similar manner with a warm environment, monitoring of urine output, mean arterial pressure and haematocrit and flap monitoring as described above. There is no place in modern anaesthetic practice for routine postoperative ventilation if surgery and anaesthesia have proceeded according to plan.

REFERENCES

1. Burns. www.who.int/mediacentre/factsheets/fs365/en/; [accessed 10.07.2016].
2. National Burn Care Referral Guidance. www.britishburnassociation.org; 2012 [accessed 1.07.2016].
3. http://www.ameriburn.org/BurnCenterReferralCriteria.pdf; [accessed 15.12.2016].
4. Kelly DA, Reynolds M, Crantford C, Pestana IA. Impact of intraoperative vasopressor use in free tissue transfer for head, neck, and extremity reconstruction. Ann Plast Surg 2014;72: S135–38.

Chapter 5.14

Thoracic Anaesthesia

Gregory McAnulty

Thoracic procedures include those performed on structures within the pleural cavity, within the mediastinum and on the chest wall including the ribs and costal cartilages, which are external to the pleural cavity.

Most operations on structures within the pleural cavity are facilitated by isolation of the lung on the nonoperative side. This allows ventilation while the lung of the operative side is collapsed to improve operative exposure. Purulent secretions may also be prevented from soiling a healthy lung, and an air leak through a bronchopleural fistula may be controlled. Many procedures, including major lung resection, may be accomplished thoracoscopically.

Operations within the mediastinum are accessed via one or other pleural cavity, or from the root of the neck, thereby avoiding the need for lung collapse.

The majority of procedures are for the diagnosis and treatment of malignancy. Other indications include correction of pectus deformities, open reduction and external fixation of rib fractures, bullectomy, cervical sympathectomy and pleurodesis or pleurectomy for recurrent pneumothorax.

Data from the Thoracic Surgery Registry (UK)[1] indicates that the frequencies of specific operations performed as a percentage of all thoracic procedures were:

- Open pneumonectomy, 1.5%
- Open partial lung resection (including lobectomy), 15%
- Mediastinoscopy and mediastinotomy, 8%
- Video-assisted thoracoscopic surgery (VATS) lobectomy, 6%
- VATS lung wedge resection, 10%
- Oesophageal resection and other oesophagogastric surgery, 1%
- VATS pleural procedures (including drainage, pleurodesis and pneumothorax surgery), 21%
- Miscellaneous bronchoscopic and gastroscopic procedures, 8.5%

ASSESSMENT OF PULMONARY FUNCTION AND ANAESTHETIC RISK

Patients in whom lung resection is proposed should have pulmonary function tests (PFTs). PFTs are more useful for the prediction of postoperative dyspnoea than mortality.

The decision to deny surgery should not be made solely on the basis of pulmonary function tests. Equally, surgery that renders a patient with insufficient respiratory capacity and an inability to clear secretions by coughing is not desirable. Patients with severe respiratory insufficiency can be further compromised by smoking-related cardiovascular disease as well as the procedure itself.

Assessment of Pulmonary Function

Preoperative evaluation of patients for lung resection should include an assessment of:

- Respiratory mechanics
- Parenchymal function
- Cardiopulmonary reserve

Spirometry measures dynamic lung volumes and provides information about airway resistance. Common measurements obtained are forced vital capacity (FVC) and forced expired volume in 1 s (FEV_1). A reduced FVC with preserved FEV_1/FVC ratio (>70%) indicates a restrictive pattern. A reduced FEV_1/FVC ratio indicates an obstructive pattern. Patients with a preoperative FEV_1 in excess of 2 L (>80% predicted) generally tolerate pneumonectomy, whereas those with a preoperative FEV_1 greater than 1.5 L tolerate lobectomy.

The diffusion capacity of the alveolar membrane is measured using carbon monoxide as a marker gas (transfer factor for lung carbon monoxide; T_{LCO} alternatively D_{LCO}). Values may be low despite normal spirometry. T_{LCO} should be measured in all patients who do not have normal spirometry and exercise tolerance. Measurements are usually reported as a percentage of values predicted for normal individuals of equivalent height and sex. Patients with preoperative results for FEV_1 and T_{LCO} that are more than 80% predicted do not require further assessment.

The risk of postoperative dyspnoea may be estimated by calculating the predicted postoperative values of PFTs. This is done by multiplying the measured values by the proportion of total lung volume (usually expressed as lobes) remaining after resection. A value as low as 30% of predicted may be acceptable. Predicted reductions in FEV_1 are not well correlated with T_{LCO} and are often overestimated. Poor PFT measurements can be tolerated by patients in whom surgery less than pneumonectomy is proposed or in whom an improvement can be expected following surgery, e.g. relief of airway obstruction by a tumour.

Patients with reduced FEV_1 (<1.5 L lobectomy; <2 L pneumonectomy) and predicted postoperative values of PFTs less than 40% should undergo assessment of cardiopulmonary function. Formal cardiopulmonary exercise testing (CPET) is the 'gold standard', but the stair climbing test is an acceptable alternative. A VO_2 max of 20 mL/kg/min (ability to climb approximately five flights of stairs) is not associated with any increased risk of complications or death. A VO_2 max of less than or equal to 15 mL/kg/min (less than three flights) is associated with a high risk of complications or death. A VO_2 less than or equal to 10 mL/kg/min (one flight) is associated with a very high risk (40%–50%) of postoperative death and nonsurgical treatment should be considered.

Arterial blood gas parameters, PO_2 less than 8 kPa (60 mm Hg) and PCO_2 higher than 6 kPa (45 mm Hg), have been used as cut-off values for pulmonary resection. Hypercapnia is not predictive of complications after resection, particularly if patients are able to exercise adequately. Oxygen saturation of less than 90% while breathing air at rest or desaturation by more than 4% from the baseline during exercise is associated with a higher risk of postoperative complications.

Assessment of Anaesthetic Risk

Thirty-day in-hospital mortality following thoracic surgery is low. Pneumonectomy for primary malignancy carries a mortality risk of 5%–6%, open lobectomy or bilobectomy approximately 2% and VATS lobectomy 0.7%–1.1%.[1]

Mortality risk can be estimated using the thoracoscore.[2] Thoracoscore is a mortality risk calculation tool based on correlates of cardiopulmonary reserve, age, sex, ASA classification, WHO performance status, dyspnoea score, extent of surgery, presence of malignancy, number of comorbidities and surgical priority.

ANAESTHETIC CONSIDERATIONS
Open Pneumothorax and Lung Collapse

The lungs are normally kept inflated by the difference between atmospheric pressure in the alveoli and the negative pressure (about -5 cm H_2O) in the potential space between the two layers of pleura. This balances the elastic recoil of the lung and the tendency of the chest wall to spring outwards.

If the integrity of the thoracic cavity is breached, the negative pressure is lost and the elastic recoil causes collapse of the lung on that side. The mediastinum, unless fixed by adhesions, shifts towards the other side, compresses the healthy lung and interferes with cardiac function. If the lung is adherent to the chest wall, these effects may not be marked. The lung collapse causes ventilation–perfusion (V/Q) mismatch, shunting, hypoxia and a high pulmonary vascular resistance in the collapsed lung. Spontaneous respiration is possible with an open hemi-thorax, but it is inefficient because only the lung on the nonoperative side expands with diaphragmatic contraction. The inspired gas for this lung comes partly from the trachea and partly from the lung on the operative side (effectively increasing dead space). This transfer of gas from one lung to the other is known as pendelluft and can be lethal. These problems are overcome with intermittent positive-pressure ventilation (IPPV) facilitated by endobronchial intubation and isolation of the nonoperative lung.

Endobronchial Instrumentation/Intubation

In adults, double-lumen endobronchial tubes are routinely used if isolation of one lung is required. Other techniques are also described below.

Double-Lumen Endobronchial Tubes

A variety of tubes have been developed to allow isolation of one lung and independent ventilation of either. They all have the essential feature of having two separate tubes, bonded together, one of which extends beyond the distal end of the other.

The longer tube has a cuff which, when correctly placed in one or other main bronchus, can be inflated to isolate that lung. This cuff is slotted or narrow, angulated and fixed just proximal to a hole in the endobronchial segment to allow ventilation of the upper lobe in most right-sided tubes. Tubes are designed to align with normal anatomy and are specifically designated for either right or left endobronchial intubation because the angle at which the right main bronchus continues from the carina is steeper than that of the left. The design also takes into account the usual shorter distance from the carina at which the upper lobe bronchus branches from the main bronchus on the right. The shorter tube is designed to open in the trachea just above the carina. A cuff proximal to the opening of this shorter tube is inflated to seal the trachea.

Tubes are manufactured in a range of sizes suitable for small to large adults and are variations on modifications (by Robertshaw and others) of the original design by Carlens. Anatomical limitations to satisfactory placement of double-lumen tubes include the laryngeal inlet (limits the diameter of tube), angulation of the carina and distance from the carina and orientation of the origin of the upper lobe bronchus. Tube size selection may be facilitated by an algorithm based on the patient height and sex.[3]

Many anaesthetists prefer to position a left-sided endobronchial tube for most procedures (other than left pneumonectomy) due to its greater stability within the longer left main bronchus. Confirmation of position using a flexible fibreoptic bronchoscope is advocated by many, especially if a right-sided tube is employed, to confirm correct side placement and bronchial cuff position (the proximal end of which should be level with the carina). The maintenance of correct cuff positioning should be reconfirmed after final patient positioning. Paediatric flexible fibreoptic instruments allow visualization through the endobronchial lumen and may be useful if ventilation of the upper lobe is in doubt.

A disposable double-lumen tube with an integral high-definition camera mounted next to the tracheal opening is available.[4]

A double-lumen tube is inserted through the laryngeal inlet under direct vision with the aid of a laryngoscope. Holding the tube so that the endobronchial part curves upwards facilitates this. Once the tip of the tube is through the cords, it is rotated approximately 120° towards the side of proposed endobronchial intubation, while the patient's head is turned in the opposite direction. A flexible bronchoscope or other suitable video imaging device may be used to identify the carina and main bronchi. A sequence for checking correct placement clinically is as follows:

- Step 1 – the tracheal cuff is inflated slowly until a seal is obtained while both lumina are employed to inflate the lungs. Bilateral breath sounds at the apices are auscultated.
- Step 2 – the tracheal catheter mount is occluded or clamped, its lumen opened to air and the endobronchial side ventilated. The endobronchial cuff is slowly inflated until no gas is heard escaping via the tracheal lumen. Unilateral breath sounds are auscultated on the appropriate side, including the apices.
- Step 3 – step 2 is repeated, except that the endobronchial side is occluded and the tracheal lumen ventilated.

Unilateral breath sounds and high inflation pressures in Step 1 usually indicate that the tube is inserted too far and both lumina are in a main bronchus. Absent apical breath sounds and high inflation pressure in Step 2 suggest that the endobronchial cuff is distal to or occluding the upper lobe bronchus.

A flexible bronchoscope may be used to ensure that the endobronchial cuff is placed just distal to the carina and, if it is a right-sided tube, that the opening of the upper lobe bronchus is not obstructed.

Most operations other than left pneumonectomy can be performed using a left-sided double-lumen tube. Although some anaesthetists prefer to use a double-lumen tube on the nonoperative side, others advocate the use of left-sided tubes in all except where there is a contraindication. Although it is easier to insert a right-sided double-lumen tube into the correct main bronchus, a left-sided tube is more stable and less likely to obstruct the upper lobe.

Endobronchial Blockers

Specifically designed balloon-tipped bronchial blockers are available and positioned with the aid of a flexible bronchoscope. They are either incorporated into a specialized single-lumen tracheal tube or require an adapted catheter mount with a port for a fibreoptic bronchoscope and a fixation device for the blocking catheter. Blockers have a lumen that allows the application of suction but are too small for the passage of a suction catheter. Balloon inflation is observed directly with the bronchoscope and the apex and base of the lung to be isolated are auscultated for the absence of breath sounds. Intra-operative collapse of the lung on the operative side is best achieved by opening the breathing circuit to air on opening of the chest with the patient paralysed. The balloon is then inflated either under direct vision with a bronchoscope or with the volume of air required to seal the main bronchus on initial positioning.

Endobronchial Intubation in Infants and Children

Lung isolation improves access for complex minimally invasive procedures. The smallest conventional double-lumen tubes are 26Fr (approximately 8.7 mm OD). These may be appropriate for children older than 8 years. In young children and infants, single-lumen tubes are most commonly used and may be advanced into one or other bronchus (rotating the bevel away from the right upper lobe bronchus may reduce the chance of it being obstructed). Smaller double-lumen tubes have been described as techniques involving the insertion of two separate single-lumen tubes.

One-Lung Ventilation

Traditionally, the same minute-volume used in two-lung ventilation was applied to the single lung with an increased inspired oxygen concentration. However, overinflation of the ventilated lung may induce barotrauma and volutrauma by producing unacceptable shear forces in the pulmonary tissue, resulting in postoperative acute lung injury (ALI), whereas high-inspired oxygen concentration may be associated with atelectasis, resulting in V/Q mismatching.

A protective one-lung ventilation strategy is associated with a reduced incidence of ALI and atelectasis with fewer intensive care unit (ICU) admissions and shorter hospital stay. This approach involves:

- Inspired oxygen concentration as low as acceptable
- Pressure control ventilation – peak inspiratory pressure less than 35 cm H_2O, tidal volume less than 8 mL/kg body weight with relatively higher ventilatory rate and beginning inspiration at FRC
- Permissive hypercapnia
- Positive end-expiratory pressure (PEEP) 4–10 cm H_2O
- Restricting pressures during re-inflation to less than 30 cm H_2O
- Frequent recruitment manoeuvres to avoid atelectasis

As an alternative, high-frequency oscillatory ventilation (HFOV) is associated with small tidal volumes, higher mean airway pressure and maintenance of a constant airway pressure. HFOV improves oxygenation but does not improve mortality.

Problems with Endobronchial Tubes and One-Lung Ventilation

- Difficulty with insertion, especially if the anatomy is abnormal or distorted. Double-lumen tubes are larger in diameter and of different conformation than conventional tracheal tubes. Laceration of endobronchial or tracheal cuffs by the patient's teeth during intubation is common, particularly with plastic tubes.

- Dislodgement – during positioning of the patient, movement of the head and neck and from surgical manipulation of the bronchus and trachea.
- Trauma – to the larynx and airways.
- Hypercapnia – seldom a problem in practice.
- Arterial hypoxaemia during one-lung anaesthesia – a higher fractional inspired concentration of oxygen (F_iO_2) is generally employed. Collapse of the upper lung and hypoxic pulmonary vasoconstriction increase its vascular resistance. Nonetheless, blood does flow through this collapsed lung and the shunt causes hypoxaemia, which is little improved by ventilation with 100% oxygen. The lower lung will be at a disadvantage too because its FRC will be reduced, with some atelectasis.

The problem can be helped by:

- Encouraging collapse of the nonventilated lung with suction or surgical manipulation
- Avoiding circumstances which promote atelectasis in the ventilated lung (prolonged ventilation with 100% oxygen, absence of PEEP, disconnection)
- Cautious application of PEEP, which can improve oxygenation in severe hypoxaemia, but may divert blood to the upper lung and reduce cardiac output, thereby worsening hypoxaemia
- Insufflating, intermittently inflating, applying continuous positive airway pressure (CPAP) or using high-frequency jet ventilation (HFJV) in the collapsed lung; in some cases, relative hypoxia may have to be tolerated because frequent re-inflation of the lung on the operative side may prolong and hinder surgery, which may present a greater risk to the patient
- Clamping the pulmonary artery when a pneumonectomy is performed

Resistant hypoxaemia may be a result of upper lobe obstruction due to too distal positioning (or migration, especially after patient positioning) of the endobronchial tube.

Pulmonary Secretions

Excessive secretions are uncommon, but occur in lung abscess, bronchiectasis, bronchopleural fistula and tumours and when infected secretions lie distal to an obstructed bronchus. Improvement may be obtained by preoperative postural drainage and antibiotics. Methods for preventing the spread of secretions into healthy parts of the lungs during surgery include the following:

- Endobronchial intubation (the most usual solution), where the healthy lung is isolated with inflatable cuffs
- Regular tracheal suction, especially after the position is changed or the lungs manipulated

- Surgical clamping of a bronchus as soon as the chest is open
- Avoiding general anaesthesia so that the cough reflex is preserved, for example drainage of empyema under local anaesthesia
- Posture – a drainage or an antidrainage posture may be employed during positioning for surgery

PRINCIPLES OF ANAESTHESIA FOR THORACOTOMY

Median sternotomy is used for access to the thymus, retrosternal goitres and anterior mediastinum; lateral thoracotomy or VATS is used for most other thoracic operations.

Endobronchial intubation is usual other than for operations on midline structures. However, many procedures (including lung resection) can be performed without this, but this requires a degree of surgical cooperation and experience. Ventilation using high-frequency oscillation (HFOV) or HFJV can provide effective oxygenation and carbon dioxide removal in the presence of an open hemi-thorax and where bronchial integrity has been breached (such as a bronchopleural fistula). This may be an option if lung isolation is not possible or desirable.

Pre-Operative Considerations

Premedication is not necessary for thoracotomy. An opioid or anxiolytic may be used, but care must be taken to avoid postoperative respiratory depression.

Patients with coexisting cardiovascular disease will require careful monitoring, but for patients undergoing open thoracotomy, invasive arterial and central venous pressure monitoring is usual anyway. Placing a radial arterial line and large-bore venous cannula in the forearm of the operative side avoids the problems of compression in the lateral position. A central venous catheter is normally inserted into the internal jugular vein of the operative side. Unless otherwise indicated, arterial and central venous cannulae are appropriately inserted after induction.

Analgesia

A functioning thoracic epidural, with the catheter tip positioned between T4 and T6 vertebrae and infusate of local anaesthetic mixed with a lipid-soluble opioid such as fentanyl, provides excellent postoperative analgesia, but an increase in mortality has been observed.[5] The combination of an intrathecal opioid, a percutaneously or intra-operatively inserted paravertebral catheter with postoperative infusate of local anaesthetic and PCA is also effective.

Nonsteroidal anti-inflammatory drugs (NSAIDs) may be prescribed in younger patients without contraindications.

Intra-Operative Considerations

Positioning

Most lung resections are performed in the lateral position. Care must be taken to avoid injuries due to pressure on the dependent arm or leg. The brachial plexus may be injured by traction on the upper arm.

Opening the Pleural Cavity

The use of a double-lumen tube or bronchial blocker will allow ventilation of the isolated nonoperative lung. The operative side lung should fall away from the chest wall. This may be delayed if there is severe COPD, or if the operative side main bronchus is obstructed by secretions or an incorrectly placed tube.

Bronchial Stapling or Suturing

Bronchial stapling/suturing is usually performed with the bronchus clamped. Use of a double-lumen tube gives control of the opposite lung and helps the anaesthetist test the bronchial stump for leaks.

Intra-Operative Hypotension

Cardiovascular instability is common during lung resection. Pressure on and distortion of the heart and great vessels may cause reduced cardiac output and arrhythmias. Vasopressors are frequently required and, occasionally, defibrillation or cardioversion. For this reason, central venous access and ensuring the proximity of a defibrillator (with internal paddles) is prudent. Hypovolaemia must always be considered even when other causes are identified.

Blood Loss

Blood loss may be considerable, but it is unusual for most lung resections. At least one large-bore cannula is essential. A central venous catheter allows venous pressure monitoring and more rapid delivery of vasopressors if required. Frequent measurement of blood loss is essential and consideration of the contribution of operative field wash volumes must be taken into account.

Closure of the Chest

If a lobectomy or pneumonectomy has been performed, the bronchial stump is normally tested for leaks. Warmed water is poured into the hemi-thorax and the operative side inflated with a continuous pressure of 20–25 cm H_2O. If no bubbles are seen, the lung is re-isolated, intrapleural drains are placed and the chest wall is sutured. The lungs should be fully expanded just before closure. The drain or drains are connected to an underwater seal, a Heimlich flutter valve and bag or an automated electric pump system.

Accidental Pneumothorax

A contralateral pneumothorax during thoracotomy may occur during mediastinal dissection or during bilateral procedures. Occlusion of chest drainage after
chest closure in the presence of a continuing air leak from the lung may cause
a pneumothorax on the operative side. It is a risk during any operation near the
pleura or where local blocks are performed in the region of the thorax (brachial
plexus block, intercostal nerves). It may be a cause of cardiovascular collapse
and be difficult to diagnose. Radiography may be useful, but often presents a
logistical challenge. Rapid insertion of a chest drain may be required to exclude
the possibility of a contralateral pneumothorax in the event of an otherwise
unexplainable haemodynamic instability.

Post-Operative Considerations

Most patients should be extubated and allowed to breathe spontaneously after
thoracic procedures. After any pulmonary resection, positive pressure ventilation places stress on the bronchial suture line.

Post-Operative Hypoxaemia

Atelectasis, sputum retention, poor pain relief and fluid overload may all contribute to postoperative hypoxaemia. Patients who have undergone a thoracotomy will require oxygen in the immediate postoperative period for up to 24 h
and chest physiotherapy. Pneumothorax should be excluded. A chest X-ray is
routine in recovery after all thoracotomies.

Cardiac Arrhythmias

Intra-operative nonsustained arrhythmias during lung resection and operations
on mediastinal structures are relatively common. The most common cardiac
arrhythmia postoperatively is atrial fibrillation (AF), the incidence of which is
18%–20% and peaks at day 2. Risk factors for postoperative AF include age
older than 59 years, male sex, intrapericardial pneumonectomy and elevated
preoperative B-type natriuretic peptide (NT-proBNP). Anti-arrhythmic prophylaxis is advocated for patients at high risk of postoperative AF, but can result in
hypotension, bradycardia and rarer complications. Patients already prescribed a
β-blocker should not have the drug discontinued abruptly preoperatively.

Torsion of Remaining Lobe

Torsion of the remaining lobe may occur after lobectomy. The presentation
may be insidious and can occur up to 2 weeks postoperatively. Chest X-ray
shows increased density of the affected lobe, which is engorged. Resection of
the affected lobe is usual.

Herniation of the Heart

Removal of pericardium together with lung resection, particularly on the
right, may allow the heart to be displaced from the mediastinum. Cardiovascular

collapse is usually profound. Chest X-ray may be diagnostic. Emergency re-exploration is required. It also may occur after traumatic pericardial rupture.

SPECIFIC OPERATIONS

Diagnostic Procedures

Bronchoscopy

Rigid Bronchoscopy

The principles of anaesthesia for rigid bronchoscopy are:

- To maintain oxygenation and CO_2 removal during the procedure
- Hypnosis and reduction of autonomic response
- Muscle relaxation to allow passage of the scope and to facilitate the conduct of tracheal and endobronchial manipulations

Total intravenous anaesthesia is commonly employed (using propofol and remifentanil or other short-acting opioids), but inhalational techniques can be used, either by using a ventilating bronchoscope (which has the proximal end sealed by a removable eyepiece and a side-arm that connects to an anaesthetic breathing system) or, less ideally, by using intermittent ventilation via a tube inserted into the open proximal end of a conventional rigid bronchoscope.

Muscle relaxation is obtained with a short-acting neuromuscular blocking drug.

Ventilation is normally maintained by the intermittent use of a high-pressure gas injector via a cannula attached to the proximal end of the bronchoscope, which is directed distally. This creates a Venturi, which entrains air into the bronchoscope. The chest and abdomen are observed as a monitor of adequate tidal volume. Care must be taken that the tubing is firmly attached to the injecting cannula because injury can occur if the injector tubing comes adrift. HFJV is an alternative, particularly if endoscopic procedures are undertaken.

Rigid bronchoscopy in infants and young children is performed using an inhalation technique and a ventilating paediatric scope which should be of a size to allow a small leak of gas through the cords.

At the end of the procedure, the bronchoscope is removed and the pharynx carefully suctioned. Ventilation is maintained with a bag and face or laryngeal mask, anaesthesia is discontinued and muscle relaxation reversed if a nondepolarizing agent has been used. The patient is normally recovered in a sitting position. Nebulized epinephrine (adrenaline; 2 mL, 1:1000 solution), intravenous dexamethasone and CPAP via a tight-fitting mask may help alleviate postprocedure laryngospasm.

Flexible Fibreoptic Bronchoscopy

Fibreoptic bronchoscopy is usually performed under topical anaesthesia and sedation with midazolam or diazepam. Opioids may be used in addition, but apnoea must be avoided. Local anaesthetic agents may inhibit bacterial growth in microbiological cultures.

A flexible fibreoptic scope may be passed via a tracheal tube or laryngeal mask airway under general anaesthesia. The diameter of the tube must be large enough to provide adequate ventilation as well as smooth passage of the instrument, and should be checked before induction. The bronchoscope will partially occlude the tracheal tube and impair ventilation, which may be a particular problem in children. A 3.6 mm diameter paediatric scope will reduce the cross-sectional area of a 5 mm internal diameter tube by almost 50%.

Removal of an Inhaled Foreign Body

Removal of an inhaled foreign body is most common in children and from the right lung. An inhaled foreign body is usually removed via a rigid bronchoscope under inhalation or total intravenous anaesthesia. Respiratory obstruction may be present and can act as a valve so that a segment of lung becomes hyperinflated. These cases can be dangerous and need experience.

An inhalational induction and maintenance of spontaneous ventilation may reduce the risk of further hyperinflation.

Oesophagoscopy

Relaxation of the postcricoid sphincter is needed for rigid oesophagoscopy and is achieved using muscle relaxants or deep anaesthesia. Suction should always be available. The anaesthetic technique should allow rapid return of reflexes. At the end of the procedure, the pharynx must be sucked clear of blood, etc. and, if not intubated, the patient turned on the inside. Otherwise, extubation after the return of protective reflexes is usual.

In obstructive lesions, regurgitation may occur from a dilated oesophagus above the lesion. Rapid sequence induction and intubation should be used.

Rigid oesophagoscopy may cause trauma, perforation and bleeding after biopsy or with oesophageal varices. Flexible oesophagoscopy has much less stimulation and may be performed under light sedation. Where aspiration of blood or gastric contents is a risk, rapid sequence induction with intubation of the trachea is advised.

Mediastinoscopy

Mediastinoscopy is performed in the supine position with a single-lumen tracheal tube. If a mediastinoscopy is planned to precede thoracotomy, a single-lumen tube should be employed first and then changed because a double-lumen tube may reduce the surgical access. In patients with obstruction of the superior vena cava and the trachea, an armoured tracheal tube may be considered. Haemorrhage can be considerable and may necessitate sternotomy.

Intrathoracic Surgery

Pneumonectomy

A right pneumonectomy removes 55% of the patient's lung tissue, and if the function of the remaining lung is compromised, the patient will be in a precarious position postoperatively. A lateral approach is usual, but prone or supine positions may also be used. Endobronchial intubation with a double-lumen tube is usual. Alternatives are a single-lumen tube (with or without a bronchial blocker) or a double-lumen tube of the same side as the operation, both of which may present a problem if the main bronchus is resected close to the carina.

Suction should not be applied postoperatively to pleural drains, which should be clamped. Intermittent transient release of the clamp (e.g. no more than 1 min every 1 h) reduces the risk of mediastinal shift, which should be suspected in the event of postoperative cardiovascular instability. Some surgeons prefer not to employ pleural drains after pneumonectomy to avoid this complication.

Arrhythmias (mostly AF) are the most common postoperative complication. Respiratory failure (due to pneumonia, bronchopleural fistula, acute respiratory distress syndrome and pulmonary aspiration) accounts for almost 60% of 30-day mortality.[6]

Serial chest X-rays are obtained to monitor a progressive rise in the fluid level in the pneumonectomy space. The time to complete obliteration is variable and may take months. Early surgical emphysema is common and is often a result of fluid accumulation forcing air into the tissues, rather than disruption of the bronchial stump. Bronchopleural fistula is a rare (<1%), but serious complication may be caused by bronchial stump dehiscence, generally as a result of infection. If very early (within 4 days of surgery), it is more likely to be due to a mechanical failure of the suture line and resuturing is more often successful. It should be suspected if a formerly rising fluid level in the pneumonectomy space is seen to fall on chest X-ray, especially if accompanied by fever and the production of purulent sputum.

The uncommon postpneumonectomy syndrome is caused by excessive lateral shift of the mediastinum into the empty hemi-thorax, most commonly after right pneumonectomy. It presents with dyspnoea and recurrent respiratory infection, which may occur weeks or even years following surgery. It may be treated by the insertion of a stabilizing prosthesis.

Lobectomy

One or (in the case of the right lung) two lobes may be resected. A VATS technique, which appears to have lower postoperative complication rates, shorter length of hospital stay and equivalent 5-year survival than thoracotomy, is used increasingly frequently. Lung isolation with a double-lumen tube is necessary for good operating conditions, but, unless a pneumonectomy is considered as a possibility, the side of the tube is a matter of anaesthetic choice.

Lobectomy is occasionally indicated for the treatment of benign conditions which are usually infective. It may also be indicated for the control of vascular abnormalities. Bronchiectasis may be associated with a large sputum load and care must be taken to avoid contamination of the normal lung.

Postoperative air leak (from lung rather than bronchus) is usually minimal but occasionally large and prolonged. Chest drains are routine and should not be clamped. Kinking or blockage of a chest drain where there is a continuing air leak can result in a tension pneumothorax and should be looked for in the event of postoperative haemodynamic instability.

Lung Volume Reduction Surgery

The principle is to reduce lung volume by resecting the worst-functioning lung tissue, allowing better function from the remaining lung tissue and improved pulmonary and diaphragmatic mechanics. Surgery is recommended for patients who are breathless and have a single large bulla on computed tomography (CT) scan and FEV_1 less than 50% predicted, or those who have severe COPD and are receiving maximal medical therapy and have measured FEV_1 and T_{LCO} more than 20% predicted, PCO_2 less than 7.3 kPa and predominantly upper lobe disease.[7]

VATS is frequently employed. Median sternotomy may be appropriate for bilateral procedures. Bilateral procedures may be accomplished sequentially, but care must be taken to avoid kinking of the dependent chest drain during the resection of the second side. The operated lung may not deflate readily due to small airway obstruction.

Postoperative analgesia with a thoracic epidural is recommended, but an intrathecal opioid may pose less risk and be as effective.

Lung Bullae and Cysts

A large bullus can compress surrounding lung tissue and may have a valvular communication with a bronchus, allowing gas to pass in more easily than out. Intermittent positive-pressure ventilation and coughing may therefore cause further distension or even a tension pneumothorax. Early isolation of the bullus from ventilation with a double-lumen tube or bronchial clamp is desirable. If bullae are bilateral, HFJV may be considered to minimize barotrauma.

Nitrous oxide may distend bullae because of its much greater solubility than nitrogen and should be avoided. Care is required to distinguish between a tension pneumothorax and distension of a bullus.

Pulmonary hydatid cysts are common in sheep-rearing communities. They can be bilateral and multiple and need excision if they become large. They may erode the bronchial wall and become infected. Preoperative treatment with a helminthicide and the use of swabs soaked in 1% formaldehyde or hypertonic saline solution avoids dissemination of the disease during manipulation.

Endobronchial intubation is indicated.

Bronchopleural Fistula

An abnormal communication between the intrathoracic respiratory system and the pleural cavity may be caused by trauma, neoplasm or infection, or arise congenitally, e.g. bullae, tracheo-oesophageal fistula. Most present after pneumonectomy, especially if right-sided, and are associated with a high morbidity and mortality. Consequences include:

● Gas leak from the lung (usually small) which may make ventilation impossible

- Collection of fluid in the pleural cavity or postpneumonectomy space which may flood the bronchial tree

If surgical repair is contemplated, isolation of the remaining lung is preferred. Following gas induction, a double-lumen tube should be inserted to isolate the opposite lung, maintaining spontaneous respiration until this is achieved. An alternative option is endobronchial intubation with an uncut single-lumen tube positioned with the aid of a fibreoptic bronchoscope, but the cuff may occlude the upper lobe bronchus. Awake endobronchial intubation may be considered. A bronchial blocker inserted into the bronchial stump may easily be pushed through the weakened suture line.

HFOV or HFJV may be valuable in compensating for a large volume gas leak.

Lung Abscess and Drainage of Empyema

Lung abscesses may be caused by aspiration, obstruction by tumour or spread from elsewhere. The vast majority respond to antibiotics alone. Radiologically guided drainage may be required. Surgery is occasionally necessary. Preoperative postural drainage, positioning so that the affected part of the lung is dependent at induction, and rapid isolation of the lung on the unaffected side may protect it from soiling with infected material.

Operations more extensive than simple drainage, such as rib resection for empyema, and those in children require general anaesthesia. The presence of a possible bronchopleural fistula will normally require a double-lumen tube. Awake intubation under local analgesia in the sitting position should be considered with a large fistula or empyema.

Other Intrathoracic Operations

Mediastinotomy

The mediastinum may be approached lateral to the sternum through the second intercostal space with the patient supine for biopsy of lymph nodes in the aortopulmonary window. As the pleural cavity is opened, endobronchial intubation will allow collapse of the lung on the operative side. Adjacent vascular structures have the potential to bleed catastrophically.

Wedge Resection, Segmental Lung Resection, Open Lung Biopsy

Isolation of the lung on the operative side greatly facilitates segmental lung resection and open lung biopsy. Thoracotomy is required where the procedure cannot be performed thoracoscopically.

Pleurodesis and Pleurectomy

Pleurodesis may be performed by instilling talc or other irritant into the pleural cavity after drainage of a recurrent (frequently malignant) pleural effusion during thoracoscopy.

Recurrent pneumothoraces are treated in the same way or with pleurectomy (with or without excision of an apical bullus). Whether performed thoracoscopically or (more rarely) as an open procedure, lung isolation is preferred. The recurrence rate is low and similar whether talc pleuradesis or pleurectomy is used.

Postoperative pain can be severe. Analgesia should be provided by a combination of local anaesthetic blocks, PCA and regular simple analgesics. NSAIDs should be avoided, as they impair the desired inflammatory response.

Decortication

Decortication is frequently a difficult and bloody procedure carried out on a patient who may be compromised by chronic infection. Haemorrhage may be a problem. Keeping the lung inflated can aid surgery. Postoperative ventilation may be necessary, but it is best avoided because a significant postoperative air leak is common. Observation in an ICU may be appropriate.

Anterior Mediastinal Masses

Most mediastinal masses arise from the organs which pass through the mediastinum, such as trachea, oesophagus, heart and great vessels. Mediastinal masses include thymic tumours, neuroendocrine carcinomas, germ-cell tumours, lymphomas, neurogenic tumours, endocrine tumours (thyroid and parathyroid tumours) and mesenchymal tumours. The majority of mediastinal tumours are benign, but 59% of the anterior superior masses are malignant.

Occasionally, mediastinal masses cause severe distal airway compression and may present a challenge to ventilation until the mass is removed. Awake fibreoptic intubation is often advocated.

Retrosternal Goitre

A retrosternal goitre may compress or distort the trachea. The surgical approach is often via median sternotomy and establishment of femoro-femoral bypass before induction may be indicated. Postoperative tracheal collapse with respiratory embarrassment is rare.

Thymectomy

The surgical approach for thymectomy is transcervical or via a median sternotomy, when one or both pleural cavities may be opened. Thymic tumours are rare, but thymic tumour or dysplasia is present in the majority of patients with myasthenia gravis. Removal may improve symptoms. A thoracoscopic approach may be possible; in which case, a double-lumen tube will be needed for lung isolation. Haemorrhage may be significant and large-bore venous access is essential.

Tracheal, Oesophageal and Chest Wall Surgery

Tracheal Stenosis and Tracheal Trauma

Tracheal stenosis may necessitate preoperative tracheal dilatation to allow passage of a tracheal tube with inflation of the cuff beyond the operation site. Rare complete tracheal rings present a considerable challenge, and homograft replacement of the segment may be considered. In tracheal trauma, placement of the tracheal tube under bronchoscopic control may be necessary. Cardiopulmonary bypass may be necessary in some cases.

Insertion of tracheal stents is managed with a rigid bronchoscope and high-pressure gas (Sanders) injector or HFJV. A bronchoscope can be used to place catheters for HFJV beyond an obstruction, although a free outflow for the gas must be provided to prevent lung distension.

The use of the neodymium–yttrium–aluminium–garnet (Nd–YAG) laser is associated with the risk of airway fire and special precautions must be taken. This includes limiting F_iO_2, using low-ignition tubes (or avoiding them altogether by jet ventilation through a rigid bronchoscope) and filling tracheal tube cuffs with saline.

Oesophagogastrectomy

The patient's general condition is often poor, owing to the lack of nutrition. Assessment and treatment to correct nutritional and electrolyte deficiencies are therefore important. A short period of enteral nutrition (or parenteral if needed) preoperatively may be of great benefit. The operation may be long and bloody and may involve opening the abdomen as well as the thorax. A minimally invasive approach to oesophagectomy may have benefit in terms of speed of recovery, 1-year survival and quality of life. Lung isolation is required for both open and minimally invasive thoracoscopic techniques. A trans-hiatal approach makes this unnecessary.

Although a thoracic epidural undoubtedly provides excellent postoperative analgesia, there is little evidence that this improves the outcome. A paravertebral catheter placed surgically may be of at least equivalent efficacy.

Pectus Correction

A relatively small proportion of patients with pectus excavatum undergo surgical correction. Surgery is undertaken towards the end of the pubertal growth spurt. Lung function should be assessed preoperatively. Intra-operative blood loss may be dramatic. Postoperative pain control may be difficult. The metal bar is removed after 6 months or so. A minimally invasive approach is now widely employed.

Lung Transplantation

Survival after lung transplantation is disappointing compared to that following heart transplantation. The International Society for Heart and Lung

Transplantation reported that the 30-day mortality in the period between 2003 and 2013 was 3%. Over the same period, 1-year survival was 88%, while 3-year survival was 61%.[8] Only a third of patients are alive 10 years after a transplant. The majority of transplants are of single lungs, but double-lung (either single lungs sequentially or as a block) and heart–lung block procedures are also performed. There is a growing interest in live donation of lung tissue, but as yet this is confined to a few centres.

Anterolateral thoracotomy in the lateral position is the standard approach for single-lung transplantation. Bilateral procedures are normally performed via a median (occasionally transverse) sternotomy. *En-bloc* procedures and, often, the second of sequential single-lung transplantations are performed using cardiopulmonary bypass.

The transplanted lung has neither normal lymphatic drainage nor autonomic innervation, and postoperative pulmonary oedema is a risk. The lowest left ventricular filling pressure compatible with adequate tissue perfusion is the target for fluid replacement.

Lung transplant recipients frequently require endobronchial or tracheal procedures to treat stenoses and tracheo- or broncho-malacia related to the airway anastomosis.

Anaesthetic Technique

Assessment of potential lung transplant recipients involves a multidisciplinary team. Assessment of the right ventricular function and the detection of pulmonary hypertension are particularly important. Severe emphysema requires care to avoid postoperative overdistension of the remaining lung in single-lung recipients. Nitrous oxide is avoided because air may remain in the graft vasculature after anastomosis.

Full invasive monitoring is established before induction. A pulmonary artery catheter is normally placed before induction, but may need to be withdrawn into its sheath before pneumonectomy. Patients may be haemodynamically unstable and difficult to ventilate adequately. Large-volume blood loss should be anticipated because pleural adhesions are common. Antifibrinolytics may be employed.

Problems

Problems of lung transplantation include:

- Haemorrhage as adhesions are separated
- Pulmonary hypertension when the pulmonary artery is clamped, in which case cardiopulmonary bypass will be needed
- Postoperative accumulation of lung water due to ischaemia before implantation, denervation and section of lymphatic drainage in new lung

THORACIC AORTIC ANEURYSM AND DISSECTION

Diseases of the proximal aorta often present acutely. The most common are aneurysmal dilatation and dissection of the media. Treatment is usually a combination of medical, endovascular and surgical strategies. Endovascular and surgical treatment still carries a high mortality and appears to be better in high-volume centres.[9]

Medical treatment aims to reduce shear forces in the vessel wall, usually with β-blockers unless contraindicated. Statins may have additional benefit. Repair of an aneurysmal ascending aorta is recommended if the diameter is more than 50 mm in patients with Marfan syndrome and more than 55 mm in others. Thresholds may be less if there are additional risk factors or aortic valve disease.[9] Depending on the pathology, the entire ascending aorta including the valve may be replaced, re-implanting the coronary arteries into the graft. It may be possible to resuspend the native valve. If the aortic root is not dilated, a graft above the sinotubular junction may be all that is required. Deep hypothermic circulatory arrest at 18°C may be employed to perform the proximal anastamosis.[9]

Thoracic endovascular aortic repair (TEVAR) has a lower peri-operative mortality and neurological complication rate than open surgery for descending aortic aneurysms but probably does not have a longer term benefit. Patients frequently have significant comorbidities. Consultation with the surgical team is needed to ensure that access is not obstructed by arterial and venous lines.

THORACIC TRAUMA

Chest trauma is often associated with multiple other injuries. Multiple rib fractures are increasingly managed with internal fixation which is associated with improved pain control and reduced need for mechanical ventilation.

Thoracic injuries can be classified as:

● Penetrating – stab, gunshot, etc.
● Nonpenetrating – blunt chest trauma, deceleration injury, barotrauma and blast injury

Nonpenetrating injuries may be associated with contusions of the myocardium, rupture of the thoracic aorta, tracheal and bronchial rupture, pulmonary contusions, oesophageal injury (rare) and diaphragmatic rupture, which may be easily missed. Hypovolaemia, hypoxia and obstructive circulatory failure due to blood loss (which may be concealed), pulmonary contusion and tension pneumothorax or cardiac tamponade may be life-threatening.

Airway obstruction or rupture, tension or open pneumothorax, flail chest, massive haemothorax and cardiac tamponade must be identified or excluded in the initial assessment of an unstable patient. A chest X-ray should be obtained early. CT scanning is indicated if there is a suspicion of complex injury. Arterial blood gases will help guide decisions to intubate and ventilate and monitor resuscitation and ventilatory management. Intubation and ventilation is indicated for the management of persisting of worsening hypoxia or hypercarbia, for the management of an associated severe head injury, for anaesthesia to facilitate transfer and for the management of other injuries and in the frail or confused. Positive pressure ventilation may exacerbate a pneumothorax causing tension and may produce instability in a hypovolaemic patient or if there is cardiac tamponade.

Pneumothorax

Spontaneous Pneumothorax

Spontaneous pneumothorax is primary (PSP) or secondary (SSP) depending on the underlying lung disease. However, most PSPs are associated with apical blebs or bullae and are more common in smokers. If symptomatic, intervention with aspiration or chest drain is indicated. Surgical intervention is indicated if the air leak is persistent or the lung fails to re-expand after drainage. Open thoracotomy may have a slightly better cure rate than VATS (1% vs. 5%). Other indications for surgery are:

- Recurrent ipsilateral pneumothorax
- Subsequent contralateral pneumothorax
- Concurrent bilateral spontaneous pneumothorax
- Associated haemothorax
- Professions at risk, e.g. pilots, divers
- Pregnancy (although less invasive management is usually adequate until after delivery)

Tension Pneumothorax

This should be considered in ventilated patients, after trauma and in patients with lung disease, especially acute asthma and chronic obstructive pulmonary disease, who have a sudden deterioration in vital signs. Patients receiving positive pressure ventilation (including noninvasive) are at risk of rapid deterioration. Patients are generally tachypnoeic, tachycardic and cyanotic. Breath sounds are usually reduced on the side of the pneumothorax, but other classical signs (tracheal deviation, hyperexpansion and hyper-resonance) may not be present. Treatment is with oxygen and urgent needle decompression using a 14G cannula inserted into the second intercostal space in the anterior clavicular line. If a hiss of air is not heard, the cannula should be re-inserted at the fifth intercostal space anterior axillary line or a chest drain rapidly placed. Formal chest drain insertion should follow.

Haemothorax

A diagnosis of haemothorax is based on the history and clinical examination. The origin of the bleeding includes punctured lung, tears of the internal mammary artery, injury to the great vessels and injury to the intercostal vessels.

Initial treatment of haemothorax is oxygen, a chest drain and analgesia. The decision to proceed to thoracotomy is based on an assessment of rate and total volume of bleeding associated with injury, as follows:

- Shock or cardiac arrest with suspected correctable intrathoracic lesion
- Specific diagnosis (e.g. penetrating cardiac or blunt aortic injury)
- Evidence of ongoing thoracic haemorrhage (drainage of 1000–1500 mL initially, >250 mL in the first hour or >1500 mL in first 24 h after the insertion of chest drain)

Cardiac Tamponade

Cardiac tamponade should be suspected in a patient with a raised systemic venous pressure (may be difficult to interpret in hypovolaemia), hypotension, pulsus paradoxus (reduction of >10 mm Hg of systolic pressure in inspiration without a change in the diastolic pressure), tachycardia or respiratory distress and a history of:

- Recent cardiac surgery
- Cardiac instrumentation
- Blunt or penetrating chest trauma
- Malignancy
- Connective tissue disease
- Renal failure
- Septicaemia
- Treatment with cyclosporin, anticoagulants or thrombolytics

Electrical alternans or nonspecific change in ST segment and/or T wave morphology may be seen on the ECG. A chest X-ray may show an enlarged heart shadow with clear lung fields.

Echocardiography may be diagnostic, but posterior tamponade can be missed on transthoracic views. If in doubt, transoesophageal echocardiography is indicated.

Pericardiocentesis is necessary to relieve tamponade in the rapidly deteriorating patient, but surgery is the definitive treatment (see Chapter 5.2).

Rupture of Descending Aorta

Traumatic rupture of the descending thoracic aorta usually occurs at the level of the ligamentum arteriosum. The adventitia holds the aorta in place; consequently, control of arterial pressure is critical. Invasive arterial monitoring (right radial will normally reflect the pressure in the aorta proximal to the injury) and administration of hypotensive agents may delay complete rupture. A CT scan, transoesophageal echocardiography or an arch aortogram is necessary to define the extent of the injury.[9] Surgical access is greatly facilitated by isolation and collapse of the left lung. Patients frequently have other serious injuries.

Endovascular repair is associated with lower postoperative mortality and fewer ischaemic spinal episodes.

REFERENCES

1. The SCTS Thoracic Surgery Audit Group. The Thoracic Surgery Registry Brief Report. Audit Years 2011-12 to 2013-14. http://www.scts.org/professionals/audit_outcomes/thoracic.aspx.

2. Falcoz PE, Conti M, Brouchet L, Chocron S, Puyraveau M, Mercier M, et al. The Thoracic Surgery Scoring System (Thoracoscore): risk model for in-hospital death in 15, 183 patients requiring thoracic surgery. J Thor Cardiovasc Surg 2007;133:325–32.

3. McAnulty G, Van Den Dyck J, Ogilvie E. Double lumen size selection: a model based on audit of successful and failed double lumen tube placement: 19AP9–3. Eur J Anaesth 2010;27:268.

4. Massot J, Dumand-Nizard V, Fischler M, Le Guen M. Evaluation of the double-lumen tube Vivasight-DL (DLT-ETView): a prospective single-center study. J Cardiothor Vasc Anesth 2015;2:1544–9.

5. Powell ES, Cook D, Pearce AC, Davies P, Bowler GM, Naidu B, et al. A prospective, multicentre, observational cohort study of analgesia and outcome after pneumonectomy. Br J Anaesth 2011;106:364–70.

6. Powell ES, Pearce AC, Cook D, Davies P, Bishay E, Bowler GM, et al. UK pneumonectomy outcome study (UKPOS): a prospective observational study of pneumonectomy outcome. J Cardiothor Surg 2009;4:41.

7. National Institute for Health and Care Excellence. Chronic obstructive pulmonary disease in over 16s: diagnosis and management. NICE Clinical Guideline 101. London: NICE; 2010. https://www.nice.org.uk/guidance/cg101.

8. Cypel M, Levvey B, Raemdonck D, Erasmus M, Dark J, Love R, et al. International Society for Heart and Lung Transplantation donation after circulatory death registry report. J Heart Lung Transplant 2015;34:1278–82.

9. Erbel R, Aboyans V, Boileau C, Bossone E, Bartolomeo RD, Eggebrecht H, et al. 2014 ESC guidelines on the diagnosis and treatment of aortic diseases. Eur Heart J 2014;35:2873–926.

FURTHER READING

Slinger P, editor. Principles and practice of anaesthesia for thoracic surgery. New York: Springer; 2011.

Chapter 5.15

Anaesthesia in Unusual Environments

Daniel Martin

ABNORMAL AMBIENT PRESSURE ENVIRONMENTS

Atmospheric Pressure

We are surrounded by air that makes up our atmosphere. This air forms an imaginary column above us that possesses a mass and is compressible. The SI unit for pressure is Pascal (Pa), and the atmospheric pressure at sea level is approximately 101 kPa, which is equivalent to 1.01 bar, 1013 mbar, 760 mm Hg or 14.7 pounds per square inch. Normally, there are only minor fluctuations in atmospheric pressure as a result of the Earth's weather systems. However, for those individuals choosing to ascend to high altitude or dive underwater, significant alterations in the surrounding pressure can have a dramatic effect on their physiology and ultimately threaten their survival.

Hypobaric Environments

High Altitude

Atmospheric pressure declines exponentially with increasing altitude; it is just over 50% of the sea level value at the base camp of Mount Everest (5300 m) and 33% at the mountain's summit (8848 m). There is also a decline in air temperature with altitude, known as adiabatic lapse rate. At the Armstrong limit or line (about 19,000 m), atmospheric pressure is 6.3 kPa, and at body temperature, this is the pressure at which free water boils spontaneously. Contrary to popular belief, the concentration of oxygen remains constant throughout the atmosphere, right up to the point at which the earth's atmosphere ends: the Karman line (about 100 km above sea level). However, the declining pressure and fixed concentration results in a decline in the partial pressure of oxygen (PO_2) at high altitude. This is described by Dalton's law of partial pressure, which states that the partial pressure of a gas in a mixture is governed by its fractional concentration multiplied by the atmospheric pressure:

$$PO_2 = PB \times FIO_2$$

Where: PO_2 = partial pressure of oxygen; PB = barometric pressure; FIO_2 = fractional concentration of oxygen

The decrease in PO_2 at high altitude affects the oxygen carriage throughout the body, resulting in hypoxaemia (a lack of oxygen in arterial blood) and a reduction in maximal exercise capacity, making exercise at high altitude feel more exhausting than at sea level. Visitors to high altitudes can also succumb to altitude-related illnesses such as acute mountain sickness (AMS), high-altitude pulmonary oedema (HAPE), and high-altitude cerebral oedema (HACE). The process of acclimatization leads to adaptation to the hypobaric hypoxia at high altitude over a period of days to weeks. Hyperventilation, tachycardia and polycythaemia contribute to restoring normal convective oxygen delivery over time.

Life-long exposure to high altitude can lead to the development of chronic mountain sickness (Monge's disease) in some individuals, a syndrome of excessive erythrocytosis, severe hypoxaemia, and pulmonary hypertension.[1]

Anaesthesia in a Hypobaric Environment

Approximately 140 million people live at an altitude of over 2500 m and each year approximately 35 million people travel to altitudes above 3000 m. Hospitals exist in a number of high-altitude areas around the world, so the delivery of care in this environment deserves consideration. Hypoxic respiratory drive at altitude is vital, and consequently respiratory depression from anaesthetic agents and opioids can be more problematic than at sea level. Where possible, patients who are not fully acclimatized should be transferred to a lower altitude.

The potency of anaesthetic gases is directly proportional to their partial pressure (rather than concentration) and this is important to consider at high altitude. It means that as the barometric pressure declines, the partial pressure (but not concentration) of the anaesthetic gas will fall, and therefore its potency will lessen. Minimum alveolar partial pressure (MAPP) is therefore more useful to consider than minimum alveolar concentration (MAC).[2]

Oxygen

At 5300 m, the barometric pressure is 54 kPa, which results in an atmospheric PO_2 of 11.1 kPa. Thus, at high altitude, patients are more likely to be hypoxaemic than at sea level, supplementary oxygen will have less of an effect, and more oxygen will need to be administered to achieve normoxaemia. At least 40% oxygen should be administered during anaesthesia and recovery at high altitude, and titrated to oxygen saturation. High-flow venturi mask systems may deliver marginally more oxygen than specified due to the lower pressure difference between the atmosphere and the negative pressure created by the jet of oxygen issuing from the nozzle.

Nitrous Oxide

Like all anaesthetic gases, potency of nitrous oxide (N_2O) is reduced at high altitude because of the decline in its partial pressure. This is such that at 3000 m, the analgesic effect of entonox (50% N_2O: 50% O_2) is minimal. Furthermore, as N_2O has a MAC of more than 100% at sea level, it has very little value as an anaesthetic agent above 3000 m given its reduced potency and the fact that more than 40%–50% oxygen will be required to maintain normoxaemia.[3]

Anaesthetic Vaporizers

Saturated vapour pressure alters with temperature, but it is unaffected by atmospheric pressure. Therefore, at a given dial setting, the partial pressure (and mass) of vapour delivered is the same whatever the altitude. However, because the density of the carrier gas is reduced at high altitude, the vapour concentration is increased. Splitting ratio is minimally affected by changes in barometric pressure. Hence, the clinical anaesthetic effect from a given dial setting is similar for all altitudes, assuming the ambient temperature is maintained constant.

Gas and Vapour Analysers

Gas and vapour analysers respond to specific properties of the gas or vapour being monitored and measure the number of its molecules, which is its partial pressure.[4] Calibration is conventionally in percentage units, in line with clinical practice at sea level. Care must be taken to interpret concentrations correctly at high altitude. For example, at 5300 m, where barometric pressure is half its sea level value, the concentration of oxygen in dry air is 20.9% (as at sea level), but its partial pressure is only 11.1 kPa. The analyser would read 11.1% oxygen if it did not compensate for the reduced barometric pressure. This is also the case for vapour analysers, all of which are responsive to partial pressure. Similar confusion may arise with capnographs if they have been calibrated in percentage at sea level.

Cylinder Pressure Gauges

Cylinder pressure gauges are reliable at altitude because the reduction in atmospheric pressure is minimal compared to cylinder gas pressure.

Flowmeters

Flowmeters (rotameters) will underestimate the actual gas flow delivered at high altitude. Gas density is proportional to atmospheric pressure; therefore, it declines with increasing altitude. At high flow rates, the space around the bobbin acts like an orifice, the flow through which is inversely proportional to the square root of the gas density, and hence of atmospheric pressure.[2] The error is approximately 20% at 3000 m. It should affect all gases equally, but this may not be true at lower flows, where laminar flow around the bobbin is governed by viscosity. Inspired oxygen monitoring is essential to ensure adequate delivery of oxygen to the patient. Respiratory peak flow meters are also inaccurate at high altitude for the same reason.

Hyperbaric Environments

Diving

Underwater, barometric pressure increases linearly by 101.3 kPa (1 atm) for every 10 m gain in depth. This increase in pressure is linear because, unlike air, water is not compressible. At 40 m depth, the pressure is therefore 5 atmospheres absolute – four underwater plus one for the atmosphere above it. Sports divers breathe compressed air to a depth limit of 40 m using self-contained underwater breathing apparatus (SCUBA). A gas mixture is inhaled through a regulator at the pressure surrounding the diver. Thus, as diver descends deeper, the gas partial pressures increase as the ambient pressure increases. At 40 m, if breathing air, the inspired PO_2 is 101 kPa, the equivalent of 100% oxygen at sea level. Dives deeper than this require different gas mixtures to avoid the hazards outlined below:

- Nitrogen narcosis – This syndrome consists of disorientation, euphoria, hallucinations, and impaired psychomotor and intellectual function. The threshold for toxicity in divers varies between individuals, but the effects are more pronounced at greater depths limiting SCUBA divers to less than 50 m. Replacing nitrogen in the gas mixture with the less lipid-soluble gas helium delays (but does not eradicate) the onset of narcosis, allowing divers to descend to even greater depths.
- Oxygen toxicity – At depths below 60 m, the partial pressure of oxygen in an air mixture can cause oxygen toxicity. The central nervous system is most vulnerable to this, usually presenting with visual disturbances, dizziness, seizures and unconsciousness.
- Decompression illness – Prolonged diving while breathing air at depth from SCUBA apparatus results in nitrogen dissolving into the bloodstream. If ascent following a dive is too rapid, this dissolved gas comes out of solution to form bubbles that may damage tissues and organs by causing emboli. This is known as decompression illness (DCI) or the 'the bends'. The treatment for DCI is hyperbaric oxygen therapy (HBOT) within a hyperbaric chamber.

Hyperbaric Oxygen Therapy

When breathing 100% oxygen at sea level, the dissolved oxygen concentration in blood is about 0.3 mL/dL; at 3 ATA (ATA is a term used to define the amount of pressurization used within a hyperbaric oxygen chamber and refers to atmospheres of pressure), this increases to 6.2 mL/dL, which exceeds the arteriovenous difference at rest (5 mL/dL) and therefore satisfies tissue oxygen demand.[5] This substantial increase in dissolved oxygen load can be of therapeutic value. Aside from the treatment of divers with DCI, HBOT is of value in the treatment of limb ulcers secondary to diabetes. It is also recommended for the treatment of severe carbon monoxide poisoning and life-threatening venous air or gas embolism. For the latter two conditions, it may be necessary to manage anaesthetized critically ill patients within a hyperbaric facility. This requires considerable skill and experience from the team involved.

Anaesthesia in a Hyperbaric Environment

Careful consideration is needed before undertaking anaesthesia in a hyperbaric environment. If HBOT is for carbon monoxide poisoning, both a primary and secondary survey of the patient are essential to ensure that there are no other injuries. Unstable critically ill patients should not be treated in a hyperbaric chamber; the enclosed space and restricted access may result in harm if problems arise. Inhalational anaesthetic agents should be avoided, as gas-scavenging systems are not possible in this environment and so an intravenous anaesthetic technique is preferred. Bradyarrhythmias have been reported in patients during compression, particularly in haemodynamically unstable critically ill patients.

Oxygen Toxicity

Increasing the ambient pressure in a hyperbaric chamber raises the PO_2 and this is further exacerbated by providing patients with 100% oxygen to breathe during a treatment. With a chamber at 3 ATA, and a patient breathing 100% O_2, the PO_2 is likely to be at least 240 kPa; this leads to a huge increase in tissue oxygenation.[6] Neurological oxygen toxicity can lead to grand malconvulsions, thought to be more common in critically ill patients. The incidence can be reduced by giving air breaks during treatments. A typical hyperbaric treatment lasts 90–120 min at between 2 and 3 ATA and includes air breaks of 5 min every 30 min.

Barotrauma

Increasing ambient pressure can damage eardrums in patients unable to equalize sufficiently (as may be the case when anaesthetized). Some centres advocate myringotomies in unconscious patients prior to HBO.

Changes in Air Temperature and Density

Raising ambient pressure increases the temperature, whereas rapid ascent (decompression) lowers the temperature. The gas breathed at depth has a higher heat capacity and is also of increased density, increasing the work of breathing. This should be borne in mind during anaesthesia in a hyperbaric chamber.

Equipment

Most standard anaesthetic equipment does not have the safety rating to be used in hyperbaric chambers. Spark generation or heat production increases the risk of fire in a high oxygen environment. In addition, it is likely that the equipment will malfunction or work incorrectly. Ventilators specifically designed for hyperbaric use are available. These are calibrated to work accurately at depth, and produce the correct tidal volumes.

The use of defibrillation in a hyperbaric chamber is controversial; equipment specifically designed for this purpose must be used. Monitoring is essential with appropriately approved equipment. Because of the change in gas volume that occurs when ambient pressure is altered (due to Boyle's law), it is advisable to fill the endotracheal cuff with water rather than air to avoid a cuff leak on descent.

REMOTE ENVIRONMENTS IN A HOSPITAL SETTING

Although austere wilderness environments are a clear challenge to an anaesthetist, there are remote areas within every hospital setting that provide their own unique challenges. Remote can be thought of as any location where an anaesthetist is required to provide anaesthesia or sedation away from the main theatre suite, where it cannot be guaranteed that help is immediately available. Examples include the radiology department, lone operating theatres, areas where electroconvulsive therapy (ECT) is provided, and the emergency department. The key to providing safe anaesthesia in these areas is self-reliance and preparation. Anticipation of problems, and having plans to resolve them, helps to alleviate the stress of working in these situations. Familiarity with the environment and facilities available is essential; visiting and assessing the area prior to providing anaesthesia can alleviate many potential hazards. A trained anaesthetic assistant must be present, preferably one familiar with that working environment. Clear communication is essential when working in a remote setting, as without this, simple problems can escalate into life-threatening scenarios. The conduct of anaesthesia should follow local and national guidelines for monitoring and safety. Being distant from the main operating department does not mean than safe practice can be disregarded.

Anaesthesia for Electroconvulsive Therapy

ECT is used to treat medication-resistant depression.[7] It is frequently administered in a remote location to elderly patients with significant comorbidity. The quality of anaesthesia can impact the effectiveness of the treatment; it must be of adequate depth without affecting treatment efficacy. During ECT, an electrical current is applied transcutaneously to the brain via electrodes placed on the skull, producing a tonic clonic seizure lasting up to 2 min. There is an initial parasympathetic stimulation, resulting in bradycardia and hypotension followed by more prolonged sympathetic activity producing tachycardia and hypertension. Arrhythmias are not uncommon and myocardial oxygen consumption increases; myocardial ischaemia can occur. Care must be taken in elderly patients or those with known coronary artery disease.

A thorough pre-assessment is essential, taking note of previous anaesthetic technique and drug doses. Relative contraindications for ECT include poorly controlled congestive cardiac failure, unstable coronary artery disease, recent stroke, untreated phaeochromocytoma, and an unstable fracture. Patients with a pacemaker should have it temporarily converted to fixed rate pacing and implantable defibrillators should be temporarily deactivated.

The patient should be starved and pre-oxygenated; tracheal intubation is unnecessary unless there are risk factors for gastric aspiration. It is important to insert a bite block to protect the patient's lips and tongue during the convulsion. Most induction agents affect seizure threshold; propofol is the commonest drug used in modern practice. A second shock may be required to achieve the required length of seizure; further boluses of induction agent may be required. A short-acting opioid can be useful in reducing the dose of induction agent required. A small dose (0.5 mg/kg) of suxamethonium is usually given. Hyperventilation should be avoided, as hypocarbia can lower seizure threshold and prolong the seizure time. If the seizure lasts longer than 3 min, it should be terminated.

Patients may be agitated or confused in the immediate postictal state. Mild headache and nausea are relatively common. Complications such as fractures or dislocations are now rare.

Anaesthesia for Magnetic Resonance Imaging

The magnetic resonance imaging (MRI) scanner poses two main challenges to an anaesthetist; its remote location and the strong magnetic field that can affect anaesthetic and monitoring equipment.[8] The strength of the magnetic field generated by the superconductors declines exponentially with distance from the magnet and Gauss lines are used to mark safe operating areas around the scanner. Equipment can be classified as MRI safe or unsafe, and it is imperative that any equipment being taken into the vicinity of the magnet is MRI safe. Unsafe equipment must stay outside the area of the magnet, with intravenous lines and anaesthetic tubing passing into the area via waveguide ports that are built into the Faraday cage design of the magnet room.

All patients (and staff) entering the vicinity of the MRI scanner require screening to determine safety risks. All foreign objects including transdermal patches must be removed and the patient should be dressed in a gown. Any medical equipment containing ferrous metallic components can produce artefact which can reduce image quality but may also become dislodged. The manufacturers of equipment or implants should provide patients and clinicians with accurate information about their MRI safety. Patients with a pacemaker or implantable cardiac defibrillator (ICD) should not go beyond the five Gauss line and consequently MRI is usually contraindicated. However, pacemaker technology is evolving and MRI-conditional pacemakers and ICDs are now produced by some manufacturers. These devices have fewer ferromagnetic components, sensors designed to resist the magnetic field and well-insulated circuitry. They may need to be reprogrammed in advance by a cardiac physiologist.

The radiofrequency currents used in the MRI scanner can induce currents and heating in monitoring leads, and severe burns can occur. MRI safe monitors use fibreoptic or carbon fibre cabling to avoid this; alternatively, foam pads can be used to insulate the cables. The ECG is prone to interference and although it can monitor rate and rhythm, it loses its ability to accurately determine ischaemic changes. When side-stream capnography is used, there will be an increase in response time, if a long sample line is used to return gas to a monitor in the control room.

Induction of anaesthesia should take place outside the five Gauss line, where standard anaesthetic equipment can be used. The patient can then have MRI-safe monitoring attached and be transferred into the scanner. Usually, the anaesthetist watches the patient and monitors from the control room, ensuring a clear view of both. If there are any anaesthetic emergencies, the scan should be terminated and the patient moved back outside of the five Gauss line before treatment is initiated.

REFERENCES

1. Rivera-Ch M, León-Velarde F, Huicho L. Treatment of chronic mountain sickness: critical re-appraisal of an old problem. Respir Physiol Neurobiol 2007;158:251–65.
2. Stoneham MD. Anaesthesia and resuscitation at altitude. Eur J Anaesthesiol 1995;12:249–57.
3. James MF, Manson ED, Dennett JE. Nitrous oxide analgesia and altitude. Anaesthesia 1982;37:285–8.
4. James MF, White JF. Anesthetic considerations at moderate altitude. Anesth Analg 1984;63:1097–105.
5. Haddon R. Anaesthesia and intensive care in the hyperbaric chamber. Curr Anaesth Crit Care 2002;5:263–9.
6. Sheridan RL, Shank ES. Hyperbaric oxygen treatment: a brief overview of a controversial topic. J Trauma 1999;47:426–35.
7. Uppal V, Dourish J, Macfarlane A. Anaesthesia for electroconvulsive therapy. Contin Educ Anaesth Crit Care Pain 2010;10(6):192–6.
8. Gooden CK. Anesthesia for magnetic resonance imaging. Curr Opin Anaesthesiol 2004;17: 339–42.

Chapter 5.16

Urological Surgery

Graeme Hilditch

GENERAL CONSIDERATIONS

Good anaesthetic practice for urological surgery, ranging from minor, short-duration day surgery to complex, major surgery, should provide safe conditions with an expeditious recovery to normality with minimal complications. Many major urological procedures involve prolonged surgery associated with significant blood loss and postoperative pain. Careful patient positioning, temperature regulation and fluid management is often required.

Patients presenting for urological surgery are frequently at the extremes of age. It is well recognized that children have particular needs (see Chapter 5.6); however, elderly patients, particularly those over 80 years, also need special consideration (see Chapter 1.2). Many patients present with multiple comorbidities, and renal impairment is common. Meticulous attention should be given to reducing risk factors for peri-operative renal failure (Box 5.16.1). For the implications of anaesthesia in patients with impaired renal function, see Chapter 1.2.

TECHNICAL CONSIDERATIONS

Pre-Operative Preparation

All patients should be fully assessed and any comorbid disease optimized before elective surgery. An assessment of functional capacity is recommended, especially for major procedures. Long-term medication should usually be continued throughout the hospital stay unless contraindicated.

Most patients do not require premedication. If they are particularly anxious, a small dose of oral benzodiazepine such as temazepam may be used.

The anaesthetist should recommend an anaesthetic technique after full discussion with the patient, including disclosure of the benefits, risks and available alternative techniques.

Patients should be adequately fasted before elective surgery.

BOX 5.16.1 Peri-operative Acute Renal Failure: Risk Factors and Principles of Prevention

Risk factors
Pre-operative renal impairment
Hypertension
Age > 65 years
Type 1 diabetes mellitus
Ascites
Congestive heart failure
Nephrotoxic agents (contrast media, NSAIDs and aminoglycosides)
Hypovolaemia
Emergency surgery
Intraperitoneal surgery

Principles of prevention
Maintain oxygen delivery
Maintain normovolaemia
Provide adequate perfusion pressure of the kidneys

NSAIDs, nonsteroidal anti-inflammatory drugs

Principles of Anaesthesia

Anaesthetic techniques will be based on the complexity of surgery, underlying comorbid disease and age of the patient, and should comply with standards for minimum monitoring.[1]

Anti-emetics should be used for patients at risk of postoperative nausea and vomiting (PONV).

Antibiotic prophylaxis will be guided by nature of surgery and local guidelines.

General anaesthesia for minor urological procedures usually entails maintenance with a volatile anaesthetic agent and the patient breathing spontaneously with a supraglottic airway device (SAD), but intubation may be required for patients at a risk of regurgitation.

Spinal anaesthesia is frequently used for some minor urological procedures, either alone or in combination with sedation. It also provides useful immediate postoperative analgesia.

General anaesthesia for major urological procedures may require additional invasive monitoring, such as intra-arterial blood pressure (IABP) and central venous pressure (CVP), goal-directed fluid management and management of blood loss (Box 5.16.2).

Analgesia

Postoperative pain can be extensive and good quality analgesia is essential. Neuraxial analgesia and regional anaesthetic techniques should be considered as part of the multimodal analgesic regimen. Low thoracic or lumbar extradural analgesia has the added advantage of helping to reduce blood loss.

> **BOX 5.16.2 Principles of Anaesthetic Technique for Major Urological Procedures[2]**
>
> Analgesia
> Management of haemorrhage
> Fluid management
> Temperature control
> Patient positioning

An understanding of the relevant nerve supply is important (Table 5.16.1).

Regional anaesthetic techniques such as rectus sheath block or transversus abdominis plane (TAP) block can be used as adjuncts for pain control for procedures with abdominal wounds. Single-shot blocks or continuous local anaesthetic infusions are suitable.

Intrathecal opioids provide effective analgesia with benefits that persist for up to 24 h. Side effects include nausea and vomiting, pruritus and respiratory depression. Contraindications include coagulopathy, recent anticoagulants, local or systemic infection and allergy to opioids.

Fluid Management

Fluid management during long cases is complex and is linked to postoperative morbidity with both excessive and insufficient fluids considered risk factors. A peri-operative plan should be developed based on the complexity of surgery and individual requirements.

During major procedures, estimating fluid status of the patient is often inaccurate; therefore, fluid management should be goal directed and guided by

TABLE 5.16.1 Nerve Supply Relevant to Epidural Analgesia for Major Urological Procedures

Location	Nerve Root	Nerve
Kidney	T10–L1	Coeliac, renal and superior hypogastric plexuses
Ureter	L1–L2	Renal and pelvic plexus
Bladder and urethra	T11–L2; S2–S4	Hypogastric and pelvic plexuses
Prostate	L1– L2, S2–S4	Pelvic plexus; pudendal nerve
Testis	T10–L1	Coeliac plexus and lesser splanchnic nerve
Penis, scrotum and distal urethra	T11–L2; S2–S4	Pelvic plexus; pudendal nerve

dynamic indices such as systolic pressure variation, pulse pressure variation, stroke volume variation or oesophageal Doppler.

A combination of balanced crystalloids and colloids is suitable.

Management of Haemorrhage

Blood loss can be considerable during long cases and some procedures are associated with sudden major haemorrhage. Anaemia should be corrected prior to surgery and all anticoagulants and antiplatelet drugs stopped at an appropriate time before surgery.

The key principle is to maintain vital organ perfusion by restoring circulating volume with crystalloids or colloids and replenishing haemoglobin with red cell transfusion.[3] Strategies to manage major haemorrhage include:

- Assessment of blood loss – weigh swabs and measure suction volumes
- Measurement of haemoglobin and clotting – using point of care (POC) devices or from blood gas analysis
- Pressurized infusion bag or rapid infusion device – for rapid, excessive bleeding
- Transfusion triggers – red cell transfusion should be considered when the haemoglobin is less than 80 g/L (may be influenced by the presence of cardiorespiratory disease, risk of further bleeding and the patient's clinical condition), transfusion is usually required when 30%–40% of the blood volume is lost
- Fresh frozen plasma – if more than six units of red cells are transfused
- Cryoprecipitate and platelets
- Tranexamic acid – 1 g by slow intravenous bolus
- Laboratory testing (haemoglobin, PT ratio, fibrinogen, platelets) – to guide transfusions of blood components

Temperature Control

Hypothermia increases the risk of complications such as wound infection, coagulopathy and myocardial ischaemia. In the postoperative period, shivering can increase oxygen consumption. During long procedures, warm air blankets, warmed intravenous fluids and temperature monitoring are essential. These strategies should be continued in the postoperative period if required.

Patient Positioning

During long, complex procedures, adequate measures must be taken to reduce the risk of superficial tissue ischaemia and peripheral nerve injuries. Careful peri-operative patient positioning, protective padding covering hard surfaces and supports, avoiding prolonged periods of hypotension with poor skin perfusion and maintaining normothermia are considered appropriate peri-operative care.

Postoperative Care

The aim of postoperative care is to encourage early mobilisation and resume normal diet. Adequate pain control reduces the surgical stress response which leads to improved recovery with fewer complications.

Oral fluids should be commenced immediately postoperatively and intravenous fluids should be restricted to minimum requirements. Following major surgery, fluid balance should be monitored by measuring hourly urine output with a target minimum of 0.5 mL/kg/h averaged over 2–4 h.

Oral diet should be encouraged and anti-emetics given to reduce nausea and vomiting, particularly for patients at risk of PONV.

Venous thromboembolism prophylaxis should comply with local guidelines.

Postoperative analgesic requirements vary with the complexity of procedures. Multimodal analgesia should be employed. Paracetamol should be considered for all cases unless contraindicated. A nonsteroidal anti-inflammatory drug (NSAID) may be used unless contraindicated (e.g. if there are risk factors for postoperative renal failure). Systemic opioids can be given either orally or intravenously using patient-controlled analgesia (PCA). Extradural anaesthesia can be useful for major procedures. Extradural infusions using a mixture of local anaesthetic and an opioid can provide good quality postoperative analgesia, but there are significant risks including high failure rate, hypotension, epidural haematoma and possible excessive fluid administration. In many hospitals, postoperative care for patients with extradural analgesia necessitates admission to a high-dependency unit.

SPECIFIC OPERATIONS

Urological procedures fall into a number of categories:

- Endoscopic procedures such as cystoscopy, transurethral resection of bladder tumour (TURBT) or prostate (TURP), ureteroscopy.
- Major surgery such as prostatectomy, cystectomy, nephrectomy and renal transplantation.
- Minor surgery such as circumcision, penectomy and vasectomy.

Paediatric reconstructive surgery for congenital abnormalities, performed in specialized centres is not considered in this chapter.

Endoscopic Procedures of the Bladder

A general anaesthetic technique for minor urological procedures is recommended.

All instrumentation of the lower urinary tract is likely to cause significant bacteraemia. Local guidelines for prophylactic antibiotics should be followed.

Cystoscopy and Transurethral Resection of Bladder Tumour

Patients with suspected bladder carcinoma require a cystoscopy or TURBT. Those who have nonmuscle invasive bladder carcinoma will require multiple follow-up cystoscopies for disease surveillance. These operations are usually performed as day-case procedures.

As bladder cancer shows a strong association with smoking, close attention must be paid to other smoking-related diseases in the pre-operative assessment.

Haematuria is common and can lead to anaemia, which if severe should be corrected before surgery.

Obstruction of the genitourinary tract can lead to renal impairment, so renal function should be checked.

A general anaesthetic technique is appropriate for minor urological procedures with the patient in the lithotomy position. Resection of tumours located on the lateral wall of the bladder can cause sudden leg movement as a result of stimulation of the obturator nerve (obturator nerve spasm). This can result in extraperitoneal perforation of the bladder wall with the resectoscope. Reducing the diathermy current helps, but muscle relaxation may be required. Alternatively, an obturator nerve block can be used.

Spinal anaesthesia is also appropriate. The block must reach at least T10 dermatome level.

Topical anaesthesia using lidocaine 1% or 2% urethral gel is usually all that is required for flexible cystoscopy and is administered by the surgeon.

Transurethral Resection of the Prostate

Benign prostatic hyperplasia is common in men older than 60 years, and TURP is common in this age group.

A detailed pre-operative assessment is required. Patients are usually elderly and with multiple comorbidities. Often there is mild renal impairment due to chronic urinary tract outflow obstruction. Cross-matched blood should be available.

A general anaesthetic technique is commonly employed. However, spinal anaesthesia up to the T10 dermatome level is the preferred technique, as it reduces blood loss and allows early identification of the symptoms and signs of TURP syndrome.

Care must be taken to move both legs simultaneously when positioning the patient in the lithotomy position. Pressure points must be padded to avoid iatrogenic injury to the common peroneal nerve where the head of the fibula rests against the leg supports. Strategies to prevent hypothermia must be followed.

Intravenous fluids should be given in small volumes due to the risk of absorption of irrigation fluids, although caution with such a conservative approach should be taken if bleeding is suspected.

During resection, blood loss is difficult to measure but is usually about 7–20 mL/g of prostate resected. It is increased by raised venous pressure (straining, excessive transfusion, excessive absorption of irrigant), prolonged operation time and release of plasminogen activators from the prostate.

The main complications are bleeding and TURP syndrome.

Transurethral Resection of the Prostate Syndrome

Transurethral Resection of the Prostate syndrome refers to the symptoms and signs associated with the excessive absorption of glycine irrigation fluid (Table 5.16.2), resulting in hypervolaemia, dilutional hyponatraemia and hyperglycinaemia. This in turn leads to cardiovascular, respiratory and renal failure along with neurological complications.[4]

Glycine has a half-life of 85 min. Metabolic products include oxalate, which may precipitate in the renal tubules if urine flow is low during the first 10 postoperative days; and ammonia, which is a cerebral depressant. Glycine is an inhibitory neurotransmitter and may cause transient blindness. The amount absorbed via the prostatic veins is typically around 700 mL (10–30 mL/min), but can reach several litres depending on the surgical skill, pressure of irrigant and duration of operation.

The main strategy should be to prevent TURP syndrome. Ensure that the irrigating fluid is not too high above the patient (less than 70 cm) and limiting the duration of procedure, preferably to less than 30 min. Ideally, TURP syndrome should be diagnosed early by close observation of the patient and monitoring the serum sodium. Regional techniques allow observation of early symptoms.

Management of TURP syndrome depends on the severity of symptoms and comprises:

- Stopping surgery promptly
- Supplemental O_2 and ventilatory support if required

TABLE 5.16.2 Symptoms and Signs of TURP Syndrome

Symptoms[a]	Signs
Nausea	Hypertension
Tight feeling in chest	Decreased conscious level
Shortness of breath	Tonic clonic seizures
Dizziness	Pupillary dilation
Restlessness	Bradycardia
Confusion	Hypoxia
Retching	ECG changes (nodal rhythm, ST changes widening QRS)
Abdominal pain	Cardiorespiratory arrest
Blurring of vision	

[a]Only observed in conscious patients.

- Checking haemoglobin, biochemistry and arterial blood gases
- Treating hypervolaemia with furosemide 20 mg
- Fluid restriction if Na^+ higher than 120 mmol/L
- Administering hypertonic saline if Na^+ less than 120 mmol/L, but ensuring slow correction (<0.5 mmol/h)
- Treating seizures with midazolam, diazepam or thiopental
- Iontropic support if required

Ureteroscopy

Ureteroscopy is used to remove kidney stones from the ureter, but also for inserting stents and investigating the upper genitourinary tract. Patients may have renal impairment secondary to obstruction, and urinary sepsis is common.

Anaesthetic considerations are the same as for cystoscopy and TURBT.

Major Urological Procedures

Open Radical Prostatectomy

Cancer of the prostate is the most commonly diagnosed cancer in men.

Traditionally, an open approach for a radical prostectomy was used for complete excision of the prostate gland, but bleeding was a major complication. Appropriate measures to manage sudden blood loss should be used.

A multimodal approach to analgesia is required and either epidural or intrathecal opioids combined with bilateral TAP blocks technique is preferred.

Early oral diet and mobilization is encouraged in the postoperative period.

Laparoscopic Radical Prostatectomy

Laparoscopic radical prostatectomy is associated with less bleeding, reduced postoperative pain and reduced length of hospital stay compared with open surgery (Table 5.16.3). The approach can be transperitoneal or extraperitoneal.

TABLE 5.16.3 Benefits of Laparoscopic and Robot-Assisted Radical Prostatectomy

Laparoscopic Compared with Open Radical Prostatectomy	Robot-Assisted Compared with Laparoscopic Radical Prostatectomy
Minimal surgical tissue trauma	Improved operative field visibility
Reduced haemorrhage	Three-dimensional imaging
Less postoperative pain	Enhanced dexterity
Faster recovery time	Improved precision
Shorter length of hospital stay	

Surgical access is either transperitoneal or extraperitoneal. For a transperitoneal approach, the patient is placed supine in a steep Trendelenburg position, but this is unnecessary for an extraperitoneal approach.

Careful positioning and protection of pressure areas is required.

The procedure can be prolonged. Active warming of the patient is recommended.

Laparoscopic surgery involves insufflation of CO_2, complications of which include surgical emphysema and venous gas embolism.

Blood loss is difficult to estimate but is usually minimal.

Postoperative analgesia is provided by a multimodal approach. Postoperative shoulder tip pain can occur due to diaphragmatic irritation.

Robot-Assisted Laparoscopic Radical Prostatectomy

Robotic surgery is an advancement in minimally invasive surgery for patients with prostate cancer and is associated with improved outcomes (Table 5.16.3).[5] The robotic systems are large and bulky, and access to the patient is limited.

The procedure can be prolonged and is performed either extraperitoneally or, more commonly, transperitoneally. The patient is positioned supine in a steep Trendelenburg position which together with the pneumoperitoneum can lead to significant cardiovascular and respiratory problems (Table 5.16.4).

The following precautions are taken:

- High levels of PEEP
- Throat pack – reduces the likelihood of contamination of the airway from regurgitation of gastric contents during steep Trendelenburg position
- Muscle relaxation – prevents patient movement once the robot has docked
- Antislip mat and legs strapped to the table, shoulder supports can be used but may cause a brachial plexus injury
- Careful protection of pressure areas
- Long extension set for intravenous fluids
- Arterial line – facilitates blood sampling if required

Appropriate measures to maintain normothermia are required.

Conservative fluid administration is preferred until urethral anastomosis is completed.

Regional techniques are unnecessary and sympathetic blockade can exacerbate the cardiovascular effects of positioning.

A multimodal analgesic regimen but avoid using NSAIDs due to the risk of renal impairment following surgery.

Early mobilization and return to normal diet is encouraged.

Abdominal Prostatectomy

This involves excision of the prostate gland when it is grossly hypertrophied.

Patients may be old and frail, so pre-operative assessment needs particular care.

TABLE 5.16.4 Problems Associated with Steep Trendelenburg Position during Robot-Assisted Radical Prostatectomy

Problem		Strategy
Positioning of patient	Patient movement	Antislip mat and leg breaks with straps
	Brachial plexus injury	Avoid shoulder supports
Cardiovascular system	Haemodynamic instability	Intra-arterial pressure monitoring
Respiratory system	Decreased FRC and $\dot{V}/Q$ mismatch	Intermittent positive pressure ventilation with PEEP
Gastrointestinal system	Regurgitation of gastric contents	Throat pack
Renal system	Reduced renal perfusion and glomerular filtration rate	Maintain normotension with vasoconstrictors
Increased dependent venous pressure	Raised intracranial pressure	Surgery contraindicated in presence of raised intracranial pressure Maintain normocapnia
	Raised intra-ocular pressure	Maintain normocapnia Ensure any glaucoma medication taken
Increased dependent hydrostatic pressure	Chemosis	Adequate eye protection
	Laryngeal oedema	Care taken during extubation

Significant bleeding is possible and appropriate measures to manage massive haemorrhage are required. Goal-directed fluid management, strategies to prevent hypothermia and careful patient positioning are necessary. A multimodal analgesic technique with systemic opioids is required.

Open Nephrectomy

Nephrectomy is mainly performed for renal cell carcinoma (RCC), although simple nephrectomies are occasionally carried out for noncancer conditions such as chronic infection or trauma. Partial nephrectomies are often performed for patients with co-existing renal impairment or small tumours. RCCs can be extremely vascular and there is a risk of significant haemorrhage. Extension of thrombus from the renal vein into the IVC occurs in up to 10% of RCCs.

Patients are generally older and often have significant comorbid disease. Smoking is one of the most common risk factors.

The operation can be performed in the supine position with a subcostal incision but is usually performed with the patient in a lateral position with a small degree of Trendelenburg tilt. This position is associated with $\dot{V}/Q$ mismatch and a reduced FRC. Development of atelectasis can lead to hypoxia.

Careful positioning and padding should be used to prevent pressure sores and nerve damage.

There is a risk of massive haemorrhage and invasive blood pressure monitoring is required. A rapid infusion device is recommended for resection of tumours with the involvement of IVC.

Tumour embolus causing collapse and cardiac arrest is an occasional complication of operations for carcinoma of the kidney. Rarely, the pleura is damaged during kidney operations. The resulting collapse of the upper lung may prove dangerous unless IPPV is employed. An underwater drain may be required.

Strategies to maintain normothermia must be used.

Epidural analgesia is appropriate, especially if a subcostal surgical incision is used, however, many anaesthetists avoid this technique due to concern regarding postoperative hypotension. Intrathecal opioids can be used as an alternative together with a thoracic paravertebral block or wound catheters.

Good quality postoperative analgesia helps prevent chest complications. Chest physiotherapy, postoperative breathing exercises and postoperative oxygen for some days may be warranted.

Laparoscopic Nephrectomy

Laparoscopic nephrectomy is increasingly popular and reduces the postoperative analgesic requirements and the length of hospital stay. However, the presence of a pneumoperitoneum and steep Trendelenburg position adds to the intra-operative concerns of an open nephrectomy.

Hypercapnia can occur as a result of the CO_2 pneumoperitoneum and minute ventilation should be increased to minimize the rise in CO_2. PEEP may be required if hypoxia is problematic.

The patient is placed in the lateral position with steep Trendelenburg tilt. Careful positioning and padding should be used to prevent pressure sores and nerve damage. Often there is a change of position intra-operatively and a review of pressure areas should be carried out.

Invasive blood pressure monitor may be helpful.

Haemorrhage can be difficult to quantify during laparoscopy.

A multimodal approach to analgesia using simple analgesia and opioids is required. Postoperative recovery should be facilitated by early oral diet and mobilisation.

Cystectomy

Bladder carcinoma that is muscle invasive or considered high risk for invasion requires removal of the bladder and dissection of the pelvic lymph nodes combined with reconstruction and urinary diversion.

As bladder cancer shows a strong association with smoking, close attention must be paid to other smoking-related diseases in the pre-operative assessment. Gross or microscopic haematuria can lead to significant anaemia. Renal function must be assessed. An assessment of functional capacity is essential to determine suitability for surgery and cardiopulmonary reserve using cardiopulmonary exercise testing is valuable in high-risk patients.

These procedures are of long duration and often involve the lithotomy position. Careful positioning and padding should be used to prevent pressure sores and nerve damage. Prevention of hypothermia is necessary. Invasive blood pressure monitoring is required.

Careful measurement of blood loss by weighing swabs and measuring suction is necessary, but urine spillage may be included in the measurements. During the resection of the bladder, it is preferable to follow conservative fluid management to reduce overfilling of the pelvic veins and minimize blood loss. Management of hypotension using vasoconstrictors rather than fluid boluses is advised. Goal-directed fluid management strategies should be used once resection of the bladder is complete and haemostasis achieved.

Management of postoperative analgesia varies. Epidural analgesia is considered effective but can lead to hypotension postoperatively. Alternatively, intrathecal opioids and regional anaesthetic techniques such as rectus sheath block or TAP block can be can be used together with postoperative morphine PCA and paracetamol. NSAIDs should be used cautiously due to the risk of postoperative renal failure.

Postoperative ileus is common, but patients should be given oral fluids immediately postoperatively and diet withheld for additional 24 h.

Renal Transplantation

Renal transplantation is considered the preferred treatment for patients with end-stage renal disease (ESRD). The peri-operative management of ESRD patients is crucial for graft survival and involves a multidisciplinary approach involving nephrologists, transplant surgeons, anaesthetists and transplant nurse specialists prior to the patient being placed on the transplant waiting list. A thorough pre-operative assessment must be carried out with particular attention given to the causes and effects of ESRD (Table 5.16.5).

The patient's renal replacement therapy must be considered and should include:

- When patient was last dialysed
- Type of dialysis (peritoneal or haemodialysis)
- Dry weight of patient - aids assessment of fluid balance
- Presence of any arteriovenous (AV) fistulae or dialysis lines

Antihypertensive medication should be continued, except angiotensin-converting enzyme (ACE) inhibitors and angiotensin-II receptor blockers, which should be stopped. Immunosuppressant therapy is commenced pre-operatively and local protocols should be followed.

TABLE 5.16.5 Common Causes and Effects of End-Stage Renal Disease

Causes	Effects
Diabetes mellitus	Anaemia
Glomerulonephritis or pyelonephritis	Platelet dysfunction
Polycystic kidneys	Accelerated atheroma and hypertension
Hypertension	Fluid and electrolyte imbalance, notably hyperkalaemia
	Metabolic acidosis
	Hyperparathyroidism
	Delayed gastric emptying
	Coagulopathy

When the transplantation involves a deceased donor, the aim is to limit the cold ischaemic time to less than 24 h, as reduced time is associated with improved outcome.

Neuromuscular blockade is necessary for surgery. Atracurium is preferred. Rocuronium and vecuronium should be used with caution, as there is a risk of prolonged duration of neuromuscular blockade. Suxamethonium should be avoided if the serum K^+ is greater than 5 mmol/L.

Vascular access, and direct arterial blood pressure monitoring if used, should be sited on the opposite arm to any AV fistulae. Arterial blood pressure should be kept within 20% of the baseline by the use of vasoconstrictors whilst maintaining normovolaemia. Measurement of central venous pressure is essential for monitoring fluid balance to achieve adequate kidney perfusion pressure. A dialysis line can be used as an alternative to a central line. A target of 10–15 cm H_2O is used. Fluid replacement with 0.9% NaCl is preferable, although balanced crystalloids can be used despite concerns about a minor rise in lactate levels.

Careful patient positioning is important, especially with respect to fistula sites which should be padded. Strategies to prevent hypothermia should be used.

Fentanyl is a more suitable systemic opioid than morphine, which is metabolized to an active metabolite, morphine-6-glucuronide, that can have a prolonged duration of action in patients with ESRD. A dose of 200–300 µg is usually required. TAP blocks are often used. Extradural and intradural analgesia are relatively contraindicated due to platelet dysfunction and the need to avoid hypotension.

Prior to reperfusion of the transplanted kidney immunosuppressants, typically methylprednisolone (1 g infused over 20 min) should be administered. Antibiotic and thromboembolism prophylaxis should be employed.

Paracetamol and fentanyl PCA (20 μg bolus, 5 min lockout) should be used for postoperative analgesia. NSAIDs are avoided. Postoperative fluid management should include 0.9% NaCl, with an hourly infusion rate equal to the previous hour's urine volume plus 50 mL. Additional boluses of fluid may be required if there is hypotension or hypovolaemia.

Minor Surgery

A general anaesthetic technique for minor urological procedures is recommended for the following procedures unless there are specific patient requirements.

Circumcision

Circumcision is the treatment for phimosis, recurrent balanitis and cancer of the penis. It is usually carried out as a day-case procedure. It is the most common paediatric urological procedure (see Chapter 5.6). Most patients are healthy.

A general anaesthetic or local anaesthetic technique is suitable. Laryngeal spasm may easily develop if general anaesthesia is too light, requiring surgery to be interrupted, the application of continuous positive airway pressure or even suxamethonium and intubation. A penile block, 10 mL 0.25% levobupivicaine can be used as the sole technique or as an adjunct for postoperative analgesia in adults.

Postoperative analgesia with paracetamol and a NSAID is suitable.

Penectomy

The incidence of penile cancer is increasing as a result of increased incidence of human papilloma virus. The extent of surgery depends on the severity of the disease and ranges from excision of the tip of penis to a total penectomy. Often, a sentinel node biopsy of the groin lymph nodes is performed with an intradermal injection of methylene blue.

If surgery is extensive, muscle relaxation and intubation is preferable. For partial penectomies, a penile block is suitable for postoperative analgesia. If a sentinel node biopsy is performed, then a penile block is inappropriate due to the interference with the spread of intradermal methylene blue. The block can be performed at the end of the procedure.

Postoperative pain varies with the extent of surgery and may require oral opioids.

Surgery of the Scrotum, Including Vasectomy

These operations may be done under local infiltration analgesia, especially vasectomy, but some surgeons prefer general anaesthesia because there is less a likelihood of haematoma formation. This may be partly due to postoperative sedation and a short bed rest. Traction on the spermatic cord may result in bradycardia or even asystole. Atropine or glycopyrrolate should be available.

Percutaneous Nephrolithotomy

Percutaneous nephrolithotomy is a minimally invasive procedure to remove kidney stones. It involves the passage of a telescope into the renal pelvis under radiological control, irrigation with saline and electrohydraulic fragmentation until the stone can be extracted. Large volumes of saline may be absorbed if the pressure in the renal pelvis is allowed to rise above 75 cm H_2O. The patient is semiprone or prone. Precautions taken for positioning the patient in the prone position include:

- Adequate number of staff to move the patient – anaesthetist to control head movement and protect airway with assistants on either side and one to control leg movement
- Body supports – should not impede chest and abdominal movement
- Head supports – to prevent pressure-related injuries, particularly to the eyes
- Protection of the airway – achieved using a securely fastened reinforced oral tracheal tube

Postoperative pain is mild and there is a low risk of pneumothorax; therefore, any respiratory symptoms should be investigated with a chest X-ray.

Extracorporeal Shockwave Lithotripsy

Extracorporeal shockwave lithotripsy fragments the stone with external acoustic shock waves. Modern lithotripters produce little pain and the procedure is undertaken with analgesics and sometimes light sedation. General anaesthesia is still sometimes required for children. This is only undertaken in specialized paediatric centres.

Lithotripsy and Lithotomy

Renal stones can be treated without open operation in many cases. Patients tend to be healthy; however, renal function should be assessed. A full blood count should be taken if there is significant haematuria. Bacteraemia is likely and prophylactic antibiotics are required.

REFERENCES

1. Association of Anaesthetists of Great Britain and Ireland. Recommendations for standards of monitoring during anaesthesia and recovery. London: AAGBI. www.aagbi.org/sites/default/files/Standards_of_monitoring_2015_0.pdf; 2015.
2. British Association of Urological Surgeons. BAUS enhanced recovery pathway. London: BAUS.: www.baus.org.uk/_userfiles/pages/files/Publications/ERP%20with%20KNB%20markups.pdf; 2015.
3. Norfolk D. Transfusion in surgery. In: Norfolk D, editor. Handbook of transfusion medicine. 5th ed. U K: The Stationary Office; 2013. p. 74–9.
4. Demirel I, Ozer AB, Bayar MK, Erhan OL. TURP syndrome and severe hyponatremia under general anaesthesia. BMJ Case Reports 2012. doi: 10.1136/bcr-2012-006899.
5. Paranjape S, Chhabra A. Anaesthesia for robotic surgery. Trends Anaesth Crit Care 2014;4:25–31.

Chapter 5.17

Vascular Surgery

Richard J. Telford

Care of the patient presenting for major vascular surgery is one of the most challenging areas of anaesthetic practice. Major vascular surgery is associated with a higher risk of adverse outcome when compared with other forms of noncardiac surgery. This is largely due to the physiological stress of the perioperative period which is associated with an increased oxygen demand of up to 40%. Meticulous preoperative assessment of vascular patients by experienced clinicians familiar with the magnitude of the physiological trespass of the proposed surgery is paramount to inform clinical decision-making, reduce risk and improve patient outcome. Major goals of the pre-assessment process are optimization of comorbidities, targeted speciality referral, choice of postoperative care facility and consideration of nonoperative management where appropriate.

RISK MODIFICATION

The following lifestyle changes may reduce the risk of vascular surgery:

- Nutritional &/or dietary – obesity is associated with morbidity after vascular surgery.
- Smoking cessation – ideally for 4–6 weeks prior to surgery, but cessation at any time prior to surgery is beneficial due to the reduction in carboxyhaemoglobin levels and consequent improvement in oxygen delivery.
- Regular exercise – graded exercise programmes can improve measured levels of physical fitness. However, evidence that this improves outcome is currently lacking.[1]

PREOPERATIVE OPTIMIZATION

Medical Optimization

Cardiovascular Disease

Referrals for elective surgery should only be accepted if documented arterial blood pressure (BP) in primary care over the preceding 12 months are less than 160 mm Hg systolic and less than 100 mm Hg diastolic. Elective surgery can proceed for patients who attend the preoperative assessment clinic without documentation of normotension in primary care if their BP is less than 180 mm Hg systolic and less than 110 mm Hg diastolic when measured in a clinic.[2]

Heart failure must be investigated and optimally treated with angiotensin-converting enzyme inhibitors (ACEIs), β blockers, aldosterone antagonists and diuretics.

There is little indication for percutaneous coronary intervention (PCI) prior to elective vascular surgery because of the necessity for a period of dual anti-platelet therapy to reduce the risk of in-stent thrombosis. Rarely, coronary artery bypass grafting (CABG) may be necessary prior to elective vascular surgery. Subsequent vascular surgery should be delayed for at least 3 months.

Heart murmurs should be investigated. Transthoracic echocardiography can give useful information on the type and severity of the heart valve lesion and information about cardiac contractility. In patients with severe aortic stenosis, valve replacement prior to major elective vascular surgery may be advisable.

Respiratory Disease

Smoking cessation is important. Bronchodilator therapy should be optimized if reversibility is demonstrated by pulmonary function testing. Underlying respiratory infection should be treated.

Renal Disease

Renal artery stenosis should be excluded as a treatable cause of renal dysfunction.

Intravenous hydration prior to aortic surgery should be considered for patients with severe renal disease.

Dialysis-dependent patients should have their dialysis optimally timed prior to elective surgery.

Diabetes

Diabetes is common in vascular surgical patients and associated with ischaemic heart disease, autonomic neuropathy and renal disease. Autonomic neuropathy predisposes to peri-operative hypotension and may be associated with silent myocardial ischaemia.

Poor diabetic control is associated with an increased length of hospital stay and an increased risk of wound infection.

Diabetic control should be optimized. Patients with an HbA_{1c} more than 70 mmol/mol (8.5%), or poor hypoglycaemic awareness, or problematic hypo-glycaemia should be referred to an endocrinologist preoperatively.

Anaemia

Anaemia is associated with an increased risk of morbidity and mortality and should be investigated and treated aggressively, aiming for a preoperative haemoglobin concentration within the normal range prior to elective surgery (females >120 g/L; males >130 g/L).

Pharmacological Optimization

Statins

Stain therapy is associated with decreased peri-operative cardiovascular morbidity and mortality. Patients presenting for major vascular surgery should be taking statins, ideally started at least 2 weeks prior to surgery. Treatment should be continued peri-operatively.

Antiplatelet Drugs

Patients presenting for major vascular surgery should be taking an antiplatelet drug to minimize the thromboembolic complications of vascular disease. Aspirin should be continued peri-operatively. Continuation of treatment with the platelet P_2Y_{12} ADP receptor antagonists (clopidogrel and prasugrel) is more contentious due to the increased bleeding risk (particularly with prasugrel). Consider switching to aspirin or alternatively, if aspirin intolerant, stop treatment 7 days prior to surgery.

β Blockers

Patients receiving β blockers should continue their medication.

In certain very high risk patients with inducible ischaemia on preoperative testing who do not fulfil the criteria for CABG, a low dose of β blocker (e.g. bisoprolol 2.5–5 mg) should be commenced 4 weeks prior to surgery and titrated to a preoperative heart rate 50–70 bpm.

ACEI and Angiotensin Receptor Blockers

Consideration should be given to stopping these 12–24 h prior to surgery unless they are being used to treat heart failure.

Anticoagulants

Warfarin should be stopped 5 days prior to surgery. Aim for a target INR of less than 1.5 on the day of surgery.

Patients who are anticoagulated to protect against the thromboembolic complications of atrial fibrillation (AF) do not need 'bridging' with heparin. Higher risk patients (e.g. patients with a metallic prosthetic valve replacement or thrombophilia) should receive bridging treatment with low molecular weight heparin (LMWH) once the INR is less than 1.5, continued up to the night before surgery.

Direct oral anticoagulants should be stopped at least 2 days before surgery.

ASSESSMENT OF FUNCTIONAL CAPACITY

Exercise capacity is a major predictor of peri-operative risk. Assessment of exercise capacity may be subjective or objective.

Subjective Assessment of Exercise Capacity

The ability to exercise is an excellent indicator of cardiovascular fitness. It is usually expressed in metabolic equivalents of task (METs) on a scale defined by the Duke Activity Status Index. One MET is the resting oxygen consumption of a 40-year-old, 70-kg male (3.5 mL/kg/min). Patients who cannot sustain 4 METs of physical activity (equivalent to climbing a flight of stairs) frequently have adverse outcomes following high-risk surgery.

Objective Assessment of Exercise Capacity

Cardiopulmonary exercise testing (CPET) is a useful risk prediction tool, particularly prior to aortic surgery.[3] Information gleaned from a CPET includes:

- A dynamic overview of cardiorespiratory fitness/reserve compared with predicted values for sex and age
- Assessment of the degree of limitation and identification of whether the cardiovascular system, the respiratory system or both are the cause of limitation
- 12-lead ECG analysis for evidence of ischaemia or arrhythmia during exercise
- Measurement of the anaerobic threshold (AT), peak O_2 consumption (VO_2 peak) and ventilatory equivalents for CO_2 at AT (VE/VCO_2) can identify high-risk individuals with an increased risk of morbidity and mortality; AT less than 10 mL/kg/min, VO_2 peak less than 15 mL/kg/min and VE/VCO_2 more than 42 indicate high risk.

SPECIFIC OPERATIONS

Abdominal Aortic Aneurysm

The abdominal aorta is aneurysmal when its diameter is more than 3.0 cm. Abdominal aortic aneurysm (AAA) is uncommon in people under the age of 60 years. In developed countries, approximately one person in 1000 develops AAA between the ages of 60 and 65, and this number continues to rise with age.

Risk factors for development of AAA include:

- Smoking – risk is directly related to the number of years smoking and decreases in the years following smoking cessation.
- Gender – men develop AAA more often than women (four to five times).
- Ethnicity – Caucasians develop AAA more commonly than people of other ethnicities.
- Comorbidity – presence of other medical conditions, such as coronary heart disease and peripheral vascular disease, increases the likelihood to develop AAA.
- Family history – the risk of developing aneurysm among brothers of a person with a known aneurysm, aged more than 60 years is nearly 18%.

The risk of rupture is related to the size of the aneurysm. Small aneurysms less than 5 cm in diameter rarely rupture (<2%), so there is no survival benefit from early surgical intervention. Patients with small aneurysms more than 3 and less than 5.4 cm in diameter should undergo regular ultrasound scanning to monitor the aneurysm size. The estimated annual rupture rate of aneurysms greater than 6 cm in diameter is 10%, rising to greater than 25% for aneurysms more than 8 cm in diameter. The 5-year survival rate of AAA more than 5 cm that are not operated on is around 20%. Current guidelines are to offer operative intervention when the aneurysm exceeds 5.5 cm, provided the patient is deemed fit enough for surgery.

Screening

In European countries, the mortality rates associated with elective AAA repair are in the order of 3%–4%. Since most aneurysms are asymptomatic, the key to reducing mortality from rupture is early diagnosis.

Population screening of men aged 65 years and over for AAA has been shown to reduce aneurysm-related mortality by almost half within 4 years of screening, principally by reducing the incidence of aneurysm rupture. Consequently, many countries have introduced AAA screening programmes. Men found to have aortic diameters of less than 3 cm are discharged. Those with aortic diameters between 3 and 5.4 cm are enrolled in a surveillance programme. Those with aortic diameters greater than 5.5 cm are referred to a vascular surgeon for consideration of surgical intervention.

Organization of Vascular Surgery

For a screening programme to be effective, it is necessary to reduce the associated peri-operative mortality to a minimum. This may be achieved by adopting the following:

● Centralization of vascular services – larger volume centres achieve better outcomes following AAA repair with reduced length of stay and improved survival after complications.
● Standardized pre-assessment – patients with AAA more than 5.5 cm in diameter should be reviewed by a multidisciplinary team (MDT) comprising a vascular surgeon, a vascular anaesthetist and an interventional radiologist after computed tomography (CT) angiography has been performed to assess the suitability for operative intervention.
● Patient information – patients considered for surgical intervention should be given consistent advice about the risks of all interventions, including information on both short- and long-term outcomes, to allow them to make an informed choice about their treatment options.
● Audit – centralized registry of data on all AAA repairs.

Surgical Techniques
Open Repair

The majority of open AAA repairs are performed via either long midline or subumbilical transverse incision. A left retroperitoneal is approach sometimes advocated if the patients have severe respiratory disease. There is an increased risk of infection with groin incisions.

The aortic graft may be a tube graft or a bifurcated ('trouser') graft.

As the abdominal aorta is a retroperitoneal structure, the peritoneum is not opened so there is less postoperative ileus and reduced postoperative atelectasis.

Endovascular Repair

Endovascular aortic aneurysm repair (EVAR) was developed as a less-invasive alternative to open repair. Modular bifurcated stent grafts are placed via open femoral arteriotomies.

EVAR is a combined surgical and radiological procedure, performed in the operating theatre or the angiography suite. Physiological disturbance is reduced, as there is no requirement for laparotomy or cross-clamping of the aorta. Patients can be transferred to the ward after a brief period of observation in a high-dependency unit. Hospital stay is reduced.

Anatomical suitability for EVAR is ascertained by CT angiogram. Approximately 75% of infrarenal AAAs are anatomically suitable for EVAR.

EVAR is associated with a 65% absolute reduction in early (30-day) mortality compared with open repair. This early survival advantage must be balanced against the risk of endograft-related complications, in particular endoleaks. After 4 years, up to 20% of patients require a secondary procedure, which if not amenable to salvage by a catheter-based approach may require open repair. This carries a high mortality.

EVAR has been used to treat patients deemed unfit for open repair, but confers no long-term survival benefit as patients succumb to their comorbidities.

Anaesthetic Management of Open Repair

The goal is to have a normovolaemic, haemodynamically stable, normothermic, pain-free patient on completion of surgery.

A balanced general anaesthetic technique (high-dose opioid with low-dose volatile agent) with a thoracic epidural for postoperative pain relief is recommended. There is some evidence that volatile anaesthetics and opioids improve tolerance of myocardial ischaemia by a mechanism similar to ischaemic preconditioning.

An effective epidural may attenuate the stress response to surgery, reducing the cardiovascular demands. It also provides effective postoperative analgesia, facilitating early extubation and reducing the incidence of pulmonary complications.

There is no evidence that epidurals reduce mortality.

Epidurals can safely be inserted in patients taking aspirin. For patients taking clopidogrel, the risk:benefit ratio should be carefully assessed. Patients should be monitored closely for the symptoms and signs of epidural haematoma.

Systemic heparinization is required prior to aortic cross-clamping. Additional heparin may be required in the presence of prolonged clamp times. Heparin can be reversed by protamine, which should be used with caution, as it may lead to myocardial depression, anaphylaxis and pulmonary hypertension.

Physiology of Aortic Clamping and Declamping

Aortic cross-clamping is necessary in open infrarenal AAA surgery. The physiological response to cross-clamping is complex and depends on myocardial function, the amount of collateral circulation present, the volume status of the patient and the function of the sympathetic nervous system. Arterial hypertension is common and due to an increase in systemic vascular resistance of around 30%. Arterial BP typically rises by 7%–10%. Cardiac filling pressures also increases as blood volume is shifted to the central veins due to reduced venous capacitance in organs distal to the clamp and because increases in cardiac workload may result in cardiac failure. This may be exacerbated by the administration of too much fluid before cross-clamping.

Cardiac output decreases by between 9% and 33% after infrarenal cross-clamping, although it may increase in some patients with good cardiac performance.

Vasodilator drugs are effective in treating hypertension and cardiac failure but risk exacerbating organ ischaemia by reducing perfusion pressure in the collateral circulation.

Release of the aortic cross-clamp may result in a dramatic reduction in BP due to the sudden decrease in systemic vascular resistance. Ischaemic metabolites and the ensuing metabolic acidosis may exacerbate myocardial depression. There may be central hypovolaemia due to sequestration of blood in the reperfused organs. The severity of hypotension is proportional to the cross-clamp time. Ensuring adequate cardiovascular filling prior to cross-clamp release and a gradual release of the cross-clamp helps to minimize declamping hypotension.

Vasodilator drugs, if used, should be discontinued before cross-clamp release.

Vasopressor drugs may be required after cross-clamp release.

Reclamping may be required if the hypotension is severe and refractory to treatment.

Intra-operative Monitoring

Direct measurement of arterial and central venous pressure, temperature and urine output is mandatory. A five-lead ECG will aid in the detection of ST segment changes.

There is some evidence that haemodynamic management to achieve an optimal value of stroke volume may reduce postoperative complication rates and shorten the hospital stay. A pulmonary artery flotation catheter (PAFC) should be considered for patients with impaired ventricular function.

Minimally invasive cardiac output monitors may provide useful information. These include arterial waveform pulse contour analysis devices and bio-impedance devices. Oesophageal Doppler monitoring may be used, but the readings obtained during the period of aortic cross-clamping are of limited value.

Peri-operative hypothermia is common in open AAA surgery because the abdomen may be open for a considerable time. Peri-operative hypothermia is associated with myocardial ischaemia and dysrhythmias, contributes to a coagulopathy and increases wound infections. Shivering can increase oxygen consumption up to six-fold, placing excessive demands on the cardiovascular system.

Forced air warming devices, fluid warmers and increased ambient theatre temperatures are important to minimize heat loss. The legs should not be actively warmed when the aorta is cross-clamped. It is important to commence heat conservation measures in the anaesthetic room.

Blood loss during elective AAA repair is highly variable with measured blood loss more than 5 L in 7% of surgery. Adequate wide-bore intravenous access is important.

A valid group-and-save is sufficient in the absence of antibodies, as most blood transfusion laboratories will issue type specific blood immediately. Homologous blood transfusion can be minimized by intra-operative cell salvage. Since vascular patients have a high incidence of coronary artery disease, the target haematocrit should be maintained at more than 27% (haemoglobin >90 g/L). Point-of-care (POC) testing devices such as the Hemocue® can provide accurate haemoglobin measurement.

Local protocols for the management of massive blood transfusion should be followed. Massive haemorrhage can produce a dilutional coagulopathy, requiring fresh frozen plasma, cryoprecipitate and platelet transfusions. Early liaison with the blood transfusion laboratory is essential if excessive bleeding occurs to ensure adequate supplies of blood and blood products. Appropriate administration of blood products is best guided by POC testing devices such as rotational thromboelastometry.

Postoperative Management

Patients require close monitoring after open abdominal vascular surgery in a critical care facility. EVAR patients can return to the ward after a short period of monitoring in recovery. Early enteral nutrition is encouraged to maintain gut mucosal integrity and reduce bacterial translocation. Good glycaemic control is important. Appropriate antacid, thromboembolic and antibiotic prophylaxis should be prescribed and early mobilization encouraged.

Following open AAA surgery patients must be closely monitored for cardiac events with serial ECGs and troponin measurements.

Concealed postoperative bleeding must be born in mind in the unstable patient, as drains are not routinely used in open infrarenal AAA surgery. Patients must be closely observed for signs of increasing abdominal distension. Deranged coagulation indices must be rapidly corrected with appropriate quantities of blood products. Rarely patients may need to return to theatre for re-exploration if blood loss continues.

Postoperative renal function should be closely monitored. The incidence of renal dysfunction after open infrarenal AAA surgery is around 5%, of which

0.6% require haemodialysis. Mortality exceeds 25% if renal failure occurs. The mainstay of renal preservation is maintenance of oxygen delivery and the avoidance of nephrotoxic drugs.

Ischaemic colitis is a rare complication after infrarenal AAA surgery (0.6%). If the collateral circulation is inadequate, the bowel may become ischaemic. Risk factors include suprarenal cross-clamp, prolonged clamp times and pre-existing mesenteric artery atherosclerosis. Ischaemic colitis presents with bloody diarrhoea, abdominal pain and unexplained fever or leucocytosis. Persistent postoperative metabolic acidosis with rising lactate concentrations that cannot be attributed to other causes should precipitate urgent surgical re-exploration.

Spinal cord ischaemia is a rare, devastating complication of open infrarenal AAA repair. It is much more common after thoracic aneurysm repairs. A flaccid para paresis with dissociated sensory loss occurs in less than 0.5% of elective infrarenal AAA repairs with higher incidence after emergency aortic surgery.

The distal circulation needs to be closely monitored. Distal atheroembolism may occur which may require exploration and possible embolectomy if the viability of the lower extremity is compromised.

Postoperative Analgesia

Postoperative analgesia in the majority of patients after infrarenal AAA surgery should be provided by an epidural infusion of low-dose local anaesthetic combined with an opioid. Multimodal nonopioid analgesia is introduced as soon as possible.

If an epidural is contraindicated analgesia of the anterior abdominal wall may be provided by rectus sheath catheters supplemented by systemic opioids administered by a patient-controlled analgesia device.

Anaesthetic Management of Endovascular Repair

The anaesthetist should consider:

- Problems of anaesthesia in remote site if the procedure is performed in the angiography suite
- Requirement for short periods of apnoea to improve the quality of the imaging
- Prolonged bilateral femoral occlusion resulting in ischaemic pain
- Risk (1%) of conversion to an open procedure

General anaesthesia with muscle relaxation and artificial ventilation provides excellent surgical conditions. Epidural, combined spinal-epidural or spinal anaesthesia are appropriate for endovascular aortic aneurysm repair. Sedation with a benzodiazepine or target-controlled infusion of propofol is usually required with local anaesthetic techniques.

Another alternative is local infiltration by the surgeon coupled with intravenous sedation. Relative contraindications include patient anxiety, previous groin surgery and obesity (body mass index >30). Ischaemic leg pain is best managed with intravenous opioids (e.g. remifentanil target concentration <2 ng/mL).

Invasive arterial BP monitoring is necessary.

Urinary catheterization is required; the high-contrast load may result in contrast-induced nephropathy.

Wide-bore venous access is required. The incidence of iliac vessel damage during EVAR is nearly 1%, although aortic rupture is extremely rare.

Anticoagulation with heparin 5000 U is recommended.

Ruptured Abdominal Aortic Aneurysm

Ruptured abdominal aortic aneurysm (RAAA) has an overall mortality rate of 65%. Patients present with signs and symptoms ranging from lower abdominal or lumbar pain in the presence of a pulsatile abdominal mass, to collapse, shock and coma. If patients are haemodynamically stable, they may be transferred for computerized tomography to confirm the diagnosis and determine suitability for endovascular repair. Free intraperitoneal rupture almost invariably results in cardiovascular collapse and death. Retroperitoneal (contained) rupture has a much better prognosis due to tamponade within the retroperitoneum, which limits further haemorrhage.

Treatment options for a patient with RAAA include:

● Immediate open repair
● Imaging with CT followed by EVAR if anatomically possible
● Imaging with CT followed by open repair if EVAR is not anatomically possible

The main advantage of immediate open repair is that further imaging is not required, and speed may save life. Conversely, EVAR is less invasive and can in most cases be performed under local anaesthesia, avoiding the life-threatening severe hypotension associated with general anaesthesia in a bleeding patient. Thirty-day mortality is similar between open repair and EVAR under general anaesthesia but lower in patients who undergo EVAR under local anaesthesia. EVAR is associated with a shorter hospital stay than open repair. However, EVAR has no survival benefit at 1 year.[4]

Preoperative Management

A rapid preoperative evaluation is required. Sometimes surgery may be inappropriate. Successful management often requires two experienced anaesthetists. A brief and targeted preoperative assessment is necessary. An operating theatre must be promptly prepared and an adequate supply of blood and blood products ensured. The Massive Haemorrhage Protocol should be triggered to alert the blood transfusion laboratory.

A restrictive resuscitation policy prior to surgical control is associated with a better outcome. It is important to maintain organ function, but not to restore a normal arterial BP. Administration of large volumes of fluid is thought to dislodge thrombus and dilute already depleted clotting factors, causing further bleeding. Red cell transfusion should be avoided unless the patient is unconscious or there is clinically significant myocardial ischaemia.

Analgesia prior to induction should be carefully titrated. In the elderly patient with haemorrhagic shock and organ dysfunction, even small doses of opioids may precipitate cardiovascular collapse. However, severe pain will cause hyperventilation and increased O_2 consumption.

Anaesthesia for Open Repair

Anaesthesia should be induced with the patient on the operating table with external warming devices connected (warming mattress, forced air warmer), the surgeon in the operating theatre ready scrubbed and the abdomen prepared before induction.

Connect large-bore intravenous access to a rapid infusion device. If possible establish invasive arterial BP monitoring and obtain a sample for blood gas analysis. Make sure an intra-operative cell salvage device is prepared. Perform a modified rapid sequence induction and be prepared for all eventualities (e.g. profound hypotension, hypertension, tachycardia, bradycardia and cardiac arrest).

Once a cross-clamp is applied and control of bleeding confirmed, aggressive resuscitation of the patient is appropriate with fluid, blood and blood products. A central venous line is inserted and noninvasive cardiovascular monitoring is employed. General haematological and biochemical goals are haemoglobin 80–90 g/L, platelets more than 100×10^9 per L, prothrombin and APTT ratio less than 1.5, fibrinogen more than 2 g/L, calcium more than 1 mmol/L and pH more than 7.35. Administration of blood and blood products is best guided by POC devices (Hemocue®, thromboelastometry).

Postoperative intensive care will be essential. Rewarming will be necessary and respiratory and cardiovascular support will be required, often for several days. Renal function, haemoglobin, coagulation and acid–base derangements all require close monitoring. Measure intra-abdominal pressures, as abdominal compartment syndrome is a frequent complication. Renal replacement therapy will be required in a significant proportion of patients. Persisting coagulopathy may require further blood product support, ideally guided by POC testing. Postoperative ileus may be prolonged and parenteral nutrition is frequently required.

Anaesthesia for Endovascular Repair

Emergency EVAR under local anaesthesia may be extremely challenging in the agitated confused patient who is experiencing severe abdominal pain. Large volumes of dilute local anaesthetic solution containing adrenaline are usually required. A supracoeliac aortic balloon may be used to control haemorrhage prior to stent-graft deployment ('radiological cross-clamp'). As with open repair, aggressive fluid resuscitation is commenced once control is obtained. The endovascular options are bifurcated EVAR or insertion of an aorto-uni-iliac

(AUI) stent and femoro-femoral cross-over graft. The latter is often performed under a general anaesthetic to permit tunnelling of the cross-over graft.

Carotid Endarterectomy

Carotid endarterectomy (CEA) is a prophylactic operation to prevent embolic stroke due to atheromatous disease around the carotid bifurcation. CEA should be performed within 14 days of a stroke or TIA when there is an internal carotid stenosis of more than 70%. The number needed to treat (NNT) to prevent one major stroke or death within 5 years is 6.

There is a high incidence of hypertension, diabetes, ischaemic heart disease and smoking-related lung disease in patients presenting for CEA. These should be optimally treated. All patients should be taking an antiplatelet drug (aspirin or clopidogrel) and a statin.

Surgical Technique

Whatever the surgical technique used for CEA, there is temporary interruption of flow up one internal carotid artery. As 80%–90% of the cerebral blood supply is delivered via the two internal carotid arteries (the remainder comes from the vertebra-basilar system), there is a potential risk of precipitating ipsilateral cerebral ischaemia, as there may be concurrent occlusive atheromatous disease in one of more vessels.

To reduce the risk of ipsilateral cerebral ischaemia, a shunt may be used. Acute complications of shunt insertion include air or plaque embolization, intimal tears and carotid dissection. The decision to insert a shunt should be based on cerebral function monitoring.

Anaesthesia for Carotid Endarterectomy

Although CEA may be performed under general or local anaesthesia,[5] there is no significant difference in peri-operative stroke or 30-day mortality between the two techniques, but myocardial infarction (MI) may be more common with local anaesthesia. However, in patients with contralateral carotid artery occlusion, local anaesthesia is associated with a significant reduction in adverse outcome (stroke, MI or death).[6]

The main aims of anaesthesia are:

- Maximize cerebral perfusion and oxygen delivery
- Minimize myocardial stress
- Maintain cardiovascular stability before, during and after surgery so as to minimize the risk of MI, neck haematoma and postoperative cerebral hyperperfusion syndrome (ipsilateral headache, hypertension, seizures and focal neurological deficit)

CEA may be performed under superficial, intermediate or deep cervical plexus block.[7] Deep cervical block is associated with the greatest risk of complications (inadvertent injection into the CSF or vertebral artery and transient phrenic nerve paralysis). It should not be used in patients with severe respiratory disease or known contralateral phrenic nerve palsy. Local anaesthesia for CEA permits the selective use of shunts guided cerebral monitoring indicated by an awake cooperative patient. However, CEA under regional anaesthesia can be stressful for the patient.

Although there are no data to favour any particular form of general anaesthetic, airway control using tracheal intubation is preferred. A light balanced anaesthetic technique permits rapid awakening and allows prompt assessment of postoperative neurological function.

Some form of neurological monitoring to guide shunt usage is useful with general anaesthesia. These include internal carotid artery stump pressure, processed ECG recording, somatosensory evoked potentials, near infrared spectroscopy and transcranial Doppler.

Intra-operative considerations include the following:

- Position the patient with the neck and head extended slightly. Patients with orthopnoea, severe respiratory disease, arthritis or degenerative spine disease may find it difficult to maintain this position if surgery is performed under local anaesthesia.
- Restrict intravenous fluids when CEA is performed under local anaesthesia, otherwise a urinary catheter may be inserted.
- Blood loss is usually minimal, but a group and save should be performed. Rarely, the surgeon may lose control of carotid artery.
- Cardiovascular lability is common, so direct arterial pressure monitoring is mandatory. Arterial BP tends to fall after induction of general anaesthesia, but an increase is common under local anaesthesia especially when the cross-clamp is applied. Postoperative hypo- and hypertension are common. A superficial cervical plexus block provides useful postoperative analgesia.

Complications of Carotid Endarterectomy

These include:

- Excessive bleeding – 2.8% of patients
- Cranial nerve damage – 1.6% of patients
- MI – 0.9% of patients
- Death or stroke within 30 days of surgery – 2% of patients

Postoperative Management

Most patients who undergo CEA can be closely monitored in the recovery ward for a period of time and then discharged to a vascular ward. Cardiovascular lability is common; the arterial BP must be closely monitored.[8] Patients must be observed carefully for the development of a neck haematoma. These occur in approximately 5% of CEAs. This complication usually develops slowly and, if unrecognized or underestimated, may be fatal.

Airway management for surgical re-exploration can be technically very difficult. Patients who have head and neck surgery have a reduction in the volume of their upper airway postoperatively due to soft tissue oedema. The additional insult of a haematoma superimposed on this oedema can further compress the airway and cause respiratory embarrassment. Oedema of the supraglottic folds makes laryngeal visualization and tracheal intubation difficult.

Evacuation of the neck haematoma under local anaesthesia is the safest option. If the operation has been performed under cervical plexus blockade and the haematoma develops early in the postoperative period, the blocks may still be effective. If the CEA has been performed under general anaesthesia or if the haematoma occurs late in the postoperative course when the local anaesthetic blocks have worn off, drainage can be performed using local anaesthetic infiltration.

Lower Limb Revascularization

Peripheral arterial disease (PAD) is caused by atherosclerosis leading to stenosis or occlusion of major blood vessels supplying an extremity. PAD includes intermittent claudication (IC), critical limb ischaemia (CLI) and acute limb ischaemia (ALI). It is a progressive disease. Some patients will require either endovascular intervention or peripheral vascular revascularization (PVR) surgery. Up to 15% of the patients with asymptomatic PAD will develop symptoms of IC or CLI and 1%–3% of them will require major limb amputation within 5 years. The development of CLI is a marker of decreased longevity; the 5-year survival for patients with CLI is 50%–60%.

IC is usually associated with gradual reduction in walking distance over months or years. Rapid exacerbation of symptoms and acute onset of IC are important warning signs for acute arterial occlusion.

CLI is a surgical emergency.

ALI may be classified as viable, threatened or nonviable with surgery planned accordingly (Table 5.17.1).

Surgical revascularization of the ischaemic lower limb is being replaced increasingly by radiological interventions (angioplasty and/or stenting). Indications for surgery are ischaemic rest pain, tissue loss (ulceration or gangrene), severe claudication with distal disease, failure of nonsurgical (endovascular) treatment and prevention of limb loss.

Clinical Management of Acute Ischaemia

Category I

These patients should be treated with intravenous heparin and analgesia. There is usually adequate time for patients to be fully investigated both surgically and medically and optimized prior to any surgical intervention.

TABLE 5.17.1 Clinical Categories of Acute Limb Ischaemia

Category	Sensation	Paralysis	Suggested Treatment
I (Viable)	No loss of sensation	None	Not immediately threatened; time to investigate
IIa (Threatened)	Minimal loss (e.g. toe)	None	Urgent treatment needed for salvage
IIb (Threatened)	More than toes and associated with rest pain	Partial	Immediate treatment needed for salvage
III (Irreversible)	Profound, anaesthetic	Profound/ rigor	Irreversible – primary amputation

Source: Adapted from Rutherford RB, Baker JD, Ernst C, et al. Recommended standards for reports dealing with lower extremity ischemia: revised version. J Vasc Surg 1997;26:517–38.

Category II

These patients also require heparinization and analgesia. Complete acute ischaemia is a medicosurgical emergency, as irreversible tissue necrosis results if perfusion cannot be restored within 6 h of the onset of symptoms.

There is minimal time for investigation. Resuscitation and preoperative optimization should not overly delay the proposed urgent intervention.

Embolectomy is usually the preferred immediate surgical management, frequently performed under local anaesthesia. Monitored anaesthesia care is recommended, as patients frequently have significant comorbidity and may be restless and in pain. General anaesthesia may be required if the patient is uncooperative or if more extensive procedures are required. Embolectomy may be followed by on-table arteriography with subsequent thrombolysis, angioplasty, stenting or arterial bypass.

Compartment syndrome secondary to reperfusion injury within the calf muscle necessitates fasciotomy in about 5% of the patients whose ALI is successfully treated. Direct pressure measurement of compartment pressures is important. A compartment pressure of 30 mm Hg or a diastolic BP less than 30 mm Hg above the compartment pressure is an indication for fasciotomy.

Patients should be closely monitored for acute rhabdomyolysis with serial creatine kinase measurements and close monitoring of renal performance. A brisk diuresis should be maintained to avoid renal failure.

Category III

These patients presenting with irreversible ischaemia may require urgent amputation. This procedure should not be delayed unduly for medical optimization so as to minimize the life-threatening systemic effects of extensive muscle necrosis in the affected limb.

Terminal care is sometimes the most appropriate option in patients with extensive tissue involvement and significant comorbidities.

Lower Limb Revascularization

The risks of peripheral vascular reconstruction (PVR) are high. Coexisting coronary artery disease (CAD) is almost inevitable, but symptoms of CAD are masked by immobility related to IC, frailty and arthritis. The ability to exercise is limited by PAD, so assessment of functional capacity is difficult. Surgery for critical limb ischaemia is often urgent with limited time for investigations. Operative duration is often prolonged with the risk of hypothermia, insidious blood loss and associated cardiovascular instability.

Anaesthesia for Lower Limb Revascularization

General anaesthesia, regional anaesthesia or a combination of the two can be used successfully for PVR. Sufficient evidence is lacking to favour one technique over the other, as there are no clinically significant differences in long-term survival whichever technique is chosen.

Regional anaesthesia has the theoretical benefit of reducing respiratory morbidity and postoperative cognitive dysfunction whilst providing good quality postoperative analgesia. It may be unsuitable for patients who are unable to lie supine due to cardiac, respiratory or musculoskeletal issues and for prolonged procedures. Some patients with CLI will be anticoagulated with systemic heparin which precludes central neuraxial blockade. The risk:benefit ratio of regional anaesthesia must be considered carefully for patients on dual anti-platelet therapy. Regional anaesthesia for PVR is achieved with either spinal anaesthesia or a combined spinal–epidural (CSE) technique. CSE techniques are useful for prolonged procedures and when epidural analgesia will be beneficial in the postoperative period.

General anaesthesia provides a theoretical benefit in high-risk patients as volatile and opioid preconditioning may provide myocardial protection against ischaemic injury. Balanced anaesthesia using positive pressure ventilation is preferable. Cardiovascular stability should be maintained throughout using fluids, vasopressors and/or positive inotropic drugs. Heparin 5000 U is usually administered before interruption of blood flow to the operative limb and graft placement.

Restoration of blood flow to an ischaemic limb following surgical reconstruction may cause transient myocardial depression and hypotension due to the release of vasoactive cytokines and metabolites from the ischaemic extremity. This can be treated with fluids, ephedrine or phenylephrine.

Whichever technique is chosen, maintenance of normothermia is vital. Active warming devices and insulation of exposed areas are mandatory. Intravenous fluids should be warmed.

Lower Limb Amputation

The indication for lower limb amputation (LLA) are:

● Primary – due to overwhelming sepsis or severe intractable pain when there is no viable arterial reconstructive option
● Secondary – after failed arterial reconstruction

The incidence of amputation is 8–15 times higher in the diabetic population compared with nondiabetic patients with 70% dying within 5 years of surgery. The 30-day mortality from LLA is between 12% and 22%, with 38%–48% of the patients dying within 1 year of surgery, reflecting the age and associated comorbidity. The risks are greater for above-knee amputation compared with below-knee amputation.

Patients requiring major amputation require careful assessment by a multi-disciplinary team and optimization of controllable risk factors.

Operative interventions should be performed promptly by a senior anaesthe-tist and surgeon on a routine operating list during normal working hours within 48 h of the decision to operate. Out of hours operating may be associated with up to a three-fold increase in mortality.

There should be formal pain management protocols in place and early access to a team of rehabilitation specialists.

Anaesthesia for Lower Limb Revascularization

Anaesthetic techniques should achieve cardiovascular stability, maintain nor-movolaemia and provide effective postoperative analgesia.

Catheter-based regional anaesthetic techniques (epidural, femoral and pop-liteal catheters) have the advantage of also providing effective postoperative analgesia with improved postoperative respiratory function and reduced post-operative cognitive decline. Central neuraxial blockade is contraindicated in patients who are anticoagulated.

REFERENCES

1. Snowden CP, Minto G. Exercise the new premed. Br J Anaesth 2015;114:186–9.
2. Hartle A, McCormack J, Carlisle J, Anderson S, Pichel A, Beckett N, et al. The measurement of adult blood pressure and management of hypertension before elective surgery: Joint Guidelines from the Association of Anaesthetists of Great Britain and Ireland and the British Hypertension Society. Anaesthesia 2016;71:326–37.
3. Hollingsworth G, Danjoux G, Howell SJ. Cardiopulmonary exercise testing before abdominal aortic aneurysm surgery: a validated risk prediction tool? Br J Anaesth 2015;115:494–7.
4. Improve trial investigators. Endovascular or open repair for ruptured AAA: 30 day outcomes from the IMPROVE randomised trial. BMJ 2014;348:f7661.
5. Howell SJ. Carotid endarterectomy. Br J Anaesth 2007;99:119–31.

6. GALA Trial Collaborative Group. General anaesthesia versus local anaesthesia for carotid surgery (GALA): a multicentre randomised controlled trial. Lancet 2008;372:2132–42.
7. Stoneham MD, Stamou D, Mason J. Regional anaesthesia for carotid endarterectomy. Br J Anaesth 2015;114:372–83.
8. Stoneham MD, Thompson JP. Arterial pressure measurement and carotid endarterectomy. Br J Anaesth 2009;102:442–52.

Section 6

Chronic Pain

Chapter 6.1

Chronic Pain

Simon Dolin

Pain has been defined by the International Association for the Study of Pain (IASP) as 'an unpleasant sensory and emotional experience associated with actual or potential tissue damage, or described in terms of such damage' (www.iasp-pain.org/taxonomy).

Chronic pain is pain that persists beyond a reasonable time in which one would expect the pain from an acute injury to settle. Three months is commonly taken as the time after which a pain becomes chronic.

The origin of the pain can be from ongoing tissue damage, such as arthritis or cancer (nociceptive), or as a result of injury to somatosensory component of neural pathways (neuropathic) or the pain can be of unknown origin. For all pain types, pre-existing psychological make-up, social factors and the psychological response to ongoing pain can make an important contribution to the clinical picture.

THE PAIN CLINIC

Pain clinics (PCs) are generally run as a multidisciplinary team usually led by anaesthetists in conjunction with other specialties, including rheumatology, neurology, neurosurgery, psychiatry and professions allied to medicine, including nursing, physiotherapy, occupational therapy and clinical psychology.

The role of the PC in patient care can be summed up as:

- To decrease subjective pain experience
- To increase general level of activity
- To optimize (mostly reduce) analgesic medication consumption
- To return the patient to work or leisure activities or improve quality of life
- To reduce use of health care resources in the longer term by developing self-management skills

Facilities required include dedicated office space, consulting rooms, space for group-based pain management, and one-to-one treatments such as transcutaneous electrical nerve stimulation (TENS) and physiotherapy. Access to X-ray imaging in a suitable facility for interventional pain procedures, with monitoring and resuscitation is also required; many PCs use day-surgery unit or similar.

Essential PC equipment includes suitable imaging, suitable monitoring for sedation, a radiofrequency lesion generator and a peripheral nerve stimulator. Access to inpatient beds is an option for those requiring complex medication changes, or therapies requiring prolonged drug administration via complex routes, e.g. epidural or intrathecal.

PC treatments, including interventional pain procedures and psychological interventions have varying degrees of evidence of effectiveness.

THE PAIN PATIENT

Chronic pain is common, affecting an estimated 20% of adults globally and increasing with age. In addition, 10% of adults are newly diagnosed with chronic pain each year. As the PC approach is essentially that of symptom control, referrals should ideally have completed diagnostic work-up and appropriate surgical and medical therapy. The most common source of referrals is from physiotherapy, rheumatology and orthopaedic clinics for musculoskeletal pain. Other sources of referrals include general medicine, surgery, neurology and palliative care. General practice referrals can be accepted as long as additional diagnostic work-up is not required.

The patient will have already tried a variety of analgesic medications, usually with only modest success. Other medications may include benzodiazepines and antidepressants. Most will have already tried physiotherapy and alternative therapies, often with limited success.

Anxiety and depression are common in chronic pain patients and can be primary problems or secondary to persistent pain. Sleep disturbance due to pain is common. Other emotions may include anger and blame.

Post-traumatic stress disorder symptoms (flashbacks, nightmares, avoidant behaviour) can be associated with chronic pain following trauma. Litigation for personal injury or medical negligence is increasingly common. The patient may be in receipt of benefits for unemployment and disability.

Many chronic pain patients are taking excessive and often ineffective analgesic medications, particularly opioids which have become increasingly widely prescribed for chronic nonmalignant pain. There are problems with long-term use of opioids in this setting, for which there is little evidence of effectiveness. Tolerance occurs relatively quickly, requiring increasing doses. This in turn can lead to opioid-induced hyperalgesia where pain pathways become sensitized by prolonged opioid exposure, especially at high doses.[1] The result is increasingly inadequate pain control combined with cumulative opioid side effects of sedation, somnolence, constipation, poor cognitive function and interference with work, leisure and social function. Other commonly co-prescribed medications such as antidepressants and anticonvulsants add to the side effects.

The combination of inadequate analgesia and excessive side effects is not in the patients' favour and detoxification of most if not all analgesic medications can transform the clinical picture. Detoxification can lead to improved pain relief and quality of life as drug-related side effects are eliminated. Many patients decide to take little or no analgesic medication in the long term in view of previous experiences.

ASSESSMENT OF PAIN

Important aspects of pain assessment are as follows:

- Site – body maps indicate the extent of pain and often request the patient to identify the primary pain site. Widespread or total body pain is a surprisingly common.
- Severity – assessed as worst pain, least pain and average pain using visual analogue pain scale (VAS), numerical rating scale (NRS) or categorical rating (none/mild/moderate/severe).
- Duration.
- Cause (and diagnosis if known) – precipitating episode or spontaneous onset. Pain of unknown aetiology is common.
- Pattern – continuous, intermittent or flare-up pattern.
- What makes the pain worse.
- What makes the pain better.
- Medications, TENS and other therapies – how effective are they.
- What words does the patient use to describe the pain.
- Depression and anxiety – sleep pattern, mood, fatigue, tearfulness, guilt feelings, future outlook and any past history of depression, how it was treated and if it was successful. Any previous contacts with mental health services.
- Past history of pain – previous investigations, surgery, interventional pain procedures and other PC treatments.
- Current activity and employment. What does the pain stop the patient from doing; How far can he or she walk or drive; Is the patient independent for dressing and bathing; Describe daily activities.
- Home situation – who is at home; Are they all well; Is the patient a carer or does he or she have a carer.
- Is litigation active.

Commonly used pain questionnaires include the Brief Pain Inventory and the McGill Pain Questionnaire. Many others have been devised for research purposes, but they are occasionally useful for clinical practice (Beck Depression Inventory, Hospital Anxiety and Depression [HAD] Scale, Somatic Perception Questionnaire). Patient pain diaries are commonly used by PCs.

PCs are not intended for diagnostic assessment. If the pain clinician is unclear of the explanation for symptoms, referral to an appropriate specialist is in order. Many complex pain problems can persist, in spite of extensive investigations and treatments. PCs often have joint clinics with other specialties, such as rheumatology, orthopaedics, maxillofacial surgery, urology, palliative care and psychiatry. Missed pathology is a problem and the pain clinician should always consider this possibility, especially if symptoms change or worsen.

Neuroimaging of Pain

There has been a recent growth in brain imaging of pain using functional magnetic resonance imaging (fMRI) and positron emission tomography (PET) which has identified key areas of brain activity in response to pain in healthy subjects and patients with chronic pain. Common activations included the thalamus, anterior cingulate cortex, insula and cerebellum. Results point towards the central role of the insular cortex and anterior cingulate cortex in pain processing, irrelevant of pain modality, body part or clinical experience. There are functional differences in pain processing between patients with chronic pain and healthy individuals.

GENERALIZED PAIN PATTERNS

Neuropathic Pain

Neuropathic pain is caused by injury to somatosensory nervous system which can be central (e.g. multiple sclerosis) or peripheral (e.g. painful peripheral neuropathy, peripheral nerve injury). Neuropathic pain presents with characteristic symptoms (pins and needles, tingling/prickling sensations, abnormal sensitivity to touch and temperature, electric shocks, burning sensations) and characteristic clinical signs, increased sensitivity to light touch (allodynia) or pinprick (hyperpathia).

Commonly used screening tools to detect the presence of neuropathic pain, based on symptoms and signs are the Leeds Assessment of Neuropathic Symptoms and Signs (LANSS) Pain Scale, Pain DETECT and DN-4.

Neuralgia is pain in the distribution of a nerve or nerves, including trigeminal and postherpetic neuralgia (PHN) and scar pain.

Painful polyneuropathies are usually symmetrical and distal, affecting the feet and sometimes the hands, common examples are diabetic, ischaemic, chemotherapy and HIV-induced neuropathies.

The mechanism of neuropathic pain is different from that of nociceptive pain. Peripheral mechanisms involve abnormal C fibre function which can become sensitized to sympathetic stimulation. Axonal sprouts develop where primary afferent neurones have been damaged which may have abnormal sensitivity to mechanical, noradrenergic and thermal stimulation and may fire independently of any sensory input. Adjacent neurones may develop abnormal connections which may be recruited into the exaggerated response to stimuli. Central mechanisms involve changes in the long-term excitability of dorsal horn cells including altered glial cells function. These are mediated in part through

N-methyl-D-aspartate (NMDA) subtype of glutamate receptor, in a process known as 'wind-up'. Damage to peripheral or central sensory neurones can lead to loss of coordination of neuronal inhibitory processes. These processes are known as peripheral and central sensitization.

Recommended treatment of neuropathic pain[2] is as follows:

- Analgesic antidepressants are the drugs of first choice; either tricyclics (e.g. dosulepin, amitriptyline, nortriptyline) or selective noradrenergic reuptake inhibitors (SNRIs, e.g. duloxetine, venlafaxine). Sedation and dry mouth are common side effects, but lower doses are generally tolerated.
- Analgesic anticonvulsants (gabapentin, pregabalin) are drugs of second choice. Other anticonvulsants such as lamotrigine, phenytoin, oxcarbazepine and clonazepam are used occasionally when other medications are ineffective or poorly tolerated. Carbamazepine is indicated selectively for trigeminal neuralgia, but rarely used otherwise. Sedation and ataxia may limit the use of these medications. Weight gain may be a problem with pregabalin.
- Sodium-channel blockers lidocaine – topical lidocaine 5% is licenced for use in painful PHN, but can be considered for localized neuropathic pain generally. Intravenous lidocaine infusions and oral mexiletine have been used, but evidence of effectiveness is lacking.
- Opioids – tramadol has been shown to be effective for neuropathic pain. Other opioids are used, but evidence of effectiveness in the long term is lacking. Risks of long-term use include accidental overdose and injury, tolerance and opioid-induced hyperalgesia.
- Capsaicin – as cream (0.75%) or patch (8%), is indicated for localized neuropathic pain for patients who wish to avoid, or cannot tolerate, oral treatments. The low strength requires multiple applications per day. The higher strength can be repeated every 12 weeks but requires topical local anaesthetic prior to use.
- Nonsteroidal anti-inflammatory drugs (NSAIDs) – generally not indicated for neuropathic pain.
- Ketamine – can be effective in the short term, but its route of administration limits its use, and it is generally not used in long term.
- Clonidine – can be used but side effects (e.g. sedation, hypotension) limit its use, and it is generally not used in long term.
- Lumbar sympathectomy (chemical or radiofrequency) – was widely used to treat ischaemic leg pain, but it was unclear whether it improved blood flow or reduced neuropathic pain. It is less commonly used now and evidence of effectiveness is lacking.
- Spinal cord or peripheral nerve stimulation – is indicated and increasingly widely used for treatment of neuropathic pain.[3]

Phenotyping of Neuropathic Pain

Medications to treat neuropathic pain are often ineffective, or relatively so. Recently attempts have been made to predict response to drug treatment, to individual patient pain symptoms and to sensory testing, in particular quantitative sensory testing. This approach is known as pain phenotyping.

Phenotypes can be defined by symptoms (tingling, pricking, burning, paroxysms of lancinating pain, numbness) and by clinical signs (mechanical or cold allodynia, pain on pressure or hyperalgesia to pinprick, mechanical hypoaesthesia, cold and warm detection thresholds). Theoretically, an optimal response in an individual would be obtained if the particular pain mechanisms as determined by phenotyping matched the mechanism of drug action. Studies are inconclusive, but research is ongoing.

Postherpetic Neuralgia

PHN is a commonly occurring neuropathic pain. The herpes zoster virus can be reactivated from its dormant state in the central nervous system following chicken pox infection earlier in life and cause injury to individual peripheral nerve including dorsal root ganglion. It causes an acute painful attack with skin lesions that gradually resolve over several weeks. In 10%–18% of cases, chronic pain and associated numbness occur in the area of the scar, more commonly in older patients.

Clinical symptoms are pain, dysaesthesia, paraesthesia, allodynia and paroxysms of lancinating pain.

The most common sites are the cranial nerves and the thoracic dermatomes.

Early recognition and prompt treatment with an antiviral agent can shorten the acute illness and reduce complications, but evidence for prevention of PHN is lacking.

Vaccination of patients older than 60 years is likely to result in a decline in PHN.

Phantom Limb Pain

Sixty to eighty per cent of individuals experience phantom sensations, the majority of which are painful, following amputation of a limb. Phantom pain has also been described following mastectomy and bowel resection. The frequency and intensity of attacks usually declines with time.

The aetiology is unclear but probably involves an imbalance of peripheral sensory input with altered spinal cord and cortical function.

The effectiveness of prophylactic treatment with local anaesthetic nerve blocks before amputation to diminish the incidence of phantom limb pain remains unproven.

Evidence of effectiveness of mirror box therapy in treating phantom limb pain remains lacking.

Other problems include painful neuromas and muscle spasms.

Central Poststroke Pain

Central poststroke pain (CPSP) affects nearly 8% of stroke patients. It originates from a lesion in the spino-thalamo-cortical pathway.

Sensory disturbance is a major component of CPSP, including abnormal temperature sensation, dysaesthesia and hypersensitivity to cutaneous stimuli.

Persistent Postsurgical Pain

Persistent post surgical pain (PPP) including scar pain can occur after any operation, but is most common after thoracotomy, sternotomy, mastectomy and inguinal hernia repair. After inguinal hernia repair, up to 30% of patients experience persistent pain with up to 10% still experiencing intrusive symptoms 1 year later.

The cause of PPP is unknown, although there may be specific peripheral nerve injury or entrapment such as ilio-inguinal and ilio-hyopgastric nerves following inguional hernia repair.

Treatment is by local infiltration of the affected peripheral nerve with local anaesthetic and steroid.

Pulsed radiofrequency lesioning of the peripheral nerve may be considered, although evidence of effectiveness is lacking.

Complex Regional Pain Syndrome

Complex regional pain syndrome (CRPS) usually affects hands or feet of one limb, but rarely can spread to involve other limbs. It is a form of neuropathic pain with associated soft tissue changes, including temperature and skin colour, oedema and sweating, decreased range of joint movement, motor dysfunction such as weakness, tremor, dystonia and hair, nail and skin trophic changes.

CRPS usually starts after a noxious event, such as trauma or surgery, is not limited to the distribution of a single peripheral nerve and is often disproportionate to the inciting event. It can occur after immobilization of the limb. In some cases, there may be no precipitating event. As diagnosis can be difficult, various sets of diagnostic criteria have been described. The most widely used are the IASP, previously known as Budapest criteria that require a combination of sufficient symptoms and clinical signs to be present. Pain, allodynia and hyperalgesia are likely to be present, as in neuropathic pain. CRPS is a diagnosis of exclusion which requires that no other condition would otherwise account for the degree of pain and dysfunction.[4]

Treatment of CRPS is similar to neuropathic pain but also may require intensive physical and psychological rehabilitation. Specialist hand physiotherapy and occupational therapy may be required. Physical rehabilitation is aimed at gentle movement and desensitization, encouraging weight bearing and functional activity. Intravenous regional block with guanethedine, local anaesthetic and NSAIDs lack evidence of effectiveness.

Further surgery on the affected limb should be avoided, as it may worsen CRPS.

Longitudinal studies suggest that the prognosis is good with many patients, making a reasonable recovery over 6–13 months, but some progress to experience chronic pain and disability.[5]

Muscle and Soft Tissue Pain

Fibromyalgia

Fibromyalgia, also known as chronic widespread pain, is a chronic pain disorder characterized by widespread musculoskeletal pain, stiffness, tenderness, fatigue and sleep disturbance. Patients may describe their symptoms as total body pain. It is similar in presentation to chronic fatigue syndrome (ME), but in the latter, fatigue rather than pain is the predominant presenting symptom. Fibromyalgia occurs most commonly in women aged 20–40 years.

On examination, there is likely to be widespread muscle tenderness on palpation.

Diagnosis can be challenging, as CRPS is a diagnosis of exclusion and requires the demonstration that other conditions do not explain better the presenting symptoms. The American College of Rheumatology criteria are the most widely used diagnostic criteria. This set of criteria was revised in 2010 to combine a Widespread Pain Index (pain in five or more anatomical locations) and a Symptoms Severity Score (fatigue, waking unrefreshed, cognitive and other somatic symptoms).

Treatment of fibromyalgia, as for many pain syndromes, involves optimization of anlagesia by use of tricyclic antidepressants and reduction and elimination of ineffective sedative opioids and banzodiazepines.

Physical reactivation is recommended. Hydrotherapy may be a useful technique. Other wise physiotherapy should be aimed at re-establishing the range of movement and at pacing activities.

Cognitive-behavioural therapy (CBT) -based pain management programmes aimed at living with and managing chronic pain as a long-term condition are recommended.

Prognosis is uncertain, as the natural history of this condition is not well described.

Myofascial Pain Syndrome

Myofascial pain syndrome is a localized pain disorder characterized by a local area of muscle tenderness, presence of 'trigger points', and a reference zone of pain that is worsened by palpation of the trigger point. Each muscle group has characteristic trigger points and pain patterns. The most common identifiable myofascial pain syndromes seen in the PC are low back pain (quadratus lumborum, gluteals, quadriceps femoris) and neck/shoulder pain (posterior cervical muscle groups, levator scapulae and upper fibres of trapezius).

Treatment is by avoidance of perpetuating factors such as repetitive muscle use, by trigger point injection and by a technique called a 'spray and stretch' which involves stretching the affected muscle group. Prognosis of this localized muscle pain syndrome is generally good.

Visceral Pain

True visceral pain is vague, diffuse and poorly defined. It often presents as midline sensation, the vagueness of which is due to the low density of sensory innervation and to visceral input within the CNS. Augmentation of symptoms can occur between different internal organs that share part of their afferent innervation. This is termed viscero-visceral hyperalgesia and is a form of central sensitization.

Patients with one chronic visceral pain may suffer from multiple comorbid conditions with pain as a common symptom, e.g. fibromaylgia. This is thought to be due to a combination of peripheral augmentation of visceral afferent signalling, central sensitization and disturbances in descending modulation which can be influenced by cognitive and emotional factors.

Examples of chronic visceral pain include:

- Functional abdominal pain syndromes such as irritable bowel syndrome
- Interstitial cystitis
- Bladder pain syndrome – painful frequent voiding
- Vulvodynia
- Chronic prostatitis

Chronic abdominal, pelvic and urogenital pain can be present despite normal gastrointestinal, urinary and gynaecological investigations.

Treatment is similar to other chronic pain syndromes including patient education, analgesic antidepressants, gabapentanoids and psychological therapies.

Transforamenal sacral nerve stimulation with an implantable neuroprosthetic device has been shown to benefit patients with chronic pelvic pain.

Pain of Advanced Cancer

Pain occurs in 70% of patients with advanced cancer. Problems related to advanced cancer are dealt with mostly by palliative care services, but there is often an overlap with PCs. Clinical features of cancer pain syndromes are as follows:

- Bone metastases from lung, breast or prostate produce multiple pain sites which worsen on movement.
- Invasion of hollow viscus (stomach, colon) by tumour produces colicky abdominal pain which worsens with eating and improves by vomiting.
- Liver metastases from bowel, lung or breast produce upper quadrant abdominal pain and hepatomegaly.
- Bladder spasm from bladder or prostate cancer produces colicky suprapubic pain. Infection or blood clots may need specific treatment.
- Ureteric colic can occur with carcinoma of the ureter or bladder and will produce loin pain radiating to the groin.
- Chest wall or rib pain occurs with carcinoma of the lung and mesothelioma.

- Abdominal metastases occur with carcinoma of the ovary and colon, and result in diffuse abdominal pain and tenderness.
- Neuropathic pain occurs when nerves are damaged by tumour, as occurs in Pancoast's syndrome or invasion of the sacral plexus.
- Headache occurs when tumours result in raised intracranial pressure and when cranial nerves are involved, such as trigeminal neuralgia associated with meningioma and acoustic neuroma.
- Spinal cord involvement can result from spinal metastases and can result in radicular pain as well as progressive sensory and motor deficit and sphincter dysfunction.
- Painful muscle spasm can result from bony metastases and following hemiplegia.
- Infection of fungating tumours produces severe pain.

Treatment of pain of advanced cancer includes active treatments such as radiotherapy (for bony metastases), chemotherapy, hormone manipulation, orthopaedic correction of pathological fractures, surgical correction of bowel obstruction and neurosurgical decompression of cranium or spinal cord. Dexamethasone is commonly used to reduce painful tissue oedema.

World Health Organization Analgesic Ladder

Analgesic therapies are based on the World Health Organization (WHO) analgesic ladder which was originally developed for pain of advanced cancer. This involves a progression from a nonopioid analgesic such as paracetamol to weak opioid preparations such as codeine–paracetamol mixtures to strong opioid such as morphine to be given by the clock.

When pain of advanced cancer is not adequately treated by active treatments or weak opioids, the following options can be used:

- Oral morphine – given as an elixir (fast acting but relatively short in duration), as tablets (also fast acting) or as modified-release tablets (either once or twice a day). Most patients manage with doses up to 200 mg/day, although some patients may require much higher doses. Alternatives include hydromorphone and oxycodone (immediate and modified release formulations) and methadone (8–12-h) which can be useful when morphine becomes less effective (known as opioid rotation). Diamorphine can also be used, but it is not available outside the UK.
- Fentanyl patch (72-h duration) and buprenorphine patch (7-day duration) – are useful alternatives to oral morphine, especially when vomiting precludes the oral route.
- Subcutaneous morphine – given by syringe driver; a commonly used technique for patients with vomiting, dysphagia and coma. Antiemetics such as cyclizine are often added when vomiting is a problem, and midazolam can also be added to treat terminal anxiety and distress.

- Coanalgesics – given to augment opioids. These include NSAIDs, tricyclic antidepressants and other drugs used to treat neuropathic pain (see above), bisphosphonates and monoclonal antibodies to treat bone pain, anticholinergics to treat bowel spasm.
- Epidural catheter – local anaesthetic-plus-opioid by continuous infusion can be used when oral opioid analgesia is unsuccessful. This can be used at home as well as in the hospice. This requires a portable pump and good coordination of staff.
- Intrathecal catheter – Using morphine, clonidine and local anaesthetic gives more widespread and better-quality analgesia than the epidural route. This can be tunnelled and externalized. This requires a portable pump; fully implantable systems are available.
- Other catheter techniques, such as interpleural, brachial and lumbar plexus infusions using local anaesthetic, have been used but require specialized expertise and good coordination of staff.

Neurolytic Techniques

A number of neurolytic techniques are in common practice for pain of advanced cancer.

Coeliac Plexus Block

Coeliac plexus block using alcohol or phenol is indicated for pain from carcinoma of pancreas, but it is also useful for pain emanating from stomach, liver and small intestine. The coeliac plexus transmits the majority of pain fibres from the upper abdomen via the splanchnic nerves and sympathetic trunks to T5–T12. The plexus lies anterior to the aorta at the level of T12/L1 vertebrae. It can be approached either posteriorly through the crura of the diaphragm or directly through the aorta, or anteriorly through the liver or stomach. The technique is usually done under X-ray fluoroscopy, but it can be ultrasound- or computed tomography (CT)-guided. Side effects include transient pain on injection, hypotension and diarrhoea.

Splanchnic Nerve Block

Splanchnic nerve blocks using phenol or alcohol are performed above the diaphragm at T11/T12 and used for a similar indication as coeliac plexus blocks.

Chemical Sympathectomy

Chemical sympathectomy, lumbar, presacral or ganglion of impar, with phenol can be used for refractory lower limb or pelvic pain.

Cordotomy

Cordotomy done via radiofrequency of the spinothalamic tract at level of C2 vertebrae is used mostly for unilateral chest wall pain from mesothelioma which can be resistant to many other therapies.

Intrathecal Neurolysis

Intrathecal neurolysis using phenol or alcohol is an occasionally used technique for trunk pain. It carries the risk of sphincter and motor paralysis. Epidural neurolysis has also been described, but results are variable.

CHRONIC PAIN BY ANATOMICAL LOCATION

Headache

Headache is primarily dealt with in general practice with specialist input from neurology. Input from the PC may be requested for interventional procedures. Headache is generally subdivided into four main categories:

- Tension-type headache
- Migraine
- Cluster headache
- Medication over use headache

Tension-Type Headaches

Consider aspirin, paracetamol or an NSAID for the acute treatment of tension-type headache. Consider a course of up to 10 sessions of acupuncture over 5–8 weeks for the prophylactic treatment of chronic tension-type headache.

Migraine

Migraine is periodic unilateral headache. The pain is described as throbbing. Associated symptoms include nausea, vomiting and diarrhoea. Photophobia is common, as is a visual aura which may precede the pain. Duration is usually about 4 h, but can be longer. Occasionally, focal neurological deficits occur. Chronic migraine is defined as headaches on at least 15 days per month of which at least 8 days are with migraine. Episodic migraine is defined as fewer than 15 headache days per month for three consecutive months.

Treatment of migraine is to abort the current attack and to prevent the occurrence of migraine in the future.[6] Abortive therapies include:

- Combination therapy with an oral triptan plus a NSAID, or an oral triptan plus paracetamol
- Monotherapy with an oral triptan, NSAID, high-dose aspirin or paracetamol for patients who prefer to take only one drug
- Oral antiemetic in addition, even in the absence of nausea and vomiting
- Nonoral preparation of metoclopramide or prochlorperazine. Consider a nonoral NSAID and/or triptan for patients in whom oral preparations are ineffective or not tolerated

- Ergotamine, previously the drug of first choice, but is contraindicated in coronary and cerebrovascular disease
- Interventional procedures have been used to terminate an attack and are listed below, but evidence of effectiveness in the acute setting is limited

Prophylactic treatment includes the following:

- Topiramate – advise female patients about the risk of fetal malformation and interference with oral contraceptive efficacy
- Propranalol
- Amitriptyline
- Acupuncture – 10 sessions over 5–8 weeks
- Riboflavin – 400 mg once daily
- Botulinum toxin A – recommended if other prophylactic treatments are not successful

Cluster Headaches

Offer oxygen and/or a subcutaneous or nasal tripan for the acute treatment of cluster headache. Use 100% oxygen at a flow rate of at least 12 L/min with a non-rebreathing mask and a reservoir bag and arrange provision of home and ambulatory oxygen.[6]

Consider verapamil for prophylactic treatment during a bout of cluster headache.

Medication Overuse Headache

Advise patient to stop taking all overused acute headache medications for at least 1 month. Stop abruptly rather than gradually. Advise that headache symptoms are likely to get worse in the short term before they improve and that there may be associated withdrawal symptoms, and provide close follow-up and support. Review the diagnosis of medication overuse headache and further management 4–8 weeks after the start of withdrawal of overused medication.[6]

Interventional Procedures for Treatment of Headaches

These are currently recommended only with special arrangements for clinical governance, consent and audit or research:

- Transcutaneous electrical stimulation of the supraorbital nerve for treating and preventing migraine
- Transcutaneous electrical stimulation of the cervical branch of the vagus nerve for cluster headache and migraine
- Transcranial magnetic stimulation for treating and preventing migraine
- Occipital nerve stimulation for intractable chronic migraine
- Implantation of a sphenopalatine ganglion stimulation device for chronic cluster headache

- Deep brain stimulation for intractable trigeminal autonomic cephalalgias
- Percutaneous closure of patent foramen ovale for recurrent migraine

Neck Pain

Cervicogenic Headache Associated with Neck Pain

Cervicogenic headache is predominantly unilateral, usually occurring with neck and arm pain. There are signs of cervical spondylosis with pain on movement and a limited range of movement of cervical spine. Pain typically starts at the back of the head, but may also involve the face, whereas migraine mostly starts at the front of the head, often centred behind the eye. When the C2 nerve root is involved, the headache is over the occiput and can be relieved by greater occipital nerve block. Injection of cervical facet joints (or medical branch blocks) can relieve pain in some circumstances and are diagnostic for radiofrequency cervical facet denervation.

Myofascial pain syndromes involving posterior cervical muscles groups and sternomastoid can present as headache and can respond to injection and stretchin.

Whiplash Injury

Whiplash injury occurs after deceleration injury to the cervical spine. Most whiplash injuries settle spontaneously within 3 months regardless of treatment. Those that persist beyond 3 months tend to become chronic. Pre-existing neck problems, including spondylosis, and speed of impact contribute to chronicity.

Structures involved in whiplash injuries are the cervical facet (zygapophyseal) joints and the intervertebral discs, with a secondary muscle pain component. The pain is predominantly unilateral, as rotation of the spine to either side often occurs during injury. Patients may also complain of headaches, arm pain and numbness, especially in the medial fingers, reflecting trauma to the nerves that contribute to the ulnar nerve where they cross the first rib.

Treatment

The following are treatment options for whiplash injury:

- Regular analgesia and TENS
- Physiotherapy
- Muscle trigger point injections with local anaesthetic and steroid
- Facet or medial branch posterior primary rami injections with local anaesthetic and steroid
- Radiofrequency cervical facet denervation of the affected facet joints: This is performed percutaneously under fluoroscopy control and involves thermocoagulation of the posterior ramus of the cervical nerves, usually C3–C5; the levels may need to be determined by selective diagnostic facet joint blocks

Cervical Radiculopathy

Cervical radiculopathy can occur with cervical disc prolapse or due to cervical spondylosis, often precipitated by minor trauma, if the intervertebral foramen is already narrowed. Cervical degenerative changes are often discophytic bulges which are a combination of disc bulge and osteophyte. Pain is typically dermatomal and neuropathic and often described as burning or lancinating. Treatment options are as follows:

- Usual medications to treat neuropathic pain.
- Cervical epidural or nerve root steroid injections via the intervertebral foramen. Dexamethasone is the preferred steroid formulation. Particulate steroids are not advised due to the risk of spinal cord ischaemia and infarction which is thought to be due to steroid suspension limiting spinal cord blood flow.
- Surgical decompression is occasionally required in refractory cases.

Face Pain

Temporomandibular Muscle and Joint Disorders

Temporomandibular muscle disorders are characterized by pain arising from masticatory muscles. This can be a variant of myofascial pain syndrome, with pain referred to distant areas. Causation is unknown.

Reproducible pain on palpation of trigger point is diagnostic. Treatment is as for myofascial pain.

Temporomandibular joint (TMJ) dysfunction is a common chronic pain syndrome, characterized by pain arising from the TMJ, with joint noise and trismus. The pain radiates widely to the temporal, mastoid and occipital areas as well as the neck. Pain is caused by arthritic changes in the joint and muscle spasm.

On examination, there is palpable and audible clicking and limited jaw opening.

Magnetic resonance imaging (MRI) is used to determine disc position and morphology and joint effusion.

Auriculotemporal nerve block may be diagnostic.

Treatment options are:

- Reassurance and simple analgesia, including NSAIDs
- Low-dose analgesic antidepressants
- Injection of local anaesthetic into the joint and associated muscle groups (masseter, temporalis and lateral pterygoid) to relieve muscle spasm
- Psychological therapies, including CBT and biofeedback
- Injection of botulinum toxin (low dose) into the affected muscle groups
- Intraoral spints
- Arthroscopy and surgery – only for severe, refractory cases

Persistent Idiopathic Face Pain (Atypical Face Pain)

Atypical face pain is continuous chronic face pain that occurs in the absence of demonstrable pathology without objective clinical signs that does not fulfil any other diagnosis. The aetiology is unknown.

A thorough diagnostic work-up is necessary to exclude oral and maxillofacial pathology.

Investigations include an orthopantogram and facial and maxillary CT imaging. Treatment options are:

● Patient education
● Analgesic antidepressants at low dose
● Analgesic anticonvulsants
● TENS
● Acupuncture
● Psychological therapies including CBT and biofeedback

Giant Cell (Temporal) Arteritis

Temporal arteritis is vasculitis causing inflammation of the walls of medium-to-large arteries of the head and neck. It can present as acute temporal pain, often with a tender inflamed temporal artery, thickening or nodularity.

The erythrocyte sedimentation rate (ESR) is high.

The diagnosis is confirmed by temporal artery biopsy.

Prompt recognition and treatment with high-dose corticosteroids (prednisolone up to 60 mg/day) is necessary to prevent blindness.

Trigeminal Neuralgia

Trigeminal neuralgia is not a specific disease but a symptom, often caused by pathology involving cranial nerve V. It may be caused by structures impinging on the nerve including a loop of artery, an aneurysm, cerebellopontine angle tumours (acoustic neuroma, meningioma) all of which are amenable to surgery as well as multiple sclerosis but most cases remain idiopathic.

● The clinical features of trigeminal neuralgia are severe episodic recurrent unilateral face pain.
● It is described as a sudden high-intensity jab or electric shock.
● It lasts a few seconds, with repetitive bursts over minutes. Frequent episodes may occur over several weeks, followed by prolonged pain-free intervals.
● It occurs in the mandibular and maxillary divisions of the trigeminal nerve; ophthalmic pain is less common.
● It is triggered by stimulation of face, lips or mouth, and patients will avoid stimulation.

Cranial nerve examination is usually normal. If a trigeminal neurological deficit is found, MRI is indicated to exclude underlying pathology, although

MRI has now become routine investigation to exclude both malignancy and neurovascular compression.

Treatment Options

Treatment options for trigeminal neuralgia are as follows:

● First-line drug therapy – carbamazepine (up to 1000 mg/day). Most cases will respond to this therapy alone. Side effects include sedation and ataxia which may limit its use in the elderly. Bone marrow suppression, liver and renal impairment occur with prolonged therapy and require monitoring.
● Second-line drug therapy – phenytoin, baclofen, clonazepam and oxcarbazepine.
● Radiofrequency trigeminal ganglion thermocoagulation.
● Injection of glycerol into the trigeminal ganglion.
● Cryotherapy of peripheral branches of the trigeminal nerve, especially mental and infraorbital nerves – repeated freezing becomes difficult because of scarring.
● Gamma knife surgery at level of nerve root – good results but may cause facial numbness.
● Microvascular decompression – The preferred interventional approach. Provides relief in 70% of patients for up to 10 years. Recommended in younger patients. Associated with morbidity and mortality not seen with the percutaneous techniques, but long-term results are better.

Thoracic Pain

Costochondritis

Costochondritis presents as pain in the anterior chest wall. Involved sites are tender to palpation without inflammation. It is a benign, usually self-limiting disorder that may respond to simple analgesia, but may require infiltration of tender points with local anaesthetic and corticosteroid.

Osteoporotic Insufficiency Fractures

Osteoporosis is a reduction in the density of bone matrix that can result in insufficiency fractures in response to minimal trauma or can occur spontaneously. It affects the thoracolumbar spine and sacrum. Osteoporosis alone does not cause pain, but fractures can produce severe pain which can take weeks to months to settle. If there is insufficient bone matrix to allow healing or if progressive fracturing occurs pain can become chronic. Insufficiency fractures increase with age, are more common in women and increase with prolonged corticosteroid therapy.

The diagnosis is confirmed by plain X-ray. Recent fractures are 'hot' on nuclear medicine bone scan and STIR sequence on MRI scan. It is important to exclude malignancy (myeloma) as a possible cause by urine and plasma electrophoresis.

Prophylaxis (bisphosphonates, oral calcium) aims to prevent the progression of the disease. Bisphosphonates can improve pain associated with the insufficiency fracture. Denosumab is now used for the treatment of established osteoporosis.

Treatment consists or oral analgesia, TENS, thoracic epidural injection at the level of the fracture and nerve root injection for root pain. Percutaneous vertebroplasty and kyphoplasty involve injecting small volumes of bone cement into the compressed vertebral body or sacrum.

Abdominal Pain

Abdominal Wall Pain

Abdominal wall pain is characterized by local tender points in the abdominal wall, particularly in the rectus abdominis muscle. Carnett's sign is elicited by asking the patient to tense the abdominal wall by lifting the legs off the couch or to attempt to sit from the supine position. Aggravation of pain confirms the muscle as the site of pain. It is probably a type of myofascial pain syndrome. It can occur adjacent to scars from previous abdominal surgery. As the diagnosis is one of exclusion, ruling out other causes of abdominal pain is essential.

Treatment is by physiotherapy and injection of tender points with local anaesthetic and corticosteroid.

Back Pain and Sciatica

Mechanical Back Pain

Mechanical back pain affects the majority of the population at some time. Although most people experience short-lived, often recurrent episodes of back pain, a small minority develop chronic back pain which increases with age. Back pain is typically worse on movement and better with rest.

Anatomy

Back pain and sciatica emanate from four possible sites in the spine:

- Lumbar facet joints – account for about 30% of back pain, increasing with age. These joints may be injured by violent rotation of the spine, such as a sporting injury or trauma. The pain is often one-sided and aggravated by extension and rotation of the spine.
- Muscle pain – a common cause of low back pain. Muscle groups may be painful to palpation and muscle spasm may be visible on examination. The most commonly affected muscles are lumbar paravertebrals, quadratus lumborum and the gluteals.
- Lumbar discs – disc degeneration is commonly seen in radiographs and MRI scans of patients with back pain. Small tears can occur in the annulus of lumbar discs, observed as high-intensity zones on T2-weighted MRI scans. Such tears may account for some back pain and also for leg pain if the tear is adjacent to a lumbar nerve root.

- Spinal nerve roots – can produce sciatica when compressed by a prolapsed intervertebral disc or hypertrophic facet joint. L3 and L4 nerve root compressions result in anterior thigh pain. L4 nerve root compression is associated with diminished knee jerk. L5 or S1 nerve root compression is associated with posterior leg pain to the foot. S1 nerve root compression is associated with diminished ankle jerk.

Spinal stenosis occurs as part of the ageing process and, combined with disc degeneration, can produce critical narrowing of the spinal canal. In the elderly, this will present as unilateral leg pain with claudication. There is usually an absence of neurological signs in the leg.

Assessment

Initial assessment is based on history and examination. STarT Back (www.keele.ac.uk/sbst/startbacktool/) is a commonly used risk assessment tool which identifies risk of acute episode becoming chronic. 'Red flag' symptoms are new onset after 55 years of age, history of trauma, nonmechanical pain and systemically unwell. They require further investigation.[7]

Although imaging of nonspecific acute low back pain is not indicated, imaging of chronic low back pain and sciatica is indicated to exclude underlying pathology such as spondylolisthesis, disc prolapse, lateral recess stenosis and spinal stenosis.

Treatment

Treatment of mechanical back pain encompasses nonpharmacological, pharmacological, invasive and surgical interventions.[7,8] Nonpharmacological interventions include:

- Self-management advice and information – encourage continuation of normal activities where possible
- Group-based exercise programme – biomechanical, mind–body or combination
- Avoid orthotics as no evidence of benefit – belts, corsets
- Manual therapies – manipulation, mobilization and soft tissue techniques, but not traction or acupuncture
- Avoid electrotherapies as no evidence of benefit – ultrasound, TENS or interferential current stimulation
- Combined physical, psychological programme for chronic symptoms
- Return to work programmes

Pharmacological interventions include:

- NSAIDs at lowest effective dose for shortest possible time
- Weak opioids, with or without paracetamol if NSAIDs are contraindicated, not tolerated or ineffective

Invasive treatments include:

- Diagnostic medial branch blocks for chronic back pain with likely facet joint component. If benefit is short lived and pain is moderate to severe, proceed to radiofrequency facet denervation.
- Epidural injection (translaminar or transforaminal) for acute sciatica but not for spinal stenosis.
- Intradiscal techniques – IDET, anuloplasty not recommended.

Surgical interventions include:

- Spinal decompression for persistent sciatica with demonstrated compressive lesion
- Spinal fusion – not recommended except for selected cases such as spondylolisthesis
- Disc replacement – not recommended

Coccydynia

Coccydynia is pain in the region of the coccyx, usually worse on sitting. It may follow a fall that results in a fracture of the coccyx, but there may also not be a history of trauma.

Treatment options for coccydynia are as follows:

- Regular simple oral analgesia
- Rubber cushions – may help distribute weight from the coccyx
- Injection of local anaesthetic and steroid into local muscle tender points
- Infiltration of local anaesthetic and steroid into the sacral nerve roots via the sacral hiatus

Surgical coccygectomy is not recommended.

Postspinal Surgery Pain

Postspinal surgery pain (failed back surgery syndrome; FBSS) represents a great challenge. Patients present with persistent back pain or leg pain, although the two often coexist. The cause can include recurrent disc prolpase, inadequate surgical decompression, scarring producing mechanical traction on nerve roots, neuropathic pain from neural injury, development of facet joint arthritis and progressive degenerative changes at levels above or below previous spinal fusions.

Treatment options for FBSS are as follows:

- Simple analgesia
- Treat as neuropathic pain – especially if leg pain is predominant and a neurological deficit is present
- Transforaminal nerve root block – injection of local anaesthetic and corticosteroid around the nerve root can provide useful symptomatic relief
- Lumbar facet denervation

- Spinal cord stimulation – recommended if pain and disability are not relieved
- Physical reactivation through a graded exercise regimen – either alone or following on from injection therapy; best done within a multidisciplinary setting with input from physiotherapy, occupational therapy and clinical psychology
- Pain management programme based on CBT – can be useful in enabling patients to better manage their symptoms and disability (see section Psychological Therapies and Pain Management Programmes)

PSYCHOLOGICAL THERAPIES AND PAIN MANAGEMENT PROGRAMMES

Psychological Therapies

Psychological therapies have much to offer to chronic pain patients. Some clinicians prefer patients to be exposed to a psychological approach from the outset, whereas others prefer to finish appropriate drug therapy, injection therapy, physiotherapy and possibly surgery first.

Psychological therapies can be either on an individual basis or as part of a group programme. A number of conditions may be worth treating with psychological therapies alone, examples include fibromyalgia and irritable bowel syndrome.

Psychological therapies include the following:

- Operant conditioning – works by removing secondary gain that may be obtained by maintaining pain behaviour. Gain can be positive, such as getting attention or permission to rest, or negative as when pain allows avoidance of unpleasant situations. This works by eliminating reward for pain behaviour and reinforcing well behaviour.
- Behavioural therapy – involves manipulating the environment by taking analgesia on a time-determined basis, physical pacing, social feedback based on achievement not pain, education about the nature of pain and relaxation training.
- Cognitive therapy – involves changing negative thoughts to more positive ones, coping skills training by stress management, relaxation and imagery and improving problem-solving skills.
- Biofeedback – uses increased awareness of physiological changes (heart rate, muscle tension) to enhance the learning of relaxation techniques. This may be particularly helpful for patients with increased muscle tension.
- Hypnosis – involves relaxation, substitution of another sensory modality that is more acceptable (warmth), displacement of perceived site pain to a more peripheral body part and dissociation to a more pleasant location (e.g. a sunny day at the beach).

Pain Management Programmes

Pain management programmes (PMPs) are well established in PCs. PMPs use CBT principles which can be applied by multidisciplinary teams involving clinical psychologists, physiotherapists and occupational therapists. Equally, principles can be applied on a one-to-one basis. There is reasonable evidence that individuals from multiple health professions can provide effective training in pain self-management to their chronic pain patients. Structured training courses exist.

General principles involve physical reactivation based on physical pacing, rationalization of drug consumption, teaching goal setting, improving coping strategies, education and reducing illness behaviour. Programmes are either inpatient or outpatient and usually run on a group basis over several weeks, although one-to-one programmes are also used. More disabled patients require more intensive programmes. PMPs are not designed to treat pain directly, but help patients to live with and manage chronic pain as a long-term condition. Many patients come to terms with their chronic pain and decide to stop being patients by no longer seeking medical assistance.

Common key elements of CBT-based PMPs are:

- Assessing problems and identifying contributing factors: biological and psychological.
- Providing information about acute and chronic pain and treatments available to gain agreement to participate in change process.
- Identifying specific behavioural goals at home, work and socially.
- Breaking down larger goals into subgoals.
- Teaching simple skills to achieve subgoals such as activity pacing.
- Developing daily activity plan incorporating specific activities and exercises relevant to subgoals, activity monitoring and pacing.
- Teaching pain self-management skills, such as options for dealing with obstacles for achieving goals, including flare-ups and unhelpful beliefs; skills include relaxation, problem-solving, challenging unhelpful thoughts such as catastrophizing.
- Reinforcing practice and application of skills and completion of daily activity plan.
- Helping problem solve difficulties between sessions and develop relapse management plan for the future.
- Terminating treatment when goals are achieved and patient confident to maintain self-management plan.

REFERENCES

1. Lee M, Silverman AM, Hansen H, Patel VB, Manchikanti L. A comprehensive review of opioid-induced hyperalgesia. Pain Phys 2011;14:145–61.
2. National Institute for Health and Care Excellence. Neuropathic pain in adults: pharmacological management in non-specialist settings. NICE Clinical Guideline 173. London: NICE; 2013. https://www.nice.org.uk/guidance/cg173.
3. National Institute for Health and Care Excellence. Spinal cord stimulation for chronic pain of neuropathic or ischaemic origin. NICE Technology Appraisal Guidance 159. London: NICE; 2008. https://www.nice.org.uk/guidance/ta159.

4. Dutton K, Littlejohn G. Terminology, criteria, and definitions in chronic regional pain syndrome: challenges and solutions. J Pain Res 2015;8:871–7.
5. Bean DJ, Johnson MH, Kydd RR. The outcome of chronic regional pain syndrome: a systematic review. J Pain 2014;15:677–90.
6. National Institute for Health and Care Excellence. Headaches in over 12s: diagnosis and management. NICE Clinical Guideline 150. London: NICE; 2012. https://www.nice.org.uk/guidance/cg150.
7. National Institute for Health and Care Excellence. Low back pain and sciatica in over 16s: assessment and management. NICE Guidance 59. London: NICE; 2016. https://www.nice.org.uk/guidance/NG59.
8. Qaseem A, Wilt TJ, McLean RM, Forciea MA. Noninvasive treatments for acute, subacute, and chronic low back pain: a clinical practice guideline from the American College of Physicians. Ann Intern Med 2017;166:514–30.

Section 7

Training, Standards and Safety in Anaesthesia

Chapter 7.1

Standards, Education, Safety and Quality Improvement

Carolyn Johnston

STANDARDS

Anaesthesia is safer than ever. Death solely as a result of anaesthesia is now incredibly rare, attributed, in part, to the introduction of safety improvements including developments in monitoring, the introduction of standards and guidelines and other system-based safety initiatives. The introduction of formalized monitoring standards has played an important role in this.[1] Guidelines and standards are used to establish and maintain good practice delivering high-quality care and enhancing patient safety. However, the standards achievable will depend upon available resources which vary from country to country. The World Federation of Societies of Anaesthesiologists aims to promote global standards in anaesthesia around the world. They have published international standards for safe practice of anaesthesia intended to provide guidance and assistance to anaesthesia professionals, professional societies, hospital and facility administrators, and governments for improving and maintaining the quality and safety of anaesthesia care.[2]

Despite these standards and guidelines, hospitals are still not as safe as we would like them to be. Clinical errors are common; 1 in every 150 patients admitted to a hospital dies as a consequence of an adverse event. Causes include human or equipment error, poor organization and lack of communication between teams. This has highlighted the need to focus on patient outcomes and quality care. Integral to this is education and training. Other tools include clinical audit, voluntary incident reporting, briefings, debriefings and checklists.

Audit

It is expected that doctors will take part in audit as part of their professional responsibilities – reviewing medical care in order to identify opportunities for improvement. Guidelines or standards have been developed for many areas of clinical practice and regular audit against these allows the detection of areas of increased risk. Where deficiencies are identified, change can be introduced and the system re-audited: 'closing the loop'. A number of well-established national audits are in place looking at clinical outcomes. These include:

- **NCEPOD** (National Confidential Enquiry into Patient Outcome and Death) – Each year NCEPOD undertakes a study on a specific topic area, such as sepsis, tracheostomy, acute pancreatitis, etc. It makes recommendations for service standards, if none exist, based on the analysis of cases submitted to the study advisory group.
- **MBRRACE** (Mothers and Babies, Reducing the Risk through Audits and Confidential Enquiries) – All maternal and perinatal deaths are reported to this audit, which also undertakes a confidential enquiry and produces recommendations. This audit has been running since 1952.
- **NAP** (National Audit Project) – Originally run by the UK Royal College of Anaesthetists, this is now led by the Health Services Research Centre. All anaesthetic departments are encouraged to participate. In the past, this has included level of consultant supervision (NAP1), complications of airway management (NAP4) and accidental anaesthetic awareness (NAP5).

Incident Reporting

An important part of safe culture is the escalation of incidents resulting in harm, or 'near miss' incidents, where harm has been narrowly averted. This allows analysis of incidents in order to detect and close any potential or actual hazards in the system. This will lead to improvements in system safety by mitigating or eliminating hazards through better design of the system, equipment or training.

Improving safety therefore relies on staff reporting safety incidents. Staff members must be free to report errors without fearing blame or negative repercussions. This is sometimes called a 'no blame' culture, but the more correct term is a 'just' culture. Staff are not blamed for errors, but performance, below expected standards, may result in corrective action.

Local incident reporting systems collate and classify incidents and 'near misses' based both on the likelihood of them happening again and the severity of harm (or potential harm). When harm occurs, or nearly occurs as in a 'near miss' incident, root cause analysis (RCA) can be used to explore all possible factors associated with the incident: by asking what happened, why it happened and what can be done to prevent it from happening again. Any errors and violations identified can then be acted upon to increase the safety of the system.

Reporting can be shared nationally, e.g. in England and Wales, data is shared with the National Reporting and Learning System database, which can identify risks on a national scale. Many health care systems have identified a specific set of harms, which are serious and should not happen in a well-designed system. These are termed 'Never Events' and must be reported both nationally and locally. This list may change periodically, but includes incidents such as wrong site surgery and retained instruments after surgery.

Duty of Candour

Hospitals have a legal obligation to tell patients or their family when a mistake has led to significant harm and to apologize. There is increasing evidence that an early apology may prevent later litigation. Regulatory bodies such as the General Medical Council have issued guidance describing the 'professional duty of candour': doctors must be open with their patients, colleagues and employers when things go wrong.

Checklists

Many high-reliability organizations (HROs) use checklists as part of a wider safety culture to reduce errors caused by lapses and improving team communication. In 2008, the World Health Organization (WHO) Global Patient Safety Challenge included implementation of a simple checklist as a low-cost, transferrable strategy to improve surgical safety worldwide. The UK National Patient safety Agency adapted the WHO checklist within the safety programme '5 Steps to Safer Surgery' guidance.

The five steps are as follows:

1. **Team briefing** – before the start of the list, the whole team meets to discuss the requirements of the list, safety concerns, staffing and equipment.
2. **Sign in** – checklist of questions before induction of anaesthesia.
3. **Time out** – checklist of questions before start of surgical intervention.
4. **Sign out** – checklist before any team member leaves the operating theatre at the end of surgery.
5. **Debriefing** – at the end of the list, the team review their performance, discuss specific concerns and take actions, including escalating concerns, to prevent any incidents from being repeated.

Many studies have investigated the effects of surgical checklists.[3] It is particularly important to the safety culture of the team that they understand the benefits and limitations of the checklist. Teams who integrate the five steps into team communication and a wider safety culture show a reduction in safety-related incidents.

EDUCATION AND TRAINING

An essential part of delivering clinical standards and quality care is to ensure that staff have the knowledge and skills to perform their role. Structured training programmes now exist with regular competency and work-based assessments. All grades of anaesthetist should maintain knowledge through continuing professional development, keeping a record of these activities. An annual appraisal process and medical revalidation requires doctors to demonstrate that they are 'up to date' and fit to practice.

Simulation

The development of medical simulation for training has provided the opportunity to improve nontechnical skills and train for rare emergencies such as anaphylaxis or failed intubation. Clinical scenarios are recreated in a realistic environment and behaviours are observed, critiqued and improved. The aim is to improve the management of critical incidents.

Human Factors

This is the scientific discipline concerned with the understanding of interactions between humans and other elements of a system (International Ergonomics Association, 2000).

Nontechnical Skills

Nontechnical skills are the cognitive and social skills that contribute to safe performance. These have been incorporated into anaesthetic training as the ANTS behavioural marker system (Fig. 7.1.1).

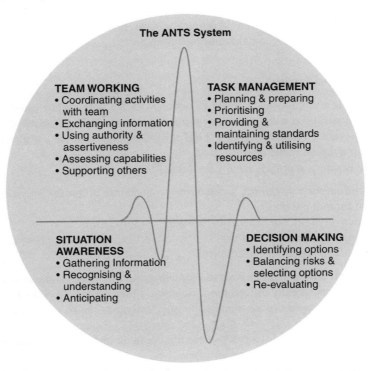

FIGURE 7.1.1 Ants behavioural marker system. With permission from Anaesthetists' Non-Technical Skills (ANTS) System Handbook v1.0, University of Aberdeen.

Human Factors Training

The ANTS system defines the core behaviours of good nontechnical skills. These fundamental safety skills are best taught by team practice focusing on nontechnical skills and behaviours, termed 'crew/crisis resource management', as the original approach was used in airline crews.

In addition to background knowledge about human factors and safety, human factors training often involves practical observation of behaviours in simulated scenarios and then feedback of performance to guide further reflection, practice and learning. The training environment may be in a clinical simulation centre, which often utilizes high-fidelity simulation. Clinical scenarios are re-created in a realistic environment and behaviours are observed and critiqued by trainers, peers and often by the participant themselves via video capture. This gives the participant a safe environment to reflect, learn and try new skills.

SAFETY

Safety is usually defined as the avoidance of injuries or harm (injury, suffering, disability or death). Health care delivery is composed of health care workers undertaking processes within a complex system, and so human error is common. These conditions contain multiple hazards.

Hazards and Errors

A hazard is a circumstance, agent or action with the potential to cause harm. Some organizations work with many hazards, but without these hazards causing adverse events. These are called 'high reliability organizations', e.g. nuclear power or aviation industries.

HROs safety approach usually includes:

- Focus on possible failure, accept error-prone nature of human activities and plan for that possibility.
- Proactively seek out hazards before they result in harm.
- Paying close attention to frontline work and safety culture where all staff feel safe to report hazards or errors.

The term error should be reserved for situations where the failure is unintentional. It is conceptually different to a violation, which is the deliberate deviation from an operating procedure, standard or rule. Violations can be subdivided into:

- Routine, habitual violations – these are common and often tolerated in the system, e.g. inadequate hand washing.
- Optimizing violations – resulting in some personal gain from breaking procedures, e.g. cutting corners to spend more time at lunch.

- Necessary violations – knowingly working around standards or rules in order to complete a task, e.g. resheathing needles because there is no sharps disposal bin nearby.

An error is the inadvertent failure to carry out a planned action as intended or application of an incorrect plan and can be subdivided according to the cognitive processes involved at the time:

- Slip – An appropriate action carried out incorrectly, e.g. puncturing the carotid artery when cannulating the internal jugular vein.
- Lapse – Appropriate action not carried out, e.g. forgetting to remove throat pack at end of surgery.
- Mistake – Decision-making failure or carrying out the wrong action, believing it to be right. This could be rule based (misapplication of correct guidelines) or knowledge based (unaware actions are a mistake).

Errors can also be considered active or latent errors:

- Active errors – An error that has immediate consequences, often at frontline of care, often termed 'sharp end', e.g. anaesthetist administering wrong drug to patient due to syringe mix up.
- Latent errors – An error that does not have immediate consequences, often occurs away from frontline delivery of care, the 'blunt end', e.g. design of ventilator placing off switch beside suction dial, inadequate time for training using new equipment.

Latent errors, active errors and violations exist throughout the system, but it is only when a number of errors or violations occur together in sequence that a hazard will result in harm. This is described in James Reason's Swiss Cheese Model (Fig. 7.1.2).

A system approach to improving safety focuses on removing errors caused by the system (usually latent errors). This is often easier than eliminating human error (as human error will always occur), or changing human behaviour. Almost 80% of errors or adverse events are system derived. In addition to a systems approach to error management, effective local and national regulation is needed to reduce unsafe violations.

A useful tool when harm occurs, or nearly occurs in a 'near miss' incident, is RCA. This process seeks to explore all the possible factors associated with an incident by asking – what happened, why it happened and what can be done to prevent it from happening again? The errors and violations identified can then be acted upon to increase the safety of the system.

Improving safety therefore relies on adequate reporting of harm and 'near miss' incidents, allowing investigation to both seek out latent errors and fix them. Staff must be able to report errors and harm without fearing that they will be blamed if the act was unintentional.

Cheese slices represent layers
of defence against error e.g.
organisational processes, staff
training, checking systems etc.

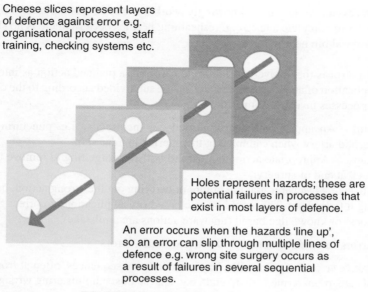

Holes represent hazards; these are
potential failures in processes that
exist in most layers of defence.

An error occurs when the hazards 'line up',
so an error can slip through multiple lines of
defence e.g. wrong site surgery occurs as
a result of failures in several sequential
processes.

FIGURE 7.1.2   Reason's Swiss cheese model.

QUALITY IMPROVEMENT

What Is Quality?

The most widely used definition of quality is the Institute of Medicine's six domains of quality:

- Safe – absence of accidental harm
- Effective – based on best evidence available producing clear benefits
- Patient centred – health care working in partnership with patients' preferences and needs
- Timely – delivered when needed, without harmful delays
- Efficient – reducing waste of supplies, time, cost, etc.
- Equitable – same care available regardless of race, gender, location, socio-economic group, etc.

What Is Quality Improvement?

Quality improvement (QI) is 'a systematic approach using specific techniques to improve these domains'. Many of these techniques are adapted from industries outside health care, such as the motor or aviation industries.

QI activity is different from audit or research, as it has different aims and focus (Table 7.1.1).

TABLE 7.1.1 Differences between QI, Research and Audit

QI	Research	Audit
Hypothesis varies, based on results of tests	Hypothesis fixed prior to testing	No hypothesis
Changing processes to improve quality	Testing a null hypothesis in experimental conditions	Assess health care performance against a set standard
Emphasis on making changes to improve service	Emphasis on creating knowledge	Emphasis on assurance or judgement

The most common model applied to structuring QI in health care is the model for improvement (Fig. 7.1.3). This takes aspects of industrial models and adapted them specifically for use in health care.

The structure emphasizes the importance of initial phase of planning, setting goals, measurement and developing a 'theory of change' before undertaking changes in an iterative change cycle.

What Are We Trying to Accomplish?

All projects should start with clearly articulating their aims: these should be based around improving a domain of quality (listed earlier) and maintain a strong patient focus. Aim statements should be SMART (specific, measurable, attainable, realistic and timely) and decided after consulting with all groups involved in the process, including patients.

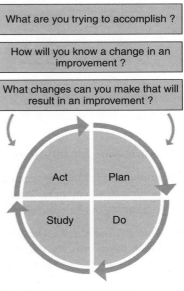

FIGURE 7.1.3 Model for improvement diagram.

How Will We Know a Change Is an Improvement?

Monitoring the correct data is vital to assess the impact of change. This also has a different emphasis to measurement for audit or research (see Table 7.1.2).

What Changes Can We Make that Will Result in an Improvement?

Evaluating and understanding the system is an important step to establish a 'theory of change' for your improvement. This is especially important in complex health care systems.

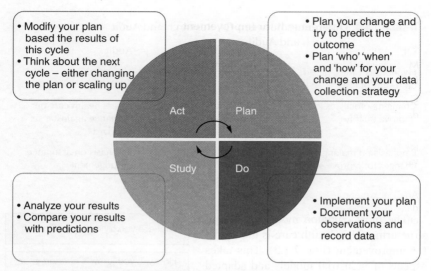

FIGURE 7.1.4   Plan-Do-Study-Act cycle.

Once these initial questions have been answered, then changes are introduced in an iterative change Plan-Do-Study-Act cycle (Fig. 7.1.4).

Measurement for Improvement

Measurement for improvement has different requirements to measurement conducted in research or audit. Some of these differences are shown in Table 7.1.2. Measurements may include the following:

- Outcome measures – These describe the outcome or end result of a process, which often involves the impact on patients, e.g. patient satisfaction with day surgery, number of surgical site infections and pain scores in recovery.
- Process measures – These measure how the process is working. A number of processes may contribute to the outcome, e.g. percentage of staff that comply with new hand hygiene protocols, number of people who complete a training course and percentage of drug charts that contain correct rescue analgesia prescriptions.
- Balancing measures – These look for potential unintended consequences, e.g. percentage of operations delayed due to new preoperative fasting guidelines and increase in nausea after changing opiate prescribing practices.

Measures can be quantitative or qualitative. It is important to choose a range of measures if possible and keep an open mind to changing metrics during the project if your experience indicates this is necessary. It is also helpful to include some measure of the impact of any improvement projects on staff and patients, even if this is as simple a subjective questionnaire.

TABLE 7.1.2 Measurement for Improvement versus Measurement for Research and Audit

Measurement for Improvement	Measurement for Research	Measurement for Audit
Sequential or continuous data collection	Single data collection period or two periods for comparison	Large summative data sample
No attempt to control for variation	Stringent attempts to control for variation	Data collected to highlight variation from standard
Analysis with time series data in run charts or SPC charts	Analysis with statistical tests describing probability of significance	Simple analysis to assess against a defined standard

Successful improvement should demonstrate change over time. This is best displayed as a run chart. Run charts usually display the median value of the data, so run chart rules can be used to interpret the data (Figs 7.1.5–7.1.7).

If the chart contains a shift or trend pattern, then these are indications of 'nonrandom' pattern of data which may be as a result of your change project.

Statistical process control (SPC) charts are similar to run charts but display a mean rather median value and have added upper and lower control lines indicating the boundaries of the variation we expect in the measurements. These use advanced statistical methods to calculate the control limits and detect when data indicate that your results have not occurred by chance (Fig. 7.1.8).

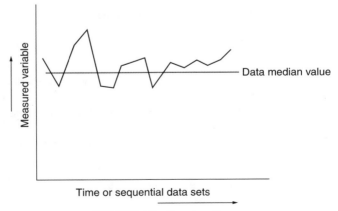

FIGURE 7.1.5 Run chart diagram.

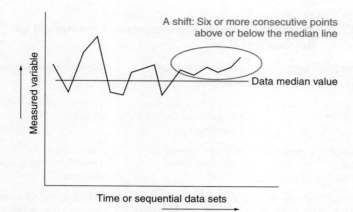

FIGURE 7.1.6 Run chart showing shift pattern.

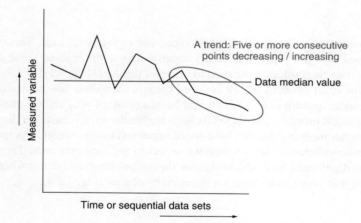

FIGURE 7.1.7 Run chart showing trend pattern.

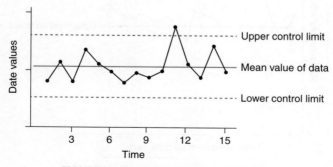

FIGURE 7.1.8 Statistical process control chart.

Systems and Processes

A system is 'a series of interconnected elements and processes which work together towards a specific aim'.

Variation in the System

Any system has average performance and some normal variation around that. We may see different results in what seems, initially, an identical process. This may be caused by the impact of things such as the variability of staff behaviour, variation in patient's physiology, wear and tear of equipment and changes in working conditions. An example of this is the cardiovascular system, which has an average cardiac output, but which may vary minute to minute. Similarly, a theatre team may be able to handle eight minor cases in a day, but this average number may increase or decrease based on patient, staff, environment and other factors.

An important part of the improvement process is to determine if this variation is the normal, random variation we always see in any complex system, or if it arises from a special circumstance that we could improve:

- Common cause or random variation – These are natural patterns or unassignable variation; the variation inherent in the system. It occurs in stable processes.
- Special cause or nonrandom variation – This is assignable variation; the variation is caused by something irregular in the system. The result is a process that acts in an unpredictable way and produces unstable results.

Special cause variation causes our processes to perform unreliably and so makes working more difficult. An example would be if there is a large unpredictable variation in the time taken for a patient to reach theatres from the ward, we cannot reasonably anticipate the next patient's arrival and so this will adversely impact on the operating theatres functions. This is 'special cause variation', there will usually be specific causes which can be corrected to make the process perform predictably, and so make the operating theatre list run more smoothly.

Understanding the System

Each system may be described by:

- Inputs – staff, equipment, patients, policies, etc.
- Processes – interconnected steps to achieve a specific outcome
- Outputs – the end result of the system, services delivered etc.

In order to improve a system, we must understand the steps and elements involved. Changes to health care systems should not be introduced on a whim but developed after time has been taken to understand what is supposed to happen and what is actually happening. This may involve a period of measurement, consultation with staff working within the system, process mapping and understanding the influences acting to disrupt the system.

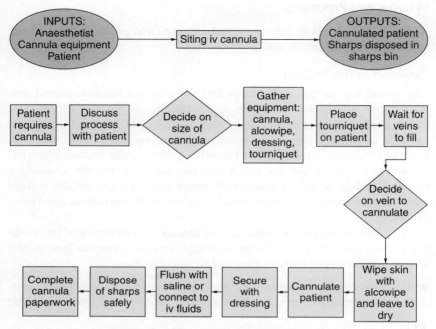

FIGURE 7.1.9   Process map for inserting a cannula.

Process Maps

A process map is a graphical representation of the steps of a process. It contains a clear scope (start and end) and all the elements and linkages in that process. It can be a large complex process such as a patient journey receiving multidisciplinary care in a specialist centre, or something more simple such as the process map of placing a cannula (Fig. 7.1.9).

Once the process is mapped out, the map can be used to highlight areas of inefficiency, high variability or waste. These can then be the targets for improvement. Each step in the process should be scrutinized to assess whether they add anything helpful to the patient's care or if they add 'value'. This is often called value stream mapping.

Driver Diagrams

A driver diagram graphically represents the primary factors influencing an outcome and the secondary factors, which influence the primary factors, so indirectly influence the chosen outcome. An example might be looking at surgical site infections (Fig. 7.1.10). Secondary drivers are often a useful focus for improvement.

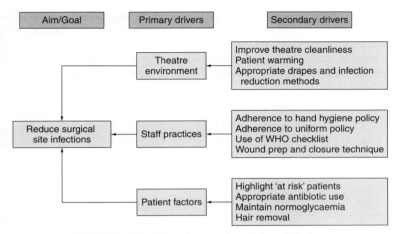

FIGURE 7.1.10 Driver diagram of surgical site infections.

A more detailed discussion of QI can be found in the further reading at the end of the chapter.

REFERENCES

1. AAGBI. Recommendations for standards of monitoring during anaesthesia and recovery 2015. http://www.aagbi.org/sites/default/files/Standards_of_monitoring_2015_0.pdf; [accessed 27.04.2017].
2. Merry AF, Cooper JB, Soyaanwoo O, Wilson IH, Eichhorn JH. International Standards for a Safe Practice of Anesthesia 2010. Can J Anesth 2010;57:1027–34.
3. Walker IA, Reshamwalla S, Wilson IH. Surgical safety checklists: do they improve outcomes? Br J Anaesth 2012;109:147–54.

FURTHER READING

The Health Foundation. Quality improvement made simple. What everyone should know about health care quality improvement. 2013. www.health.org.uk/publication/quality-improvement-made-simple; [accessed 10.10.2016].

Kohn LT, Corrigan JM, Donaldson MS, editors. To err is human: building a safer health system. Committee on Quality of Health Care in America, Institute of Medicine. Washington, DC: National Academy Press; 1999.

Langey GJ, Moen RD, Nolan KM, Nolan TW, Norman CL, Provost LP. The improvement guide: a practical approach to enhancing organizational performance. San Francisco, CA: Jossey-Bass; 2009.

Berwick DM. The science of improvement. JAMA 2008;299:1182–4.

Goldmann D. Ten tips for incorporating scientific quality improvement into everyday work. BMJ Qual Saf 2011;20:i69–72. doi:10.1136/bmjqs. 2010.046359.

Porter ME. What is value in health care? N Engl J Med 2003;363:2477–81.

Flin R, O'Connor P, Crichton M. Safety at the sharp end. A guide to nontechnical skills. Farnham: Ashgate Publishing; 2008.

Dixon N, Pearce M. Healthcare quality quest. Guide to using quality improvement tools to drive clinical audits. Health quality improvement partnership. 2011. www.hqip.org.uk/public/cms/253/625/19/193/HQIP-Guide-to-using-Quality-Improvement-Tools-to-drive-CA-2011. pdf; [accessed 10.10.2016].

Dixon-Woods M, McNicol S, Martin G. Ten challenges in improving quality in healthcare: lessons from the Health Foundation's programme evaluations and relevant literature. BMJ Qual Saf 2012;21:876–84.

Appendix 1

Dictionary of Adult Medical Disorders

This appendix catalogues some of the unusual medical disorders that may present in adults. The key features and anaesthetic implications are outlined for each disorder. Of necessity the descriptions are brief and the reader is directed to the list of useful websites at the end of this appendix to obtain more comprehensive information. (AV, atrioventricular; BP, blood pressure; CPAP, continuous positive airway pressure; DVT, deep venous thrombosis; ETT, endotracheal tube; GA, general anaesthetic; IPPV, intermittent positive-pressure ventilation; PA, pulmonary artery; SAD, supraglottic airway device; SVR, systemic vascular resistance.)

Name	Description	Anaesthetic Implication
Achalasia	Degeneration of myenteric neural plexus Dilated oesophagus Treated by Heller's operation (myotomy)	Dysphagia Aspiration Risk of regurgitation
Acromegaly	Pituitary adenoma Excessive growth hormone	Large tongue Difficult intubation Impaired glucose tolerance
Addison disease	Destruction of both adrenals Hyperpigmentation May be debilitated	Hypotension Hypoglycaemia Hyponatraemia
Alport syndrome	May present in young adult	Renal failure Hypertension in pregnancy
Alveolar hypoventilation Central alveolar hypoventilation Ondine's curse	Poor central respiratory drive May be cervical cord pathology	Respiratory failure Need for postoperative support

Name	Description	Anaesthetic Implication
American trypanosomiasis	See Chagas disease	
Amyloidosis	Abnormal protein deposits Due to chronic infection, or multiple myeloma, or autoimmune disease	Large tongue May affect heart valves, conduction and ventricular function Renal failure Peripheral neuropathy
Amyotrophic lateral sclerosis Motor neurone disease	Progressive degeneration of motor neurons Commoner in men	Bulbar weakness Respiratory weakness Suxamethonium causes dangerous hyperkalaemia
Anorexia nervosa	Morbid fear of obesity Much commoner in young women Weight up to 60% below normal	Temperature loss Bradycardia and hypotension Long QT interval Heart block Delayed gastric emptying Care with fluid and electrolytes Hypoalbuminaemia
Ankylosing spondylitis Bamboo spine	Vertebral ankylosis Mainly in men May cause respiratory failure	Difficult laryngoscopy Aortic regurgitation Pulmonary fibrosis Very difficult spinal anaesthesia
Asbestosis	May develop mesothelioma May develop carcinoma of lung Lung fibrosis	Pleural effusions Respiratory failure
Autonomic hyperreflexia	In response to skin or visceral stimuli below spinal cord lesion Hypertension and tachycardia	Need deep anaesthesia or adequate regional analgesia
Behçet syndrome	Iritis, mouth and genital ulcers Polyarthritis May be CNS lesions	May be taking corticosteroids Mouth ulcers complicate airway management
Beri-beri See Wernicke encephalopathy	Thiamine (B_1) deficiency	Peripheral neuropathy Autonomic neuropathy High-output cardiac failure

Name	Description	Anaesthetic Implication
Buerger disease Thromboangiitis obliterans	Peripheral vascular disease Young male smokers Emphysema and bronchitis	Lung disease Difficulty measuring BP Cuff measurement over-reads
Central alveolar hypoventilation	See alveolar hypoventila-tion	
Chagas disease American trypanosomiasis	Parasitic infection in Central and South America Can cause achalasia (see above in this appendix)	Cardiomyopathy Conduction abnormalities Risk of aspiration
Charcot–Marie–Tooth disease Peroneal muscular atrophy	Sensory and motor periph-eral neuropathy Hereditary (dominant) Presents in teens	Phrenic nerves may be involved Avoid suxamethonium (risk of hyperkalaemia)
Christmas disease Haemophilia B	Factor IX deficiency Sex-linked recessive	Ensure factor IX >60% normal Give factor IX fraction Liaise with haematologist
Congenital analgesia	Abnormal cutaneous sensation	Maintain temperature Care with positioning
CREST syndrome Scleroderma variant	Calcinosis Raynaud phenomenon Sclerodactyly Telangiectasia	Regurgitation risk Lesions in heart and lungs
Creutzfeldt–Jakob disease	Progressive loss of coordination Ataxia Variant disease caused by prions	Poor nutrition Use disposable instruments for airway management
Crohn disease	Inflammatory bowel disease Young adults Causes diarrhoea and fistulae	May be severely toxic Anaemia May be taking corticosteroids
Dermatomyositis Polymyositis	Proximal muscle weakness Arthritis May affect lungs	Regurgitation risk Poor mouth opening Anaemia Sensitive to relaxants
Eaton–Lambert syndrome	See myasthenic syndrome	
Eosinophilic granuloma	Adult version of histiocy-tosis X Localized lung lesion	Anaemia May be taking corticoste-roids

Name	Description	Anaesthetic Implication
Erythema multiforme See also Stevens–Johnson syndrome	Papules and bullae on skin and mucous membranes Sulphonamides can be the cause	Laryngeal oedema at extubation
Factor V Leiden mutation	Resistance to anticoagulant effect of protein C	High risk of DVT and PE
Fibrosing alveolitis Hamman–Rich syndrome	Cyanosis, cor pulmonale	Respiratory failure May be taking corticosteroids
Gaisböck syndrome	Polycythaemia due to reduction in plasma volume Seen in men Smokers, obese, hypertensive	Cardiovascular disease Risk of DVT Venesection may be needed
Glomus jugulare tumours	In middle ear or posterior fossa	Very vascular tumours May secrete 5-HT
Glucagonoma	Malignant tumour of α cells in pancreas Glucagon causes diabetes mellitus	Control blood sugar and ketosis Handling releases glucagon Prone to DVT and PE
Goodpasture syndrome	Autoimmune disease Young adults Severe lung haemorrhages Glomerulonephritis	Microcytic anaemia Hypertension Assess renal function May be immunosuppressed Large ETT facilitates suction
Gorham syndrome	Bone destruction Pathological fractures Teenagers or young adults	Cervical spine may be affected Respiratory involvement
Haemochromatosis	Iron deposits in liver, pancreas, joints, skin, heart Liver dysfunction	Diabetes mellitus, possible heart failure
Haemolytic uraemic syndrome	Haemolysis, renal failure Thrombocytopaenia	Renal dysfunction Anaemia
Hamman–Rich syndrome	See fibrosing alveolitis	
Hartnup disease	Tryptophan malabsorption Pellagra (see below in this appendix) and ataxia	Responds to nicotinamide
Henoch–Schönlein purpura	Bruising, abdominal pain Nephritis Seen in adolescents	Renal dysfunction

Name	Description	Anaesthetic Implication
Hereditary spastic paraplegia	See Strumpell disease	
Huntington chorea	Progressive chorea Autosomal dominant inheritance	Regurgitation risk Poor nutrition May be pseudocholinesterase deficient
Hydatid disease	Infection with the dog tapeworm *Echinococcus granulosus* Cysts in liver, lungs or muscle	Rupture during excision may cause severe anaphylaxis
Hypokalaemic familial periodic paralysis	Potassium moves into muscle cells Attacks provoked by meals	Postoperative respiratory failure Arrhythmias Sensitive to relaxants
Idiopathic thrombocytopaenic purpura	Autoimmune disease Often treated by splenectomy	Possible airway bleeding May be taking corticosteroids Avoid heparin, aspirin Rebound thrombosis after splenectomy
Infectious mononucleosis	Epstein–Barr virus Rarely can cause splenic rupture	Tonsils obstruct airway
Insulinoma	Hypoglycaemia after fasting and exercise May metastasize to liver	Continual glucose monitoring Hyperglycaemic rebound
Jervell and Lange-Nielsen syndrome	Autosomal recessive inheritance Nerve deafness Long QT interval	Tendency to ventricular tachycardia
Lentiginosis	Small brown skin macules	May also have hypertrophic obstructive cardiomyopathy
Leprosy	*Mycobacterium leprae* infection Peripheral neuritis Thickened nerves	Often given corticosteroids for neuritis Analgesia in limbs Muscle wasting
Lingual vein thrombosis	Severe upper airway obstruction	Awake fibreoptic intubation Heliox may be useful

Name	Description	Anaesthetic Implication
Ludwig angina	Infection of submandibular space Usually anaerobic (*Actinomyces*)	Upper airway obstruction Indurated floor of mouth Trismus, unaffected by relaxants
Lyme disease	Tick-borne *Borrelia* infection Named after Lyme, Connecticut Skin lesions	Can progress to: Meningoencephalitis Myocarditis Peripheral neuropathy
Meig syndrome	Pleural effusion Ovarian cyst (often carcinoma)	Drain effusion May be malnourished
Mikulicz syndrome	Enlargement of salivary and lachrymal glands May be due to sarcoidosis	May make intubation difficult Avoid anticholinergic drugs
Motor neurone disease	See amyotrophic lateral sclerosis	
Moya Moya syndrome	Stenosis or occlusion of internal carotid arteries Collaterals at the base of brain More common in Japanese	May deteriorate after anaesthesia Avoid straining (e.g. in labour) Maintain cerebral perfusion
Multiple myeloma See Waldenström macroglobulinaemia	Bone marrow infiltration Often affects cervical spine	Anaemia Renal dysfunction Hypercalcaemia Unstable cervical spine
Myasthenic syndrome Eaton–Lambert syndrome	Autoimmune prejunctional disorder Usually with small cell lung carcinoma Weakness of proximal muscles May be associated with bulbar muscle weakness	No response to anticholinesterases Autonomic dysfunction Sensitivity to all relaxants Increased twitch during tetany
Neurofibromatosis	See Von Recklinghausen disease	
Ondine's curse	See alveolar hypoventilation	
Ovarian hyperstimulation syndrome	Excessive vasoactive peptides	May cause acute lung injury

Name	Description	Anaesthetic Implication
Paterson–Brown–Kelly syndrome Plummer–Vinson syndrome	Oesophageal web Anaemia and angular stomatitis	Risk of regurgitation Anaemia
Paraplegia	Level of cord lesion should be known	Autonomic hyperreflexia (see above in this appendix) Suxamethonium may cause dangerous hyperkalaemia if used between 1 and 2 days and 6 and 12 months after injury
Parkinson disease	Tremor, rigidity and dyskinesia Loss of dopaminergic neurones in substantia nigra May be associated with autonomic dysfunction	Continue therapy perioperatively Risk of regurgitation Postoperative chest infection common Postoperative confusion possible
Pellagra	Niacin (nicotinamide/nicotinic acid) deficiency Dementia, diarrhoea, dermatitis	Confusion and excitement Responds to intravenous nicotinamide
Pemphigus vulgaris	Autoimmune bullous eruption Affects skin and mucous membranes Epidermis separates with friction forces	Avoid skin traction and friction Scarring and narrowing of larynx Avoid airway trauma Small ETT may be better than SAD May be fluid and electrolyte losses
Peroneal muscular atrophy	See Charcot–Marie–Tooth disease	
Pharyngeal pouch	Usually above cricopharyngeus Can lead to aspiration during the night	Ask patient to manually empty it Cricoid pressure ineffective Use awake fibreoptic intubation
Pickwickian syndrome	Gross obesity, hypoventilation Cor pulmonale, polycythaemia	Regional anaesthesia preferred Need IPPV or CPAP after GA Avoid respiratory depressant drugs High risk of DVT

Name	Description	Anaesthetic Implication
Plummer–Vinson syndrome	See Paterson–Brown–Kelly syndrome	
Pneumatosis cystoides intestinalis	Gas-filled cysts in submucosa of gut Usually in large bowel May cause bowel obstruction	Avoid nitrous oxide
Polyarteritis nodosa	Autoimmune, commoner in men Widespread effects, especially lungs, kidneys, skin, heart, CNS, joints	Evaluate lung and renal function Heart failure from coronary arteritis
Polymyositis	See dermatomyositis	
Post-poliomyelitis syndrome	Weakness developing many years after original infection May affect bulbar/respiratory muscles	Regurgitation risk Possibility of ventilator failure
Primary pulmonary hypertension	Unknown aetiology Mainly in young women	Dangerous condition Invasive monitoring Consider PA catheter No hypoxia or cardiac depressant drugs
Pulmonary cysts (bullae)	Emphysematous space over 1 cm diameter Present with breathlessness	Minimize peak airway pressure Beware of tension pneumothorax Avoid nitrous oxide
Pulseless disease	See Takayasu disease	
Reninoma	Very rare benign tumour of juxtaglomerular cells Young adults Autonomous secretion of renin	Hypertension Hypokalaemia Careful monitoring of CVS
Romano–Ward syndrome	Autosomal dominant inheritance Prolonged QT interval	Tendency to ventricular tachycardia
Sarcoidosis	Multisystem granulomatous disease Lung nodules and lymphadenopathy Neuropathy, including cranial nerves Eyes often affected	May have laryngeal involvement Hypercalcaemia Renal function may be impaired

Name	Description	Anaesthetic Implication
Scleroderma	Lung fibrosis Raynaud phenomenon common Rarely can affect heart and kidneys See CREST syndrome	Limited mouth opening Risk of regurgitation Hypovolaemia Difficult venous access Regional anaesthesia preferred
Scurvy	Vitamin C deficiency Bruising and petechiae	Loose teeth, swollen gums Anaemia Excessive surgical bleeding
Sheehan syndrome	See Simmond disease	
Simmond disease	Hypopituitarism Due to tumour or after surgery Necrosis of anterior lobe after obstetric haemorrhage is called Sheehan syndrome	Depends on exact hormone deficiencies Hypoglycaemia, hypothermia Water and electrolyte balance
Sjögren syndrome	Dry eyes, diminished salivary secretion Usually with rheumatoid arthritis Multisystem involvement common	Avoid anticholinergics Humidify inspired gases Impaired airway access due to swollen salivary glands
Stevens–Johnson syndrome See erythema multiforme	Most severe form of erythema multiforme Can be fatal	May need intravenous fluids May need intensive care
Strumpell disease Hereditary spastic paraplegia	Progressive degeneration of spinal cord Usually only affects legs Varying inheritance pattern	Avoid suxamethonium
Systemic lupus erythematosus (SLE)	Autoimmune vasculitis, mainly women Affects skin, kidneys, heart, lungs May cause peripheral neuropathy Antiphospholipid antibodies cause thrombosis Thrombocytopaenia or antibodies to clotting factors cause bleeding defect	Cardiac and renal involvement Anaemia Assess clotting status Avoid hypothermia (Raynaud)

Name	Description	Anaesthetic Implication
Syringomyelia	Cavities in spinal cord Muscle weakness and scoliosis Can cause respiratory failure	Bulbar palsy Autonomic hyperreflexia Sensitive to muscle relaxants Avoid suxamethonium (hyperkalaemia)
Takayasu disease Pulseless disease	Mainly in Asian girls Occlusive arteritis Affects aorta and large vessels May affect cerebral arteries	Hypertension if renal arteries involved Use invasive BP monitoring Maintain cerebral perfusion Neuraxial block useful to reduce SVR
Thromboangiitis obliterans	See Buerger disease	
Urine drinking	In psychiatric disorders	Hyponatraemia needs correction
Von Recklinghausen disease Neurofibromatosis	Autosomal dominant inheritance Café-au-lait spots and neu-rofibromas CNS tumours (benign and malignant) Acoustic neuromas are common	Laryngeal tumours may occur Often kyphoscoliosis Relaxants may have pro-longed effect 1% have associated phaeo-chromocytoma
Waldenström macro-globulinaemia See multiple myeloma	Related to multiple my-eloma Presents in elderly men	Anaemia Bleeding tendency Cardiac failure
Wegener granulomatosis	Midline granulomas Ulcers in nose, palate, larynx and trachea Large nodules in the lungs Glomerulonephritis	Assess airway by preopera-tive indirect laryngoscopy Intubation may cause bleeding and possible respi-ratory obstruction Occasionally diagnosed by the anaesthetist
Wernicke encephalopathy See Beri-beri	Acute thiamine (B_1) deficiency Common in alcoholics	Confusion Ataxia and nystagmus Korsakoff psychosis Treat with intravenous thiamine

Name	Description	Anaesthetic Implication
Wolff–Parkinson–White syndrome	AV accessory path (bundle of Kent) Re-entrant tachycardias	Short PR interval Delta wave at start of QRS Avoid digoxin
Wolfram syndrome	Autosomal recessive Pituitary diabetes insipidus Diabetes mellitus Optic atrophy and deafness	Fluid balance

FURTHER READING

Fleischer L. Anesthesia and uncommon diseases. 4th ed. Philadelphia: WB Saunders; 2012.

USEFUL WEBSITES

http://www.nlm.nih.gov/
https://www.rarediseases.org
https://www.ncbi.nlm.nih.gov
http://www.omim.org/

Appendix 2

Dictionary of Paediatric Medical Disorders

This appendix catalogues some of the unusual medical disorders that may present in infancy and childhood. The key features and anaesthetic implications are outlined for each disorder. Of necessity the descriptions are brief and the reader is directed to the list of useful websites at the end of this appendix to obtain more comprehensive information. (AS, aortic stenosis; ASD, atrial septal defect; IHD, ischaemic heart disease; PDA, patent ductus arteriosus; VSD, ventricular septal defect.)

Name	Description	Anaesthetic Implication
Aarskog–Scott syndrome Faciodigitogenital dysplasia	Mainly affects male infants Stunted growth, broad facial features, genital abnormalities and mild mental retardation	Intubation problems
Achondroplasia	Short-limb dwarfism Prominent forehead with protruding jaw Respiratory problems due to narrowed nasal passages	Intubation problems Extradural anaesthesia safe
Acquired neuromyotonia	See Armadillo syndrome	
Acrocephalosyndactyly	See Apert syndrome	
Adrenogenital syndrome	Defect in adrenal synthesis of corticosteroids resulting in aldosterone and cortisol deficiency Female virilization due to overproduction of androgens	Check electrolytes Corticosteroids if salt-losing

Name	Description	Anaesthetic Implication
Aglossia–adactylia syndrome	See Möbius syndrome	
Albers–Schönberg disease Marble bone disease Osteopetrosis	Similar to osteogenesis imperfecta Brittle bones, pathological fractures Hepatosplenomegaly	Anaemia Care with positioning
Albright–Butler syndrome	Renal tubular acidosis with hypokalaemia Renal calculi	Correct electrolytes Renal impairment
Albright osteodystrophy Pseudohypoparathyroidism	Ectopic bone formation Mental retardation	Hypocalcaemia ECG conduction defects Neuromuscular problems Convulsions
Alport syndrome	Nephritis and nerve deafness Renal failure in later life	Renal impairment
Alström syndrome	Obesity, deafness and blind by 7 years of age Diabetes mellitus and renal failure after puberty	Obesity Diabetes mellitus Renal impairment
Amyotonia congenita Kugelberg–Welander disease Werdnig–Hoffmann disease Infantile muscular atrophy	More severe infantile muscular atrophy than Welander Spinal muscular atrophy with anterior horn cell degeneration, death before puberty Chronic respiratory problems due to muscle weakness	Sensitivity to intravenous anaesthetics Avoid respiratory depressants Avoid muscle relaxants
Amyotrophic lateral sclerosis	Degeneration of motor neurones	Avoid suxamethonium (excessive potassium release) Avoid respiratory depressants
Analbuminaemia	Almost absent albumin	Sensitive to protein-bound drugs
Andersen disease	See glycogen storage disease IV	
Andersen syndrome	See cystic fibrosis	

Name	Description	Anaesthetic Implication
Anderson disease	Hereditary hypocholester-olaemic syndrome, characterized by intestinal fat malabsorption	No anaesthetic problems reported
Andre syndrome	See Otopalatodigital syndrome	
Angelman syndrome	Microcephaly	Seizures Cardiac anomalies
Angio-osteohypertrophy	See Klippel–Trenaunay syndrome	
Anhidrotic ectodermal dysplasia	See Christ–Siemens–Touraine syndrome	
Apert syndrome Acrocephalosyndactyly	Craniosynostosis and micrognathia Congenital heart defects (e.g. VSD)	Intubation problems Raised intracranial pressure Cardiac anomalies
Armadillo syndrome Isaacs syndrome Acquired neuromyotonia	Arises in childhood or adult life Spontaneous myokymia of arms and legs with increased tone Muscle activity persists throughout sleep, but is abolished by carbamazepine and phenytoin	Muscle activity persists during general and regional anaesthesia Muscle activity suppressed by muscle relaxants
Arthrogryposis multiplex	Scoliosis, myopathy, congenital contractures Micrognathia, cervical spine and/or jaw stiffness Congenital heart disease in 10% of patients	Difficult venous access Airway problems Sensitivity to intravenous anaesthetics Cardiac anomalies Malignant hyperpyrexia risk
Asplenia	Absent spleen Bilateral visceral right-sidedness Complex cardiovascular anomalies with cyanosis and heart failure	Cardiac anomalies
Ataxia–telangiectasia	Cerebellar ataxia Skin and conjunctival telangiectasia Defective immunity with decreased serum IgA and IgE	Recurrent chest and sinus infections Bronchiectasis

Name	Description	Anaesthetic Implication
Barlow syndrome	Click-murmur mitral valve prolapse Bradycardia resistant to atropine Arrhythmias responding to β-blockade Thromboembolism	Avoid excessive tachycardia and anxiety Antibiotic prophylaxis
Bartter syndrome	Hyperplasia of juxtaglomerular apparatus Onset in infancy or early adolescence	Electrolyte abnormalities
Beckwith syndrome Wiedemann syndrome	Infantile gigantism Macroglossia Persistent severe neonatal hypoglycaemia	Airway problems Hypoglycaemia
Blackfan–Diamond syndrome	Congenital idiopathic red-cell aplasia Hypersplenism Congenital cardiac defects (e.g. VSD)	Corticosteroid therapy Anaemia Thrombocytopaenia Cardiac anomalies
Bloom syndrome	Defect in DNA management	Restrict X-ray exposure
Bournville disease	See tuberous sclerosis	
Bowen syndrome Cerebrohepatorenal syndrome	Hypotonia, hepatomegaly and neonatal jaundice, polycystic kidneys Hypoprothrombinaemia Associated congenital heart disease	Renal impairment Cardiac anomalies
Branched-chain ketonuria	See maple syrup urine disease	
Cardio-auditory syndrome	See Jervell and Lange-Nielsen syndrome	
Carpenter syndrome	Cranial synostosis with small mandible Congenital heart disease – PDA and VSD	Intubation problems Cardiac anomalies
Central core myopathy	See amyotonia congenita	
Cerebrocostomandibular syndrome	Cleft palate, micrognathia, microthorax, tracheal abnormalities, vertebral anomalies	Intubation problems Respiratory problems

Name	Description	Anaesthetic Implication
Cerebrohepatorenal syndrome	See Bowen syndrome	
CHARGE association	Micrognathia, cleft palate, choanal atresia Microphallus and cryptorchidism Congenital heart disease in 70%	Intubation problems Cardiac anomalies
Chediak–Higashi syndrome	Partial albinism Hepatosplenomegaly and immunodeficiency	Recurrent chest infections Corticosteroid therapy Thrombocytopaenia
Cherubism	Macroglossia with tumorous lesions of mandible and maxilla cause airway obstruction and respiratory distress	Intubation problems Urgent tracheostomy Profuse surgical bleeding
Chondroectodermal dysplasia	See Ellis–van Creveld syndrome	
Chotzen syndrome	Craniosynostosis Renal failure	Intubation problems Renal impairment
Christ–Siemens– Touraine syndrome Anhidrotic ectodermal dysplasia	Defective thermoregulation due to absent sweat glands Heat intolerance and recurrent chest infections No hair or teeth	Intubation problems Cooling mattress Avoid atropine
Chronic granulomatous disease	Inherited disorder of leucocyte function Recurrent infections Hepatomegaly	Poor pulmonary function Strict asepsis
Cockayne syndrome	Progressive mental and physical retardation, deafness, blindness, bony malformations	Intubation problems
Congenital myopathy	Central core disease Ventilation problem due to muscle weakness	Sensitive to muscle relaxants Malignant hyperpyrexia risk
Conradi–Hunermann syndrome	Chondrodystrophy and mental deficiency Associated congenital heart disease and renal anomalies	Airway problems Cardiac anomalies Renal impairment

Name	Description	Anaesthetic Implication
Cretinism	Congenital hypothyroidism Muscle weakness may cause respiratory problems Cardiomyopathy Corticosteroid therapy may be required	Airway problems Cardiac anomalies Sensitive to intravenous anaesthetics Hypoglycaemia Electrolyte abnormalities
Cri-du-chat syndrome	Microcephaly, micrognathia and macroglossia Associated congenital heart disease (ASD and VSD) in 25% of cases	Airway problems Intubation problems Cardiac anomalies
Crouzon disease	Craniosynostosis Cranial operations can be very bloody Coarctation of aorta	Intubation problems Postoperative respiratory obstruction
Currerino triad	Sacral agenesis, presacral mass and anorectal malformation	Avoid caudal analgesia
Cutis laxa	Elastic fibre degeneration Fragile skin, blood vessels, etc. Pendulous upper airway mucosa causes respiratory obstruction Emphysema and cor pulmonale	Frequent chest infections Difficult to maintain intravenous access
Cystic fibrosis Andersen syndrome Fibrocystic disease	Intrinsic lung disease characterized by inspissation of secretions, airway obstruction and chronic obstructive pulmonary disease Postural drainage prevents accumulation of secretions Also associated with malnutrition, liver dysfunction and bleeding tendency	Humidification Antibiotics Bronchodilators Intubation facilitates bronchial suction Hypoxia poorly tolerated Hypotension poorly tolerated Avoid dehydration Avoid atropine
Dandy–Walker syndrome	Cerebellar malformation Hydrocephalus	Airway problems
Diastrophic dwarfism	Micrognathia and short neck	Intubation problems

Name	Description	Anaesthetic Implication
DiGeorge syndrome Third and fourth arch syndrome	Absent thymus – immunodeficient and increased susceptibility to infection Absent parathyroids results in hypocalcaemia and tetany Aortic arch anomalies with cardiac failure	Stridor Recurrent chest infections Susceptible to blood transfusion-induced graft-versus-host reaction
Down syndrome Mongolism Trisomy 21	See trisomy 21	
Dubowitz syndrome	Microcephaly and micro-gnathia Hypertelorism	Intubation problems
Duchenne muscular dystrophy	Commonest muscular disorder of childhood – usually die in second decade Progressive muscular weakness and scoliosis, leading to chronic respiratory failure Frequent cardiac muscle involvement, with occasional cardiac arrest	Minimal drug dosage Avoid muscle relaxants Avoid respiratory depressants Postoperative ventilatory support often necessary Cardiac problems Malignant hyperpyrexia risk
Dutch–Kentucky syndrome	See Hecht–Beals syndrome	
Dyggve–Melchior–Clausen syndrome	Short trunk dwarfism Mental retardation, short neck, macroglossia	Intubation problems
Dysautonomia	See familial dysautonomia	
Dystrophia myotonica	See myotonica dystrophia	
Ebstein anomaly	Tricuspid valve disease	Supraventricular tachycardia during induction
Edwards syndrome	See trisomy 18	
Ehlers–Danlos syndrome	Collagen abnormality – hypermobility of joints and fragility of skin, blood vessels and tracheal mucosa Spontaneous rupture of blood vessels associated with aneurysms Mitral regurgitation Bleeding diathesis of unknown cause	Difficult to maintain intravenous access Intubation may cause severe tracheal bruising Spontaneous pneumothorax ECG conduction abnormalities

Name	Description	Anaesthetic Implication
Eisenmenger complex	Pulmonary hypertension, intracardiac shunts, hypoxia Decreases of systemic vascular resistance increase the shunt Vasoactive agents, hypercapnia and further hypoxia exacerbate pulmonary hypertension	Strong tendency to asystole Very slow equilibration with inhaled gases Ketamine may be useful
Ellis–van Creveld syndrome Chondroectodermal dysplasia	Ectodermal defects with skeletal anomalies Associated congenital heart defects (usually septal) in 50% of cases	Poor lung function Respiratory failure due to chest wall defects Cardiac anomalies
Epidermolysis bullosa	Skin and mucous membranes easily blistered, resulting in extensive scarring	Avoid skin trauma Ketamine recommended Corticosteroid therapy Check for porphyria (similar skin lesions)
Eulenburg disease	See paramyotonia congenita	
Fabry disease	Lipid storage disease Lipid build-up results in myocardial infarction, stroke and renal failure	As for adults with IHD Renal impairment
Faciodigitogenital dysplasia	See Aarskog–Scott syndrome	
Fallot tetralogy	Cyanotic congenital heart disease comprising VSD, pulmonary stenosis, overriding aorta and right ventricle hypertrophy	Avoid fall in SVR which causes further desaturation
Familial dysautonomia	See Riley–Day syndrome	
Familial periodic paralysis	Muscle disease characterized by hyperkalaemia and attacks of quadriplegic paralysis	Monitor serum potassium Avoid thiopental Avoid muscle relaxants
Familial unconjugated hyperbilirubinaemia	See Gilbert disease	
Familial xanthomatosis	See Wolman disease	
Fanconi anaemia	Defect in DNA regeneration	Sensitive to X-rays

Name	Description	Anaesthetic Implication
Fanconi syndrome Renal tubular acidosis	Proximal tubular defect usually secondary to other disease and characterized by acidosis, potassium loss and dehydration	Correct electrolytes Correct acid–base abnormality Monitor renal function
Farber disease Lipogranulomatosis	Sphingomyelin deposition Widespread visceral lipogranulomas involving CNS, heart and kidney	Intubation problems Cardiomyopathy Renal impairment
Favism	Glucose-6-phosphate-dehydrogenase deficiency Haemolytic anaemia Haemolysis induced by oxidant drugs (e.g. sulphonamides, aspirin)	Avoid oxidant drugs
Felty syndrome	A form of idiopathic thrombocytopenic purpura Anaemia, neutropaenia and susceptibility to infections	Corticosteroid therapy
Femoral hypoplasia syndrome	Unusual facies with micrognathia Femurs hypoplastic or absent	Intubation problems
Fibrocystic disease	See cystic fibrosis	
Fibrodysplasia ossificans	See myositis ossificans	
Focal dermal hypoplasia	See Golz–Gorlin syndrome	
Forbes disease	See glycogen storage disease type III	
Freeman–Sheldon syndrome	Craniofacial abnormalities with microstomia and scoliosis	Intubation problems
Friedreich ataxia	Cerebellar degeneration, progressive ataxia and myopathy Myocardial degeneration with failure and arrhythmias, respiratory failure, diabetes, and peripheral neuropathy Treatment as for amyotrophic lateral sclerosis	Atracurium safe Heart failure

Name	Description	Anaesthetic Implication
G syndrome	See Opitz–Frias syndrome	
Gardner syndrome	Multiple polyposis, bony tumours, sebaceous cysts and fibromas	No anaesthetic problems described
Gargoylism	See mucopolysaccharidosis I	
Gaucher disease	Cerebroside accumulation in CNS, liver, spleen, etc. Pseudobulbar palsy	Pulmonary aspiration Anaemia Thrombocytopaenia Neutropaenia
Gilbert disease Familial unconjugated hyperbilirubinaemia	Jaundice precipitated by minor upsets, including starvation	
Glanzmann disease Thrombasthenia	Reduction in platelet ADP resulting in abnormal function Abnormal haemorrhage, platelet infusion rarely effective	Corticosteroid therapy
Glycogen storage disease type I Von Gierke disease	Hepatomegaly, enlarged kidneys Severe attacks of hypoglycaemia	Monitor blood glucose Monitor acid–base balance Diazoxide for hypoglycaemia
Glycogen storage disease type II Pompe disease	Muscle deposits, severe hypotonicity and neuromuscular weakness Macroglossia and respiratory problems due to muscle weakness Massive cardiomegaly and heart failure Rarely survive infancy	Extreme care Avoid respiratory depressants Avoid cardiac depressants Avoid muscle relaxants Airway problems
Glycogen storage disease type III Forbes disease	Deficiency of debrancher enzyme with onset in early childhood Mild growth and mental retardation, hepatomegaly, cardiomegaly and muscle weakness	Hypoglycaemia

Name	Description	Anaesthetic Implication
Glycogen storage disease type IV Andersen disease	Glycogen deposition in liver and spleen resulting in hepatosplenomegaly and progressive liver failure	Hypoglycaemia Hepatic failure
Glycogen storage disease type V McArdle disease	Myopathy due to glycogen accumulation in muscles Weakness, respiratory problems and cardiomyopathy	Care with cardiac depressants Atracurium safe Avoid suxamethonium
Glycogen storage disease type VI Hers disease	Onset in infancy and early childhood Sometimes so mild that syndrome may pass undetected Moderate growth retardation	
Glycogen storage disease type VII Tarui disease	Muscle weakness with exercise intolerance and myoglobinuria	
Goldenhar syndrome Oculo-auriculo-vertebral syndrome Hemifacial microsomia	Unilateral facial hypoplasia Small mandible, micrognathia with unilateral cleft defect unilateral maxillary hypoplasia, cervical vertebral defects Associated congenital heart defects (Fallot and VSD) in 20% of cases	Airway problems Intubation problems Atropine-resistant bradycardia Cardiac anomalies
Golz–Gorlin syndrome Focal dermal hypoplasia	Dental and facial asymmetry and stiff neck Associated congenital heart defects (AS and ASD) Renal anomalies	Difficult airway Cardiac anomalies
Gorlin syndrome	Basal cell naevi Skeletal anomalies	No anaesthetic problems described
Groenblad–Strandberg disease Pseudoxanthoma elasticum	Degeneration of elastic tissue in skin, eyes and cardiovascular system results in fragile blood vessels with frequent rupture and bruising Thromboses	Difficult to maintain intravenous access

Name	Description	Anaesthetic Implication
Guerin–Stern syndrome	Hypertension due to pro-renin/renin Production See also arthrogryposis multiplex	Airway problems Cardiac problems
Guillain–Barré syndrome	Muscle weakness due to acute idiopathic progressive polyneuritis May involve cranial nerves with autonomic dysfunction, bulbar palsy, hypoventilation and unstable circulation Usually self-limiting in up to 6 weeks	Avoid suxamethonium for up to 3 months (hyperkalaemia) Plasmapheresis may be used
Haemorrhagic telangiectasia	See Osler–Weber–Rendu syndrome	
Hallermann–Streiff syndrome	Micrognathia, brittle teeth, hypoplastic nares	Intubation problems
Hallervorden–Spatz disease	Rare progressive disorder of basal ganglia occurring in late childhood and leading to death Dementia, myotonia and muscular rigidity with trismus	Intubation problems Dystonic posturing temporarily relieved by general anaesthesia
Hand–Schüller–Christian disease	See histiocytosis X	
Hanhart syndrome	See Möbius syndrome	
Hay–Wells syndrome	Maxillary hypoplasia	Intubation problems
Hecht–Beals syndrome Dutch–Kentucky syndrome	Trismus and various skeletal abnormalities	Airway problems
Hemifacial microsomia	See Goldenhar syndrome	
Hepatolenticular degeneration Kinnier–Wilson disease	Defect in copper metabolism, hepatic failure, epilepsy, trismus, weakness	
Hermansky syndrome	Albinism and thrombasthenia Bleeding diathesis with bruising and platelet abnormality	Platelet infusion may be required

Name	Description	Anaesthetic Implication
Hers disease	See glycogen storage disease type VI	
Histiocytosis X Hand–Schüller– Christian disease Letterer–Siwe disease	Histiocytic granulomas in bones and viscera – laryngeal and pulmonary infiltration, cor pulmonale, hepatic involvement, hypersplenism and diabetes insipidus Clinical course as for acute leukaemia	Gingivitis Intubation problems Anaemia Pancytopaenia Electrolyte disturbance Corticosteroid therapy
Holt–Oram syndrome Hand–heart syndrome	Upper limb abnormalities Congenital heart disease – usually septal defects Sudden death	Cardiac anomalies
Homocystinuria	Deficiency of cystothionine synthetase Thromboembolic phenomena, lens dislocation, osteoporosis, kyphoscoliosis, mental handicap, hypoglycaemia and renal failure	Increased blood viscosity Increased platelet adhesiveness Hypoglycaemia Renal impairment
Hunter syndrome	See mucopolysaccharidosis II	
Hurler syndrome	See mucopolysaccharidosis I	
Hutchinson–Gilford syndrome	See progeria	
Hypospadias dysphagia syndrome	See Opitz–Frias syndrome	
I-cell disease	See Mucopolylipidosis II	
Ichthyosis X-linked ichthyosis	Dry, fish-like scales on the skin's surface Condition often begins in early childhood	Difficult skin fixation of intravenous cannulae, etc.
Idiopathic infantile hypercalcaemia Supraventricular aortic stenosis syndrome William–Beuren syndrome	Hypercalcaemia and mental retardation Abnormal facies with stellate blue eyes Congenital stenosis of aortic and pulmonary valves	Airway problems Cardiac anomalies Monitor serum calcium

Name	Description	Anaesthetic Implication
Infantile muscular atrophy	See amyotonia congenita	
Isaacs syndrome	See armadillo syndrome	
Ivemask syndrome	Asplenia, situs inversus, dextrocardia, cyanotic heart disease	Cardiac anomalies
Jervell and Lange-Nielsen syndrome Cardio-auditory syndrome	Cardiac conduction defects, arrhythmias, prolonged QT interval and enlarged T wave Deafness	Syncope Cardiac arrest Consider pacemaker insertion
Jeune syndrome	Lung problems due to chest wall deformity	Chronic respiratory infection
Kallman syndrome	Hypothalamic disorder associated with delayed puberty, anosmia and brittle bones	
Kartagener syndrome	Dextrocardia, sinusitis, bronchiectasis, immunoin-competence See also asplenia syndrome	Chronic respiratory infection
Kasabach–Merritt syndrome	Rarely survive more than a few weeks from birth Enlarging haemangioma with thrombocytopaenia and haemorrhage	Blood and platelet transfusion Corticosteroid therapy
Kawasaki disease	Risk of coronary and other aneurysms Treatment with γ-globulin within 10 days	Risk of myocardial infarction
Kearns–Sayer syndrome	Mitochondrial cytopathy Cardiomyopathy Chronic external oph-thalmoplegia, retinitis pigmentosa, deafness and seizures	Sudden complete heart block during anaes-thesia Normal response to muscle relaxants
King–Denborough disease	Noonan syndrome-like skeletal abnormality with dysmorphic facies and myopathy	Malignant hyperpyrexia risk
Kinnier–Wilson disease	See hepatolenticular degeneration	

Name	Description	Anaesthetic Implication
Klinefelter syndrome	Chromosomal aneuploidy Crush fractures of osteoporotic vertebrae May be very large in adult life	Care with positioning
Klippel–Feil syndrome	Congenital fusion of cervical vertebrae Cleft palate, neurological defects, scoliosis and VSD may coexist	Airway problems Intubation problems Cardiac anomalies
Klippel–Trenaunay syndrome Angio-osteohypertrophy	Cleft palate, short wide neck and inability to extend neck Arteriovenous fistulae, high-output failure Thrombocytopaenia	High-cardiac output state Thrombocytopaenia
Kneist syndrome	Neck stiffness	Difficult intubation
Kugelberg–Welander muscular atrophy	See amyotonia congenita	
Kwashiorkor	Pterygoid fibrosis	Intubation problems Electrolyte abnormalities Low serum cholinesterase
Larsen syndrome	Connective tissue defect Multiple joint dislocations, unstable neck, pulmonary infections	Difficult intubation Chronic respiratory problems
Laryngomalacia	Upper airway obstruction	Airway problems
Laurence–Moon–Biedl syndrome	Obesity, polydactyly, mental retardation Associated congenital heart disease and renal failure	Cardiac anomalies Diabetes insipidus
Leber disease	Congenital optic atrophy Idiopathic hypoventilation with sensitivity to diazepam and mild analgesics	
Leopard syndrome	Multiple leopard skin spots, hypertelorism, congenital heart disease	Severe pulmonary stenosis
Leprechaunism	Severe mental retardation Endocrine disorders including hyperinsulinism Renal tubular defects	Hypoglycaemia Renal impairment

Name	Description	Anaesthetic Implication
Lesch–Nyhan syndrome	Mental retardation Hyperuricaemia Renal failure before puberty	Renal impairment
Letterer–Siwe disease	See histiocytosis X	
Lipodystrophy	Generalized loss of all body fat Portal hypertension, hypersplenism, nephropathy Diabetes mellitus	Hepatic impairment Anaemia Pancytopaenia
Lipogranulomatosis	See Farber disease	
Lowe syndrome Oculocerebrorenal syndrome	Affects males only Mental retardation, hypotonia, renal acidosis, osteoporosis	Hypocalcaemia Renal impairment
McArdle disease	See glycogen storage disease type V	
McKusick–Kaufman syndrome	Hydrocolpos, syndactyly and cardiac abnormalities	Cardiac anomalies
Macroglossia, acute		Airway problems Intubation problems
Mafucci syndrome	Enchondromas, fragile bones and haemangiomas	Labile blood pressure Sensitive to vasodilator drugs Anaemia
Mandibulofacial dysostosis	See Treacher Collins syndrome	
Maple syrup urine disease Branched-chain ketonuria	Metabolic disease involving accumulation of keto and amino acids Severe neurological damage and respiratory disturbances	General supportive measures Blood sugar abnormalities Electrolyte abnormalities
Marble bone disease	See Albers–Schönberg disease	
Marchiafava–Michaeli syndrome	Autoimmune haemolytic anaemia with paroxysmal nocturnal dyspnoea Venous thromboembolism	Corticosteroid therapy

Name	Description	Anaesthetic Implication
Marfan syndrome Arachnodactyly	Congenital connective tissue disorder Kyphoscoliosis, pectus excavatum, joint instability Aortic, pulmonary and mitral valve involvement and dissecting aneurysms Emphysema and lung cysts	High anaesthetic risk Airway problems Pneumothorax Cardiac anomalies
Maroteaux–Lamy syndrome	See mucopolysaccharidosis VI	
Meckel syndrome Meckel–Gruber syndrome	Microcephaly, encephalocoele, micrognathia and cleft palate Congenital heart disease Polycystic kidneys with renal failure in infancy	Intubation problems Cardiac anomalies Renal impairment
Median cleft face syndrome	Varying degrees of cleft face Frontal lipomas	Difficult intubation
Meckel–Gruber syndrome	See Meckel syndrome	
Metaphyseal dysplasia	See Pyle disease	
Miller–Diecker syndrome	Microcephaly Death in infancy or childhood	Airway problems Intubation problems
Möbius syndrome Hanhart syndrome Aglossia–adactylia syndrome	Rare congenital abnormality of the cranial nerves Congenital facial diplegia, micrognathia and associated limb deformity	Intubation problems Recurrent aspiration
Mongolism	See Down syndrome	
Morquio–Ullrich syndrome	See mucopolysaccharidosis IV	
Moschkowitz disease	A form of thrombotic thrombocytopenic purpura Neurological damage and renal disease Treated by splenectomy	Corticosteroid therapy
Mucopolylipidosis I	Like early MPS I	Airway problems

Name	Description	Anaesthetic Implication
Mucopolylipidosis II I-cell disease	Lysosomal storage disorder causing vacuolization of bone, cartilage and fibroblasts Musculoskeletal abnormalities, including chest wall deformities – also cardiac valvular lesions Death within first decade	Airway problems Intubation problems Frequent chest infections Cardiac anomalies
Mucopolysaccharido-ses (MPS)	Hereditary metabolic disorders with deposition of abnormal amounts of mucopolysaccharides in body tissues resulting in permanent progressive cel-lular damage	
MPS I Hurler syndrome Gargoylism	Chest infections, pulmo-nary hypertension, valve lesions, cardiomy-opathy and heart failure Death before puberty	Upper airway obstruction Difficult intubation Frequent chest infections Cardiac anomalies
MPS II Hunter syndrome	Stiff joints, dwarfism Macroglossia with laryn-geal and pharyngeal involvement and increased secretions Thoracic skeletal abnor-malities Valve lesions, cardiomy-opathy	Upper airway obstruction Cardiac anomalies
MPS III Sanfilippo syndrome	Mental retardation, agitation and dementia	No anaesthetic problems reported
MPS IV Morquio–Ulrich syndrome	Severe kyphoscoliotic dwarfing with atlantoaxial instability Chest wall deformity leading to respiratory and cardiac failure by second decade Aortic incompetence and cardiomyopathy	Intubation problems Cardiac anomalies Cervical spinal cord damage

Name	Description	Anaesthetic Implication
MPS V Scheie syndrome	Considered to be a mild form of MPS I – can live to adulthood Hernias, joint stiffness, aortic valve involvement	See MPS I
MPS VI Maroteaux–Lamy syndrome	Myocardial involvement with heart failure by the age 20 Kyphoscoliosis, chest infections and respiratory failure Hepatosplenomegaly	Anaemia Thrombocytopaenia Cardiomyopathy Poor lung function
MPS VII Sly syndrome	Extreme fluid retention Moderate mental retardation, hydrocephalus Survival into teenage or young adult years	Frequent chest infections
Multiple endocrine adenomatosis (MEA) type I Wermer syndrome	Hyperparathyroidism, pancreatic and pituitary tumours Occasionally bronchial carcinoid tumours	Hypoglycaemia Hypercalcaemia Renal impairment Carcinoid
Multiple endocrine adenomatosis (MEA) type II Sipple syndrome	Pheochromocytoma, thyroid carcinoma, parathyroid adenoma, CNS tumours, mediastinalschwannoma and Cushing disease	Pheochromocytoma
Multiple mucosal neuroma syndrome	MEA type IIB Marfanoid features Onset during first decade	Intubation problems
Myalgia encephalitica	Postviral weakness In extreme cases reduction of myocardial muscle	Caution with muscle relaxants
Myasthenia congenita	Like adult myasthenia gravis	Preoperative plasmapheresis Isoflurane safe
Myositis ossificans Fibrodysplasia ossificans	Bony infiltration of tendons, fascia and muscle Stiff neck, reduced thoracopulmonary compliance with respiratory failure	Airway problems Intubation problems Corticosteroid therapy

Name	Description	Anaesthetic Implication
Myotonia congenita Thomsen disease	Decreased ability to relax muscles after contraction	Avoid muscle relaxants
Myotonica dystrophia Dystrophia myotonica	Weakness and myotonia Pulmonary complications due to impaired ventilation and poor cough Cardiac involvement with conduction defects	Avoid respiratory depressants Avoid suxamethonium Nondepolarizing relaxants may not relax myotonia Regional techniques may not relax myotonia Malignant hyperpyrexia risk
Nager syndrome	Abnormality of development of first and second branchial arches	Airway problems
Nemaline myopathy	Inadequate ventilation due to muscle weakness	Sensitive to nondepolarizing relaxants Malignant hyperpyrexia risk
Neonatal hypoglycaemia (idiopathic)	Symptomatic hypoglycaemia, mental retardation and convulsions	Hypoglycaemia Diazoxide effective Corticosteroid therapy
Neurofibromatosis	See Von Recklinghausen disease	
Niemann–Pick disease	Diffuse infiltration of sphingomyelin and cholesterol in CNS, lungs, etc. Epilepsy, ataxia and mental retardation	Anaemia Thrombocytopaenia Pulmonary insufficiency
Noack syndrome	Craniosynostosis and digital anomalies Obesity	Intubation problems
Noonan syndrome	Male Turner syndrome Micrognathia, short, webbed neck, pectus excavatum Congenital heart disease Renal hypoplasia, hydronephrosis	Airway problems Cardiac anomalies Renal impairment
Oculo-auriculovertebral syndrome	See Goldenhar syndrome	

Name	Description	Anaesthetic Implication
Oculocerebrorenal syndrome	See Lowe syndrome	
Ollier disease	Multiple chondromas within bones Pathological fractures	Care with positioning
Opitz–Frias syndrome Hypospadias dysphagia syndrome G syndrome	Genital and craniofacial abnormalities	Airway problems
Orofaciodigital syndrome	Cleft palate, lobed tongue, hypoplastic maxilla and mandible Hydrocephalus Polycystic kidneys	Airway problems Intubation problems Renal impairment
Osler–Weber–Rendu syndrome Haemorrhagic telangiectasia	No coagulation defect Pulmonary arteriovenous (AV) fistulae	Difficult to control bleeding Epistaxis Cardiac anomalies Recurrent chest infection
Osteogenesis imperfect fragilitas ossium	Fragile teeth and bones, pathological fractures Respiratory problem due to chest wall deformity	Care in positioning Subcutaneous haemorrhage Malignant hyperpyrexia risk
Osteopetrosis	See Albers–Schönberg disease	
Otopalatodigital (OPD) syndrome Rubinstein- Taybi syndrome Andre syndrome	Predominantly affects males Microcephaly, micrognathia and hypertelorism Two subtypes – OPD I Rubinstein- Taybi syndrome OPD II Andre syndrome	Airway problems Intubation problems
Paramyotonia congenita Eulenburg disease	Weakness and myotonia induced by exposure to cold Derangement of serum potassium	See myotonica dystrophia Electrolyte abnormalities
Patau syndrome	See trisomy 13	
Pendred syndrome	Deafness and goitre	Check euthyroid Otherwise as for cretinism

Name	Description	Anaesthetic Implication
Pfeiffer syndrome	Craniostenosis, syndactyly	Airway problems Haemorrhagic surgery
Phenylketonuria	Phenylalanine hydroxylase deficiency Hypertonia, convulsions, mental retardation	Hypoglycaemia Seizures Sensitivity to CNS depressants
Pierre Robin syndrome	Micrognathia, hypoplastic mandible with glossoptosis, cleft palate and small epiglottis Respiratory obstruction tends to disappear after 2 years of age Associated congenital heart disease	Intubation problems Nurse in prone position Cardiac anomalies
Polycystic kidneys	Associated cysts in other organs Cerebral aneurysms in 15% of cases	Renal impairment
Polycystic liver	Associated cysts in other organs Hepatic impairment occurs late	
Polysplenia	Bilateral visceral left-sidedness Associated with complex congenital heart disease See also asplenia	Cardiac anomalies
Pompe disease	See glycogen storage disease type II	
Porphyria	Paralytic crises precipitated by wide variety of drugs Autonomic imbalance Abdominal pain	Avoid 'trigger' agents
Potter syndrome	Renal agenesis, typical facies and pulmonary hypoplasia Also maternal oligohydramnios	Ventilation may be impossible even if intubated

Name	Description	Anaesthetic Implication
Prader–Willi syndrome	Hypotonia and absent reflexes in the neonate Later polyphagia and extreme obesity, mental retardation, hypogonadism and sometimes cardiovascular abnormalities May be very large in adult life	Obesity Airway problems Cardiac failure
Progeria Hutchinson–Gilford syndrome	Premature ageing starts 6 months to 3 years Adult cardiac disease – myocardial ischaemia, hypertension, cardiomegaly, etc.	As for adults with IHD
Progressive external ophthalmoplegia (PEO)	Mitochondrial myopathy similar to Kearns–Sayer syndrome	Care with induction agents
Prune belly syndrome	Agenesis of abdominal muscles Poor cough due to muscle weakness, causes respiratory problems Renal anomalies	Recurrent respiratory infections Treat as 'full stomach' Avoid muscle relaxants Renal impairment
Pseudohaemophilia	See von Willebrand disease	
Pseudohypoparathyroidism	See Albright osteodystrophy	
Pseudoxanthoma elasticum	See Groenblad–Strandberg disease	
Pyle disease (Spondylo) metaphyseal dysplasia	Craniofacial abnormalities – mandibular prognathia	Airway problems
Reiger syndrome	Similar to dystrophia myotonica and other myopathies Maxillary hypoplasia, abnormal teeth, mental retardation	See amyotonia congenita and dystrophia myotonica
Renal tubular acidosis	See Fanconi syndrome	

Name	Description	Anaesthetic Implication
Rett syndrome	Affects females Dementia, autism, movement disorders and abnormal respiratory control	Cardiac anomalies
Riley–Day syndrome Familial dysautonomia	Deficiency of dopamine hydroxylase with autonomic instability and increased sensitivity to adrenergic and cholinergic drugs Hypersalivation, regurgitation, poor temperature control and unexplained fluctuations of blood pressure	Labile blood pressure Insensitive to CO_2 Avoid respiratory depressants Reduced sensitivity to pain
Ritter disease	Fragile skin	Difficult venous access
Robinow syndrome	Fetal face syndrome Achondroplasia	Airway problems
Romano–Ward syndrome	Congenital delay of depolarization with prolonged QT interval	Sudden death during induction May require transvenous pacing or stellate ganglion block
Rubinstein–Taybi syndrome	Microcephaly, mental retardation Swallowing abnormality with frequent chest infections Associated congenital heart disease	Chronic lung disease Cardiac anomalies
Russell–Silver syndrome	See Silver syndrome	
Saethre–Chotzen syndrome	See Chotzen syndrome	
Sanfilippo syndrome	See mucopolysaccharidosis III	
Scleroderma	Diffuse cutaneous stiffening with contractures	Airway problems Intubation problems Difficult venous access Corticosteroid therapy

Name	Description	Anaesthetic Implication
Sebaceous naevi disease	Linear naevi from forehead to nose Hydrocephalus and mental retardation Congenital heart disease – coarctation, hypoplastic aorta	Airway problems Cardiac anomalies
Sheie disease	See mucopolysaccharidosis V	
Shprintzen syndrome	Micrognathia, deafness and congenital cardiac abnormalities occur	Intubation problems Cardiac anomalies
Shy–Drager syndrome	Diffuse degeneration of central and autonomic nervous systems Cardiac arrhythmias Hypersensitivity to epinephrine (adrenaline) and angiotensin	Labile blood pressure Ephedrine effective
Shy–Magee syndrome	Central core disease Myopathy and myotonia	Malignant hyperpyrexia risk
Silver syndrome Russell–Silver syndrome	Short stature, skeletal asymmetry, micrognathia, macroglossia, café-au-lait spots, sweating and mental deficiency Abnormal sexual development	Airway problems Intubation problems Hypoglycaemia
Sipple syndrome	See multiple endocrine adenomatosis type II	
Smith–Najer syndrome	Mandibulofacial dystonia	Airway problems
Smith–Lemli–Opitz syndrome	Mental retardation, micrognathia, skeletal and genital anomalies and intrinsic lung disease Hypoplasia of thymus with increased susceptibility to infection	Airway problems Intubation problems
Sotos syndrome	Nonprogressive cerebral gigantism Normal intracranial pressure	Airway problems

Name	Description	Anaesthetic Implication
Spondylometaphyseal dysplasia	See Pyle disease	
Sprengel deformity	Congenital elevation of scapula with scoliosis and torticollis Associated with Klippel–Feil syndrome	Intubation problems
Stickler syndrome	Progressive arthro-ophthalmopathy Myopia, retinal detachment, secondary glaucoma, pain and stiffness of joints with hypotonia, kyphoscoliosis, maxillary hypoplasia Occasional cleft palate, deafness	Intubation problems
Still disease	Juvenile chronic polyarthritis Limited movement of jaw and of cervical spine Atlantoaxial subluxation may be present	Difficult airway Fibreoptic intubation Ketamine may be useful
Sturge–Weber syndrome	Cavernous angioma of face Intracranial calcification, convulsions and progressive neurological deficit	Cardiac problems
Supravalvular aortic stenosis syndrome	See idiopathic infantile hypercalcaemia	
Tangier disease	Analphalipoproteinaemia Splenomegaly, low serum cholesterol and neurological abnormalities in 50% of cases Premature coronary disease	Care with muscle relaxants Anaemia Thrombocytopaenia
Thrombocytopaenia with absent radius (TAR) syndrome	Episodic thrombocytopaenia Congenital heart disease in 30% of cases – commonly Fallot tetralogy Death within first year in up to 40% of cases	Avoid surgery in first year Cardiac anomalies
Tarui disease	See glycogen storage disease type VII	

Name	Description	Anaesthetic Implication
Tay–Sachs disease	Gangliosidosis CNS degeneration, blindness and progressive dementia	No anaesthetic problems reported
Taybi syndrome	See otopalatodigital syndrome	
Thomsen disease	See myotonia congenita	
Thrombasthenia	See Glanzmann disease	
Tourette syndrome Gilles de la Tourette syndrome	Repetitive, rapid sudden movements (tics) and coprolalia Prolonged QT interval syndrome associated with pimozide treatment	Motor aspects may be confused with seizure-like activity
Treacher Collins syndrome	Mandibulofacial dysostosis Micrognathia, maxillary and mandibular hypoplasia, microstomia and ear deformities, but less severe than Pierre Robin deformity Coexistent congenital heart disease	Airway problems Intubation problems Cardiac anomalies
Trisomy 4	Complete trisomy 4 is lethal	
Trisomy 6	Craniofacial abnormalities, unusually short webbed neck, flexion contractures Growth and psychomotor retardation	Airway problems Intubation problems
Trisomy 8	Dysmorphic facies, micrognathia, musculoskeletal abnormalities, congenital heart disease and hydronephrosis	Intubation problems Cardiac anomalies Renal impairment
Trisomy 13 Patau syndrome	Mental retardation Microcephaly, micrognathia and cleft palate Dextrocardia and congenital heart disease (e.g. VSD) Usually fatal by 3 years of age	Intubation problems Cardiac anomalies

Name	Description	Anaesthetic Implication
Trisomy 18 Edwards syndrome	Micrognathia, short sternum, renal malformations, clenched hands, low-set ears Associated congenital heart disease (VSD, patent ductus, pulmonary stenosis) in 95% of cases Usually die in infancy	Intubation problems Cardiac problems Renal impairment
Trisomy 21 Down syndrome Mongolism	Microcephaly, atlantoaxial instability, hypotonia Hypersalivation Associated congenital heart disease (especially septal defects) in 50% of cases	Airway problems Intubation problems Cardiac anomalies Hypoglycaemia
Trisomy 22	Death before or shortly after birth due to severe malformations, including microcephaly and cardiac abnormalities	Cardiac anomalies Hypoglycaemia
Tuberous sclerosis Bournville disease	Adenoma sebaceum of skin – ash leaf and café-au-lait spots Intracranial calcification, epilepsy and mental retardation Hamartomas in heart, lungs and kidneys	Cardiac anomalies Arrhythmias Renal impairment
Turner syndrome	Micrognathia with short webbed neck Aortic and pulmonary stenosis, coarctation and aneurysms of aorta Renal anomalies	Intubation problems Cardiac anomalies Renal impairment
Urbach–Wiethe disease	Mucocutaneous hyalinosis – a type of histiocytosis Hyaline deposits in larynx and pharynx	Intubation problems
Vater syndrome	VSD and intrinsic pulmonary disease Renal failure occurs	Cardiac anomalies Renal impairment
Velocardiofacial	Cleft palate, congenital heart defects	Airway problems Cardiac anomalies

Name	Description	Anaesthetic Implication
Von–Gierke disease	See glycogen storage disease type I	
Von–Hippel–Lindau syndrome	Haemangioblastomas in posterior fossa and spinal cord Associated with pheochromocytoma, hepatic and renal cysts	Pheochromocytoma risk Hepatic pathology Renal impairment
Von Recklinghausen disease Neurofibromatosis	Tumours in all parts of CNS Fibromas of pharynx, larynx and heart Kyphoscoliosis, multiple lung cysts and renal artery dysplasia Increased incidence of pheochromocytoma	Airway problems Cardiac problems Pheochromocytoma risk
Von Willebrand disease Pseudohaemophilia	Defective platelet adhesiveness with factor VIII deficiency Also capillary abnormality	Correct coagulopathy with: Tranexamic acid Desmopressin (DDAVP) Fresh frozen plasma Avoid salicylates
Weaver syndrome	Rare developmental condition with unusual craniofacial appearance and micrognathia May be very large in adult life	Airway problems Intubation problems
Weber–Christian disease	Chronic nonsuppurative panniculitis with widespread fat necrosis including peritoneal, pericardial and meningeal Adrenal insufficiency, constrictive pericarditis	Avoid trauma to fat
Welander muscular atrophy	Peripheral muscular atrophy	Sensitive to muscle relaxants Sensitive to opiates
Werdnig–Hoffman disease	See amyotonia congenita	
Wermer syndrome	See multiple endocrine adenomatosis type I	

Name	Description	Anaesthetic Implication
Werner syndrome	Premature ageing, diabetes mellitus, early cataracts, mental retardation in 50% of cases Hypercalcaemia, bony lesions like osteomyelitis and myocardial ischaemia See also progeria	Anaesthesia as for adults with IHD
Wiedemann syndrome	See Beckwith syndrome	
Williams–Beuren syndrome	See idiopathic infantile hypercalcaemia	
Wilson disease	Hepatolenticular degeneration Decreased caeruloplasmin causes widespread abnormal copper deposition	Hepatic failure Muscle relaxants ineffective Renal impairment
Wilson–Mikity syndrome	Prematurity – <1500 g birth weight Severe chronic lung disease with fibrosis, possibly due to oxygen toxicity	Recurrent chest infections Corticosteroid therapy Right heart failure
Wiskott–Aldrich syndrome	Primary immunodeficiency with thrombocytopaenia All have low platelet count, anaemia and clotting problems Eczema and asthma	Anaemia Thrombocytopaenia Susceptible to transfusion-induced graft-versus-host reaction Susceptible to infection Cardiac anomalies
Wolf–Hirschorn syndrome	Associated with poor intrauterine growth, severe psychomotor retardation, characteristic facies and various midline fusion abnormalities	Malignant hyperpyrexia risk
Wolman disease Familial xanthomatosis	Adrenal calcification Resembles Niemann–Pick disease with hepatosplenomegaly, hypersplenism and clotting problems	Anaemia Thrombocytopaenia
X-linked ichthyosis	See ichthyosis	

FURTHER READING

Lerman J, Steward DJ, Coté CJ, editors. Manual of pediatric anesthesia: with an index of pediatric syndromes. 6th ed. Philadelphia: Churchill Livingstone; 2009.

USEFUL WEBSITES

https://medlineplus.gov/encyclopedia.html
http://www.medicinenet.com
https://www.gpnotebook.co.uk
http://www.whonamedit.com

Index